Principles and Practice of
Child and Adolescent
Forensic Psychiatry

Principles and Practice of
Child and Adolescent
Forensic Psychiatry

Edited by

Diane H. Schetky, M.D.

Elissa P. Benedek, M.D.

American **P**sychiatric Publishing, Inc.

Washington, DC
London, England

Manufactured in the United States of America on acid-free paper
06 05 04 03 02   5 4 3 2 1
First Edition

American Psychiatric Publishing, Inc.
1400 K Street, N.W.
Washington, DC 20005
www.appi.org

Library of Congress Cataloging-in-Publication Data
Principles and practice of child and adolescent forensic psychiatry / edited by Diane H. Schetky,
   Elissa P. Benedek. – 1st. ed.
        p. ; cm.
   Includes bibliographical references and index.
   ISBN 0-88048-956-1 (alk. paper)
   1. Forensic psychiatry. 2. Child psychiatry. 3. Adolescent psychiatry. I. Schetky,
Diane H., 1940– II. Benedek, Elissa P.
   [DNLM: 1. Forensic Psychiatry. 2. Child Abuse. 3. Child Custody. 4. Child Welfare. 5.
Commitment of Mentally Ill. 6. Juvenile Delinquency. 7. Violence. W 740 P9575 2002]
RA1151.P6736 2002
614´.1–dc21

                                                                        2001041367

British Library Cataloguing in Publication Data
A CIP record is available from the British Library.

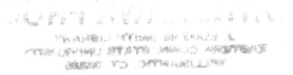

Contents

Contributors

Cheryl S. Al-Mateen, M.D.
Associate Professor, Departments of Psychiatry and Pediatrics, Medical College of Virginia, Virginia Commonwealth University, Richmond, Virginia

Marc Amaya, M.D.
Assistant Professor Emeritus, Department of Psychiatry and Behavioral Sciences, Duke University, Durham, North Carolina; Clinical Associate Professor, Department of Psychiatry, University of North Carolina at Chapel Hill

Peter Ash, M.D.
Associate Professor, Department of Psychiatry and Behavioral Sciences, Emory University, Atlanta, Georgia

Richard Barnum, M.D.
Director, Boston Juvenile Court Clinic; Assistant Clinical Professor of Psychiatry, Harvard Medical School, Boston, Massachusetts

Elissa P. Benedek, M.D.
Clinical Professor of Psychiatry, University of Michigan Medical Center, Ann Arbor, Michigan

Paul M. Brinich, Ph.D.
Clinical Professor, Departments of Psychology and Psychiatry, University of North Carolina at Chapel Hill; Associate Consulting Professor of Medical Psychology, Department of Psychology and Behavioral Sciences, Duke University, Durham, North Carolina

Catherine F. Brown, Ed.M.
Executive Editor, *Psychiatric News* (Newspaper of the American Psychiatric Association), Washington, D.C.

Maggie Bruck, Ph.D.
Associate Professor, Division of Child and Adolescent Psychiatry, Department of Psychiatry and Behavioral Sciences, Johns Hopkins School of Medicine, Baltimore, Maryland

W. V. Burlingame, Ph.D.
Clinical Professor, Department of Psychology, University of North Carolina at Chapel Hill; Assistant Consulting Professor of Medical Psychology, Department of Psychiatry and Behavioral Sciences, Duke University, Durham, North Carolina

Stephen J. Ceci, Ph.D.
Helen L. Carr Professor of Developmental Psychology, Department of Human Development and Family Studies, Cornell University, Ithaca, New York

Beth K. Clark, Ph.D., A.B.P.P.
Private Practice, Forensic Psychology, Ann Arbor, Michigan

Charles R. Clark, Ph.D., A.B.P.P.
Private Practice, Forensic Psychology, Ann Arbor, Michigan

Dewey G. Cornell, Ph.D.
Clinical Psychologist and Professor of Education, Curry School of Education, University of Virginia, Charlottesville, Virginia; Director, Virginia Youth Violence Project, Charlottesville, Virginia

Debra K. DePrato, M.D.
Associate Professor of Clinical Public Health and Preventive Medicine; Chief, Section of Forensic Medicine; Program Director, Louisiana State University Health Sciences Center Juvenile Corrections Program, Louisiana State University Health Sciences Center, School of Medicine, New Orleans, Louisiana

Leah J. Dickstein, M.D.
Professor and Associate Chair for Academic Affairs; Director, Division of Attitudinal and Behavioral Medicine, Department of Psychiatry and Behavioral Sciences; Associate Dean for Faculty and Student Advocacy, University of Louisville, Louisville, Kentucky

Yvonne B. Ferguson, M.D., M.P.H.
Private Practice, Child Psychiatry, Santa Barbara, California

Thomas G. Gutheil, M.D.
Professor of Psychiatry, Harvard Medical School, Boston, Massachusetts

Melvin J. Guyer, J.D., Ph.D.
Professor of Psychology, Department of Psychiatry, University of Michigan, Ann Arbor, Michigan

Jill Hayes Hammer, Ph.D.
Assistant Professor of Clinical Psychiatry, Department of Psychiatry, Louisiana State University Health Sciences Center, School of Medicine, New Orleans, Louisiana

James C. Harris, M.D.
Director, Developmental Neuropsychiatry, and Professor of Psychiatry and Behavioral Sciences, Pediatrics and Mental Hygiene, Johns Hopkins University School of Medicine, Baltimore, Maryland

Angela M. Hegarty, M.B., B.Ch., B.A.O. (NUI)
Clinical Assistant Professor, Department of Psychiatry, New York University School of Medicine, New York, New York

Diane E. Heisel, M.D.
Treatment Services Director, Center for Forensic Psychiatry, Ann Arbor, Michigan

Stephen P. Herman, M.D.
Associate Clinical Professor of Psychiatry, Mount Sinai Medical Center, New York, New York

Robert J. Levy, J.D.
William L. Prosser Professor of Law, University of Minnesota, Minneapolis, Minnesota

JoAnn Macbeth, J.D.
Partner, Crowell and Moring, Washington, D.C.

Carl P. Malmquist, M.D., M.S.
Professor of Social Psychiatry, University of Minnesota, Minneapolis, Minnesota

Philip Merideth, M.D., J.D.
Forensic Psychiatrist, Mississippi State Hospital and University of Mississippi Medical Center, Jackson, Mississippi

Steven Nickman, M.D.
Clinical Associate Professor of Psychiatry, Harvard Medical School, Boston, Massachusetts

Donna M. Norris, M.D.
Private Practice, Child Psychiatry, Boston and Wellesley, Massachusetts; Senior Associate in Psychiatry, Children's Hospital Medical Center; Assistant Clinical Professor, Harvard Medical School, Boston, Massachusetts

Kathleen M. Quinn, M.D.
Director of Training in Child and Adolescent Psychiatry, Cleveland Clinic, Cleveland, Ohio

Bruce D. Perry, M.D., Ph.D.
Director, Child Trauma Academy, Houston, Texas; Medical Director, Provincial Programs in Children's Mental Health, Alberta Mental Health Board, Calgary, Alberta, Canada

Alvin Rosenfeld, M.D.
Private and Consulting Practice, New York, New York, and Greenwich, Connecticut

Diane H. Schetky, M.D.
Private Practice, Forensic Psychiatry, Rockport, Maine; Clinical Professor of Psychiatry, University of Vermont College of Medicine at Maine Medical Center, Portland, Maine

Herbert A. Schreier, M.D.
Chief of Psychiatry, Children's Hospital Oakland, Oakland, California

Charles L. Scott, M.D.
Assistant Clinical Professor of Psychiatry and Director of Forensic Psychiatry Training, Department of Psychiatry, University of California at Davis, Sacramento, California

Jon A. Shaw, M.D.
Professor of Psychiatry and Pediatrics and Director, Division of Child and Adolescent Psychiatry, Department of Psychiatry and Behavioral Sciences, University of Miami School of Medicine, Jackson Memorial Medical Center, Miami, Florida

C. J. Voight, M.D.
Unit Director, Center for Forensic Psychiatry, Ann Arbor, Michigan

Saul Wasserman, M.D.
Clinical Associate Professor of Child Psychiatry, Stanford University Medical School, Stanford, California; Private and Consulting Practice, San Jose, California

Foreword

A Voyage of Discovery

Thomas G. Gutheil, M.D.

In the late nineteenth century into the early part of the twentieth, a popular amusement involved looking at drawings to discover the outlines of hidden pictures of children concealed among leaves, plants, and other pastoral details. This image well captures the notion that childhood itself could be seen as hidden for some time in the shadows of ignorance and inattention. Early artists failed even to see the differing proportions of children and sketched them as though they were diminutive adults.

Sociologists have noted that childhood as a phenomenon and a developmental stage was also discovered relatively recently: children were not merely small adults nor parental property, but evolving organisms with unique cognitive, moral, and social development as well as vulnerabilities. Awareness of these truths led to interest in the ways children develop and the ways in which they needed legal protections, such as child labor laws.

But here, too, attention and understanding came relatively late to the game. The case of *In re Gault*, for example, which was among the earliest cases to establish a number of legal protections for children, appeared only a handful of decades ago. We might thus conclude that we are still relatively early in the discovery of the legal and forensic contexts in which children appear.

Fortunately for the success of this ongoing voyage of discovery, the present work is edited by two recognized giants in the specialized field of child forensic psychiatry. Drs. Schetky and Benedek have achieved a quantum leap in a subject that has been largely preoccupied with concerns regarding adult issues. From the more shallow pool of child forensic specialists, the editors have drawn the very best as authors, to present a text that is not only comprehensive but rich in both historical detail and practical guidance for the clinician. Laudably, the thrust of this text always favors evidence-based research rather than political correctness.

Discoveries in child forensic psychiatry are complicated by the same pendulum swings of fashion that bedevil other fields of knowledge. Consider sexual abuse of children. First it was unrecognized; then it was overdiagnosed by any amateur with an "anatomically incorrect" doll; finally, rational approaches to uncontaminated assessment began to be identified and employed. The subject is illuminatingly explored in this text.

Child violence is another emerging area of concern. Children at increasingly younger ages seem to be seizing all-too-available guns and shooting their teachers, classmates, and random passersby. These vital matters are also explored herein.

The editors employ the highly successful format of previous clinical handbooks, a format which melds the clinical and legal issues into an easily followed sequence; case examples are actively employed, pitfalls are identified, including those of countertransference, and a practical action guideline helps the clinician find out rapidly just what to do. In the book as a whole, after a review of the history of the child forensic field and some basic instruction on interacting with the legal system, the editors explore child custody, child abuse, youth violence, juvenile offenders, and legal issues such as commitment of children and treatment of minors. Beyond these fundamental issues, the parts contain some chapters addressing vital current matters never or rarely addressed before, such as vicarious traumatization in clinicians working with children; Munchausen syndrome by proxy; children's access to weapons; and aspects of sexual harassment in school-age children.

You hold in your hands a classic in the making. This textbook represents the high-water mark of the subject for this millennium. Every clinician who works with children and adolescents should read this through and then keep it on a handy shelf for repeated ready reference; child forensic psychiatrists should memorize it. The subject will also be of great interest and utility to psychologists and attorneys working in this field. And it is no prediction at all—it is a certainty—that this will become the definitive work for training programs everywhere. The editors are to be congratulated for bringing light to a shadowed and undiscovered country; their fortunate readers may now share the voyage of discovery.

Preface

Diane H. Schetky, M.D.
Elissa P. Benedek, M.D.

This volume replaces our previous book, *Clinical Handbook of Child Psychiatry and the Law,* which is now out of print and outdated. In the 10 years that have elapsed since its publication, we have seen a dramatic expansion in the field of child and adolescent forensic psychiatry and heightened interest in training in this area. This volume covers the same basic issues addressed in our previous book, with expanded and updated material and increased emphasis on issues related to adoption, youth violence, and juvenile offenders. We introduce new topics, including vicarious traumatization of the clinician, parenting assessments, transracial and transcultural adoptions, sexual harassment, child pornography, sexually aggressive youth, the neurodevelopmental impact of violence in childhood, and telepsychiatry. In addition to clinical chapters, we have included more background material on law and more research in important areas such as the suggestibility of child witnesses and the effect of violence on children. Extensive references are provided that reflect current developments in the area of child and adolescent forensic psychiatry.

We have followed a similar format to that used in our previous book. Each chapter follows the same basic outline to provide easy access to the material. Case examples take the reader into the real world of child and adolescent forensic psychiatry. The examples are designed to get the reader to think about the issues and link the material in the chapter to actual clinical situations. Some of the cases are fictional, some are composites, and some are actual cases with the identities of the parties involved disguised. The cases also point to the vast array of issues that the forensic examiner may confront. Like the children and adolescents who enter the family courts and juvenile justice system, the reader is embarking on a voyage with many interesting turns.

This volume is intended for a wide audience including, but not limited to, practicing clinicians, forensic examiners, attorneys, and judges who may wish to use it as a reference book and trainees in child and adolescent psychiatry or psychology who may use it as a basic text. In addition, clinicians will find it useful in preparing for board certification in forensic psychiatry.

ACKNOWLEDGMENTS

Dr. Schetky wishes to thank Rod Hook for his ongoing technical support with her computer crises. Without his ready availability and patience, she might still be writing and editing this text. Special appreciation is also extended to our authors for putting up with seemingly endless editing and for adhering to deadlines in spite of other pressing issues in their lives (such as being held hostage in Turkey, as recently happened to one of our authors). Finally, many thanks to Pam Harley of American Psychiatric Publishing for her diligent help with the final editing of this text.

PART I

Basics

Part I introduces the reader to the principles of law and provides a basic framework for approaching forensic evaluations. In Chapter 1, Dr. Schetky traces the burgeoning development of the specialty of child and adolescent forensic psychiatry and changing views of children and their rights. Chapter 2 introduces the reader to the legal system and its unique terminology. In user-friendly language, attorneys Guyer and Levy describe the history of the American legal system, the hierarchy of the American court system, standards of proof in civil and criminal cases, and the differences between civil and criminal cases.

Dr. Schetky sets the stage for forensic work by reviewing the ethical principles that guide the practice of forensic psychiatry in Chapter 3. Common ethical issues are covered along with the methods used to handle ethical complaints. As with most of the chapters that follow, pitfalls are discussed and guidelines offered. In the following chapter, Dr. Schetky delineates the differences between the ordinary child psychiatric evaluation and the forensic evaluation. The reader will become acquainted with the perils of wearing two hats, a theme that is reiterated throughout this text.

Dr. Benedek walks the reader through the often confusing world of depositions and courtroom testimony in Chapter 5. She provides a step-by-step discussion of what to anticipate and advises on how to maintain one's professional integrity and not be intimidated under cross-examination. In Chapter 6, Drs. Clark and Clark provide a comprehensive overview of psychological testing including specialized tests used in forensic evaluations. They discuss the validity of some of the newer forensic tests that clinicians may consider requesting at the onset of an evaluation, if the forensic psychologist feels they are appropriate.

The potential for vicarious trauma is always present when participating in child and adolescent forensic evaluations. The traumatized child can tug at our heartstrings or infuriate a normally objective clinician. Forensic evaluators must confront man's inhumanity to man on a regular basis. As noted by Dr. Hegarty in Chapter 7, if one does not deal with the feelings invoked by vicarious trauma, fatigue, nightmares, compassion fatigue, and burnout may result from participating in forensic evaluations.

CHAPTER 1

History of Child and Adolescent Forensic Psychiatry

Diane H. Schetky, M.D.

Forensic psychiatry is a subspecialty of psychiatry in which scientific and clinical expertise is applied to legal rather than therapeutic issues and ends. These legal contexts may include civil, criminal, or legislative matters. In addition, there is a growing body of research within the field. In the latter part of the twentieth century, child and adolescent forensic psychiatry emerged as a sub-sub-specialty, and interest in this area continues to grow along with demands for experts in this field. Although the roots of child and adolescent forensic psychiatry go back a century to the founding of the first juvenile court, it is only within the past few decades that residency programs have offered any didactic training in this area and only recently has some exposure to the area become a training requirement in psychiatry and child psychiatry.

THE EVOLUTION OF CHILDHOOD

Childhood, as we know it today, is a relatively new concept. Demause (1974) reminds us that "the history of childhood is a nightmare from which we have only recently begun to awaken." The further back in history one goes, the lower the level of child care was and the more likely children were to have been killed, abandoned, beaten, terrorized, and sexually abused. He notes that terrorizing children was common, the practice of farming children out to wet nurses interfered with parental empathy, and parents in general lacked empathy and emotional maturity. In addition, high infant mortality rates undoubtedly affected the extent to which parents

became emotionally invested in their children. We know that the sexual abuse of children has been widespread throughout history and that severe beatings of children were common until the nineteenth century, when the practice of punishing them by putting them in dark closets gained popularity over beatings. Infanticide and exposure of infants, particularly females, were practiced until the fourth century, as was child sacrifice in some cultures.

The notion of childhood as a separate period in life began to emerge in the sixteenth century in response to changes in the adult world. Two notable influences were the teachings of the Jesuits and the invention of the printing press. The Jesuits stressed schooling of children, shame, childhood innocence, and the need to protect children from adult secrets. There followed campaigns against the sexual abuse of children, although child prostitution continued to flourish into the Victorian era. The invention of the printing press contributed to a separation between adults and children in that, as a result of it, adults gained access to information that children did not have. Ironically, the mass media, in particular television and the Internet, now threatens to erode these boundaries.

THE EARLY TREATMENT OF CHILDREN UNDER THE LAW

In order to appreciate the many changes that have occurred in how the legal system and society respond to children in need or in trouble, we need to recall that prior to the twentieth century children were for the most part treated as the property of their parents. Early custody disputes reflect that children were valued not so much for themselves but rather for the labor they might provide, and they were fully exploited in the labor market prior to laws prohibiting child labor. Children charged with misconduct were subject to the same criminal proceedings and sanctions as adults and even jailed with them. Exceptions existed for children under age 7, who along with the insane were considered to lack the capacity for reason, which is necessary to form criminal intent; hence, they were not brought to trial. Under English common law, children under age 7 continued to be exempted from criminal proceedings and those 14 years and older were subject to the same penalties as adults. However, there are records of children as young as 8 years old being executed in the early nineteenth century in England and the United States for crimes as minor as theft (Platt 1977).

There were no laws protecting children from abuse or neglect, and the first prosecuted case of child abuse had to be taken to the Society for Prevention of Cruelty to Animals, because the Society for Prevention of Cruelty to Children, founded in 1875 in New York, had not yet been established. Foster care as we know it now did not exist at that time, although under Charles Loring Brace trainloads of children from the slums of New York City were placed with farm families in the Midwest. Brace (1872) believed that given a change in circumstance, "many of their vices [would] drop from them like the old and verminous clothing they left behind." Some of these children thrived, whereas others were terribly exploited. The distinction between dependent and delinquent children was often blurred, and they were treated in similar fashion in terms of placements. Institutional care developed as an alternative to almshouses, and children could be placed there by their parents or the courts although racist practices often excluded minorities.

DEVELOPMENT OF THE JUVENILE JUSTICE SYSTEM

The nascent field of criminology was dominated by European writers and English law, and various theories abounded as to the causes of delinquency, including moral or physical inferiority, hereditary factors, urban living, and economic instability (Platt 1977). Under the influence of social reformers in the late nineteenth century, a rehabilitative ideal emerged that was to change the way in which juvenile delinquents were handled. A medical model was adopted that stressed multidisciplinary evaluations, the prevention of delinquency, and treatment rather than dwelling on pathology. This reform movement culminated in the establishment of the first juvenile court in 1899 in Chicago; other states soon followed suit.

The juvenile court assumed an attitude of benevolence and attempted to decriminalize the children who passed through its doors, but in doing so, it deprived them of due process rights. With the help of medical and mental health professionals, it sought to understand the total child and respond to him "as a wise, merciful father handles his own child whose errors are not discovered by the authorities" (Mack 1909). The American Orthopsychiatric Association formed as an interdisciplinary forum for understanding the causes and treatment of delinquency. For those youths needing placement, training centers were established that aimed to remove children from corruptive influences. Many of these centers were sectarian and emphasized religion, moral training, discipline, labor, and industrial training.

Disillusionment was soon to follow as the early juvenile court was not able to live up to its promises. Dispositional and treatment components of clinics were severely lagging, and there was inadequate funding to sustain programs. In addition, the benign atmosphere of the court failed to curb the behavior of more hardened delinquents. In *In re Gault* Justice Fortas charged that "in most juvenile courts the child receives the worst of both worlds: that he gets neither the protection accorded to adults nor the solicitous care and regenerative treatment postulated for children." Stone (1976) lamented that "the court's only function in many cases is to funnel children from unsuitable homes to unsuitable placements." In the 1960s, President Johnson's Commission on Law Enforcement attempted to improve the juvenile justice system. The Commission's report noted the failures of the juvenile courts and stressed the need for prevention through community-based diversion programs aimed at predelinquents. The effort failed to have any significant effect on hard-core delinquents. We continue to struggle with how best to intervene with this difficult segment of the population, and the law has recently moved toward treating juveniles who commit serious crimes more like adults and removing the former protections of the juvenile court. The increase in the number of adolescents committing violent crime has created a demand for more adolescent forensic psychiatrists to consult with schools and courts.

CHILD CUSTODY

Under Roman law "the father had absolute control over his children and could sell or condemn them to death with impunity" (Derdeyn 1976). English law stressed the father's absolute right to the child in as much as the child was viewed as property. Similar concepts prevailed in the United States, and it was assumed that in return for support a father was entitled to the child's services. Only gradually did the notion evolve that the custody of children involved not only support but also responsibility for the care of children. In the late nineteenth century, the father custody presumption gave way to the tender years presumption, which deemed maternal care to be necessary for the young child. The pendulum swung to favoring mother custody and remained there (except in cases of moral unfitness) until the introduction of shared custody arrangements in the 1980s. The concept of the child's best interests did not emerge until 1881 in the case of *Chapsky v. Wood*. In this decision, the judge awarded custody of a 5-year-old girl to her grandmother over her father citing the paramount concern of the welfare of the child. In 1925, Judge Benjamin Cardozo specified that the court's role is to serve as *parens patriae* and do "what is in the best interests of the child" (*Finlay v. Finlay* 1925). (The term *parens patriae* originally referred to the king's guardianship over people legally unable to act for themselves.) Impetus for the involvement of mental health professionals in custody decisions was provided by Goldstein, Freud, and Solnit (1973) in *Beyond the Best Interests of the Child*, which applied psychoanalytic principles to the resolution of custody disputes. As no-fault divorces became more common, courts began paying more attention to the needs of the involved children. Custody issues have since taken on new dimensions with the advent of surrogacy, adoptions by gay and lesbian parents, and international and transracial adoptions.

ABUSED AND NEGLECTED CHILDREN

The sexual abuse of children has been documented since the sixth century B.C., but society's response to the problem has been slow. Mandatory reporting laws for child abuse did not go into effect until 1974. As a result of this federal legislation and increased media attention to both physical and sexual abuse, reporting of allegations continues to soar and reports of suspected sexual abuse now outnumber reports of physical abuse. Clinicians are increasingly being asked to help differentiate valid claims of abuse from undocumented or false ones. The demands of the court in this regard sometimes exceed our ability to differentiate true from false allegations of abuse, and new research on children's memories and suggestibility sounds a note of caution in this regard.

Foster care emerged in the early twentieth century as an alternative to institutional care for children, but it has traditionally favored Caucasian children. Children were often lost in the foster care system, their physical and mental health needs neglected, and little effort was made to find permanent placement. Placements often broke down, and multiple placements with ensuing attachment disorders were common. Much has been done to change this situation in recent years with more emphasis being put on avoiding placement through providing in-home services. Time limits are now put on duration of foster care, and permanent placement has become a top priority with either return to the home or adoption. Another change has been the increased use of kinship placements and focus on the child's needs rather than the parents'. Agencies have become much more aggressive in locating adoptive homes for hard-to-place children and have relaxed their former rigidity regarding only placing children with "traditional" families. Forensic practitioners are often asked to confer on questions of placement, parental reunification, and termination of parental rights.

CIVIL LITIGATION

In the past, the courts did not allow recovery for damages that were purely psychological in nature. Changes in the law have opened the way for claims invoking posttraumatic stress disorder (PTSD), and child and adolescent forensic psychiatrists are becoming involved as experts in these cases. Many of them are second-generation sexual abuse cases with adults abused as children now suing their perpetrators. Some states have removed statutes of limitation for sexual abuse cases, which leaves a long window of time in which a victim can bring about a civil suit. Research on PTSD and greater public awareness of this condition have led to more litigation by plaintiffs who have experienced or witnessed trauma. Sexual harassment has become a new area of litigation and schools may now be held liable for failure to address the problem.

Experts may also be involved in malpractice cases against physicians with litigation typically involving boundary violations, suicide of a patient, or adverse outcomes to medication. The 1990s have seen a spate of suits against therapists for failing to diagnose sexual abuse or falsely diagnosing it and inducing their patients' recollections of abuse.

ETHICS

As the specialty of forensic psychiatry grows, so does the need for ethical guidelines.

Many psychiatrists have flocked to the field as the last refuge from managed care, and if they have not done forensic fellowships, they may lack grounding in basic principles of forensic ethics. Child and adolescent forensic psychiatry, even more so than adult forensic psychiatry, falls through the cracks, as neither the American Academy of Child and Adolescent Psychiatry (AACAP) nor the American Academy of Psychiatry and Law (AAPL) has adequate guidelines to address its unique issues.

TRAINING

Currently there are 34 one-year fellowships in forensic psychiatry in the United States that are certified by the Accreditation Council on Graduate Medical Education (ACGME) and 5 Canadian fellowship programs. Some offer more training than others in child and adolescent forensic issues; information about these programs may be obtained from the AAPL Web site (www.aapl.org). In 1994, the American Board of Psychiatry and Neurology began offering certification in the subspecialty of forensic psychiatry, thereby replacing the board certification previously offered by the American Board of Forensic Psychiatry. A 1-year forensic fellowship from a program certified by the ACGME is now a requirement to be eligible to take the board exam for added qualifications in forensic psychiatry.

Many other opportunities abound for getting exposure to forensic psychiatry short of doing a fellowship. AAPL, which was founded in 1969, is a growing and thriving organization that holds annual meetings each fall. Increasingly, the programs contain sessions and courses dealing with child and adolescent forensic issues, reflecting the growing number of child and adolescent psychiatrists who have joined AAPL. It also publishes an excellent quarterly journal and a newsletter. AACAP has published practice parameters on forensic issues and also offers programs dealing with forensic psychiatry at its annual meetings. Working in youth correctional facilities offers a good immersion course in issues of juvenile crime and justice and does not require a forensic fellowship. Mentorship with a more experienced forensic clinician is another way of getting started with some forensic cases in a private practice.

REFERENCES

Brace C: The Dangerous Classes of New York and Twenty Years' Work Among Them. New York, Wynkoop & Hallenbect, 1872

Demause L: The History of Childhood. New York, The Psychohistory Press, 1974, p 1

Derdeyn A: Child custody in historical perspective. Am J Psychiatry 133:1369–1375, 1976

Finlay v Finlay, 148 NE 624 (NY 1925)

Goldstein J, Freud A, Solnit A: Beyond the Best Interests of the Child. New York, Free Press, 1973

In re Gault, 387 US 1 (1967)

Mack J: The Juvenile Court, 23 Harvard Law Rev 104–122 (1909)

Platt A: The Child Savers: The Invention of Delinquency. Chicago, University of Chicago Press, 1977

Stone A: Mental Health and the Law. New York, Jason Aronson, 1976, p 156

CHAPTER 2

Introduction to the Legal System

Melvin J. Guyer, J.D., Ph.D.
Robert J. Levy, J.D.

INTRODUCTION TO THE LEGAL SYSTEM

We address this chapter to those with no formal training in law or the legal system. But most of you read the newspaper, watch *The Practice* and *NYPD Blue*, and occasionally indulge in a novel about lawyers. Moreover, you are probably acquainted with at least some legal proceedings: impeachment, to be sure, and rules of evidence—*Daubert* and *Fry* admissibility rules, perhaps. Some of you may have had experience with criminal procedure: "Mirandizing" suspects or the "not guilty by reason of insanity" defense. But such contacts with the legal system must have been ambiguous at best.

We will assume, with your permission, that you know little about the topic. We set out the legal system's basic framework in a sort of basic civics course style to help you as mental health clinicians in your many and various interactions with the courts, legal agencies, legal actors of several kinds, and, especially, with your patients who are also lawyers' clients. The concepts and definitions to which we introduce you may well make your professional contacts more comfortable and your contributions more useful.

We address the following topics: structure of the court system; types of legal proceedings; pretrial proceedings; and a potpourri of important (and sometimes very arcane) legal niceties and doctrines, such as appeals and appellate courts' roles in the legal system (and how such cases are "cited," that is, found in judicial reports), judicial treatment of clinicians (e.g., are you always con-sidered an expert?), judicial decision making, and evidence doctrine dynamics.

STRUCTURE OF COURTS

History

The origins of the American legal system trace to ancient English principles and the emergence of modern nation-states from their medieval antecedents close to a millennium ago. (The "King's," or "national," courts and national legal doctrines, the "common law," over time replaced the local magistrates and idiosyncratic doctrines imposed by previously all-powerful nobles on serfs and renters in their fiefdoms.) These historical roots eventually produced the doctrines controlling the contracts you now sign with your employers and employees and the law determining whether you can sue or be sued by the angry therapy patient who rear-ended your car in the parking lot. More importantly, from these roots grew the foundations of the system of courts in which you will testify, the formal substantive rules for adjudication of the civil disputes for which you will provide clinical expertise, and the "adversary" procedures that favor jury decision in civil and criminal cases and permit a lawyer for litigants opposed to your patient's or client's claim or defense to cross-examine. This adversarial system is governed both in procedure and substantive doctrine by adherence under most circumstances to established principles determined by previous, sometimes even ancient, decisions (called *precedents*). The policy of such adherence is described by an ancient term, *stare decisis*.

The same ancient tradition tracing to the emergence of nation-states contains the roots of modern American criminal procedure, shaping and sometimes controlling several of the frequently controversial constitutional rights afforded criminals, such as the right to be presumed innocent until proved guilty, trial by a jury of peers, the right to confront and cross-examine witnesses, and protection from self-incrimination.

Hierarchies

State court systems are arranged as hierarchies: the "lower" courts functioning as trial courts and "higher" courts providing "appellate" review, a supervisory function for trial court decisions. Such review typically includes the trial court's procedure, as well as the merits of decisions. With some exceptions, trial courts exercise general jurisdiction—the authority to hear and decide all types of cases, civil and criminal, that the state legislature, the ultimate source of all judicial jurisdiction, has authorized. The one exception to this rule of state legislative hegemony derives from the United States Constitution's decree that the "Great Writ," the writ of habeas corpus, which frees any person from illegal imprisonment, "shall not be suspended except in cases of invasion or rebellion." The constitutional provision governs the states because of the Constitution's Supremacy Clause, designed to prevent the states from evading constitutional principles. Every state legislature also provides a system of specialized courts, or courts of limited jurisdiction, for cases of less importance (e.g., misdemeanors rather than felonies, small monetary claims) and cases in which special training for judges is thought to be necessary (e.g., juvenile delinquency and neglect, housing, "commitment" of those who cannot take care of themselves, decedents' estates and wills).

Federal Courts

The U.S. Congress has authorized a parallel system of federal trial and appellate courts to decide cases arising under the Constitution and specifically enacted federal statutes. The Congress has also enacted rules for federal court jurisdiction of civil cases if the parties are residents of different states. Appeals from federal trial courts are heard by one of nine U.S. Courts of Appeal. And, of course, the nine justices of the U.S. Supreme Court may exercise their appellate jurisdiction and review any decision by one of the Courts of Appeal. The often arcane rules governing federal jurisdiction lie far beyond the intended scope of this chapter. Because of the centrality of federal-state relations in the American judicial and political system, the United States Constitution specifi-

cally authorized U.S. Supreme Court appellate jurisdiction to review any final state judicial decision. This review most often occurs when a state supreme court holds that a state statute passes federal constitutional muster and when a citizen's constitutionally protected rights may have been abridged by a state statute or some state official. U.S. Supreme Court decisions of appeals of such "state action" cases occur in criminal proceedings when defendants claim some denial of the individual protections afforded by the Constitution's Bill of Rights.

Specialized Courts

As we have indicated, some state courts are specialized and exercise jurisdiction constrained by subject matter or by the special character of particular cases. The example most of you will recognize is the juvenile court, which usually has authority over matters relating to minors: *delinquency* (any act which if committed by an adult could be prosecuted as a criminal offense), and *dependency* and *neglect*—any child who is at risk due to caretaker inability, dangerous inattention, abuse, or abandonment. These sources of judicial jurisdiction, if proved, allow supposedly specially trained or assigned judges to exercise authority over the problematic behavior of minors and the care of such minors by their parents, even if the behavior of the minor and the care of the parent are not criminal. Suppose a child regularly refuses to obey the reasonable demands and instructions of his or her parent or a parent refuses to provide his or her child with essential food or medical care. The child could be adjudicated neglected or dependent, the judge could order the child removed from the family and placed in foster care, the family could be ordered to provide the needed services, the child could be ordered to obey his or her parents, or the parents' *parental rights* could be terminated. In short, under this legal regime, at least during the child's minority, judges are given enormous power to determine the circumstances of the child's family relationships and upbringing.

Surrogate, probate, and orphans' courts are different names for another type of specialized tribunal, exercising authority over such matters as the financial affairs of persons who are legally or otherwise vulnerable, the young and the aged, the infirm, and the mentally ill. These courts conduct "civil commitment" and "guardianship" proceedings, grant adoptions, supervise the administration of estates and trusts and their trustees, and decide contested wills. From ancient times, such courts, acting as *parens patriae* (the community's parent, originally the king), exercise authority and responsibility to protect those who cannot protect themselves. Specialized courts of the kinds described often call on clinical professionals for advice and testimony. A probate court might ask for mental health professional testimony as to the ability of a patient with Alzheimer's disease to handle his own finances; parents whose parental rights the state is seeking to terminate may ask a child clinician for an opinion that they are capable in the future of taking adequate care of their children despite one parent's drug addiction or mental illness. The litigation contexts in which requests for clinical advice and testimony may be requested are multifarious, and the roles of the professional will vary with the client and the context. The clinician must understand how these variations affect his or her role and responsibility. The bulk of this book focuses on these contextual and role variations and the professional and ethical double binds these variations can cause the unwary.

TYPES OF LEGAL PROCEEDINGS

Courts of general jurisdiction hear both civil and criminal cases. For civil cases, a forum is provided to resolve the enormous variety of disputes that can arise between two litigants, plaintiff or defendant, third-party intervenors, cross-plaintiffs, and cross-defendants. Each of these legal actors is called a *party*—the generic label for any entity asserting a legal claim. A party may be an individual, a corporation, or indeed even a large class of individuals who share a common legal grievance or defense. An example of such a class is all women with silicon breast implants who claim injury and illness caused by the implants; another such class is all patients who develop tardive dyskinesia after years of compelled psychiatric medication.

Dynamics of Legal Proof

The essence of most cases can be explored by asking and answering three fairly simple questions:

1. **What must be proven?** Each type of civil lawsuit requires, if the plaintiff is to prevail, that specific assertions, known as the *elements* of the *cause of action*, be proved (similarly with a defendant's defenses, such as self-defense as a response to a lawsuit for assault and battery).
2. **Who must prove the elements?** In a civil suit, the plaintiff, that is, the person lodging the legal complaint, must prove the elements of the cause of action. This duty is expressed, in legal jargon, as the

burden of proof. In criminal cases, because of the "presumption of innocence" (remember the old saw: "It's better that ten guilty defendants go free than that one innocent defendant be convicted"), the state has the burden of proving the elements of the crime charged against the defendant. Despite these cautions designed to protect defendants in criminal cases, burdens of proof can and do shift for strategic and efficiency reasons. For example, if a criminal defendant claims the defense of not guilty by reason of insanity, in at least some states the defendant must carry the burden of introducing sufficient evidence of insanity to make a *prima facie* case (one that has offered evidence sufficient to allow a jury verdict favorable to the plaintiff)—only then does the burden of proof shift and require the prosecution to prove that the defendant is not insane.

3. **How much proof must be offered?** In most civil cases, the plaintiff, who has the burden of proof, must prove his case by a "preponderance of the evidence." But in some cases, again for practical or efficiency or fairness reasons, the more stringent "clear and convincing evidence" is required. This burden is imposed in some cases where the state is plaintiff or where the case involves some measure of punishment or stigma for the defendant. Paternity suits, terminations of parental rights, and commitments to mental hospitals have all been identified (occasionally by constitutional decree) as situations in which the more onerous burden of proof is required. In criminal cases, for reasons we have already mentioned, the burden of proof required is the even more stringent *beyond a reasonable doubt*.

Civil Cases

Civil disputes are usually categorized generically: contract claims, property and financial disputes, *torts*, including such subtypes as negligence, medical malpractice, libel, and slander, and various nonphysical invasions of the plaintiff's person or interests claimed to cause mental or physical injury and/or financial loss. An example of the last category is a claim by a child's parent or other relative for "pain and suffering" caused when the defendant killed or seriously injured the child.

Civil disputes typically involve a plaintiff asserting a financial loss because of the defendant's behavior and a request for a legal remedy for the loss—either a financial recovery or an *injunction* that the defendant must "cease and desist" from continuing the behavior causing the plaintiff injury. A contract claim, for example, must assert the legal elements of the cause of action; these include that one of the parties made an offer to the other, that the offeree made a valid acceptance of the offer, that the resulting agreement contained adequate consideration (the financial inducement for acceptance of the agreement), and that the defendant had breached the agreement to the plaintiff's financial disadvantage. Contract claims are typically set in the world of business dealings; but many contract lawsuits involve personal relationships in which finances are secondary considerations. For centuries marriages were considered contracts and their validity (in annulment proceedings) was determined as business contracts are still assessed; divorce was considered the remedy for breach of the marriage contract, with damages assessed against the breaching party. This is only one small way in which ancient concepts and the elements of causes of action conceived hundreds of years ago, under very different social and legal conditions, continue to affect social relationships and the development of legal remedies.

Tort actions are probably the most common form of civil action and the one most familiar to nonlawyers. A plaintiff asserts that the defendant owed her a "duty of care" and acted in a negligent manner, causing the plaintiff a foreseeable harm, loss, or injury. Personal injuries from car accidents, medical malpractice, and product liability claims are all examples. That the defendant owes the plaintiff a duty of care is sometimes clear and settled from statutes or judicial precedents: the physician's responsibility to her patient, for example, or the landlord's to his tenant. In some instances, however, especially when a novel cause of action is being asserted, the duty issue may be doubtful. The action for damages filed by the states against the tobacco companies affords a timely example. Another is the recent spate of suits by parents of adult patients against therapists for assisting patients to recover "memories" of childhood abuse. The duty of care issue is whether a therapist whose patient's relatives have been injured by the patient's false allegations can be liable to the relatives for negligent therapy. Courts have reached different conclusions about the issue.

Procedure and Evidence in Civil Cases

Civil suits follow a fairly standard course, governed by formal rules of "civil procedure" and codified "rules of evidence." These rules provide in very specific detail for every aspect of a lawsuit; where the suit can be filed, time deadlines for filing (called statutes of limitations), and methods of serving notice of the suit to the defendant are all specified in rules. Deviations may result in dismissal of the suit before the merits are reached.

Pretrial and Discovery in Civil Cases

"Rules of civil procedure," unique to each state but everywhere closely following the rules adopted in federal courts, allow and encourage full pretrial (i.e., preliminary to court hearings) exploration by each party of the opposing party's legal claims or defenses. The rules typically require full disclosure by each party of facts that conceivably bear on the cause of action or defenses to it. The parties are permitted to seek and obtain information through a variety of specified methods. The process is called *discovery*. It can include a variety of techniques.

Depositions. Depositions involve the taking of sworn testimony of the opposing party and any other person thought by the deposing party to have some knowledge of facts pertaining to the issues in the lawsuit. Depositions of clinicians are often taken if they have examined a child during the period preceding filing of a divorce or custody case.

Interrogatories. This technique involves a written deposition, usually questions requiring a written answer under oath, submitted to a party by the opposing litigant. The information sought can be far-reaching and extensive. In a suit claiming personal injury, for example, the plaintiff may be asked to set out the name and location of every health care provider ever visited, the reason for the visit and any diagnosis or treatment received.

Subpoenas. A subpoena is a court order (prepared and served by a lawyer) requiring the appearance of a witness for deposition or trial. A demand for the appearance of a witness or party with his or her records is known as a *subpoena duces tecum* (the Latin persists because lawyers, unlike clinicians, dislike giving up any of their ancient, mystifying vernacular). A request for record production may be very broad and general, such as when a company is asked to produce all phone logs, e-mails, and interoffice memos having any bearing on a case. Such requests for documents are open-ended and deemed continuing at least during the discovery phase of the case. The party seeking records or testimony does not need to know what the records contain before making a blanket request for production.

Examination of evidence. The rules of discovery permit examination and testing, where appropriate, of evidence produced. Documents may be analyzed and tested for authenticity, origin, and age. Similarly, plaintiffs who seek damages for physical and/or emotional loss—as well as any person, such as a custody contestant, whose mental state is "in issue"—may be required to submit to an independent medical and/or psychological examination

(IME), conducted by an examiner of the demanding litigant's choosing. In damage actions, the defendant is permitted to test the claims of loss or injury made by the plaintiff before the case proceeds to trial. The expert conducting an IME may be deposed by the opposing party concerning background, training, experience, and values. Typical deposition questions might include: "Doctor, have you ever done an IME of a defendant, or do you restrict your practice to testifying against injured plaintiffs?" "Isn't it true that the child psychiatry training program at [your university] has been suspended by the AHA?" "Isn't it true, Doctor, that you wrote an article for the *Psychological Bulletin* arguing that children [here fill in anything awful]?" Of course, the expert's opinions can also be explored and questioned. If a trial occurs, the IME examiner may expect to be called as an expert witness and to be examined and cross-examined by the litigants, and reference can be made to the expert's prior deposition for purposes of impeachment (i.e., to cast doubt on the reliability of the testimony).

Evidence disclosure. The parties may be required, before trial, to disclose the witnesses whom they intend to call, the nature of the witnesses' testimony, as well as any documents or physical evidence that might be introduced in evidence at trial. Expert witnesses' claimed expertise, education and experience, and the nature of their opinions must be disclosed so that the opposing party can prepare a defense, can perform a *voir dire* of the expert (an examination to prove, if the opponent wants to and can, that the expert is not in fact qualified as an expert), and can prepare to rebut the expert's testimony by calling an opposing expert as a witness.

Free discovery was introduced into the rules of procedure as a way of guaranteeing that the parties to a civil suit would approach trial knowing what evidence their opponent would introduce and be prepared to rebut it. Most observers believe that liberal pretrial discovery has produced earlier and fairer settlements and trials based on the merits rather than "surprise" and "ambush." But it has also made it possible for wealthier litigants to intimidate their less-well-off opponents through extensive discovery, raising their opponents' legal costs to sometimes unbearable amounts.

Civil Trials

If a civil case goes to trial, it may be heard by a jury, or if both parties agree, by the judge, acting as the fact finder. Some cases, those that traditionally were considered equity (or injunction) causes of action, are heard and decided only by a judge. The first element of a trial by jury is for the litigants, with the judge's supervision, to

impanel a jury after the voir dire of a jury panel. This exercise, consisting of questioning of jurors either individually or in groups by either the lawyers or the judge (depending on the jurisdiction), is designed to ensure that no juror biased about a particular litigant or a particular cause of action will be permitted to sit in judgment. Thus a juror who has been robbed at gunpoint would be excused from a prosecution for armed robbery, as would a relative of one of the case's parties.

At trial, the plaintiff puts his or her case on initially, setting out the facts that support the claim. Evidence is presented in the form of witness testimony and exhibits, which may be documents, photographs, charts, and so forth. The introduction of evidence is governed by formal rules of evidence. These are complex and codified rules applied by the judge to proffered testimony—but only at the request of the party against whose interest the testimony is proffered. These rules and the judge's application of them determine what the jury will be permitted to know about the case. When an objection is made to a proffer of evidence, the judge must rule on admissibility. These trial objections, always sharpening interest in dramatized trials or "Court TV," are obviously attempts by one party to influence the fact finder's view of the evidence and the case by precluding attention to some bit of evidence. "Speculation," "hearsay," "irrelevant," "repetitious," and "no foundation" are among the many objections you are likely to find familiar.

Each of the party's witnesses can be cross-examined by the opposing party. When the plaintiff's presentation of her case is complete (she "rests"), the defendant will usually make a motion to dismiss on grounds that the plaintiff has not proved a *prima facie* case. If this motion is denied, the defendant will then proceed to introduce her defenses and rebuttals to the plaintiff's witnesses. The trial now proceeds for the defendant as it did for the plaintiff. Then, before closing argument and the judge's "charge" to the jury, the plaintiff has a chance to introduce witnesses in rebuttal of the defendant's case. Rebuttal witnesses are often used against expert witnesses; they may challenge the opposing expert's knowledge, experience, or training or simply testify that the expert's testimony is based on some kind of factual or theoretical error.

The rules of evidence provide for the use of expert witnesses if it can be shown that by reason of scientific training, educational experience, or specialized knowledge, the expert has an understanding that ordinary persons do not possess and if the expert's testimony can be shown to aid the jury's deliberation in any fashion. As this phrasing indicates, the rules of evidence are generally oriented toward admissibility of expert testimony, subject to cross-examination and rebuttal "for what it's worth." In many states, though, expert testimony is still frowned on when the testimony "usurps the role of the jury"—for example, is directed to the *ultimate issue*, that is, answers the question that is the jury's responsibility to decide, as in "I believe the defendant was not guilty by reason of insanity," or "I conclude that the child was sexually abused." Once qualified by the court as an "expert," the expert witness may offer learned opinions and explanations derived from his special knowledge. Lay witnesses are usually restricted to testimony about what they have directly experienced.

After completion of the case presentations, the judge instructs ("charges") the jury on the law to be applied to the facts the jury finds proved from the testimony presented. The jury is told that it can make credibility judgments about the testimony of the various witnesses but that it is bound by the facts as presented and may not seek additional or external data to resolve its uncertainties. The jury is also instructed on the burden of proof, a topic we discussed earlier.

The judge's charge informs jurors of the legal elements of the cause of action and reminds them to ignore any testimony they heard to which proper objection was made. Although such testimony is typically struck from the record, it remains both in the transcript and, many contend, in the memories of jurors. Indeed, some social psychologists' laboratory research with mock jurors has shown that objections only call evidence more dramatically to jurors' attention and make the objectionable evidence more salient than at least some of the testimony to which no objection was made! Jury instructions these days are generally standard text material, prepared by professional groups and called *JIGs* and *CrimJIGs* (Jury Instruction Guides and Criminal Jury Instruction Guides). Interestingly, jurors quizzed on judges' instructions often display little understanding of the law they have applied or even recollection of what they have been told. Jurors do know that they have to decide who wins, and if it is the plaintiff, how much money must be awarded to provide compensation for the losses they have found the plaintiff incurred. In recent years, efforts to compel jurors to follow the law more—rather than only their rough sense of justice—in particular cases have led many jurisdictions to adopt the practice of requiring "special verdicts." These are verdict forms delivered when the jury begins its deliberations that require the jurors collectively to answer specific questions. The notion is that jurors' discretion will be constrained by compelling greater adherence to the legal elements of the case; in the event that special verdict forms show that the jury wanted the plaintiff or the defendant to win

despite contrary factual findings (an inconsistent verdict), the judge is in a better position to correct the jury's error.

Juries can award plaintiffs their actual losses, of course, and, in some instances, *punitive damages* as well. Excessive punitive damage awards in some recent highly publicized civil actions have led to a new legislative and even constitutional movement, approved by the U.S. Supreme Court, to constrain the imposition of punitive damages.

Criminal Cases

Criminal cases invoke the community's direct and vital interest in protecting the safety of its citizens and their values and community order (and, sometimes, what legislators believe should be their morals). Forbidden behaviors are legislatively codified in criminal statutes, providing citizens with advance notice of what acts by individuals are subject to societal sanction. Criminal sanctions can be imposed on behavior of minor significance, such as traffic infractions, or on behavior of substantial consequence and taboo, such as intentional homicide. As a consequence of this enormous variety in rule-breaking behavior, sanctions imposed on persons convicted of a crime can vary enormously, from small fines and community service to capital punishment, with great discretion left to judges to address the individual circumstances of individual defendants. In recent years, however, at least for major crimes, there has been a movement to adopt sentencing guidelines, designed to lessen judicial discretion and to equalize punishment for similar crimes and for similarly situated defendants. Sentences, and the proper method of punishing those who commit criminal acts, have become highly emotional issues. Sentencing guidelines have lessened the importance of clinical analysis and prediction by probation officers and clinicians in individual cases; they have also led to enormous increases in public costs and populations of prisons. Crime and the punishment for crimes will be among the major social and political issues in the next decades.

Procedure in Criminal Cases

Criminal justice is characterized by the constitutional and legislative imposition of a variety of formal procedures intended to protect a defendant from the vast powers the state has at its disposal in prosecuting defendants. Defendants' procedural rights usually derive from ancient English law, some of it codified in England in the Magna Carta, centuries of parliamentary statutes and judicial decrees, and other concepts derived from colonial reactions to the abuses of power of the Inquisition and the "Star Chamber." Many of the most well-known criminal procedural protections were codified in the Bill of Rights (the first ten amendments to the United States Constitution). These rights include: protection from compelled self-incriminating testimony, prohibition of illegal searches and seizures of evidence, a right to help from an attorney and a free attorney for the indigent, trial by jury, ability to confront and cross-examine opposing witnesses, a right to call witnesses in defense, and a bar against cruel and unusual punishment on conviction. The rights enumerated in the Bill of Rights now apply to state criminal prosecutions by virtue of the Due Process Clause of the Fourteenth Amendment. The general trend of decisions over time has expanded defendants' procedural rights—but the course has been neither smooth nor always in the same direction. For example, it took 40 years after the U.S. Supreme Court first declared that indigent criminal defendants are entitled to a free attorney until the Court held that all such defendants are entitled to counsel in both state and federal courts, and even today, indigent defendants are entitled to assigned counsel only if they are threatened with imprisonment rather than financial sanction alone. In short, constitutional protections for criminal defendants are controversial and subject to continuing shaping and trimming by state and federal courts.

Pretrial proceedings.   After a suspected criminal is arrested, a series of formal steps, some of them imposed by constitutional decree, must follow. The person arrested must be advised of his or her legal rights (Miranda warnings); the defendant must be formally notified of the charges and must be given an opportunity to plead to the charges and, with a few exceptions in cases of violent crimes, offered an opportunity to be released under conditions that offer some assurance (usually money, called *bail*) that the defendant will appear at subsequent proceedings.

The next stage requires the prosecutor to make some formal showing, either to a grand jury, which can issue an indictment, or, in some jurisdictions, to a judge in a preliminary hearing requested by the defendant after an "information" has been filed alleging the crime, that there is a threshold measure of evidence (probable cause to believe) that a crime has been committed and that the defendant committed it. The prosecutor need not put on the full measure of evidence available on these occasions, only enough to convince the grand jury or the preliminary hearing judge that probable cause exists. If the defendant is "bound over" for trial (and he almost always is), security arrangements to assure the defendant's attendance are reviewed.

In most states the prosecutor is obligated to share her file on the case with the defense, allowing the defendant to peruse reports from the police, witnesses' statements, and physical and other evidence. Constitutional precedents require the prosecutor to make available to the defendant any exculpatory evidence known to her. The U.S. Supreme Court has ruled that if the prosecutor fails to disclose exculpatory evidence, the prosecution must be dismissed.

Pleas and jury verdicts in criminal cases.   If a criminal case does not settle, the trial is governed by formal rules of procedure and the usual rules of evidence with some special intricacies adapted to the criminal context. Most prosecutions do not reach trial because defendants and their lawyers justifiably believe that a negotiated agreement, a *plea bargain*, is likely to get the defendant a better deal, for example, conviction of a lesser offense with a less onerous penalty, than she might obtain if she "rolls the dice" by going to trial. The defendant is entitled to a jury trial, which can be waived. The defendant is not required to take the stand in her own defense (a requirement that would violate the self-incrimination prohibition). Conviction of the defendant leads to a sentencing hearing and imposition of a sentence by the judge.

SUMMARY

This account of a vital and dynamic legal system, whose edges (if not its underlying principles) are under continuing examination and reflection, is necessarily elementary. When you come into contact with lawyers and the legal system, you will discover many idiosyncrasies of law and practice (and often many idiosyncratic practices of lawyers and judges) that might make you wonder about the accuracy of this account. Nonetheless, one lesson we hope you will not doubt: Lawyers, judges, and court systems all have one great (but not always attainable) goal—to do justice in individual cases without disrupting the orderliness and fairness of the legal system and of the community the system seeks to serve.

APPENDIX—LEGAL CITATIONS

Clinicians are often confronted, either in the courtroom while testifying or in consultations with lawyers, with questions such as: "Well, Doctor (occasionally pronounced with slight, forensic scorn), isn't it true that in the Jones case (alternatively, in *Jones v. Smith*), the court rejected your theory in a case identical to this one? You can find the case at 21 Ark [Arkansas Supreme Court Reports] 496, 375 SW2d [West's Southwest Reporter Second Series] 1025." Needless to say, such questions are designed, at least in part, to intimidate the forensic mental health expert, because he usually doesn't have his own lawyer nor does the expert's client's lawyer care in the slightest about the expert's comfort level. And the lawyer is often successful because the expert doesn't know the case or how to distinguish it from the case at hand and no clue as to the meaning of the numbers or the books to which the lawyer is referring.

The following short description is not designed to give clinicians law library research skills. Indeed, it seems sensible initially to warn readers that when situations of the kind described in the previous paragraph occur, they should seek legal help rather than relying on their own case-finding or, even more important, case-reading skills. Nonetheless, some awareness of what judges and lawyers mean when they talk such numbers mumbo jumbo may help experts to keep their cool. Appellate (but not trial court) decisions in every state are recorded and retrieved according to a volume numbering system originally conceived and currently maintained by the West Group, a large and dominant legal publishing house. (Today, all cases can also be retrieved electronically either through Lexis, a system maintained by a West Group competitor, or through WestLaw, a computerized service of the West Group.) At one time, every state maintained official reports of all decisions by its supreme court (and sometimes of decisions of its intermediate courts of appeal). For cases reported officially as well as by the West service, the citations are typically reported in a parallel fashion. Therefore, a decision's citation in a brief might look like this:

Jones v. Smith, 225 Mass 75, 410 NE2d 513 (1994)

In ordinary language, this citation means that a reader who wants to read the *Jones v. Smith* case can find it in volume 225 of the official Massachusetts Reporter at page 75 or in volume 410 of the West Northeast Reporter, second series, at page 513, and that the case was decided in 1994.

If the case had been in the Massachusetts intermediate appellate court, the citation would have looked like this:

225 Mass App 75, 410 NE2d 513 (1994)

To an ever-increasing extent, state judicial systems are forgoing their own official publications and relying solely on the West system. Thus the citations for the cases referred to would look like this

410 NE2d 513 (Mass 1994) (the Massachusetts Supreme Court decision)

or

410 NE2d 513 (Mass App 1994) (the intermediate appellate court decision)

For decision reporting purposes, the West system arbitrarily divides the country into seven areas: Atlantic (A and A2d—including Pennsylvania, Delaware, etc.), Northeast (NE and NE2d—including New York, Massachusetts, etc.), Southeast (SE and SE2d—including Virginia, North Carolina, etc.), Southern (So and So2d—including Mississippi, Kentucky, etc.), Southwestern (SW and SW2d—including Texas, Oklahoma, etc.), Northwestern (NW and NW2d—including Minnesota, Iowa, etc.), and Pacific (Pac and P2d—including California, Oregon, etc.).

There are additional mystifying idiosyncrasies with which we can bore you. Some state courts are known by unusual names and sometimes (but not always) the names affect citation forms. For example, the highest court in New York is known as the New York Court of Appeals, but the citation form is not affected; on the other hand, unlike court designations in any other state, the New York trial court is known as the supreme court, and official citations to its decisions, for reasons unknown to your otherwise expert authors, come in the form 27 Misc 424, 525 NY Supp (or NYS2d) 1002; the New York intermediate appellate court is known as the Supreme Court, Appellate Division.

The federal courts have their own designations and citation forms. The U.S. Supreme Court cites its own decisions in three different citation styles, although commentators usually refer only to one official set of reports and one unofficial set. We could go on—but those of you who are not bored must be bewildered—and here your education into (some of the easier to understand) legal research intricacies must pause.

REFERENCES

Burnham W: Introduction to the Law and Legal System of the United States, 2nd Edition. St. Paul, MN, West Group, 1999

Friedman LM: American Law: An Introduction, 2nd Edition. New York, WW Norton, 1998

Llewellyn KL: The Common Law Tradition: Deciding Appeals. Boston, MA, Little, Brown, 1960

Mauet TM: Trial Techniques, 4th Edition. Boston, MA, Little, Brown, 1996

CHAPTER 3

Forensic Ethics

Diane H. Schetky, M.D.

Case Example 1

Dr. Domingo has been treating Pedro Del Gado in psychotherapy for conduct problems for the past 6 months. Mrs. Del Gado informs him that she is no longer putting up with her abusive husband and that she has filed for divorce and is seeking sole custody of Pedro. A few months later, Dr. Domingo receives a subpoena to come to court with his records to testify at the divorce hearing on behalf of Mrs. Del Gado. He calls her attorney who says, "Doc, we really need you. You know more about this family and Pedro's needs than anyone else does."

Case Example 2

Mrs. Gluck, M.S.W., considers herself to be an expert on child sexual abuse and testifies for the state in a highly publicized case involving alleged sexual abuse at a day care center. She invokes both the "sexually abused child" and "sexual abuse accommodation" syndromes to fortify her argument that many of the plaintiffs have been sexually abused, even though they show no physical findings of abuse and their statements about alleged sexual abuse are equivocal at best.

Case Example 3

Dr. O'Reilly is hired by the defense to review a case in which two young male plaintiffs allege sexual abuse by a priest. The case is out of state, and she does not know anything about the referring attorney. She reviews a large amount of discovery material but does not have access to the plaintiffs. Based on what she has read, she sees a trail of behaviors in the priest and the boys that is highly suggestive of sexual abuse. She shares her impressions verbally with the attorney and says she does not think she can be of much help to the defense. The attorney thanks her, and she assumes she is off the case.

GUIDING ETHICAL PRINCIPLES

Controversy exists within the field of psychiatry as to whether a separate code of ethics is needed for the practice of forensic psychiatry. The guiding principle in the practice of medicine, since the time of Hippocrates, has been *primum non nocere*, first do no harm. Medicine stresses beneficence, helping the patient, along with nonmaleficence, not doing harm. If these values were given primacy in forensic settings, they would lead to the expert skewing data in order to help the examinee and would make it impossible to conduct an objective forensic assessment. The situation is further complicated in child custody cases in which the forensic examiner is guided legally by what is in the child's best interests. In contrast, no such advocacy role exists when evaluating a child or adolescent in criminal or civil proceedings, other than custody. Rather, the expert's duty becomes that of the truthful reporting of findings to the court to aid in the court's deliberations. Diamond (1988) proposes that the forensic psychiatrist's role is that of a fiduciary to the court and that, unlike the treating psychiatrist, he holds no fiduciary duty to the patient.

The traditional doctor-patient relationship assumes confidentiality and patient advocacy, which do not exist in forensic settings yet; the American Psychiatric Association (APA) and the American Academy of Child and Adolescent Psychiatry (AACAP) make no exceptions for forensic psychiatrists in their ethical guidelines. Forensic psychiatrist Paul Appelbaum (1997) suggests that the primary value in forensic psychiatry should be justice that is based on the ethical principles of truth-telling and respect for persons. He reminds us that clinical obligations are abrogated in other medical specialties besides forensic psychiatry and offers the example of the research physician for whom truth holds primacy over any duty to the patient. It is the ability to tell the truth in court that allows us to render credible and useful testimony. Honesty may entail discussing the limitations of the basis of one's testimony and even altering one's opinion in the face of new contradictory evidence. Appelbaum (1997) defines respect for persons as "acting to negate the risks associated with one's role." For instance, the examinee may perceive an empathic forensic examiner as being there to help him and might in turn disclose information that is not in his best interest. The examiner may need to remind the examinee of the examiner's role. Respect for persons also involves protecting the confidentiality of forensic exams beyond the judicial setting.

The American Academy of Psychiatry and the Law (AAPL) (1995) has established ethical guidelines governing the conduct of forensic evaluations that stress honesty and strive for objectivity, confidentiality, and consent. It does not address the overarching issue of the primacy of the APA guidelines. Interest in clarifying this issue is high in both organizations, particularly because APA or AACAP membership is a prerequisite for membership in AAPL. The AAPL guidelines do not deal with issues unique to child and adolescent forensic psychiatry. AACAP has published practice guidelines for conducting custody evaluations and evaluations for suspected child sexual or physical abuse, but neither contains much discussion about ethical issues (AACAP 1997a, 1997b).

The American Psychological Association (1994) offers very specific guidelines regarding role clarification and separating forensic evaluation from treatment. Their Ethics Code also stresses that if a therapist is compelled to testify about a patient, that he or she only do so as a fact witness. The Code speaks to the need to recognize boundaries of particular competencies and the limits of expertise (American Psychological Association 1992).

PITFALLS

Role Confusion

Clinicians need to be clear about whether their role with a patient is that of one who treats or that of a forensic examiner. The patient needs to be apprised of this at the onset. Roles may become blurred when legal issues arise in the course of therapy if, for instance, a young patient discloses sexual abuse or a patient's parents divorce. It is very easy for therapists to get drawn into legal issues, and focus on those issues may derail therapy. Therapists may

naively assume that they are in a position to help the court because of their long-term relationships with the litigating parties and their insights into family dynamics. It is their very involvement that prevents them from being objective evaluators. Furthermore, much of what they know about a family is based on narrative truth, that is, as perceived by the patient, as opposed to corroborating evidence and facts that a forensic evaluator would consider in rendering an opinion. Therapists are less likely to question what their patients tell them, whereas forensic psychiatrists tend to be more skeptical, considering motives, the possibility of secondary gain, and malingering.

The therapist who is subpoenaed to testify in court faces many perils. Her credentials may be challenged before the patient's family, and they may learn things about her that affect her anonymity. They may see her attacked for being less than objective; she may be forced to reveal things about parents that they did not know were in her records, or she might have to reveal hurtful comments made by a child about a parent. Involvement in the often hostile climate of a child custody battle may adversely affect her opinions about her patient's parents and compromise her ability to work with them. Opinions she offers the court about a parent may be based primarily on what a child or parent has told her rather than on direct observation. The therapist's testimony may also be tainted by her wish not to hurt her patient. Finally, in custody disputes, one side often emerges unhappy and that parent may have no incentive to support ongoing therapy for the child.

Problems also arise if a forensic examiner becomes a treating clinician. If he refers the patient to himself, this may appear self-serving. There is risk that treatment may become an extended forensic evaluation and that the patient, knowing the therapist has testified once, is likely to have concerns about future confidentiality. Exceptions may exist in underserved areas where therapists and forensic examiners are scarce.

Impartiality

Impartiality implies that the examiner enters into a forensic case with no preconceptions, stereotypes, biases, or agendas and that she is able to approach the case with an open mind.

Using the terms *perpetrator* and *victim* prior to any findings of fact may indicate bias. Examiners who have an agenda may tailor questions to the desired responses and ignore disconfirming statements or evidence. They may also invoke offbeat theories to support their unique opinions, even though they are not currently accepted in the profession. Such behaviors amount to intellectual dishonesty. Prior ties, be they social or professional, to any of the parties in the case may also affect the outcome of a forensic evaluation. Even if the examiner feels he will not be biased by them, a jury may decide otherwise.

Diamond (1973) argues that "there is no such thing as an impartial witness; the objectivity of the expert witness is largely a myth; the solution is to drop all pretense of impartiality and allow the trier of fact to clearly see the biases and values of the witness." Being court-appointed may confer the outward appearance of neutrality, but it does not mitigate against unconscious bias and issues of countertransference, which may affect opinions and recommendations. An expert might identify with the particular lifestyle of foster parents and favor them over the parents of a child in their care, even though returning home to impoverished parents might be preferable for the child. Judges are not without biases and may appoint experts with similar views to evaluate a case.

Conflicts of Interest

Conflicts of interest should preclude involvement in forensic cases. A forensic examiner might be treating a relative of a plaintiff whose attorney is seeking his services. In such a case, he needs to decline, citing conflict of interest without giving the specifics. Other potential conflicts of interest might include classmates of the examiner's children, prior patients, and persons in the examiner's social or professional circles.

Confidentiality and Consent

Information contained in forensic reports is subject to rules of confidentiality with the exception of their use by attorneys involved in the case and the court. Subjects of forensic exams should be informed of the purpose of the evaluation, who has retained you, and the limitations of confidentiality. Once an expert has testified in open court on a matter, her testimony is public record except in juvenile cases in which courtrooms may be closed to the public and records are sealed.

The Limits of Prediction

Forensic examiners are often asked to predict future violence in persons they have examined. This question comes up in commitment hearings, decisions about removing an abused child from an abusive home, whether or not to pursue parental reunification, waiver, presentencing evaluations, and cases involving preventative detention. The Supreme Court in the case of *Schall v. Martin* (see Chapter 25, "Overview of Juvenile Law," for case description) allowed for preventative detention of potentially dangerous juveniles. Early research warned that mental health professionals were ill equipped to predict future violence. Grisso and Appelbaum (1992) challenge this assumption and argue that in certain situations such testimony is not necessarily unethical. They opine that it may be ethical if the predictive testimony has adequate scientific support and note that the research in this area is becoming more sophisticated. They note the need to consider the "ethically significant nature of the predictive testimony, the foundation of the predictive testimony, and the legal consequences of the prediction." However, in most cases, the expert is better off outlining risk factors for potential violence along with mitigating factors, rather than making absolute predictions.

Death Penalty Cases

The American Medical Association (1995) prohibits physicians from participating in legally authorized executions, and the APA has endorsed this position. Many believe that it is unethical for psychiatrists to take any part in actions that might lead to the death of an inmate, and the APA (1990) has argued that physicians should not be involved in medicating an inmate with the purpose of restoring competency so that he or she can be executed, nor should they participate in evaluations regarding the competency to be executed. Instead, it recommends commuting the sentence to life imprisonment and then treating the inmate's mental illness.

The U.S. Supreme Court in *Thompson v. Oklahoma* (1988) banned the execution of persons who committed their crime prior to age 16. It reasoned that juveniles have less culpability than adult offenders and that capital punishment as a form of retribution should not be applied to them. However, executions of persons age 17 or 18 at the time they committed their crimes are permitted, and there are currently 70 inmates in this category on death row. Many states are attempting to curb crime rates by restoring the death penalty in the belief that it acts as a deterrent, although the basis for this belief has never been proven. More juveniles are being waived to adult courts and receiving harsher punishments. It is conceivable that we may soon see some states arguing for the execution of juveniles who have committed heinous crimes.

Hired Guns

Pejorative terms such as *hired guns* or *courtroom whores* have been applied to expert witnesses who "sell their testimony instead of time" (Gutheil 1998). They may be easy to spot by the fact that they always offer the same opinion, for example, finding sexual abuse or recommending paternal custody. They may be arrogant and unwilling to speak to the limitations of their examinations or to admit that they might be wrong. The incentive to engage in this sort of behavior may be purely financial, the expert may have difficulty holding ground in the face of the hiring attorney's efforts to shape his or her opinions and testimony, or he or she may have a personal agenda. Although the extent of the hired gun problem may be exaggerated by the media, it nevertheless exists and does not help the public image of forensic psychiatry. We are also seeing a backlash in which critics of repressed memory theory have invoked these terms to attack the credibility and integrity of reputable clinicians and researchers who have testified in cases of posttraumatic stress disorder.

Fees

It is always unethical for the forensic examiner to accept a contingency fee because it creates a vested interest in the outcome of a case. In contrast, attorneys whose roles are adversarial commonly take contingency fees in tort litigation cases. If an examinee is truly indigent, the forensic examiner can offer to do the case pro bono or refer it to a forensic clinic, if one exists in the area.

Billing in forensic cases can become quite complex, particularly if one is on the road and doing cases back-to-back. Gutheil and colleagues (1998) provide an interesting discussion of this matter and billing units, along with the problem of the temptation to overbill.

It is a mistake to go into forensics merely because it is potentially a lucrative field. It may be lucrative, but it is also intellectually and ethically challenging, and the expert's behavior is very public and subject to scrutiny. Ethical integrity is essential if the expert wishes to stay on top. It is important to have other sources of income to fall back on, such as consulting work, a salaried job, or a part-time therapy practice, so that you can be selective about the cases in which you choose to become involved.

REPORTING ETHICAL VIOLATIONS

Appelbaum (1992) notes that the courts have inadequate mechanisms for controlling the quality of testimony, that they often fail to adequately qualify potential expert witnesses, and that rarely do they invoke penalties for witnesses who perjure themselves.

Neither the AACAP nor the AAPL has a forum for hearing ethical complaints. Ethical complaints must be handled through the district branches of the APA, where they most likely will be heard by members who have little grounding in the principles of forensic psychiatry. The members hearing a complaint will turn to the APA's *The*

Principles of Medical Ethics With Annotations Especially Applicable to Psychiatry (American Psychiatric Association 2001), which offers little guidance for forensic practices. However, members of the AAPL Ethics Committee are available to district branch ethics committees to assist in cases involving forensic psychiatry issues. Alternatively, complaints may be brought to state licensing boards. Ethical complaints against forensic psychologists are heard either by state licensing boards or by state psychological association ethics committees.

Aggrieved parties may also file civil suits against forensic examiners. There have been cases in which experts were sued for failing to find sexual abuse and for falsely diagnosing sexual abuse. In one particularly troubling case, *Althaus v. Cohen* (1998), a child psychiatrist was sued for believing her patient's allegations of abuse and failing to conduct a forensic evaluation. The judge instructed the jury that the psychiatrist held a duty of care to the parents of her teenage patient, who was no longer in the custody of her parents. The jury concluded that the psychiatrist violated this duty by failing to meet with the patient's parents. The case was appealed and the Pennsylvania Supreme Court ruled that the trial court had erred in imposing such a duty upon Dr. Cohen. This case is discussed in more detail in Chapter 33, "Psychic Trauma and Civil Litigation."

As is evident in this discussion, there are currently no adequate mechanisms in place for handling complaints about the ethical conduct of forensic psychiatrists. Developing the means to handle ethical complaints within subspecialty associations is extremely costly. It seems unlikely that the APA Principles of Medical Ethics, which is a derivative of the American Medical Association Code of Ethics, will expand to encompass forensics. However, the APA periodically publishes *Opinions of the Ethics Committee on the Principles of Medical Ethics With Annotations Especially Applicable to Psychiatry* (American Psychiatric Association 2001), which does take up forensic questions. The best remedy to the matter of complaints is to practice prevention, including better training in forensic psychiatry and the use of continued medical education, expanded practice guidelines, peer review, and consultation with more experienced forensic psychiatrists.

CASE EXAMPLE EPILOGUES

Case Example I

Although Dr. Domingo would like to be helpful to the court, having read this chapter, he realizes that his testimony may not be helpful to Pedro and might even compromise his therapy with him. He also realizes that he is biased in favor of Pedro's mother, with whom he has spent more time than with Pedro's father, about whom he lacks much firsthand information. He follows the advice of Strassburger et al. (1997) and responds to the subpoena stating, "Having observed the patient only from the vantage point of a treating clinician, I have no objective basis for rendering an expert opinion, with a reasonable degree of medical certainty, on a legal as opposed to a clinical question" (p. 454).

Case Example 2

Mrs. Gluck is being less than honest with the court when she infers that the "sexually abused child syndrome" and the "sexual abuse accommodation syndrome" are reliable means of diagnosing child sexual abuse and that they are accepted psychiatric diagnoses. She is misusing concepts to satisfy her agenda of proving sexual abuse. Numerous cases have been overturned because syndrome testimony of this sort was admitted into evidence. In her eagerness to prevail, she has done a disservice to the justice system and the child plaintiffs, and she has also compromised her integrity.

Case Example 3

Dr. O'Reilly has not heard the last of this aggressive attorney, who calls her 6 months later shortly before trial requesting that she testify only to the physical improbability of the plaintiffs being sexually abused in the positions they described. She does not wish to be in a position of helping acquit someone whom she believes to be guilty. Furthermore, testifying in such a narrow scope would not be a full or honest reflection of her opinions in the case. She refuses. The attorney is not happy but goes on to retain one of her colleagues who testifies at the trial. The priest is convicted.

ACTION GUIDELINES

Avoid Dual Roles

If forensic issues arise in treatment cases, insist on an outside forensic evaluation. Therapists who are compelled to testify should do so in as narrow a way as possible and refrain from offering opinions or recommendations.

Perform Integrity Checks

The contrary quotient asks: "How often do I give the side that hired me what they want?" If you are always offering the desired opinion, this raises questions about your ethical integrity (Schetky and Colbach 1982). Another useful check is to read your reports from the vantage point of the other side, looking for omissions, bias, or weakness in your arguments. It is useful to ask, "How might my report have differed had I prepared it for the opposing side?"

Utilize Peer Review and Consultation

AAPL has established a program of peer review of reports and transcripts of depositions or hearings, which is open to members at the annual meeting. This has proven to be a very popular teaching forum. Informal peer review with more experienced forensic colleagues is another way in which you can seek opinions on difficult ethical issues.

Avoid Offering Opinions on Parties Not Seen

This issue may arise in unilateral child custody evaluations in which the examiner needs to refrain from making any comparisons of parents or offering opinions on a parent he has not seen. It also arises when the expert is attempting to respond to media inquiries about high-profile cases or celebrities. Any comments should be prefaced with the comment: "As a child and adolescent psychiatrist, I cannot comment about people I have not personally examined, but I would be glad to discuss the issue in general with you."

Respect Boundaries

Respect boundaries and avoid social or sexual encounters with any parties or relatives of parties you have seen in a forensic context.

Do Not Exceed Your Area of Expertise and Stay Current

Be familiar with and stay abreast of changes in your professional ethical codes. Take advantage of continued medical education courses dealing with forensics and ethics. AAPL also offers an excellent 3-day board review course that covers ethical issues along with other topics.

REFERENCES

Althaus v Cohen, 729 A2d 1124 (Pa Sup Ct 1998)

American Academy of Child and Adolescent Psychiatry: Practice Parameters for Child Custody Evaluations. Washington, DC, American Academy of Child and Adolescent Psychiatry, 1997a

American Academy of Child and Adolescent Psychiatry: Practice Parameters for the Forensic Evaluation of Children and Adolescents Who May Have Been Physically or Sexually Abused. Washington, DC, American Academy of Child and Adolescent Psychiatry, 1997b

American Academy of Psychiatry and the Law: Ethical Guidelines for the Practice of Forensic Psychiatry, Revised. Bloomfield, CT, American Academy of Psychiatry and the Law, 1995 [www.aapl.org/ethics.htm]

American Medical Association: Current Ethical Opinions of the Council on Ethical and Judicial Affairs. Chicago, IL, American Medical Association, 1995

American Psychiatric Association: Death row inmates shouldn't be made to become competent. Psychiatry News 25(15):2, 1990

American Psychiatric Association: Opinions of the Ethics Committee on the Principles of Medical Ethics With Annotations Especially Applicable to Psychiatry, 2001 Edition. Washington, DC, American Psychiatric Association, 2001

American Psychiatric Association: The Principles of Medical Ethics With Annotations Especially Applicable to Psychiatry, 2001 Edition. Washington, DC, American Psychiatric Association, 2001

American Psychological Association: American Psychological Association Code of Ethics. Washington, DC, American Psychological Association, 1992

American Psychological Association: Guidelines for Child Custody Evaluations in Divorce Proceedings. Am Psychol 49(7):677–680, 1994

Appelbaum P: Forensic psychiatry: the need for self-regulation. Bulletin of the American Academy of Psychiatry and Law 20(2):153–162, 1992

Appelbaum P: A theory of ethics for forensic psychiatry. J Am Acad Psychiatry Law 25(3):233–246, 1997

Diamond B: The psychiatrist as advocate. Journal of Psychiatry and Law 1:7–19, 1973

Diamond B: The psychiatrist: consultant vs activist in legal doctrine. Paper presented at the annual meeting of the American Academy of Psychiatry and the Law, San Francisco, CA, October 20, 1988

Grisso T, Appelbaum P: Is it unethical to offer predictions of future violence? Law Hum Behav 16:621–633, 1992

Gutheil T: The Psychiatrist as Expert Witness. Washington, DC, American Psychiatric Press, 1998, p 7

Gutheil T, Slater F, Commons M, et al: Witness travel dilemmas: a pilot study of billing practices. J Am Acad Psychiatry Law 26(1):21–26, 1998

Schall v Martin 467 US 253 (1984)

Schetky D, Colbach E: Countertransference on the witness stand: a flight from self? Bulletin of the American Academy of Psychiatry and Law 10(2):115–122, 1982

Strassburger L, Gutheil T, Brodsky A: On wearing two hats: role conflict in serving as both psychotherapist and expert witness. Am J Psychiatry 154(4):448–456, 1997

Thompson v Oklahoma 4887 US 815 (1988)

SUGGESTED READINGS

Appelbaum P: The parable of the forensic psychiatrist: ethics and the problem of doing harm. In K Law Psychiatry 13:249–259, 1990

Ciccone R, Clements C: Forensic psychiatry and applied clinical ethics: theory and practice. Am J Psychiatry 141(3):395–399, 1984

Griffith E: Ethics in forensic psychiatry: a cultural response to Stone and Appelbaum. J Am Acad Psychiatry Law 26(2):171–184, 1998

Kermani E, Kantor K: Psychiatry and the death penalty: the landmark Supreme Court cases and their ethical implications for the profession. Bulletin of the American Academy of Psychiatry and Law 22(1):95–108, 1994

Rossner R, Weinstock R (eds): Ethical Practice in Psychiatry and the Law. New York, Plenum, 1990

Schetky D: Ethics and the clinician in custody disputes. Child Adolesc Psychiatr Clin N Am 7(2):455–465, 1998

Stone A: The ethics of forensic psychiatry: a view from the ivory tower, in Law, Psychiatry, and Morality. Edited by Stone A. Washington, DC, American Psychiatric Press, 1984, pp 57–76

CHAPTER 4

Introduction to Forensic Evaluations

Diane H. Schetky, M.D.

Case Example 1

Dr. Bartoli is doing a custody evaluation on a family with three children. The father has agreed to pay for the evaluation in installments with the final payment due prior to the release of her report. The court date is approaching, and Dr. Bartoli, being compulsive and conscientious, has her report ready to release pending the final payment. She receives a phone call from the father saying he and his wife have decided to reconcile and they do not need her report.

Case Example 2

An attorney refers his client to a child and adolescent psychiatry clinic for a forensic evaluation of her parenting skills. The state has filed a petition to terminate her parental rights, and he is requesting an independent evaluation. The attorney insists his main concern is with what is in the best interests of his client's children. Dr. Gould, a resident, is assigned the case and reviews records, meets with the mother, and observes her with her young children. He produces a very comprehensive report in which he raises serious concerns about the mother's parenting skills. He is irate because the attorney does not like his findings and chooses not to use his evaluation.

Case Example 3

An attorney calls Dr. Wolf requesting an urgent evaluation of her client's two children, who are refusing to return to their mother after a 2-month summer visitation with their father, the client. The children are alleging physical abuse by their mother and verbal abuse by their stepfather.

LEGAL ISSUES

Dealing With Attorneys

Initial Involvement With a Case

Attorneys contact forensic examiners because of mental health– or disability-related issues in their cases, which, according to one survey of attorneys and judges, arose in one-seventh of their cases and in one-third of juvenile cases (Mossman and Kapp 1998). The same survey found that the most important factors attorneys consider in selecting expert witnesses are their knowledge, ability to communicate, and their local reputation. The importance of obtaining a favorable opinion from the expert ranked only fifth—above previous experience with the expert. Attorneys are also interested in the integrity of a potential witness and whether or not he or she will stand by his or her opinion.

Most often, forensic referrals come directly from an attorney, the guardian *ad litem* for the child, or the expert is appointed by the court. Requests for parenting assessments may also come from protective services. Those requests that come directly from parties involved in a legal matter should always be funneled through their attorneys to clarify legal issues and determine that they, in fact, have legal representation. It is wise to ascertain whether a psychiatric or psychological examination is being requested, as some attorneys and judges do not understand the difference.

In the initial contact, the attorney will want to know something about your background. It is customary to send your curriculum vitae; however, this alone does not reflect your forensic experience. The latter may be kept in a separate file and should include the names of the cases in which you have testified or been deposed, docket numbers, court jurisdiction, dates of cases, types of cases, places of testimony, and names of retaining attorneys. A computer database is a good way of keeping track of forensic cases. The retaining attorney may request this list, as may the attorney for the other side once the examiner's name has been produced as a potential witness. You should be aware that attorneys also have ready access to any prior testimony you have given through computer databases such as WestLaw and Lexis-Nexis, and they may read any relevant publications you have authored.

It is important to clarify which party the contracting attorney represents, and it is useful to know who the parties and other attorneys are to rule out any possible conflicts of interest. For instance, the author was once requested to do a visitation assessment by an attorney representing a father who lived in Alaska who said the children in question lived "somewhere in the midcoast area of Maine." Somewhere in midcoast Maine turned out to be a block away from her home, which was too close for comfort, and she withdrew from the case.

Determining the Purpose of the Evaluation

As the legal issue at hand will be the focus of the evaluation, it is critical to know what it is and what the pertinent legal standard is; be certain that you understand the meaning of the wording. Attorneys may not always be sure at the onset of a case how they plan to defend it. They may be seeking the views of an expert to see if, for instance, mental illness is grounds for an insanity defense or in civil cases whether damages have ensued as a result of psychic trauma. It is useful to request a cover letter in which they articulate their particular questions about the case.

In child and adolescent forensic psychiatry, cases typically involve issues of child custody, personal injury, criminal issues, presentencing evaluations, occasional malpractice cases, and rarely, the insanity defense. These issues will be discussed in subsequent chapters. The distinctions between civil and criminal cases are major. The former involve a lower standard of proof (preponderance of evidence), and the issue at stake is usually money. The latter involve potential loss of liberty and require a higher standard of proof (beyond a reasonable doubt). In practical terms, civil and custody cases often take years to settle. Criminal cases are settled more swiftly and are usually heard on a trailing docket, which means the expert may be called to testify on short notice.

Spelling Out Ground Rules

Forensic examiners should never give premature assurances about the nature of their potential testimony until they have had a chance to complete their evaluation. It is advisable to tell the referring attorney that you will call the case as you see it, which may not necessarily be to his or her liking. Examiners should make it clear from the onset that their ethics and objectivity will not be compromised. It is not possible—nor is it ethical—to offer opinions on a particular party one has not personally evaluated. However, experts may be retained for other purposes such as critiquing prior evaluations, testifying about theoretical issues, or advising the attorney on trial strategy.

Deciding Whether to Accept a Case

Your Qualifications

The expert needs to ask whether she has sufficient expertise in the area in question, because credentials will be reviewed in court as part of qualifying the expert. If she has doubts, these should be shared with the referring attorney and she might even suggest a more experienced colleague. Neophytes should not be embarrassed by paucity of credentials; inexperience may often counter the image of being a hired gun. For instance, knowledge of forensic principles and the ability to do a thorough, objective assessment may be more important than being able to boast of having seen two dozen juvenile arsonists. It is always appropriate to seek consultation on difficult cases at any stage in one's career.

The expert also needs to be open regarding any skeletons in his closet that might preclude his involvement in a case, such as a pending malpractice suit, prior ethical complaints, or even a recent arrest for speeding or driving under the influence, if relevant to the case.

Merits of the Case

Considering the time and energy that goes into a forensic evaluation, it is useful at the onset to ask whether the case merits such an investment on your part. Is this an issue about which you feel strongly? Is there enough data available to permit an in-depth evaluation? If a party is claiming false allegations of abuse, is there sufficient doubt to warrant examining the records or parties?

Time and Distance Limitations

It is almost always ill advised to accept a case on short notice. Rarely is there time in which to do adequate preparation, and such referrals often indicate that a witness has backed out of the case at the last minute or that the attorney is poorly organized.

Given the paucity of child and adolescent forensic examiners, requests for evaluations from out of state are not uncommon, particularly if the expert has a national reputation or area of special expertise. One needs to weigh the impact of time lost to travel on one's practice and family.

Trials may not proceed on schedule, and the expert may spend many long hours waiting to testify or stuck in airports. Travel time need not be lost time and can be put to good use reviewing the case, reading, or enjoying audiobooks. Geographic desirability and novelty-seeking genes also enter into the equation. A word of caution: accepting a case in Florida in the depths of winter may be appealing, but the case is likely to come to trial in the heat of summer.

Conflicts of Interest

Dual agency occurs if one has a duty to two different parties, such as the therapist who tries to simultaneously act as forensic examiner, as was discussed in Chapter 3, "Forensic Ethics." With forethought, such duality can be avoided in most situations.

Sometimes an expert may be contacted by the opposing side when she has already discussed the case with the other side's attorney. This is almost always grounds for refusing to become involved, even if the side that first contacted her did not hire her, because she is now tainted and privy to confidential information and considered part of the first attorney's team. If this situation arises, the forensic examiner should cite a conflict of interest without going into details. Unfortunately, some attorneys engage in what Berger (1997) refers to as preventive contracting, in which they contact a potential witness—with no intention or using him or her—merely to prevent the other side from retaining that person.

Another conflict of interest might involve a vested interest in the outcome. For example, you might happen to hold stock in a discount department store that is being sued by the parents of a 5-year-old who was injured when a large, poorly stacked box fell from a shelf and landed on her head.

Any prejudices the examiner holds that could be related to the case should also be shared, such as strong feelings about sexual preference or custody arrangements.

Is the Attorney Someone With Whom You Can Work?

This may not be possible to assess until you have embarked on the evaluation. In some instances, you can ask around about the attorney's reputation and speak to others who might have worked with her. Qualities to look for include legal acumen, ethical conduct, respect for clients, organizational skills, and good communication skills. It is important that attorneys be accessible, maintain good lines of communication with their experts, and not withhold important information. Attorneys who are unduly familiar or attempt to seduce you with flattery or money should give you reason to think twice about accepting referrals from them.

Liability of the Expert Witness

Can an expert witness be sued for what he says in his report or on the witness stand? In most jurisdictions, if the expert is court appointed, he is considered to be acting in a quasi-judicial capacity and accordingly is entitled to the protection of absolute immunity. Courts have expanded the doctrine of absolute judicial immunity to include those persons involved in an integral part of the judicial process. This enables them to act freely without the threat of a lawsuit and encourages them to act with disinterested objectivity. Less clear is the liability of the expert who is acting without a court order.

Out-of-State Cases

In 1998, the American Medical Association (AMA) passed a resolution stating that "expert witness testimony is the practice of medicine." This has raised the unresolved question of whether licensing should be required in each state in which the expert testifies. If requested to perform a forensic evaluation in a state where you are not licensed, it is prudent to ascertain that the laws of that state permit you to perform an evaluation and/or testify there. If not, one might be disqualified to testify and could face civil or criminal actions as well as disciplinary actions (Simon and Shuman 1999). Reid (2000) provides a useful list of state licensure requirements for out-of-state forensic psychiatric examinations. Yet another issue to be aware of is that you may not be covered by your liability insurance if you are conducting an evaluation in a state where you do not hold a license and that state requires licensure for forensic evaluation. Alternatively, you may have the examinee come to a state where you are licensed to perform the evaluation.

It is important to become familiar with the legal standards of the examinee's state and the interpretation of these standards, particularly if they differ from those in the state in which you work. For instance, within the United States there are three different standards for the insanity defense and the wording of the standards varies from state to state.

CLINICAL EVALUATIONS

Structuring the Evaluation

Fees

Fees should be discussed at the onset. Rates vary regionally and by experience and are customarily much higher than the reimbursement one would receive for psychotherapy. Justification for higher rates includes added training and skills, the demanding nature of the work, and the often disruptive effect these cases have on one's practice and life. Most experts charge by the hour. Gutheil (1998) recommends choosing a fee that you would not be embarrassed to state in court. Exorbitant fees may alienate jurors and lead them to believe your opinion has been bought. Flat fees are not a good idea because one can never anticipate exactly how much time might be involved in a case. The amount of material to be reviewed in civil cases often mushrooms as the cases mature and as parties and their experts are deposed; the expert may be asked to review hundreds of pages of depositions.

In out-of-state cases, it is customary to request a per diem rate in addition to reimbursement for travel, lodging, and meals. It is not proper to bill for time spent sleeping. When possible, a retainer fee should be requested at the onset, which covers estimated time to be spent reviewing records, interviewing parties and collaterals, conferring with the attorney, and preparing a report. Retainers are not possible when doing defense cases for the state, that is, for a public defender or protective services, and oftentimes there is a cap on what they are willing to pay. Reimbursement in state cases is usually lower, but the cases are often of interest and good for the learning curve.

Some forensic experts charge more for time spent testifying. The amount of time spent in court is but a small fraction of the time devoted to the case, and jurors may raise eyebrows at what they view as excessively high fees for courtroom testimony.

Contracting With the Attorney

It is advisable to develop a service agreement with the retaining attorney. This should cover the nature of the services to be provided, your hourly rate, and policies on billing for phone calls, missed appointments, or appointments canceled at the last minute. In addition, it should cover per diem rates, travel policies, and expectations of reimbursement for portal-to-portal travel and waiting time when called to testify. A statement that failure of the party to pay the attorney does not relieve that attorney of obligation to pay fees related to the referral should

be included. The agreement should be signed by the attorney and a copy returned to the examiner. Providing the attorney with your tax ID number will expedite payment.

Access to Parties and Information

Having agreed to participate in the case, the examiner should state which parties he wishes to see, discuss which records to review, and anticipate approximately how much time will be involved. Attorneys can be very helpful in amassing and even indexing discovery material such as school records, prior psychiatric evaluations, medical records, and hospitalizations. Physicians are not the best judges of what material is legally relevant, nor are attorneys the best judges of what materials are clinically relevant. Therefore, it is often necessary to sift through a great deal of information, some of which may not be relevant. The other rationale for reviewing all of the material is to make sure the attorney has not withheld records unfavorable to her client. However, there may be cases in which it would be prohibitively expensive to expect the expert to read all of the documents that do not appear to be relevant to the forensic issue in question.

Deadlines

Attorneys, in contrast to psychiatrists, work under a variety of deadlines. Discovery dates refer to the deadline for listing one's experts and allows each side time in which to review data, depose experts, and explore strategies prior to trial. Written reports need to be submitted prior to trial in time to allow both sides to review them. It is important to inquire whether or not the referring attorney wants a written report and, if so, by what date.

Determining Need for Further Consultation

Early into the evaluation it is usually apparent what additional consultations will be needed. For instance, psychological testing often helps bolster the examiner's opinions and may be useful in ruling out faking good in parenting assessments or faking bad in tort litigation. Neurological or other medical assessments may be indicated in some children, and these should be obtained in time to incorporate results into your report.

Scheduling

Berger (1997) recommends that referring attorneys schedule the evaluation and offers a twofold rationale for this: If the patient fails to show or arrives late, this becomes the attorney's problem and he is liable for paying for the scheduled time; in addition, it avoids the problem of prior contact with the examinee, which might affect the examiner's objectivity. On the other hand, direct contact with the parties might ensure that they know how to find your office, and some of these early interchanges may be quite telling and could be considered part of the evaluation.

Obtaining Consent

At the onset, you need to clarify with the parties to be examined who retained you and for what purpose. The fact that the examination is not therapy should be stated and may need to be reiterated in the course of the evaluation. Examinees must be apprised of the limited confidentiality and told who will have access to the report. The above discussion provides the basis for informed consent to the forensic evaluation. Forms should be signed indicating consent to the evaluation and waivers for release of information.

If there is any question about capacity to give consent, you need to refer to the court or counsel and have a guardian appointed. For instance, the author was once asked to do a parenting assessment regarding possible termination of parental rights on a blatantly psychotic woman who denied giving birth to the child in question.

Meeting With the Parents

In ordinary diagnostic evaluations, one assumes that parents are being straightforward and acting out of concern for the child. In contrast, in forensic evaluations, parents' presentations may be colored by the nature of the legal issue, skewed memories, and their motives. In custody or visitation disputes, parents will often offer information that is self-serving and withhold information that might put them in a bad light. Parents in the throes of crisis or divorce may demonstrate regressive behavior that is not representative of their usual level of functioning. Occasionally, parents will reveal extremely damaging information about themselves that may raise concerns about their motivation for custody and their judgment. Forensic examiners need to be more aggressive than therapists in looking for contradictions and inconsistencies and probing for more detail.

If parents are not living together, it may be necessary to obtain their respective accounts of the child's history and current functioning. Contradictions may abound and leave examiners feeling as if they are on a seesaw. It is critical to hear both sides in order to obtain a balanced picture of what is going on and to treat them with parity. This involves spending approximately equal amounts of time with each parent and asking them similar questions. The forensic examiner is not expected to play detective, and many areas of disparity will have to be resolved by

the court. Assessment of parental capacity will be covered separately in Part II, "Child Custody."

Meeting With the Child or Adolescent

It is always interesting to ask a child or adolescent what their understanding of the purpose of the evaluation is and whether anyone has told them what to say. The child or adolescent needs to be told at the onset the purpose of the interview, with whom it will be shared, and that it is the judge or jury, not the examiner, who is the ultimate decision maker. With young children you might say that your job is to help the judge understand how they are doing, how they have been affected by something, such as divorce or trauma, and what their needs are. Most evaluations of a child can be accomplished within 2 to 4 hours over several visits, depending on the nature and complexity of the case. If the visits are lengthy, as may occur if the child is coming from a great distance, he should be offered a break. The risk of extended evaluations is that the child or adolescent may perceive them as a demand for more information and begin to confabulate either for attention or to appease the examiner. In addition, the more involved the examiner becomes, the easier it is to slip into a therapeutic stance.

The interview should be tailored to the legal questions at hand. With young children you can use standard playroom tools such as puppets, drawing, and a dollhouse. However, it is also necessary to take a more structured approach that includes assessment of cognitive functioning, reality testing, ability to differentiate pretend from fantasy, and memory for past and current events in their lives. As will be discussed in Chapters 13, "Developmental Aspects of Memory in Children," 14, "Reliability and Suggestibility of Children's Statements," and 15, "Interviewing Children for Suspected Sexual Abuse," the use of narrative recall will yield the most accurate statements from children, and multiple-choice, either/or, and leading questions should be avoided whenever possible. With very young children or those lacking in cognitive maturity, it may be impossible to avoid using some leading questions.

The interview should be recorded in some form, and there is no problem-free way of doing this. Audiotapes do not capture nonverbal behavior and may not always be audible. Videotapes are excellent as teaching tools and for the examiner to review what has transpired. However, it is difficult to keep young children in one place, they may feel intimidated by the camera, and if they have been subjects of child pornography, there is risk of re-traumatizing them. Other concerns about videotapes include the risk that they may be shown in court out of context, used to coach a witness, or that they may fall into the wrong hands. Taking notes during the interview may distract the child but is an effective way of recording, assuming your handwriting is legible. It is important to not only record the child's responses to questions but also how the question was phrased. The examiner should be aware that the opposing attorney may request to see these notes, and if they are illegible, she may request that they be dictated. Handwritten notes should not be discarded; it is perfectly acceptable for the opposing attorney to request to examine them.

At closure, the child should be praised for effort or cooperation but not for content of what is disclosed. It is important not to give the child any premature assurances about the outcome of the case.

Rarely, a third party—parent, guardian, or attorney—may request to sit in on the evaluation. This is usually awkward, and there is a risk that the third party may influence or inhibit the examinee or, by their very presence, imply that the examiner is not to be trusted. This practice should be discouraged unless the examinee is a very young child with separation problems, one who is terrified of the evaluation and needs a support person, or an interpreter is needed. You might want to check state laws applicable to this situation.

Observations of the Parent-Child Relationship

Observing children with their parents is an important part of any evaluation involving custody or visitation. Exceptions might be an infant removed at birth who has no relationship with the parent or children who are not having ongoing visitation with their parents. Observing interactions between parent and child is an excellent tool for assessing attachment and parenting skills, which are discussed further in Chapters 8, "Child Custody Evaluations," and 9, "Parenting Assessment in Cases of Neglect and Abuse." These observations may be made through a one-way mirror, with the examiner sitting in but not participating in the visit in her office, or during home visits. These evaluations are also useful for the unconscious material that emerges that a parent does not ordinarily volunteer, such as seductive, intimidating, or overly controlling behavior.

Corroborating Information

Much more effort goes into corroborating information in forensic evaluations than in diagnostic evaluations. If we err in the initial diagnosis of a patient we are treating, we have the opportunity to reassess and make adjustments in our treatment plan and usually no serious harm ensues. In

contrast, we do not have the luxury of extended time in forensic evaluations and much more is at stake concerning the outcome of legal proceedings. For instance, if a father is wrongfully acquitted of child sexual abuse, the victim and other potential victims remain at risk. On the other hand, if a father is erroneously convicted of sexual abuse, irreparable harm is done to his child's relationship with him, not to mention his reputation, career, and the possibility of incarceration.

Because credibility is often an issue in forensic evaluations, care needs to be taken in cross-checking what the child has said to others, when possible. Police reports obtained immediately after disclosure are helpful. Although children's descriptions of abuse may shift over time, the core features usually remain consistent. Results of physical examinations are helpful in determining whether injuries are consistent with allegations. However, you should heed the dictum that absence of physical findings does not mean absence of sexual abuse. Verbal reports from teachers, day care providers, and babysitters help complete the picture of how a child is functioning.

Other sources of valuable data include school reports, past psychological testing, and previous psychiatric evaluations. These may be used to document prior levels of functioning relevant to a particular trauma or event. They also provide cross-checks on the reliability of the history given by parents. Not uncommonly, parents may ascribe all of a child's symptoms to a particular event, but a check of the records indicates similar behaviors prior to the trauma being litigated or other traumas not volunteered by the parents.

Housekeeping Issues

Keeping track of all the discovery material that accompanies a case is challenging. Attorneys will often want to know at what point materials were received and whether they were read before or after the forensic examination. Berger (1997) offers a useful system for labeling documents, in which the first packet is labeled A, with the date on it, and lowercase letters are used for the individual documents, followed by numbers, indicating the number of pages in the document, for example, Ab 1–3. The next packet received would be Ba 1–5, Bb 1–10, and so on. Mailings are usually accompanied by cover letters listing the enclosures. It is important to cross-check to see that no pages are missing.

Sometimes material arrives nicely indexed in a binder. At other times, there may be no apparent order. It is helpful to begin by reviewing the complaint, then the police or the medical and psychiatric reports in chronological order, saving the opinions of other experts or professionals until the end so as not to be biased by them. It is tempting to use highlighting markers in reviewing documents, but the risk is that the other side may request to see the materials you reviewed and question the meaning of highlighted material. Alternatively, you can make notations on a separate piece of paper or a laptop computer as you go along, indicating the pages to which you are referring. It is very useful to construct a timeline of significant events, which will help to organize the chronology of the case and may also accentuate inconsistencies in the history.

It is not unusual to end up with several crates of materials on a case, and storage soon becomes a problem. Records need to be kept until a case has settled, and it is prudent to hold onto your own report until the statute of limitations has expired. With juveniles this does not begin to toll until they have reached the age of majority. It is best to check with the attorney before disposing of other documents related to the case. Disposal of records should be done in such a way that there is no risk of them falling into the wrong hands or flying around the town dump on a windy day. Burning or shredding works well, and the latter may be composted or disposed of with trash. Alternatively, there are services that will destroy records on location.

THE WRITTEN REPORT

Function of the Written Report

The well-written report often becomes a bargaining chip in reaching an out-of-court settlement. Should the case go to court, the report becomes the basis for your testimony and will serve to refresh your memory. The cross-examining attorney will attempt to discredit your report, and it is useful to anticipate the weaknesses of the report at the time of writing and rectify them if possible. The report is also your work's product and should not contain anything that might embarrass you in years to come. Usually attorneys want a preliminary verbal report, and if it is not favorable, they may not want a written report. Sometimes attorneys may request that a report be modified. This is ethically permissible if changes have to do with errors of fact, misinterpretations, rewording of the conclusion to be consistent with statutes, or shortening or elaborating the report. It would be unethical to comply with requests to alter facts or change your opinion.

The report should be directed toward the legal question at issue. The length of the report will depend on the complexity of the issues and sometimes the age of the child. The report should contain the building blocks that provide the foundation for your opinion. It should demonstrate that you have attempted to rule out other possible causes for the examinee's behaviors or symptoms. Psychodynamic formulations and speculations should be kept to a minimum, because they are difficult to prove in court. A carefully documented history of child neglect, its impact on the child, and a mother's failure to avail herself of services will provide more ammunition for terminating parental rights than will psychoanalytic interpretations about her ambivalence toward her child.

Diagnoses are usually not included in custody evaluations. In contrast, they are more relevant in parenting assessments for protective services and tort litigation that focuses on damages.

Language of the Report

Your report is likely to be read by attorneys from both sides, their clients, the judge, and experts hired by the opposing side. It should be free of psychiatric jargon and intelligible to a lay person.

Tact is required and pejoratives or judgmental statements should be avoided. For example, it is easy to substitute "he states" for "he claims" and "he was suspicious and mistrustful" for "he was paranoid." The report should strive for balance—addressing strengths as well as weaknesses. Direct quotes are very helpful for bringing the report to life and allowing the parties to speak for themselves. A mother's statement that she is a good mother because her "kids ain't torched the house yet," tells a lot about her concept of parenting. Vague or speculative statements should be avoided along with terms such as "obviously" or "clearly," which may not be so to others reading the report.

Proofread the report ever so carefully for typos and content. Computer spell checks are wonderful but do not pick up on transposed names, wrong numbers, and homonyms. Finally, do not overlook the envelope in which the report is sent. The author once used a new typist who sent a report to "The Horrible Judge Gil." Fortunately, Judge Gil had a sense of humor.

Organization of the Report

The report should bear your letterhead, and the title of the report should reflect that it is a forensic evaluation. It is useful to have the examinee's birth date among identifying information so that when you go to court months or years later, you can remember how old the child was when examined. It also helps to orient the reader. The report might be organized as follows:

Circumstance of the evaluation. This indicates who retained you and for what purposes.

Sources of information. This section includes both first-hand and secondhand information that was relied on in reaching your conclusion and recommendations. The report should reflect where, when, and for how long you saw the parties. If records were requested but never received, this should be stated.

Purpose of evaluation. This section should state the legal issue and what was requested of you.

Informed consent. This part of the report should begin with comments that the purpose of the evaluation has been discussed with the examinee along with discussion regarding who might have access to your report.

History. In relating the history, it should be clear from whose perspective it is coming, that is, "according to the mother" rather than presenting data as factual. History that is not relative to the issue may be excluded or abbreviated.

Observations and foundations for opinions. Direct observations provide a strong bulwark for opinions and should be carefully detailed. The patient's manner should be described in terms of degree of cooperation, defensiveness, rapport, and so forth, that may have bearing on the material elicited. Whether to include a formal mental status exam will depend on the nature of the legal question being asked. In custody evaluations, which parent brought the child may have bearing on that session. Children's drawings may be amended to reports, but caution should be exerted in how much interpretation to offer. Often they will speak for themselves. Inasmuch as they may be admitted into evidence, you should make a copy so as not to be left empty-handed.

Other sources of information. Those sources of information relied on in forming your opinion may be briefly summarized and may include police, school, medical and psychiatric records, and other collateral parties with whom you have spoken.

Formulation and recommendations. Any conclusions must be supported by data in the report, including the history, direct observations, and records reviewed. Courts are likely to ask whether opinions are fair and reasonable and whether recommendations are feasible. In some cases, it may not be possible to arrive at an opinion, for example, whether or not a child's allegations of sexual abuse are credible. In such cases, one can state the pros and cons, the limiting factors that make it difficult to resolve the questions, such as young age of child at time of alleged abuse, or contaminated interviews. The examiner can still be helpful to the court by coming up with recommendations to safeguard the child.

PITFALLS

Psychiatrist-Related Pitfalls

Myopia

The expert may be overly focused and, for instance, only see the world through the lens of child sexual abuse. She is not troubled by the nonspecificity of the sexually abused child syndrome and fails to consider that enuresis in a child of divorcing parents might just be stress-related. She tends to cling to her views, is not open to other interpretations for a child's behavioral changes, and fails to do an in-depth evaluation.

Bias

Closely related to myopia is the problem of bias. As noted in Chapter 3, "Forensic Ethics," the examiner may not even be aware of it. Perhaps the worst sort of bias is the expert's conviction that he is not biased. Notes Judge Bazelon (1974): "Like any other man, a physician acquires an emotional identification with an opinion that comes down on one side of a conflict: he has an inescapable, prideful conviction in the accuracy of his own findings."

Duel Agency

It is very easy to fall into this trap if not vigilant about your role. Remember that you cannot wear two hats and you cannot serve two masters.

Inadequate or Faulty Database

Taking shortcuts usually backfires and may end up embarrassing the evaluator. For instance, a guardian *ad litem* wrote off a father based on information obtained solely from the mother. She went through a cursory home visit, spending a total of 15 minutes with him, and had nothing good to say about him in her report. She was quite embarrassed in court when a neutral child development specialist who had spent ample time observing both parents with their toddler countered many of her negative assertions.

Nonmedical clinicians may misinterpret physical findings, for example, equating yeast infections or urinary tract infections with child sexual abuse. If in doubt, they should confer with the physician who treated the child in question.

Quoting the Literature

It is tempting to bolster your opinions by citing the literature. This is usually a losing gambit, because the other side will come up with tomes countering yours and make you look foolish when you have not heard of the impressive texts from which they are quoting. If they happen to quote something you have written, make sure that it is in context and ask to see it.

The Need to Please

Forensic psychiatrists may succumb to the need to please the referring attorney. This may occur out of the wish to be liked or fear of turning off a good referral source.

Inflating Credentials

Do not try to inflate a meager curriculum vitae with courses you have taken, lectures attended, or media interviews. Do not imply you are board certified if you are only board eligible. Do not be apologetic about your status, but do draw on your cumulative learning and training and remember that even the most respected forensic psychiatrists once stood in your shoes.

Patient-Related Pitfalls

Noncompliance

If an examinee fails to appear or appears but refuses to participate in the evaluation, his attorney should be notified. In some cases, a limited report may be submitted based on record review alone. Failure of the examinee to cooperate should be noted.

You've Been Had

Getting taken in by a con man or skilled psychopath is a learning experience. He may be very charming, use the right buzzwords, and even feign sincerity and remorse. His charm is usually skin deep, and when he doesn't get his way, he shows his true colors and can become intimidating and threatening. History usually points to externalizing behaviors, lack of conflict, and antisocial behaviors.

Harassment

Harassment may occur in the form of threats to one's person, obscene phone calls, or calls in the middle of the night with no one on the other end. Such calls should be reported, although the phone company is not always helpful. A female psychiatrist complained about obscene phone calls she was getting at her office and was told to get an unlisted number. She solved the problem on her own by getting caller ID. Stalking behaviors should be reported to the police. A more likely form of harassment is the filing of complaints without merit against you with licensing boards or ethics committees. Some examinees arrive with a long history of litigious behavior, which should put the forensic examiner on notice.

Attorney-Related Pitfalls

Coercive Tactics

This lawyer has trouble hearing no and may try to get you to alter your report or testimony. If he is behaving unethically, this is grounds to withdraw from the case (Gutheil and Simon 1999).

Withholding of Information

Lawyers need not send you all of the relevant discovery material they have. If they withhold critical pieces of information such as the fact that a mother has lost custody of two previous children, this is a problem. The lawyer may attempt to defend her actions, saying she did not want to bias you. However, if she is not being honest with you, it will be difficult to work with her. Furthermore, it is preferable to hear damaging information from her than be confronted with it for the first time while being cross-examined.

Boundary Violations

Attorneys, like mental health professionals, are not immune to boundary violations. They may occur with clients, expert witnesses, or both. If an attorney you have never met calls you at home on the weekend, addresses you by your first name, and is unduly familiar, this should raise red flags. You might do well to avoid contracting with him.

The Unprepared

This attorney often requests an expert "under the wire," sounds disorganized and inarticulate, and is not entirely clear about what he wants from you. If he is like this with you, you need to wonder how he will present himself in court.

Poor Communication

If an attorney is too busy to return your calls, you have to wonder if the case is important to him and whether he will devote adequate time to it. Mental health professionals can also be faulted for not returning calls. However, with answering machines, fax machines, and e-mail, there is no excuse for notifying an expert, just before he was scheduled to testify, that a case had settled when the attorney has known this for a week. Experts also appreciate follow-ups on the outcome of court cases and feedback, both good and bad, on their testimony.

CASE EXAMPLE EPILOGUES

Case Example 1

Not only is Dr. Bartoli's report not needed, but the father refuses to pay for the time she spent preparing it, stating that the lawyers in the case have depleted his funds. She is left with the options of taking him to small claims court, paying for her attorney to write him a letter, handing the account over to a collection agency, or overlooking the bill. She resolves to work only on retainer in future custody cases and to have a formal contract regarding payment with the retaining attorney.

Case Example 2

Dr. Gould has become too invested in his evaluation and the outcome. He has forgotten that he did the evaluation for the attorney, not the children, and that it is protected as the attorney's work product. The attorney ethically is bound to represent his client's interests and wishes, in spite of telling Dr. Gould that he only wants what is best for the children.

Case Example 3

Dr. Wolf, who is a seasoned forensic psychologist, immediately asks what the custody arrangement is and learns that the mother has sole custody of the boys. He informs the attorney that he cannot see the children without the mother's permission and offers the attorney several suggestions, including 1) getting consent from the mother, 2) contacting protective services, and 3) petitioning the court for an order to change custody.

ACTION GUIDELINES

Strive for Honesty and Objectivity

Do not be afraid to admit that you do not know something. Take time to self-reflect and examine the basis for your opinions. Ethical integrity will help maintain your reputation and that of your profession.

Maintain Control of the Evaluation

Be firm about your terms, and do not allow anyone to force you into doing something that you feel is unethical or against the law.

Learn to Live With Ambiguity

Avoid premature closure, and wait for pieces of the puzzle to fall in place. Try to look at issues from all sides, and steer a middle course based on what seems most reasonable. Reconcile yourself to not being able to resolve all contradictions.

Learn to Critique Your Report From the Other Side

Ask yourself: "How will this statement stand up under cross-examination?" Try to anticipate where you are vulnerable and consider how you will deal with the weaknesses in the case.

Know Your Limitations

Do not overload yourself with too many forensic cases or too many cases of one kind. Avoid exceeding the limits of your database when offering opinions. Be cautious about making predictions, and recognize that past behavior is usually the best predictor of future behavior. Pace yourself and take good care of yourself.

Seek Consultation

When in doubt, turn to a more experienced colleague. Utilize peer review. Legal consultation may be available from a hospital's attorneys or your liability insurance plan carrier. Effective use of consultation also provides some protection in the event that one is sued.

Keep Current and Stay Involved

Do not allow fears of the legal system or malpractice litigation to restrict your practice. Read the forensic literature, take courses, attend annual meetings, stay involved, and learn from each case you see.

REFERENCES

American Medical Association: Report of the Board of Trustees on Expert Witness Testimony. Board of Trustees Report 18-1-98. Chicago, IL, American Medical Association, 1998

Bazelon D: Psychiatrists and the adversary process. Scientific American 230(6):18–23, 1974

Berger S: Establishing a Forensic Psychiatric Practice. New York, WW Norton, 1997

Gutheil T: The Psychiatrist as Expert Witness. Washington, DC, American Psychiatric Press, 1998

Gutheil T, Simon R: Attorneys' pressures on expert witnesses: early warning signs of endangered honesty, objectivity and fair compensation. J Am Acad Psychiatry Law 27:546–553, 1999

Mossman D, Kapp J: Courtroom whores—or why do attorneys call us? findings from a survey on attorney's use of mental health experts. J Am Acad Psychiatry Law 26:27–36, 1998

Reid W: Licensure requirements for out-of-state forensic examinations. J Am Acad Psychiatry Law 28:433–437, 2000

Simon R, Shuman D: Conducting forensic examinations on the road: are you practicing your profession without a license? J Am Acad Psychiatry Law 27:75–82, 1999

CHAPTER 5

Testifying:
The Expert Witness in Court

Elissa P. Benedek, M.D.

Case Example 1

An attorney requests that the psychiatrist review the documents of his client, a 16-year-old girl who was severely burned after her flannel nightgown caught on fire. The attorney requests that the psychiatrist review the records, including mental health records, and render an opinion as to the extent of mental and emotional damages. During the telephone conversation, the attorney insists that there is no need for the psychiatrist to see his client and emphasizes that the medical records will speak for themselves.

Case Example 2

An attorney requests a consultation with Dr. Mehta, a child and adolescent forensic psychiatrist, regarding the effect of a below-the-knee amputation that a young schizophrenic boy has undergone in either causing or exacerbating a psychosis. After reviewing the history and seeing the young boy, there is no support for the attorney's theory that the amputation precipitated or exacerbated the patient's psychotic episode. In fact, the episode occurred before the injury and amputation. The attorney insists that "common sense" would make it clear to a jury that for a young boy an amputation must affect mental functioning and indeed did precipitate another psychotic episode. She refuses to accept Dr. Mehta's opinion and argues with her and pressures her to change her opinion and testify that the boy's illness was exacerbated by the amputation.

Case Example 3

A psychiatrist who has written extensively on child custody, divorce, and visitation is testifying with regard to the most appropriate placement of minor children. During the course of testimony, he is asked about a colleague's reputation, skill, and integrity by an attorney. He personally believes there were gross inadequacies in the conduct of the other expert's evaluation, but he declined to offer an opinion in court. He consults you as a forensic psychiatrist as to whether he is "doing the right thing."

The involvement of psychiatrists, psychologists, social workers, nurses, nurse clinicians, and mental health clinicians in the legal arena continues to grow and remains highly controversial. Expert testimony by mental health professionals at depositions and administrative hearings alters many lives—the lives of plaintiffs, defendants, and the experts. It has been estimated that mental health clinicians participate in up to 1 million legal cases per year, and that the number grows each year. The appropriate role of a mental health professional in the courtroom as an expert witness has been debated by numerous authors. While the debate rages, mental health professionals continue to participate as expert witnesses and as consultants to attorneys and courts. This chapter addresses the broad role of the expert witness from a psychiatrist's point of view.

LEGAL ISSUES

The Basis of Expert Testimony

Mental health professionals may be called to testify as fact witnesses or as expert witnesses. As a fact witness, a witness testifies about matters that he or she has perceived or witnessed. As a fact witness, the witness is treated as other witnesses. As a mental health professional, the fact witness would be asked to provide information from their practice (e.g., What is the patient's diagnosis? treatment plan? prognosis?). If a patient puts his emotional and mental health in the record as a possible cause of damage, the treating psychiatrist is at risk for being called as a fact witness. The psychiatrist may attempt to dissuade an attorney from calling him by suggesting that a review of treatment goals and objectives, response to treatment, diagnosis, and other information may not be helpful to a patient's case. For example, if a patient alleges emotional damages subsequent to sexual harassment during the course of employment, it would not be helpful to that patient if her medical records revealed intensive psychotherapy and psychopharmacology three years prior to the alleged incidents. This tactic is ordinarily more persuasive than suggesting to an attorney that testifying in court will disrupt the doctor-patient relationship or may be harmful therapeutically to a patient. Unfortunately, for many attorneys the "case" is more important than the patient's mental health. If the patient's attorney insists on the treating psychiatrist's testimony, the psychiatrist might call his or her own attorney to ask for advice. As a last-ditch effort, a psychiatrist may attempt to contact a judge personally; however, this tactic rarely works.

An expert witness differs from a fact witness in that an expert may testify to matters of special learning, knowledge, and opinion. A mental health clinician may be qualified as an expert on the basis of special training or education (a degree, board certification, or attendance at a seminar) or, less commonly, special experience, skills, or education. The expert's testimony must be relevant to the matter in dispute, be reliable (have a scientific basis), and be based on some special expertise not otherwise available to judge or jury. The testimony must be deemed to do more good than harm, that is, probative value should be greater than prejudicial value. An expert witness may draw conclusions from his or her own database (examination) or others' database (medical records). For example, the expert may review school records, past medical records, and past therapy records; speak with family members; speak with schoolteachers about the behavior of a patient; and request that psychological testing be done. Information gathered by others and communicated to the experts via depositions, medical records, interviews, psychological testing, and other laboratory testing may be useful in formulating a final opinion. After reviewing and analyzing the other opinions, the expert may be allowed to formulate an opinion using "hearsay"

material (material that has not been gleaned from a first-hand discussion with the patient).

The expert's job is not to empathize with the patient or treat or help a patient, but rather to inform and teach a judge and jury regardless of whether the expert's testimony helps or harms the attorney's client. The expert's client is the attorney or the court that asks for her consultative expertise. The underlying theory of the American legal system and the adversary system of justice is that each side presents its best version of a case without perjury or manufactured evidence. All expert testimony is subject to cross-examination and rebuttal. In many cases, an expert's testimony is helpful, and in others, it is essential and required. For example, in standard-of-care or medical malpractice cases, only an expert in a particular medical specialty can offer testimony about standard of care. An obstetrician is not generally accepted as an expert with regard to depression and suicidal ideation.

Without expert testimony, a court will not entertain certain forms of litigation. For example, in Michigan, in a medical malpractice case without an expert agreeing that there are legitimate grounds for a suit (in a written affidavit), the court will not entertain a malpractice action. Additionally, the advent of advanced technology in the mental health field has a resulted in increasingly complex litigation and has intensified the use of psychiatrists and psychologists to explain to the court sophisticated tests and procedures and their meaning, for example, the Millon Clinical Multiaxial Inventory (MCMI) and computed tomography (CT) or magnetic resonance imaging (MRI) scans.

In criminal cases, failure to engage an expert may constitute ineffective assistance of counsel and result in the reversal of a conviction. For example, in death penalty cases in which ingestion of drugs are involved prior to the commission of a crime, failure to call a psychopharmacologist or an addiction specialist may constitute grounds for an appeal, based on ineffective assistance of counsel, and result in grounds for an appeal and a possible reversal. Accordingly, in *Ake v. Oklahoma* (1985), a murder case that involved possible mental illness, no psychiatrist was called to testify; the U.S. Supreme Court overturned a conviction on the grounds that the defendant, Ake, should have had access to psychiatric assistance in preparing an insanity defense. The court stated, "We note that when the defendant has had a preliminary showing, his insanity at the time of offense is likely to be a significant factor at trial. The Constitution requires the State provide access to a psychiatrist's assistance on this issue if the defendant cannot otherwise afford one."

Tort Reform

One of the areas in which expert mental health testimony is used the most is the issue of expert testimony in the arena of civil litigation, or torts. A *tort* is a civil wrong, which addresses wrongs done to one person by another and the mechanisms for compensation for the resultant injury. Throughout the United States, there has been a movement for tort reform in an attempt to control the use of professional experts or "hired guns." A succinct definition of a hired gun is that offered by Gutheil (1998): "A hired gun is an expert witness who sells testimony instead of time." Hired guns are willing to testify to opinions favorable to the attorney and his client, regardless of its clinical validity. It is possible to recognize hired guns, because they often testify only for the defense (plaintiffs) and often testify in areas in which they have no known expertise.

In an attempt at tort reform, in Michigan, for example, the state senate passed a bill that required an expert to devote no less than 50% of his or her professional time to active clinical practice in the same specialty as the physician who is identified as a defendant in a medical malpractice action, or to be an instructor in that specialty in a medical school. The bill allows for a combination of clinical practice and teaching responsibilities. Mental health professionals are routinely queried during voir dire examinations with regard to the amount of time they spend in clinical practice and are disqualified as experts if they no longer practice clinical medicine/psychiatry. For example, one well-known psychiatrist, who primarily testified as a plaintiff's expert, admitted that he had last visited with a patient 10 years prior to testifying as a psychiatric expert in a high-profile case with regard to use of medication in a psychiatric patient. The court opined that his experience was no longer current nor was it applicable. Most states also require that experts state their opinion as being "of reasonable medical certainty," which is standard jargon that is shorthand for "more likely than not" or 51% certainty with regard to an opinion. This is lower than an absolute certainty standard, the "beyond a reasonable doubt" standard used in criminal cases, or the intermediate standard of "clear and convincing evidence," which is sometimes described as 75% certainty.

Exceptions to Expert Testimony

The three most common exceptions to the broad admissibility of expert testimony are: 1) eyewitness reliability, 2) truthfulness of a witness, and 3) syndrome or profile testimony. For the most part, psychologists are called as experts to testify with regard to the reliability of eyewitness testimony. This testimony generally focuses on psychological research bearing on the fallibility of eyewitness memory and the role of such factors as the effects of stress on the witnesses, the problems associated with cross-racial identification, and the effects of post-event misinformation (i.e., information learned by an eyewitness after the event in question). The legal arguments that have been offered against expert testimony on eyewitness evidence include the following: 1) mental health professionals do not have special expertise concerning eyewitness behavior; 2) the evaluation of the credibility of testimony by a witness is a province of the trier of fact and therefore not appropriate testimony for an expert; 3) the findings of eyewitness research have not "gained general acceptance in a particular field to which it belongs," (the *Frye*, or *Daubert*, test will be discussed later); 4) the findings of eyewitness researchers are common sense, and therefore, there is no need for an expert to inform the court of results; and 5) an expert opinion may have undue influence on jurors, who can sort out credibility issues for themselves.

In eyewitness identification cases, it is generally the defense who wishes to use the expert. In the United States, legal opinion is currently divided about the value of expert evidence on eyewitness testimony, but case law has been moving in the direction of admitting such evidence. In Canada, courts have been resistant and consistently reject such testimony.

The second area in which expert testimony is often disputed is the area of truthfulness, or credibility, of other witnesses. Testimony regarding credibility of other witnesses is offered in cases that deal with child abuse, sexual abuse, malingering, or feigning of mental illness. Traditionally, common law did not permit direct testimony by an expert on the truthfulness of another witness, that is, one who has not been directly examined but simply observed in the courtroom.

Frye Test

There is still considerable resistance in courts to accept syndromes or diagnoses not included in the latest edition of the *Diagnostic and Statistical Manual of Mental Disorders*. Such syndrome testimony might include battered wife syndrome, brain trauma syndrome, violent parent syndrome, brainwashing, or syndromes surrounding sexual abuse. In the past, courts have held that these profiles or syndromes do not meet the *Frye* test. This standard or test is derived from language in *Frye v. United States*, and it was known as the general acceptance rule. The *Frye* test dates back to 1923, when an opinion provided by the district court of appeals in the murder conviction of James A. Frye was affirmed (*Frye v. United States*, 1923). The *Frye* test poses a rule that mandates that any scientific or professional opinion expressed by an expert witness must represent generally accepted thinking by a *significant* membership of that discipline or that profession. The inquiry that gave rise to the *Frye* test centered around an attempt to determine if Mr. Frye had been truthful. An expert witness attested that the systolic blood pressure taken during a polygraphic exam was a definite way to determine if a subject was lying. If the subject were lying, according to the expert, systolic blood pressure would be elevated; if not, it would remain normal. The trial court did not accept the expert's testimony nor did the appellate court.

It is not enough that an expert is prepared to testify that the technique and procedure are valid or that a court believes that the evidence is helpful or reliable. Testimony must meet a standard of general scientific acceptance in the scientific community. The *Frye* test allowed radar evidence, public opinion surveys, breathalyzers, psycholinguistics, trace metal detection, bite mark comparison, and blood spatter analysis into the courtroom; but when used, on rare occasion, it has been a mechanism for denying polygraphic testing results, spectrographic voice identification, voice stress test, and hypnosis as a means of refreshing a witness's memory.

In 1993, the U.S. Supreme Court established a new standard for the admissibility of scientific evidence in federal court cases in *Daubert v. Merrill Dow Pharmaceuticals, Inc.* (1993). The court rejected the *Frye* rule that had required that scientific evidence be "generally accepted as reliable" in the relevant scientific community as a prerequisite to such evidence's admissibility. The standard adopted by the *Daubert* court was based on Federal Rule of Evidence 1102, and it appears to be, at first blush, more permissive than the *Frye* test. It actually provides trial judges an important tool to prevent introduction of conjuncture or "junk" science into evidence under the guise of expert scientific testimony. *Junk science* can be defined as little more than the unsubstantiated conjecture of a quasi or self-proclaimed expert.

Daubert involved the attempt by a plaintiff in a products liability case to introduce expert testimony that the drug Bendectin could cause birth defects. The district court ruled such testimony inadmissible, because all prior studies had concluded that Bendectin did not cause birth defects. The court reasoned that the lack of published studies supporting the plaintiff's expert's position indicated that their position was not generally accepted within the scientific community. The court of appeals

affirmed the district court's opinion. The Supreme Court reversed, however, holding that the proper standard for admissibility is contained in Federal Rule of Evidence 702, which superseded *Frye* and which provided: "if scientific, technical, or other specialized knowledge will assist the trier of fact to understand the evidence or to determine a fact or issue, a witness qualified as an expert by knowledge, skill, experience, training, or education may testify thereto in the formative opinion or otherwise. Whether the expert's theory or test is generally accepted within the relative scientific community is only one factor to be considered by the court in applying Rule 702, but it is not the only criteria." Testimony has been allowed under *Daubert* with regard to the connection between mental illness and subsequent behavior. The *Daubert* court also read Rule 702 to require that an expert's testimony must amount to "scientific knowledge" to be admissible. It specified that "scientific" implied a grounding in the *methods* and *procedures* of science and knowledge that was "more than a subjective belief or unsupported speculation." The *Daubert* court further maintained that cases involving scientific evidence with regard to evidentiary reliability (for the purposes of admissibility under Rule 702) would be based on scientific validity. Scientific validity was construed to mean that the theory or technique that was at the heart of the expert's opinion could be tested.

Daubert thus required that when faced with an offer of expert scientific testimony, it was in the trial judge's province to determine whether 1) the offered testimony was scientifically valid and 2) whether it would assist the trier of fact to understand or determine a fact of issue. As the *Daubert* court put it, this entails a preliminary assessment of whether the testimony is scientifically valid and whether the reasoning and methodology properly can be applied to the facts issued. These preliminary matters must be established by *a preponderance of the evidence prior to the introduction of such testimony before a jury.* An anonymous legal commentator observed, "Before *Daubert*, the trial judge had to ask, What do the relevant scientists think of this? The judge had to decide, Has the proponent of this evidence shown that scientists agree with her?" After *Daubert*, the trial judge had to decide, Is this good science or junk science?

Daubert thus places the trial judge in the role of gatekeeper, charged with weighing the evidence to determine whether expert testimony is scientifically valid before such testimony is permitted to reach the jury. For example, a judge can decide whether one molecule of a potentially carcinogenic chemical touching a plaintiff's skin could reasonably cause a plaintiff to have a fear of cancer.

The role of the judge as gatekeeper of the trial court is designed to prevent juries from being persuaded by "expert testimony." The credentials of the expert may seem impressive and a novel theory plausible, but both the expert and the science may be worthless. Unfortunately, although the Supreme Court in *Daubert* gave trial judges this role, it did not provide them with concurrent instructions on how to open or close the gate. It provided a list of factors for trial courts to consider, such as whether the expert's methodology could be tested, whether it had been subject to peer review and publication, the known or potential rate of error of methodology, and whether methodology is "generally accepted" within the relevant scientific community, but it did not weigh these factors nor did it note whether all of them needed to be satisfied in a particular case. One commentator on *Daubert*, Kozinski, was not impressed by the expert's credentials in determining science. The judge observed, "Something doesn't become scientific knowledge just because it is uttered by a scientist, nor can an expert's self-serving assertion that his conclusions were derived by the scientific method be deemed conclusive." The court's task, then, is "to analyze not what the experts say, but what basis they have for saying it" (43 F3d [9th Cir 1995], pp. 1315–1316).

With regard to the acceptance of expert testimony, *Daubert* may prevent testimony from hired gun experts who lack sufficient training and experience in clinical diagnosis of mental illness. Most recently, a nurse clinician with two months' rotation on a psychiatric ward was barred from testifying with regard to the effect a possible rape may have had on a female psychiatric inpatient. The court noted that her "experience" was really inexperience and she could not be deemed an expert. *Daubert* hopefully will prevent testimony from experts who lack sufficient training and experience in the clinical diagnosis of mental illness. Additionally, it may bar testimony from experts who, although possessing the requisite training and experience, fail to employ standard diagnostic techniques. Their testimony is often little more than a support of conjecture. Finally, it may prevent experts from basing their opinions solely on the body of academic "research" that suggests a causal link between a particular event and significant psychological injury.

CLINICAL ISSUES

Negotiation With Retained Attorney

Chapter 4, "Introduction to Forensic Evaluations," discusses the necessity for conducting a forensic clinical evaluation before agreeing to participate in a case or as an expert witness. It is clear that the process of becoming an expert witness begins the moment one accepts a telephone call from an attorney or court and agrees to review the case material and to possibly become involved in litigation. It continues through evaluation to report writing and may culminate in testifying in court. However, at its broadest definition, being an expert witness involves evaluation, consultation, and possible testimony, despite the fact that this chapter deals predominately with testifying.

Preparation

Subsequent to a clinical evaluation discussion with an attorney and completion of a written report, if a clinician becomes aware that testimony at a deposition or trial or answers to interrogatories will be necessary, it is sensible to contact the attorney to discuss these potential issues at a pretrial conference. It is important to confer with regard to answers to interrogatories and possible pretrial affidavits. Finally, it is important to review the written report and its conclusions, and their meanings, with the referring attorney. This formal meeting allows a clinician an opportunity to educate an attorney about the clinical answers in the case, as the clinician understands them. The meeting allows the attorney and the clinician to define medical terminology and legal standards in nontechnical terms. Such a meeting is also valuable for understanding the attorney's trial strategy, anticipating questions in a deposition, and anticipating a possible sequence of direction and cross-examination. In addition, clinicians and attorneys have an opportunity to meet one another and to become apprised of the strengths and weaknesses of each other and of the case. The clinician has an opportunity to evaluate the attorney and vice versa. It is helpful to know and understand all the actors in the courtroom drama before the drama begins.

Interrogatories and Depositions

Interrogatories

Interrogatories are similar to depositions. That is, their purpose is to discover information about the opposed expert and his or her proposed testimony. Interrogatories as part of the discovery process are written responses under oath to a series of standardized questions from the attorney on the other side. In some circumstances, interrogatories may be substituted by a letter or report from the expert. In other cases, the expert will draft the answers to the interrogatories, and in some others, the attorney will draft answers and the expert will review and criticize them. It is important to not simply accept an attorney's summary of your expert opinion in an interrogatory. As knowledgeable as attorneys are, they do not understand how a specific choice of words or medical terms may affect or change an opinion. In addition, attorneys may either overstate or understate an expert's qualifications to testify in a specialized area. Thus, although it is a temptation to allow an attorney to draft a response to an interrogatory and not review it, it is important to remember that it is a form of sworn testimony.

Depositions

A deposition has been described as a dress rehearsal for a trial. No judge or jury is present at a deposition. However, attorneys, a court reporter, and a plaintiff or the plaintiff's family may be present. Depositions are taken for discovery purposes in order to preserve testimony or for cross-examination at the time of a trial to impeach the credibility of a witness. Originally, depositions were done solely for the purpose of preserving testimony at a trial. For example, a potential witness might be unavailable at the time of a trial because of conflicting obligations or even death. Deposition testimony of an expert witness may be used at the time of trial because of the unavailability of the witness. Expert witness depositions are often taken *de bene esse* ([for the time being] prior to the trial without judge or jury) and may be videotaped and used at trial. Most attorneys prefer live testimony at a trial rather than deposition testimony, as most witnesses present as more interesting and credible live as compared to on videotape.

The second purpose of a deposition is to discover what a potential witness may say at a trial and the style and manner of the witness's presentation. Here all the expert's opinions and the basis for such opinions are explored by opposing counsel. Opposing counsel also has an opportunity to observe firsthand how an opposing witness will hold up under the stressful circumstances of cross-examination at a trial. Infrequently, experts change their opinions during the course of questioning during a deposition. This may occur when attorneys ask if the expert is familiar with a particular piece of evidence or testimony. A change in opinion or waffling of an opinion is, of course, always helpful to opposing counsel. Infrequently, after the rigors of a deposition, an expert may decide not to testify if called at trial.

The third purpose of a deposition is to impeach the credibility of a potential witness. In this situation, an attorney uses material in a deposition during the trial to demonstrate there is a difference between an expert's answer in a deposition and the opinion she expresses at trial or between an expert's answer at deposition and

information that the expert has published previously. Statements from a deposition may be quoted out of context in order to support or bolster opposing counsel's position. Clinicians should be aware that attorneys share old depositions in trial transcripts and that it is not unusual to have one's opinion from an old deposition or trial be used to impeach a new opinion in a similar but distinct case. This is especially so since the advent of the Internet, which allows attorneys to communicate with other attorneys via e-mail. The expert may be surprised at how much data counsel has accumulated with regard to prior testimony. Some transcripts of old depositions are also available on the Internet.

The site for a deposition is the expert's choice, and it can be held in a clinician's office, in an attorney's office, or at a court reporter's office. In many states, the plaintiff or defendant has a right to be present during a deposition. This occurs despite the fact that the expert may feel uncomfortable in the presence of a plaintiff or defendant during a deposition. Friends or family members of a plaintiff or defendant may also be present to provide support for the defendant/plaintiff even though he or she will not be questioned. The proceedings in a deposition are recorded by a court reporter.

In preparing for a deposition, there is no substitute for reviewing all materials that have been furnished previously and being familiar with them. The subpoena contains the time and place of the deposition. It also notes what material should be brought to the deposition. This may include a curriculum vitae of the expert, copies of the expert's previously published scientific papers, a text that the expert has relied on in formulating an opinion, and other miscellaneous items. All material requested (except the attorney's work products, such as letters) is open to opposing counsel and may be inspected by him or her and attached to the record of the deposition as exhibits. These materials include clinical notes, summaries of the case, and notes that the expert has generated and written on medical records, and even other depositions. An expert may be called on to explain why he or she has underlined material in a deposition, made a marginal comment, or used a sticky note to find or summarize material.

Because a judge is not present to rule on objections, attorneys do exercise more latitude in the range of questions. An attorney may offer an objection to a question posed by the opposing counsel, but many attorneys object infrequently and let the deposition proceed with no questions. If the behavior of one attorney is too objectionable to the expert, too hostile or too demeaning, or ranges too far and wide, opposing counsel may choose to terminate the deposition and ask for a ruling from a presiding judge with regard to whether to continue; however, termination of a deposition is rare. The expert may request to receive a copy of the deposition to be proofread for typographical errors or errors of content. This deposition copy should always be read carefully and corrected. It is advisable to insist on a copy of the deposition and not waive the right to review it. It is important to know what one has said in a deposition prior to trial and to have this written record available to review prior to trial.

It is also important to clarify payment for a deposition prior to the actual taking of the deposition. If there is reason to believe opposing counsel will not be responsible for payment, it is both ethical and common practice to ask for payment before the deposition. The firm that deposes the expert generally pays for the deposition, although it is also prudent to clarify in advance who is responsible for payment. It is also permissible to charge for the time spent in proofreading the deposition.

In preparation for a deposition, it is ethical and wise to discuss with counsel the form of answers she prefers. Some counsels advise experts to always answer "yes," "no," or "I don't know" or only reply in short narratives. Others encourage experts to discourse extensively in answer to queries to frighten opposing counsel, to prepare the grounds for settlement, and to discourage trial. Ultimately, it is the expert's choice with regard to style. However, the expert should always remain cool, calm, and collected. If attorneys become enraged and act in outrageous fashions, the rule to follow is to be impartial and objective and not to enter into the fray.

Courtroom Testimony

If a clinician has never visited a courtroom, either as an expert or a defendant, it is helpful to visit the courtroom prior to testifying. A courtroom can be a strange and bewildering, foreboding place to the uninitiated. The role and function of courtroom personnel are unclear, and the mere atmosphere may feel hostile to a novice. It is always helpful to ask a colleague sophisticated in forensics to observe testimony prior to an actual testifying experience and to critique the content of proposed testimony. It is also sensible for a novice to ask that the colleague accompany the novice expert witness to court. A more experienced colleague provides a support system and is available to critique the novice's performance subsequent to actual testimony.

Dress and demeanor are important in testifying; body language is also important. For example, do not slouch or lean back. It conveys the message that you are anxious or nervous. It is inappropriate to dress in blue jeans and a turtleneck or not to remove an overcoat, scarf, and boots prior to testifying. It is important to dress in a neat and conservative, nonflamboyant fashion and in a manner that does not detract from your testimony. Attorneys are occasionally flamboyant, wearing cowboy boots or extravagant jewelry, but they are allowed more latitude than expert witnesses, and drama and flamboyance may enhance rather than detract from their performance. Dress is a clear way of showing respect for one's self and for the legal process in preparation for trial.

Trial

The first key to a successful and tension-free court appearance is to review in preparing for the trial. The expert must review all relevant material, including all prior *preparation*. In addition, reviewing the entire database available and conferring with counsel about expected testimony and cross-examination is important. The second key is planning—not only planning for proposed testimony but planning ahead with regard to such mundane matters as knowing where a courtroom is located, knowing how to get into a courtroom, where to park, and advance planning and concern about who will care for your patients when you are unavailable. The third key is practice. Gutheil (1998) advises practicing testimony and being familiar with visual aides in a courtroom, such as blackboards, video machines, slide projectors, and examples you hope to use to convey your points to a judge and jury with assistance of counsel.

The fourth key to a successful court appearance is a pretrial conference. Before the expert testifies, there is often additional information that has been presented to the court by other witnesses. This is information that has not been gleaned from medical records, deposition testimony, or other documents. Counsel may be surprised by the style, demeanor, and actual testimony of prior witnesses. This pretrial conference may be used to emphasize particular points that a plaintiff/defendant has made by underscoring how the plaintiff/defendant's historical narrative in the evaluation process differs from the narrative he or she has presented during deposition and trial testimony. This bears on a plaintiff/defendant's credibility indirectly. It is wise to get a synopsis of the trial testimony to date before being on the stand. Finally, a pretrial motion may limit the scope of the proposed expert testimony. An expert may not be allowed to testify in certain areas because of a ruling made by the judge before or during the trial.

The fifth key is to be aware of pitfalls. By the time testimony is necessary at a trial, it is apparent to both the attorney and consultants that there are weaknesses in the expert's opinion. Opinion testimony by another expert may have been presented. It is important to notify the attorney what are possible pitfalls in testimony and how these will be handled. The sixth and final key is presentation. Presentation encompasses appearance, demeanor, and factors that support an opinion, including notes and material from the patient's clinical history, materials from the clinician, or testimony of the patient or treating physician that will buttress the opinion the expert plans to testify to.

Qualification of Experts

The qualification of experts is called *voir dire*. When one is called as an expert witness, the first step in the testimony process is that the attorney leads a witness through a standard set of questions designed to provide the foundation for the expert's credentials. These questions include relevant aspects of education and training, such as medical school, residency, and fellowships. These questions also cover any special qualifications of a particular expert, including membership and offices held in local and national organizations, publications, presentations, awards, and special consultations.

Following the recital of credentials, the opposing counsel has an opportunity to cross-examine further. Opposing counsel's emphasis will be on the weakest areas of the witness's experience and training, such as lack of board certification or special qualifications, limited contact with a particular population, and short duration (that is, the length) of a particular evaluation. There may be an attempt to discredit the expert witness. Wise attorneys often skip cross-examination during voir dire, as it allows the expert once again to reemphasize his or her credentials. Voir dire is generally not particularly difficult or dramatically challenging. On occasion, it may feel like a personal attack, and in fact, it may be designed to embarrass or discomfort the expert. However, the best witnesses remain calm and dispassionate and recognize that such behavior is just another attempt to discredit, a tactic used by opposing counsel.

Direct Examination

During this portion of the testimony, a witness will be asked first to identify the defendant/plaintiff and to explain the facts and conclusions on which an opinion is based. It is important that the expert present all relevant data in a clear, logical, and coherent fashion. This data may include information that is not helpful to a particular plaintiff or defendant. It is important to present a balanced picture. It is equally important that the expert

avoid using technical jargon; terms such as illusions, delusions, hallucinations, affect, and loosening of associations must be avoided and nontechnical terms used. If a technical term is used, the expert should carefully define what the term means and spell it for the benefit of the court transcriptionist. In addition, any laboratory tests or psychological tests and their significance must be explained. Data might be elicited from each test, and which tests are currently considered valid and reliable could be noted. Judges and jurors have no innate understanding of psychological tests, and they tend to think of psychological testing as objective and clinical evaluations as subjective. On occasion, it is important to articulate that the interpretation of a particular neuropsychological test is as subjective as the interpretation of a clinical evaluation.

Attorneys may attempt to use clinicians to establish the credibility of their client. Most courts today do not allow testimony in regard to client credibility from experts, believing that this invades the province of a judge or jury. Questions about credibility generally raise legal objections, which are upheld. With any objection, the clinician should allow counsel to argue the merits of an objection and the court to rule upon it. A clinician has no expertise in regard to the validity of a legal objection. Although it is tempting to engage in the legal debate, it is inadvisable.

Testimony is resumed when the judge rules on an objection. A novice may find it difficult to remember that an objection is not personal and is not an objection against the clinician. It is an objection based on legal precedent or legal grounds. When an objection is sustained, if witnesses do not attempt to modify their testimony to comply, they may be chastised from the bench. For example, a judge may sustain an objection to extensive narrative testimony in an area and insist that the expert reply with a yes or no answer. Being scolded by a judge in open court does not make a favorable impression on the jury.

The attorney may decide prior to the onset of a trial whether to use the direct examination to elicit material that is unfavorable to a client and that may be inconsistent with the expert's findings. Material may be a prior statement by the patient, the patient's medical history, or comments by another expert. If such material does not come out on direct examination, it most likely will come out on cross-examination. The ultimate decision in regard to trial strategy is, of course, always the attorney's, despite the fact that an expert may feel that he or she is more experienced than a particular attorney (and may be) or that an attorney's decisions will lead to disaster for the client; the conduct of the case is ultimately the attorney's responsibility. Second-guessing an attorney is poor clinical judgment. Although on occasion it may be tempting, more often than not it leads to disaster.

Cross-Examination

The behavior of attorneys that arouses the greatest anger among mental health professionals is that exhibited during cross-examination. The purpose of cross-examination is to discredit or impeach a witness, that is, to contribute to the stated purpose of a trial: seeking truth. However, in practice, cross-examination may seem to the novice witness to be less concerned with elucidation of the truth than with embarrassing and humiliating the expert. The opposing attorney's primary examination in cross-examination, ordinarily, is to mitigate the impact of testimony given by a witness in direct examination. Some attorneys go to great lengths to suggest bias or expose uncertainty in a witness's testimony. Some attorneys attempt to malign or distort a witness's testimony or to misconstrue it to a judge or jury. The primary goals for an expert during cross-examination may seem simple, but they may also be difficult to observe.

1. Always be honest. Remember that mental health professionals not only have an ethical responsibility to be honest, but in a courtroom, we are also under a sworn oath.
2. Admit it when you do not have certain information. That information may not be in the database or in an expert's fund of knowledge. This information may include specific information about a patient or literature related to a disputed area in the case.
3. Take time to think. Occasionally, attorneys in cross-examination attempt to lead witnesses in a hostile fashion, asking questions at a machine-gun pace. A witness always should take time to think. If being pushed to answer a question, a witness can request time from the court.
4. Do not speak for other experts. An expert can only provide his or her expert opinion and cannot speculate on what other experts might write or say.
5. It is important not to be critical of other experts. Such criticism is ultimately not valid, because it is impossible to know all the material, data, skills, and experience that another expert took into consideration in formulating an opinion. Criticizing another expert is not looked on favorably by the bench or the jury.
6. Just as in deposition, it is important not to talk too much. An expert can be boring if too pedantic. On occasion, it is tempting to elaborate, or rather filibuster, with the rationalization that one is educating the judge or jury. Instead, the judge and jury may become bored and become inattentive during lengthy, ponderous, unnecessary explanations.

Redirect and Recross

At this stage of the trial, the experts, attorney, and opposing counsel have an equal opportunity to elaborate challenge points that may have emerged during direct examination and cross-examination. Only material that has emerged on direct and cross-examinations may be referred to during redirect and recross. Opposing counsel will object if new material is introduced during this stage of the proceedings. A judge will have to make a ruling as to whether the material is new. The objection is upheld, sustained, or overruled.

Attorneys and psychiatrists are divided with regard to whether clinicians should answer the so-called ultimate issue question in the case. This would mean directly addressing the legal issue in question, for example, whether a person is incompetent, insane, or committable, whether a child has been sexually abused, whether parental rights should be terminated, or which parent serves the best interest of a child. These are but a few examples of the ultimate question that an expert may be asked to answer. Some commentators would suggest that mental health experts should only testify with regard to evaluation and diagnosis, treatment, and potential outcome. Still others would allow testimony with regard to the ultimate issue. Such testimony will be subject to cross-examination in the adversarial process. To date, no one has suggested that responding to all requests for testimony on the ultimate issue is unethical.

When testimony is completed, the witness may be excused by the judge. The witness must then decide if he or she wishes to remain in the courtroom to listen to other expert testimony and witnesses or leave. On occasion, the witness may be sequestered prior to testimony and asked to leave the courtroom after testimony. Leaving does make a witness seem less involved, more objective and impartial, and less invested in the outcome of the case. On occasion, attorneys may request that an expert sit at counsel's table and act as a personal coach to that attorney while other witnesses are being questioned. Although on rare occasions this may be acceptable, it is better to prepare the attorney for cross-examination of other witnesses ahead of time or during pretrial conferences. Sitting at a counsel's table may make the expert appear nonobjective and too involved in the outcome of a particular case.

PITFALLS

Psychiatrist-Related Pitfalls

The psychiatrist must attempt to be objective when evaluating forensic cases. Such objectivity needs to be carried over into the courtroom. The psychiatrist is not the advocate for the plaintiff/defendant. He or she merely presents data and conclusions based on a database.

Inadequate database. It is important to insist on access to all available materials in the attorney's files.

Inadequate literature review. Relevant clinical literature must be reviewed before giving testimony. Although one cannot hope to review all the literature in a given area, it is prudent to refer to scientific material written by other authors in the area in question. It is also prudent to review deposition testimony that might have been given in that area and to review any material an expert may have written in that area.

Hired gun. A psychiatrist who always testifies for the prosecution or for the defense (plaintiff or defendant, respectively), will become quickly known in her community or nationally as nonobjective, a hired gun. Additionally, one who testifies regularly outside his area of expertise may also be tagged as a hired gun.

Testifying outside one's area of expertise. It is seductive to be called an expert, and it is easy to be trapped by that appellation into testifying outside of one's area of expertise.

Attorney-Related Pitfalls

Coercion. Attorneys are adept at persuasion, and they may attempt to overtly coerce or seduce a clinician into changing an opinion. Remember that attorneys are prepared to evaluate and destroy the other side of the case and may attempt to do that with an expert to coerce an expert into changing an opinion.

Lack of preparation. Attorneys may come to court without adequate preparation. This is disconcerting for the expert. A pretrial conference with the attorney helps the expert to determine the degree of the attorney's preparation and to make suggestions regarding mental health areas that the attorney should know. In addition, many skilled attorneys are unfamiliar with mental health issues and unfamiliar with the materials mental health experts use, such as standard textbooks, the *Diagnostic and Statistical Manual of Mental Disorders*, and the *Physician's Desk Reference*.

Communications. Attorneys may not be skilled in communicating legal standards in a nontechnical way. It is important to continue to ask for clarification.

Patient-Related Pitfalls

Dual agency. The clinician should decide which role he or she may accept with regard to individuals. One cannot assume the roles of forensic expert and treating clinician without falling into the trap of dual agency. As noted in Chapter 3, "Forensic Ethics," it is difficult, if not impossible, to retain the objectivity necessary to be an expert when treating a patient, and in addition, there are ethical prohibitions spelled out in the psychiatrist's code of ethics (American Psychiatric Association 2001) with regard to dual agency.

CASE EXAMPLE EPILOGUES

Case Example 1

The psychiatrist informs the attorney that she will not be able to render a diagnosis nor will she be able to discuss the extent of his client's mental and emotional damages without examining his client. In this situation, the medical records do not speak for themselves. Medical records are useful when one discusses whether a psychiatric or psychological examination has been conducted properly. They are also helpful when discussing what a particular syndrome or diagnosis means. However, you cannot evaluate psychological damage without a hands-on evaluation of an individual.

Case Example 2

It is always bad news when an attorney attempts to argue with a psychiatric opinion. Dr. Mehta informed the attorney prior to the evaluation that she will "call things as she sees them." The attorney agreed with the conditions of the evaluation and then proceeded to abrogate the contract, deciding that a written report would not be necessary. Attorneys are skilled at presenting their position or side of the case. Dr. Mehta held firm and decided that this would be the last case she would evaluate for this particular attorney. The attorney had told Dr. Mehta several times at the onset of the case she wanted a valid opinion, not a hired gun.

Case Example 3

You note that on occasion it is appropriate to discuss the conduct of another colleague's psychiatric or psychological evaluation. You caution the psychiatrist not to make an ad hominem attack on his colleague. However, you remind him that medical professionals do criticize other colleagues on their conduct of an internal medical examination, a surgical procedure, or the reading of an X ray. Thus, although the general psychiatrist is doing what is comfortable for him (that is, not criticizing his colleague's reputation, skill, and integrity), it is ethical and professionally acceptable to criticize the conduct of an examination.

ACTION GUIDELINES

A. Go to court before acting as an expert and observe a skilled, ethical expert in action.
B. Take advantage of other useful training techniques, such as participating in a mock trial at a training institution or law school. If a novice can survive the challenge of a mock trial, the trial may seem tame in contrast. Participants are often surprised at their performances during mock trials and learn a great deal from their errors. Videotapes of mock trials or real trials are also useful for critique training.
C. View Court TV as a way of desensitizing yourself.
D. Seek feedback from peers who have observed your testimony with regard to accuracy and style of testimony; this helps to correct blind spots all experts suffer from.

REFERENCES

Ake v Oklahoma, 470 US 68 (1985)

American Psychiatric Association: The Principles of Medical Ethics With Annotations Especially Applicable to Psychiatry, 2001 Edition. Washington, DC, American Psychiatric Association, 2001

Appelbaum PS: Evaluating the admissibility of expert testimony. Hospital and Community Psychiatry 45:9–10, 1994

Appelbaum PS: The role of the mental health professional in court. Hospital and Community Psychiatry 36:1043–1046, 1985

Bank SC, Poythress NG: The elements of persuasion in expert testimony. Psychiatry and Law 10:173–204, 1982

Benedek EP: Testifying in court, in Child and Adolescent Psychiatry: A Comprehensive Textbook. Edited by Lewis M. Baltimore, MD, Williams & Wilkins, 1996, pp 1150–1154

Daubert v Merrill Dow Pharmaceuticals, Inc. 113 S Ct 2786 (1993)

Frye v United States, 293F 1013, 34 ALR 145 (DC Cir 1923)

Gutheil TG: Psychiatrist as Expert Witness. Washington, DC, American Psychiatric Press, 1988

Gutheil TG: The Psychiatrist in Court. Washington, DC, American Psychiatric Press, 1998

Harrol PA: A new lawyer's guide to expert use: prepare your expert so you don't have to prepare for disaster. The Practical Lawyer 39:55–63, 1993

Poythress NG: Coping on the witness stand: learned responses to learned treatise. Professional Psychology 11:169–179, 1980

Quen JM: The psychiatrist as expert witness, and the psychiatrist in the courtroom, in Selected Papers of Bernard Diamond. Edited by Quen JM. Hillsdale, NJ, Analytical Press, 1994, pp 233–248

Resnick PJ: Perceptions of psychiatric testimony: an historic co-perspective on an hysterical invective. Bulletin of the American Academy of Psychiatry and Law 14:203–219, 1986

Strassburger L, Gutheil T, Brodsky A: On wearing two hats: role conflict in serving as both psychotherapist and expert witness. Am J Psychiatry 154:448–456, 1997

Weinstock R, Leong G, Silva A: Opinions by the AAPL forensic psychiatrists on controversial ethical guidelines: a survey. Bulletin of the American Academy of Psychiatry and Law 19(3):237–248, 1991

Ziskin J, Faust D: Coping With Psychiatric and Psychological Testimony. Venus, CA, Law and Psychology Press, 1981

CHAPTER 6

Psychological Testing in Child and Adolescent Forensic Evaluations

Beth K. Clark, Ph.D., A.B.P.P.

Charles R. Clark, Ph.D., A.B.P.P.

Case Example 1

The local department of social services contacts a psychologist requesting an evaluation of a single-parent family to determine whether to terminate parental rights. The children, a 6-year-old boy and an 8-year-old girl, have been in foster care for about a year because of neglect. During this time they have had sporadic supervised visits with the mother. The children were described by their foster parents as "hyperactive" and undersocialized when they first came into their home. Though they have settled down, the foster parents are concerned that they revert to their old behavior after each visit with the mother. The mother is described by the social services worker as seeming "spaced out," and the worker wonders whether she might be "a little crazy." However, she also describes her as attached to her children and wanting them back.

The psychologist conducts extensive interviews with the mother and the children, and they are observed interacting. The mother is given a battery of psychological tests, which includes an intelligence test, projective techniques, and standardized psychological inventories. She is also given a series of behavior rating scales in order to assess her perception of the adaptation and behavior of her children. The foster parents are interviewed and also given the same rating scales. Both children are given intelligence tests, age-appropriate projective tests, and an instrument that measures academic functioning. The older child is given a personality inventory. Test data are integrated into interview data and history.

The data indicate that the mother may be impulsive and unable to tolerate stress, and they raise some question about her potential for alcohol or drug abuse.

There are suggestions of antisocial attitudes and very poor interpersonal skills, accompanied by strong narcissistic needs; these appear to be long-standing, chronic problems. The mother gives an extremely different account of the children's behavior on the rating scales from that given by the foster parents. Test data on the children suggest significant intellectual deficits. The older child appears to be well behind her peers in academic skills. There are some alarming indications of cognitive disorganization and distortion of interpersonal relationships. The younger child appears withdrawn from adult figures and experiences them as unable to help him. The psychologist compares this test data with information received from her interviews, observations, and from external sources. Interview data confirm that the mother has a drug problem. The psychologist prepares to write her report.

Case Example 2

A bitter custody dispute is referred by the court for evaluation. Three children, ages 2, 5, and 7, are involved. The psychologist has each child draw pictures of his or her family and gives the two older children a Wechsler intelligence test. The mother and father are given the Rorschach. In light of complaints by the mother, which raise questions of psychopathology or personality disorder in the father, he is given the Minnesota Multiphasic Personality Inventory—2 (MMPI-2). In the report, the psychologist includes the computer printout from the MMPI-2 scoring. He notes that the mother is the more nurturing parent, because she reported more people-oriented percepts on the Rorschach. He also notes that this test shows that she has healthily resolved her Oedipal conflict. The father, he notes, is not to be trusted and may be a sociopath, because the MMPI-2 Scale 4 (Psychopathic Deviate) is elevated; he does not indicate the extent of the elevation. He also expresses concern that the father has seen human figures on Card III of the Rorschach as having both breasts and penises; he offers that this response is indicative of confusion of sexual identity and fits a sexual abuser profile. He also notes that one of the children has drawn a figure without hands, which the psychologist maintains indicates possible conflict over aggression or sexuality, which in turn suggests that this child has been a victim of sexual abuse. The examiner recommends that sole custody be awarded to the mother and that parenting time with the father be suspended until he has entered psychotherapy because of his clear potential for sexual abuse.

Case Example 3

An 11-year-old boy and his 9-year-old sister are present when the boy's clothing is ignited by contact with an electric heater; the boy is severely burned on his face and hands. The parents sue the maker of the heater and the store that sold it. Among the damage claims is the psychological trauma to the boy as a result of the burns and to his sister from witnessing the event. A psychiatrist/psychologist team is asked to evaluate the children. Interviews are conducted with the children and their parents. The boy will say little about the injury and seems withdrawn; the parents are concerned about the withdrawal but say he has always been a child who does not talk about his problems. He was tested in school prior to the injury because of these concerns. The daughter freely discusses the experience without much difficulty and says that she feels sorry for her brother, but she is not very worried about it. The parents indicate they have been able to talk at length with the daughter about the situation.

A battery of tests is given to each child. The daughter responds within normal limits on all of the tests. She shows healthy problem-solving abilities and good overall adjustment. The son's test results, on the other hand, show pervasive concerns about body integrity. Images of fire are everywhere, and projective stories primarily consist of children being injured or in grave danger. There are test indications of marked social withdrawal and anxiety.

The chief issue before the courts in years past was whether medical training or methodology was necessary for expert testimony regarding mental and emotional conditions; the general response has been that it is not. Where psychologist qualifications have been mentioned in appellate decisions discussing the admissibility of testimony based on testing, they have included factors such as the possession of a doctorate, licensing, teaching experience, publication in professional journals, membership in the American Psychological Association, and certification by the American Board of Professional Psychology. Medical credentials as such have not been specified as necessary, nor has medical supervision of psychological work.

A secondary controversy regarding the admissibility of testimony based on psychological testing pertains to the scientific acceptability of test findings in general and of particular test instruments. As indicated below, all tests are not created equal in regard to reliability and validity, and some tests are more applicable to legal issues than are others. On this question, courts have generally upheld the admissibility of psychological testing, leaving open the question of the weight that might be accorded to it. Testing in general and certain instruments in particular—those deficient in psychometric foundation—remain subject to challenge in court, in the voir dire of the proposed psychological expert or in cross-examination. This is no different, however, from the legal challenges any mental health testimony is liable to face.

A related issue, and one which also concerns all expert testimony, is the extent to which psychological testimony should embrace opinions on the so-called ultimate issue—the factual and legal question on which the trier of fact must rule, such as the best interest of the child or the presence of negligence and damages. Rules of evidence adopted by the federal and state courts differ in regard to the limits placed on the scope of expert opinion testimony. Where opinions on ultimate issues are permitted, the adequacy of claimed bases for those opinions, whether psychological test data or other evaluative information, is subject to legal challenge.

LEGAL ISSUES

Psychologists in the United States have testified on a variety of legal issues since the 1920s, either on the basis of research findings or on the results of psychological testing. Controversies concerning the admissibility of clinical psychological testimony based on testing have in almost all jurisdictions been resolved in favor of broad latitude to psychological expert testimony.

CLINICAL ISSUES

Indications for Psychological Testing

Contribution to the Overall Evaluation

Forensic questions about children can place clinicians in a position of tremendous responsibility. Because of the difficulty and importance of helping the court to decide such things as how a child's life will be structured, whether to permanently terminate a parental relationship, or how damaged a child might be from abuse, the evaluation must be extensive and thorough. Although psychological testing should never be used alone in making recommendations, it is often useful and sometimes essential to a comprehensive evaluation.

Psychological testing permits observation of each subject under controlled conditions. Ideally, tests are given to each subject in a uniform fashion: the same questions are asked; and each subject is under the same expectations to respond. A relatively objective view of the subject is possible, in that the tests are constructed so as to minimize any influence or bias the examiner might bring to the evaluation.

Additionally, testing adds normative information to the picture. Psychological tests compare the performance of an individual to the performance of the general population or to a more specific population, such as psychiatric patients. This statistical comparison adds objective data not available simply from a clinical interview. Although clinicians are sometimes frustrated that tests cannot speak specifically enough to the issues involved in child forensic work to dictate definitive answers to legal questions, testing can provide information that augments that gathered from other assessment methods.

Finally, the use of psychological tests permits the examiner to measure and evaluate the subject's approach to the assessment itself. Understanding an individual's set or general approach to the evaluation—candor and insight, guardedness and deception, repression and denial—can be essential to accurately evaluating the assessment data as a whole. Some tests, such as the MMPI, used with adults and adolescents (MMPI-2 and MMPI-A, respectively [Butcher and William 1992]), have built-in measures that provide significant information about whether a subject may be trying to underestimate or exaggerate difficulties or may be trying to present himself or herself in a biased manner. Close attention to a child's approach to testing can provide data regarding whether the child may have been coached or influenced by a parent. For example, in a custody dispute, if a child were to give rote answers to every card on the Rorschach (Exner 1995), and these answers all had the theme of a bad man, one might wonder whether the child had been told to make sure that that thought was conveyed. Continuation of this set throughout the interview, interaction, and observation portions of the evaluation would reinforce this concern.

Choice of Tester

The administration and interpretation of psychological tests require specific training, not only in personality theory, psychological development, and psychopathology but also in test construction and quantitative research methodology. Although some tests can be administered by a technician, the interpretation should not be done by anyone other than a psychologist fully trained and experienced in all of the instruments given. As will be further explained below, responsibility for the interpretation of testing cannot be left to a computer program alone. Finally, because of important issues regarding role, clinicians who are providing ongoing treatment to a child should usually avoid evaluating and testing that child in conjunction with a legal proceeding (Greenberg and Shuman 1997).

When to Use Testing

Many, if not most, child evaluations can benefit from psychological testing. Its research base and standardized administration make it particularly useful in forensic settings in which clinicians are called on to carefully ground and explicate their findings. Clinicians should be sure to use the most current versions of available tests, as they typically are revised periodically to include up-to-date norms. Properly employed tests can be a useful adjunct to the evaluation, providing information that converges with other sources of information or that raises by itself useful hypotheses to be explored. Following is a list of particular forensic areas, with recommendations of whom to test and what type of questions testing may be of use in answering. More specific information about each type of test is included in a subsequent section of this chapter, "Selection of Tests and Their Relative Utility."

Abuse and neglect. There are three general areas where testing can be of particular help with questions of abuse and neglect. First, especially in regard to sexual abuse, there are often questions of the reliability of the child's report. Second are questions of the effects of abuse and neglect on the child. Third, there may be questions pertaining to an adult involved, either as an alleged perpetrator of abuse or in terms of parenting ability in the case of neglect. It is important to note here that although testing should be used with caution in any forensic setting, it and other assessment techniques should be used extremely carefully in the area of sexual abuse, in which the focus is often on a question of fact: whether sexual abuse occurred or not. Whatever information it may provide about behavioral traits or conditions, neither testing nor any other clinical assessment technique can provide an actual answer to a question about a fact in dispute. Case Example 2 shows a situation in which the misuse of testing created serious effects in a custody dispute.

Testing can contribute to judgments of a child's reliability. Intelligence tests can, for example, provide information on whether the child is intellectually capable of being able to remember details, understand, and coherently report an incident. In addition, knowledge of the child's intellectual functioning, cognitive and developmental level, and view of his or her world can provide a context for the clinician to evaluate the child's report. Specific references to abuse are not commonly encountered in the testing situation. However, comparison of less direct themes in the child's productions with interview data can help in assessing reliability. Some of the newer rating scales and personality inventories contain validity scales, which give information about the child's approach to the test situation.

Testing can also provide information about the effects of abuse and neglect. Physical abuse or neglect can in itself cause decrements in intellectual functioning and learning disabilities. Testing can elucidate these issues, as well as such effects as trauma- or anxiety-induced problems in attention and concentration. Thematic content of some tests can provide data on the effects of abuse. A sexually abused child who tells more stories than the norm about being physically damaged or terrorized by adults on the Roberts Apperception Test (Roberts 1994) may lead the evaluator to more strongly consider whether serious damage has occurred. Similarly, bland and affectless test responses from a child who suffered abuse may signal maladaptive emotional blunting and withdrawal. Information on the coping styles and interpersonal skills of the child can add important data to the consideration of placement when that becomes necessary. With respect to cases in which the adult disputes an allegation of abuse or neglect, testing of the accused adult may have value in contributing to a clearer total picture of the individual, which may be helpful to the trier of fact. It is important to underscore, however, that psychological testing is not capable of identifying the guilty or the innocent or of establishing the credibility or truthfulness of a person. Any conclusion based on test data that an accused individual is or is not a sexual abuser is a conclusion that goes beyond the data. As is true of other assessment strategies, there is no reliable test-based profile of offenders or any pattern of test results that would indicate truthfulness. Test indications of intentional distortion of the person's presentation—denial, exaggeration, guardedness, or malingering—may shed light on the individual but cannot be brought to bear directly on a question of guilt or innocence.

Termination of parental rights.   Evaluation of the adults involved in the question of termination of parental rights is obviously as important as that of the children themselves. Although there is often data in social services

records on both parents and children, frequently a forensic evaluation is not considered until very late in the termination process. Often data of a mental health nature are from therapists who are in the difficult position of both treating the child or parent and providing evaluation information for the court or social services. An evaluation that includes concrete information from testing of the presence or absence of character disorder or frank psychopathology of the parents, their intelligence and cognitive integrity, and their social skills and personality can be of great use to the court. It can help to generate hypotheses about a parent's insight and ability to use psychotherapeutic or educational and social intervention. Treatment issues, goals, and impediments may be identified, increasing the likelihood of success when a strategy of intervention is attempted.

In addition, testing the children in cases in which termination of parental rights is at issue can provide information on their level of functioning and attachment to the parent, which can be woven together with interview, observation, and history to determine whether further contact with the parent would be beneficial or detrimental. The complex question of how the parents' and child's temperaments, strengths, and weaknesses interact can be addressed by considering test results. Case Example 1 describes a case in which relatively vague speculations by foster parents and social service workers were initially the only data regarding the psychological function of the children and mother in this case. The testing that accompanied the evaluation provided information on the chronicity of the mother's problems and her intellectual limitations, as well as finding a complexity in the problems of the children that might tax even the most able parent. This led to the synthesis and recommendation that are reported in the epilogue at the end of the chapter.

Delinquency and criminal proceedings.   Testing is frequently used in cases of juvenile delinquency commitments to identify personality variables, treatment foci, and academic and social skill levels. Assessments are ordered by courts to determine whether adolescents charged with serious felonies, particularly murder and rape, ought to be tried not as juveniles but as adults, subject to the full range of adult sentencing provisions. Where the binding over of juvenile defendants to adult jurisdictions is not automatic, that is, simply based on factors such as age, provisions for the waiver of juvenile court jurisdiction to an adult court differ across the states. Many considerations taken into account by the courts, such as the seriousness of the offense, the juvenile's criminal record, or the welfare of the community, are not assessment questions open to psychological or psychiatric assessment. Though in practice frequently outweighed by those considerations, juvenile waiver provisions commonly involve an assessment of the juvenile's character and amenability to treatment or rehabilitation in a juvenile facility. On those issues, psychological testing can serve as another source of information about personality functioning, insight, and treatment motivation.

At times in particular jurisdictions, questions of competency to stand trial, criminal responsibility, and insanity are raised in respect to juveniles. Whereas it is debatable whether adult standards of competency and criminal responsibility are appropriate to juveniles, when juveniles are tried as adults, it is the standard legal tests of competency and insanity that are used. A full discussion of the role of testing in regard to what are essentially adult issues goes beyond the scope of this chapter.

Clinicians and courts may be tempted to use psychological testing as a means to predict the potential for violence or sexual aggression in children and adolescents. To date, no psychological test has been validated for this purpose, and because of statistical problems associated with predicting relatively rare events such as school shootings, as well as a lack of any clear current understanding of what leads to violence, valid tests of dangerousness are unlikely to be developed soon. Testing is as problematic in this regard as other clinical predictive methods that have been tried. Using even an instrument that is sensitive to signs of character pathology or aggressive conduct, such as the MMPI, specifically for this purpose is far more likely to result in false positives—the erroneous identification of youngsters as dangerous—than accurate predictions.

Child custody.   As with termination of parental rights, child custody questions require thorough evaluations of both adults and children, including interview, observation of parent-child interaction, and consideration of testing. When a dispute has reached an impasse that requires a custody evaluation, parental animosity may be expected to be high, together with concern by the parents that their points of view be fully heard. Testing can contribute to the thoroughness of the evaluation as well as add an objective comparative standard to the process. Testing also enhances the clinician's ability to compare and contrast parental strengths and weaknesses in relation to those of their children. Parent rating scales can be compared with interview data as a measure of how accurately a parent understands the children. Testing of the children can lend important information about any special needs or problems they have, how children view adult figures, how they perceive the family, and whether and how the divorce process has affected them.

Civil damages.   Civil suits brought because of injury to a child have more and more often required the evaluative services of a forensically trained clinician. These can include claims of psychological effects of a physical injury, emotional stress because of disasters or toxic exposure, and psychological trauma resulting from sexual or physical abuse. At times, parents are also named as plaintiffs in these suits. For example, in the case of sexual abuse occurring at a preschool, a parent may enter the suit because of claims of psychological stress caused by having to deal with the trauma experienced by his or her child.

In assessing psychological damage to plaintiffs, testing may help identify or rule out preexisting conditions, which may have continued unchanged or may have been exacerbated by the events in question. Testing can help answer questions of malingering or unreliability, which often need to be considered in situations in which large amounts of money are at stake. Comparisons of current and past testing, when available, can point to changes in psychological functioning.

The intrusion of the traumatic event into test data may indicate how pervasive the response to the injury is. For example, the boy in Case Example 3, a burn victim, became anxious, tearful, and could not respond to Card IX of the Rorschach, which is frequently seen as smoke and fire, illustrating the claims made on his behalf regarding traumatic symptoms. A general picture of personality functioning and coping skills will aid in the difficult task of attempting to predict future effects of the trauma. It is worth considering testing parents of children involved in civil litigation, even if the parents are not named plaintiffs, although this may not be allowed in some cases. Research has shown the importance of addressing the aftermath of trauma by adults and institutions (Friedrich 1990). Information on the parents' functioning as well as that of the children provides a systematic picture of the experience of the family unit. At the very least, appropriate parent inventories and child behavior scales should be administered to parents whose children are plaintiffs in civil suits.

Selection of Tests and Their Relative Utility

Most often a battery of tests, rather than a single instrument, are administered. Individual tests should be selected for inclusion in an assessment strategy to provide information about specific problems at issue in the case. The most commonly used tests and their relative utility in child forensic work are listed next. Included are test instruments used with adults, who will be the focus of assessment in many cases involving children, particularly in child custody questions.

Adults

Intelligence tests. The most common adult intelligence test in use today is the Wechsler Adult Intelligence Scale—3rd Edition (WAIS-III; Wechsler 1997), although the Stanford-Binet, which has a lower "floor" or more sensitive measurement of impaired intellectual functioning, is especially useful with the developmentally disabled. The WAIS-III, like its counterparts for children, provides measures of a variety of abilities taken to be associated with what is commonly referred to as intelligence. It especially assesses abilities important to academic and occupational achievement, rather than for social skills and creativity, and a variety of specific intellectual capabilities. Cognitive impairment of various types can be identified in WAIS-III performance, as can areas of strength and comparative skill. Many psychologists tap the WAIS-III for useful information regarding personality factors, which is similar to the information obtained from projective testing. Although the Wechsler can be helpful in this way, tests of intelligence would usually not be administered unless there was some concern about the adult having an intellectual deficit or significant cognitive impairment.

Personality inventories. Well-researched personality inventories are very commonly given; they have considerable reliability and provide quantified results that may be readily interpreted in light of published norms. Such tests are "paper-and-pencil" instruments that require endorsement by the subject of various statements pertaining to beliefs, emotions, and behavior, for example, by marking them true or false or by rating their applicability to the test subject. Among the instruments developed for use with nonclinical populations are the California Psychological Inventory (Gough 1987), the Sixteen Personality Factors Questionnaire (Cattell et al. 1993), and the NEO PI—Revised (Costa and McCrae 1992). The MMPI-2, for some years the most commonly administered psychological test, is designed to assess significant functional disorders in the neurotic, characterological, and psychotic spectra but is also sensitive to subclinical personality factors or traits. The Millon Clinical Multiaxial Inventory—3rd Edition (Millon 1994) was specifically designed to assess DSM-IV (American Psychiatric Association 1994) personality disorders, although it is normed on individuals who are in the early stages of treatment and may provide an overestimate of problems in other populations. The Personality Assessment Inventory is also being increasingly used to assess adult psychopathology.

Although they are often called *objective* tests, the personality inventories, no less than other tests, require clinical skill to use and are therefore susceptible to some subjectivity in interpretation. Undue reliance on the score profile from such instruments in reaching diagnostic conclusions, let alone recommendations on matters such as custody or sexual abuse, without considering the psychometric properties of the instruments together with a variety of data obtained elsewhere, invites error. The instruments are *objective* in the relative sense that they sharply reduce subjective factors, particularly those produced in the interaction between examiner and subject, which are present in other assessment methods. Although somewhat time-consuming for subjects to complete, they allow for efficient and inexpensive use of examiner time.

Projective tests. Projective tests require responses by the subject to ambiguous stimuli. A wide variety of such instruments have been developed, though few are in common use currently. The Rorschach inkblot technique is perhaps the best known and most widely used of these instruments; 10 cards are presented in sequence to the subject, who is asked to indicate what the inkblots on the cards might be; inquiry follows as to where on the card the percept was seen and what made it appear to the subject in the way that it had. It can provide information on psychopathology or its absence. It is also used to examine the subjects' usual response or coping style, how they approach ambiguous situations, and how emotions are handled. Comparison of the Rorschach summaries of various members of a family can help generate hypotheses about how the styles of various members might interact with those of others in the family.

Most clinical psychologists view projectives as adding information to the examination not otherwise available. Unlike the self-report inventories, the manifest content of projectives gives little clue as to what a "good," or desirable, response might be.

This aspect of these techniques is particularly valuable in forensic settings in which subjects are not disinterested in the outcome and recommendations and in which they may feel strong needs to present themselves in particular ways. Projectives also permit an observation of a subject's response to an ambiguous and unfamiliar task.

Projective tests vary in the extent to which they have been subjected to the empirical study of their psychometric properties. Generally, when examined, such instruments appear to have, relative to the "objective" personality measures of tests of ability and aptitude, poor reliability and uncertain validity. These problems are sometimes compounded by the lack of standardization in administration, scoring, and interpretation. As test instruments, projective techniques are more vulnerable than other types of testing to examiner error and bias, because they typically require a great deal of subjectivity in interpretation, if not in scoring and administration. Used carelessly, they may be more tests of the examiner than of the subject. In the case of the Rorschach at least, considerable work has been done by Exner and his associates (Exner 1995) on improving standardization and reliability, quantifying scoring, and identifying from empirical research personality and behavioral correlates of test data; as a result, Exner's Rorschach shares more in common with objective personality instruments than do other projectives. Tests such as the Thematic Apperception Test (Murray 1971), Draw A Person techniques (Goodenough and Harris 1950), and non-Exner Rorschach systems (Exner 1995), although perhaps useful in some types of assessments, lack the psychometric properties necessary for forensic evaluation and are thus not recommended for use, especially in light of the availability of other more rigorous measures.

Parenting inventories.   If parental attitudes and abilities are in question, such as in child custody and parental fitness evaluations, there are psychometrically valid instruments available to aid in such an assessment (Heinze and Grisso 1996). The Parent-Child Relationship Inventory (Gerard 1994) assesses parental attitudes toward parenting and their children. Data are obtained regarding the similarity of the parent's responses to those parents who display attitudes consistent with good parenting. The Parenting Stress Index (Abidin 1995) aids in the identification of potentially stressful parent-child relationships by screening for reported parental stress. The Child Abuse Potential Inventory (Milner 1986) was developed in order to assess a parent's risk of physically abusing a child. It measures a set of risk factors that are compared to norms of parents who have physically abused their children.

Children

Intelligence and adaptive behavior.   Intelligence testing for children can be helpful even if there is no question of serious intellectual difficulties. This testing can give significant information about the child's cognitive abilities, especially his or her ability to understand the current legal or familial situation, to report events accurately, or to interpret events. The Wechsler Intelligence Scale for Children—3rd Edition (WISC-III; Wechsler 1997), the Wechsler Preschool and Primary Scales of Intelligence—Revised (WPPSI-R; Wechsler 1989), and the Kaufman batteries (Kaufman and Kaufman 1983) are most commonly used. For very young children, the Bayley Scales of

Infant Development—2nd Edition (Bayley 1993) and the Miller Assessment for Preschoolers (MAP; Miller 1982) are available. Inventories such as the Vineland Adaptive Behavior Scales (Sparrow et al. 1984) use structured interviews to help determine the functioning level of developmentally disabled children.

Personality inventories.   There have been several personality inventories developed in recent years that are geared to children. These have similar advantages to adult inventories in that they have scales that provide information on the child's approach to the test itself, as well as the ability to compare scores with nonclinical and psychiatric normative populations. The MMPI-A is available for teenagers 14 years or older, and the MCMI-III has its counterpart in the Millon Adolescent Clinical Inventory (Millon 1993). For younger children, the Personality Inventory for Children (PIC; Lachar 1989) and the Behavior Assessment System for Children (BASC; Reynolds and Kamphaus 1990) are inventories with reading levels and norms for children ages 8 through 18.

As most clinicians are aware, children are not always the most accurate reporters of their emotional state and behaviors. To supplement children's reports, there are a number of instruments available that allow parents and others to report. The PIC has a counterpart, the Personality Inventory for Youth (Lachar and Gruber 1995), which is completed by parents regarding their children. In addition to parent rating scales, the BASC also includes scales for teachers. The scales can be integrated to form a comprehensive picture of the child. Although it does not have validity scales, the Child Behavior Checklist (Achenbach 1991) can be useful in making comparisons of the way each parent in a custody dispute, for example, sees the children and the extent to which this may or may not coincide with the evaluator's hypotheses about the children. Parents in custody disputes may be quite discrepant in their views of the children, and both may underestimate the effect of the dispute on their children. In other situations, such as termination of parental rights, the scales can be compared to those filled out by teachers and other significant adults such as foster parents. In cases of civil damage, comparisons of ratings by parents or others may indicate the reliability with which certain features of behavior appear. This type of concrete information about the parents' own assessment of their children and how it relates to those of others can be an asset in making recommendations.

Projective testing.   Discovering how children, especially young children, feel and think about events in their lives is not an easy task. In forensic evaluations the issue is particularly sensitive. Most would agree that it is not appropriate to directly ask young children about their preference for one parent or the other in a custody evaluation or to ask leading questions in an evaluation of sexual abuse. Most children, no matter their age, are exquisitely aware of why they are being evaluated and may feel anxious about what they say to an evaluator in light of how it may affect their parents or the decision of the court. Projective testing provides a forum a step removed from direct discourse and can skirt a child's conscious intentions and permit reasonable inferences about the child's needs and fears. Case Example 3 shows how testing can reveal serious difficulties in a child who is uncomfortable in an interview situation.

As mentioned above, poorly validated child projective tests, such as the Children's Apperception Test (Bellak 1986), should be avoided in child forensic evaluations. An Exner Rorschach, however, will give information about a child similar to that previously mentioned in regard to adults. Validated projectives, such as the Roberts Apperception Test for Children (RAT-C; Roberts 1994) and the Tell Me a Story Test (Costantino et al. 1988), are particularly useful in forensic cases. Both tests have children make up stories about sets of pictures representing typical situations and possible problems in child and family life. The tests are then quantitatively scored and compared with a general population of children.

Projective drawings are sometimes used by clinicians. Great care should be taken in the selection and especially the interpretation of drawings. As is the case with adults, it has been charged that tests such as the Draw a Person (Goodenough and Harris 1950) are too far removed from the referral question and too indefensible in court to be of much utility. However, the Kinetic Family Drawing (Burns 1982), which asks the child to draw a picture of his or her family doing something, appears to be quite directly related to the issues involved in much child forensic work. How the child describes the picture and answers questions about it may provide useful clinical information, even if it does not yield test scores comparable to normative values. Who is and is not included in the picture, the activity depicted, and the interaction among family members may help generate hypotheses about the child's view of the family. For younger children, there are a number of structured play techniques in the literature (e.g., Gardner 1982; Lynn 1959, as found in Palmer 1983), which take the child though a series of vignettes, during which the type of play is observed and noted. It is important to note that these techniques are not psychological tests. They may indeed be more properly considered as clinical observation tools.

Inferences made from a child's performance on these tasks must be very cautiously made and be integrated with interview and other observational data. It would be inappropriate to base important conclusions or recommendations solely or largely on such inferences.

Tests of academic functioning. It is often helpful to determine whether and how a child's school performance has been affected by events at issue. The Wide Range Achievement Test—3rd Edition (Wilkinson 1993) and the Wechsler Individual Achievement Test—II (Wechsler 2001) are quick tests of such basic areas as reading, spelling, and mathematics skills. For a broader picture of a child's academic abilities, the Woodcock-Johnson Psychoeducational Battery—Revised (Woodcock and Johnson 1989) provides data on a number of skills in relation to the child's age and grade level. With these tests, the evaluator can determine a child's academic rank relative to peers and can use this information in conjunction with the intelligence scales and teacher and parent reports to look at overall adaptation of the child. There are also numerous tests related to specific learning disabilities that can be used if indicated.

Neuropsychological testing. In some cases, such as personal injury cases involving head trauma or toxic tort litigation, tests of the child's memory and other neuropsychological functioning may be required. Selected tests or comprehensive batteries, such as the Halstead-Reitan Neuropsychological Test Batteries for Children (Reitan and Davison 1974) and the Nebraska Neuropsychological Children's Battery (Golden 1986), are often used. Specific tests of memory in children have only recently been designed. These include the Children's Memory Scale (Cohen 1997) and the Test of Memory and Learning (Reynolds and Bigler 1994).

Attention-deficit/hyperactivity disorder (ADHD) is a differential diagnostic question that occurs with some regularity in forensic evaluations of children. There are a number of tests and rating scales that can be of use in screening for ADHD. The Test of Variables of Attention or Connors' Continuous Performance Test are computerized assessments of the ability of a child to pay attention. The revised Conners' Rating Scales and a number of scales developed by Barkley (1998) are typically used in the assessment of ADHD.

Tests addressing specific forensic issues. There are several specific issues that frequently arise in child forensic evaluations that have been addressed by equally specific tests. The Trauma Symptom Checklist for Children (Briere 1996) is a self-report instrument that purports to measure posttraumatic stress in children. The Child Sexual Behavior Inventory (Friedrich 1997) is a parent-report measure that compares the behavior of the child being assessed to normative sexual behavior of children of the same age. Whereas both of these inventories are psychometrically sound and have validity scales, they should be carefully used in the forensic arena because they are quite "face" valid, with "open content." Unlike the MMPI or the Rorschach, for example, what the test purports to measure may be quite obvious to the test-taker. Thus, these measures may be somewhat more vulnerable to exaggeration or to defensiveness by a plaintiff who may have an interest in presenting a certain way. The validity scales incorporated into the instrument may not identify particular instances of response bias related to litigation. This is even truer for simple checklists, which are sometimes misleadingly called tests. Most checklists have no validity scales and are highly susceptible to deceptive responding by subjects in forensic evaluations.

There have been other efforts to develop tests that are designed specifically for use in child custody evaluations. The Bricklin Scales (Bricklin and Elliot 1997) and the Ackerman-Schoendorf Scales for Parent Evaluation of Custody (Ackerman and Schoendorf 1992) are examples of this genre. Although such scales invite strong and even exclusive reliance by examiners and the court on their results, empirical research to date does not justify such reliance, and none can be recommended as substitutes for full consideration of the wide variety of data obtained in standard evaluations.

The prosecution of youngsters, both as juveniles and adults, is an emerging issue. To date, instruments addressing competency to stand trial that are valid for youth offenders are not available. Grisso's Instruments for Assessing Understanding and Appreciation of Miranda Rights (Grisso 1998) are based on research with children as young as 10. The Grisso Miranda Instruments are not designed to yield an overall score and do not purport to actually measure competency to waive Miranda rights; however, they can be a useful adjunct to an evaluation of this competency.

Interpretation of Test Data

The results of psychological tests do not stand alone but must be carefully interpreted in light of the information obtained in the rest of the evaluation. Test interpretation is inherently inferential, and care should be taken to stay as close to the actual data as possible. Although it may be interesting to make wide-ranging dynamically oriented hypotheses about test responses when evaluating a person for treatment planning, it is inappropriate to do so in the forensic arena where the evaluator must be able to

clearly account for the basis on which conclusions and recommendations are made. Speculations about repressed Oedipal content as seen on the Rorschach are much less helpful to the court than clear statements about how such a conflict may be expressed in personality style, behavior, and parenting abilities. Misidentifying remote and speculative inferences from testing as *findings* and *indications* may be seen as a misuse of testing and a disservice to the individuals affected. The examiner bears grave responsibility for affecting the lives of others and must strive to ground recommendations in actual data rather than speculation.

Integration With Other Evaluation Data

In Case Example 2, the psychologist has made an important error in interpretation. He has taken several isolated responses from the test data and has extrapolated from them evidence of sexual abuse. There is no single response on any test instrument that warrants such an accusation; test data need to be considered as a whole, and individual responses have little significance by themselves.

Interpretations of test responses should not go beyond what the tests themselves can measure. In a thorough evaluation, each test should be carefully scored and interpreted. The information gained from the tests should be integrated into hypotheses about persons and how they interact with one another, if that is relevant to the legal question. These hypotheses can then be considered in light of the other data from the evaluation, including document review and clinical interview. Interpretive hypotheses from testing can help objectively confirm what the clinician has found and enrich an understanding of otherwise unexplained facts. They serve also to point out discrepancies or other avenues to pursue. As can be seen in Case Example 1, testing indicated that the mother could have substance abuse problems. This led the psychologist to interview her in depth about drug abuse, which she then admitted. Rather than simply reporting an inference from test data, the psychologist now had clear, direct evidence that could be used in her report.

Use of Computer-Scored Interpretation

Many psychological tests have computer programs available that not only score them but also provide clinical interpretations based on the test data. It may be tempting for the clinician not trained in testing or psychometrics to consider these printouts a finished interpretation and include them verbatim in reports without further investigation. As most manuals for these tests point out, this is not the intended use for the automated interpretations. Computerized interpretation may help the clinician, especially one inexpert in testing, to generate hypotheses that, again, must be carefully integrated with other data. However, many of the statements generated by computer programs may not be completely accurate descriptions of the person being evaluated, because the programs do not take into account the richness of the full evaluation, or even all possible data from the test itself, and instead generate hypotheses on the basis of actuarial data. The resulting interpretive statements are derived from aggregate data; within normative groups, each individual's behavior, characteristics, or score occupies a place around a group average or other measure of group tendency. To conclude from an individual's score on an instrument that he or she is typical of the normative group neglects the fact of variance. Without referring to other data, the extent to which a person fits the picture of the group to which he or she is assigned by virtue of a score cannot be known. Computerized interpretations are in actuality more or less accurate for particular individuals, depending of a variety of factors. It is necessary that these factors be identified and considered by the examining clinician. The introduction into court proceedings of uninterpreted computerized interpretations may lend testing a false importance that leads to more attention by the court to small parts of the testing than to the rest of the data.

Reporting of Test Data

In reporting test results in the forensic setting, there needs to be attention to accountability; nothing should be reported as opinion in written work or in testimony that cannot be supported by data and reasoned inference. It should be clear from the written report which data were considered and the way in which conclusions were reached. Unlike consultation reports read by colleagues in the mental health field, results and opinions should be presented in clear language rather than in jargon. A treatment of testing results that is overly technical mystifies rather than elucidates for the basis of opinions and may mask an absence of any adequate basis for an opinion. Excessive detailing of raw test data may indicate lack of expertise, because it is no substitute for clear and accurate summarization of the results of testing.

Release of Raw Test Data

There has been some controversy over the appropriateness of releasing raw test data, that is, score sheets and computer-generated data, directly to attorneys. Psychologists must be careful to protect test security so that test materials are not rendered useless by their exposure to the general public. They also must be sure that tests are not misinterpreted or misused by untrained parties. If clinicians are concerned about any of these issues, they may take steps such as seeking a protective order to maintain test security or agreeing to give the raw data only to another professional able to interpret it.

Balanced Reporting

Clinicians who use psychological tests, as well as those who conduct forensic evaluations, sometimes forget that attention needs to be paid to the relative strengths of each person being evaluated. Custody disputes in particular should not ordinarily be battles of pathology, with attempts to demonstrate which of the parties is the more disturbed. The court needs to know what they do well. It also needs to know not only how a child has been and might be affected but also the positive aspects of how she is coping with a stressful situation. When reporting on deficits, psychopathology, or personality problems, attention should be paid to the comparative extent of these problems, especially because children involved in forensic cases are often not from traditional clinical populations.

Nonselective Reporting

It may be tempting for the clinician, who has already formed some hypotheses about a subject from the interview, to report test findings that only support these hypotheses. In Case Example 2, the psychologist neglected to report his observations of the father and children, which indicated a warm and loving relationship. Also, he neglected to mention that he had never interviewed the children about possible abuse. Instead, he had selectively used some test responses to confirm his hypothesis of sexual abuse. Test data that are discrepant with the clinician's overall hypotheses should be reported and explained candidly. In the long run, it will be left to the trier of fact and not the clinician to determine which of the data are most compelling.

PITFALLS

Failure to Administer Tests in a Standard Fashion

Psychological tests should be administered in the standardized way they are intended, as provided by their manuals. Administering a few subscales of the WISC-III or a couple of Rorschach cards is poor practice in general, but never more so than in forensic settings. Such administration outside testing protocols results in nonvalid findings that have no clear and interpretable relationship to group norms.

Anything that might allow the test-taker to appear to be or be influenced by outside sources should not be permitted in forensic evaluations. Tests should not be sent home with subjects for completion, nor should interested parties be present in the room when tests are given. In some settings, attorneys or parents may want to monitor or observe the evaluation. This is problematic, especially because children may alter their responses if they are being observed. For example, a child who knows that his parents are watching may be uncomfortable telling a story on the RAT-C that reflects family problems. In extenuating circumstances, unobtrusive video- or audio-taping, or the use of one-way mirrors, may permit observation while reducing the chances of outside influence. However, they are not optimal.

Careless test administration leaves the clinician open to questions about the accuracy of conclusions and the quality of recommendations. Similarly, lack of control over choice of tester, when testing is delegated, or the way in which testing is conducted damages the actual and perceived reliability of reported test findings.

Misuse of Testing by Attorneys or the Court

Laypersons, including lawyers and judges, may attempt to misuse or misinterpret psychological testing in court in several ways. Testing can present an aura of complete objectivity and can seem to be the most important piece of data rather than an integrated part of a whole evaluation. In particular, computerized reports may give a false sense of scientific certainty and may be unduly impressive to a nonclinician. Attorneys sometimes try to use individual responses or tests selectively. For example, an often-encountered line of questioning in testimony about the MMPI-2 involves asking how a client responded to particular items. Clinicians who fail to correct this approach support a mistaken view that a single scale or score, taken out of context, can be considered meaningful. It is the responsibility of clinicians to do their best to see that those involved understand the proper use of testing.

gathered. On the basis of her familiarity with the laws of her state regarding termination of parental rights, she concludes that the children have extensive, serious, and complicated problems that will require intensive attention and monitoring by a parent, as well as long-term treatment. She concludes that the mother's concern about her children seems only to reflect her own needs. Her drug problem and long-standing interpersonal difficulties do not allow her to provide the level of care required by her children, and the psychologist recommends termination of parental rights.

Case Example 2

The psychologist in this case has gone far beyond the test data by making speculative statements that have little grounding in objective data. His use of interpretations of the projective tests and drawings as clear-cut signs of an actual occurrence is inappropriate. On the basis of these insufficient and faulty data, the court moves to cut off the father's access to his children. The children are extremely upset at this and begin to show symptoms of depression and anxiety. The father's attorney calls in a new evaluator, who does extensive interviewing and testing of the father, but who is denied access to the mother or the children now in her custody. The new evaluator concludes that there is an insufficient basis to arrive at a finding of sexual abuse in this case. The judge, having ruled, is not swayed; citing the earlier court-ordered evaluation of all parties, parenting time with the father is not reinstated. The father files a malpractice suit and an ethics complaint against the first psychologist.

Case Example 3

The psychologist carefully reviews the previous test battery given to the son. She notes that there was some concern about the boy's social skills and that his level of anxiety appears to have increased. The concerns about body integrity and danger so prominent in the current assessment were not apparent in the earlier testing. Academic functioning has shown marked impairment; as tests show, he has fallen behind his classmates in most areas. She and the psychiatrist can identify no other life events that may have contributed to this change, and they conclude that what the child is experiencing appears to have occurred after being burned. Neither interview nor test data support a claim of damage to the daughter, who appears to be dealing successfully with the accident and is functioning normally.

CASE EXAMPLE EPILOGUES

Case Example 1

The psychologist prepares an extensive report that includes a separate section on test results and integrates the results with the rest of the information

ACTION GUIDELINES

A. Know the law.

B. Use a qualified evaluator.

C. Select and administer appropriate tests.

1. Give a battery of tests.
2. Use tests appropriate to ages of children and to issues involved in the evaluation.
3. Administer tests uniformly to all parties.
4. Administer tests in a standardized fashion within protocols provided by manuals.
5. Use tests that are well researched and documented.
6. Avoid tests without adequate validation or that too clearly telegraph their intent.

D. Interpret cautiously.

1. Integrate data with other clinical findings and documentation.
2. Do not rely solely on computerized interpretations.
3. Avoid overinterpretation of single scores or responses.
4. Keep interpretations close to the data, avoiding remote inferences.

E. Report responsibly.

1. Provide a balanced view of each party.
2. Include all relevant data, even data that do not support conclusions and recommendations.
3. Assume subjects will have access to the report.

REFERENCES

Abidin RR: Parenting Stress Index. Odessa, FL, Psychological Assessment Resources, 1995

Achenbach R: Conceptualizations of developmental psychopathology, in Handbook of Developmental Psychopathology. Edited by Lewis M, Miller S. New York, Plenum, 1991, pp 3–14

Ackerman MJ, Schoendorf K: ASPECT: Ackerman-Schoendorf Scales for Parent Evaluation of Custody—Manual. Los Angeles, CA, Western Psychological Services, 1992

American Psychiatric Association: Diagnostic and Statistical Manual of Mental Disorders, 4th Edition. Washington, DC, American Psychiatric Association, 1994

Barkley RA: Attention Deficit Hyperactivity Disorder, 2nd Edition. New York, Guilford, 1998

Bayley N: Bayley Scales of Infant Development—2nd Edition. San Antonio, TX, Psychological Corporation, 1993

Bellak L: The Thematic Apperception Test, the Children's Apperception Test, and the Senior Apperception Technique in Clinical Use. Orlando, FL, Academic Press, 1986

Bricklin B, Elliot G: Critical Child Custody Evaluation Issues: Questions and Answers. Test Manual Supplement for the BPS, PORT, PASS, PPCP. Furlong, PA, Village Publishing, 1997

Briere J: Trauma Symptom Checklist for Children. Odessa, FL, Psychological Assessment Resources, 1996

Burns RC: Self-Growth in Families: Kinetic Family Drawings Research and Application. New York, Brunner/Mazel, 1982

Butcher JN, William CL: Essentials of MMPI-2 and MMPI-A Interpretation. Minneapolis, MN, University of Minnesota Press, 1992

Cattell RB, Cattell AK, Cattell HEP: Sixteen Personality Factors Questionnaire. San Antonio, TX, Psychological Corporation, 1993

Cohen M: Children's Memory Scale. San Antonio, TX, Psychological Corporation, 1997

Costa PT, McCrae RR: NEO PI Manual. Odessa, FL, Psychological Assessment Resources, 1992

Costantino G, Malgady RG, Rogler LH: Tell-Me-A-Story: Manual. Los Angeles, CA, Western Psychological Association, 1988

Exner JE: The Rorschach: A Comprehensive System, Vols I–III. New York, Wiley, 1995

Friedrich WN: Psychotherapy of Sexually Abused Children and Their Families. New York, Norton, 1990

Friedrich WN: Child Sexual Behavior Inventory. Odessa, FL, Psychological Assessment Resources, 1997

Gardner RA: Family Evaluation in Child Custody Litigation. Caskill, NJ, Creative Therapeutics, 1982

Gerard AB: Parent-Child Relationship Inventory. Los Angeles, CA, Western Psychological Services, 1994

Golden CJ: Manual for the Luria-Nebraska Neuropsychological Battery: Children's Revision. Los Angeles, CA, Western Psychological Services, 1986

Goodenough FL, Harris DB: Studies in the psychology of children's drawings: II. Psychol Bull 47:369–433, 1950

Gough HG: The California Psychological Inventory Administrator's Guide. Palo Alto, CA, Consulting Psychologists Press, 1987

Greenberg SA, Shuman DW: Irreconcilable conflict between therapeutic and forensic roles. Professional Psychology: Research and Practice 28:50–57, 1997

Grisso T: Instruments for Assessing, Understanding, and Appreciation of Miranda Rights. Sarasota, FL, Professional Resource Press, 1998

Heinze MC, Grisso T: Review of instruments assessing parenting competencies used in child custody evaluations. Behavioral Sciences and the Law 14:293–313, 1996

Kaufman AS, Kaufman HL: Interpretive Manual for the Kaufman Assessment Battery for Children (K-ABC), 1983

Lachar D: Personality Inventory for Children. Los Angeles, CA, Western Psychological Services, 1989

Lachar D, Gruber CT: Personality Inventory for Youth. Los Angeles, CA, Western Psychological Services, 1995

Lynn DB: Structured Doll Play Test Manual of Instructions. Boulder, CO, Test Developments, 1959

Miller LJ: Miller Assessment for Preschoolers. San Antonio, TX, Psychological Corporation, 1982

Millon T: MACI Manual. Minneapolis, MN, NCS, 1993

Millon T: MCMI-III Manual. Minneapolis, MN, NCS, 1994

Milner JS: The Child Abuse Potential Inventory: Manual. Webster, NC, Psytec, 1986

Murray HA: Thematic Apperception Test Manual. Los Angeles, CA, Western Psychological Services, 1971

Palmer JO: The Psychological Assessment of Children, 2nd Edition. New York, Wiley, 1983

Reitan RM, Davison LA: Clinical Neuropsychology: Current Status and Applications. Washington, DC, Winston, 1974

Reynolds CR, Bigler ED: Test of Memory and Learning. Austin, TX, Pro-Ed, 1994

Reynolds CR, Kamphaus RW: Handbook of Psychological and Education Assessment of Children, Vol I: Intelligence and Achievement; Vol II: Personality, Behavior and Context. New York, Guilford, 1990

Roberts GE: Interpretive Handbook for the Roberts Apperception Test for Children. Los Angeles, CA, Western Psychological Services, 1994

Sparrow SS, Balla DA, Cicchetti DV: Vineland Adaptive Behavior Scales: Survey Form Manual. Circle Pines, MN, American Guidance Service, 1984

Wechsler D: Wechsler Preschool and Primary Scales of Intelligence—Revised. San Antonio, TX, Psychological Corporation, 1989

Wechsler D: WAIS-III Administration and Scoring Manual. San Antonio, TX, Psychological Corporation, 1997

Wechsler D: Wechsler Individual Achievement Test—Second Edition Manual. San Antonio, TX, Psychological Corporation, 2001

Wilkinson GS: Wide Range Achievement Test—3 Administration Manual. Wilmington, DE, Wide Range, 1993

Woodcock RW, Johnson MB: Manual for the Woodcock-Johnson Psychoeducational Battery—Revised. Allen, TX, DLM Teaching Resources, 1989

CHAPTER 7

Vicarious Traumatization

Angela M. Hegarty, M.B., B.Ch., B.A.O.

Case Example 1

Dr. Berry, a psychiatry resident, was in danger of being terminated from her program because she had shown up at work, on several occasions, with alcohol on her breath and had been caught drinking alcohol in her office at the hospital. She had been experiencing symptoms of posttraumatic stress disorder (PTSD) for over a year and was using alcohol to cope with her distress, yet her supervisors had no idea what was going on.

She had been working with a victim of torture in outpatient therapy and had to testify at his deportation hearing. She failed to tell her supervisor that she frequently dreamed of the horrific events described by her patient, nor did she mention her desire to leave psychiatry. Rather, she went to her supervisor to discuss issues of confidentiality, privilege, and risk management. As she awaited the court's decision on the case, she could not eat or sleep and called in "sick" at work.

Case Example 2

Mr. Bell, a social worker specializing in working with victims of domestic violence, was pleased when a woman he saw in individual therapy initiated divorce proceedings against her abusive husband. The patient was delighted when Mr. Bell agreed to testify on her behalf in court at the custody hearing. Mr. Bell remained unconcerned that he had never spoken to Mr. Bell or to others involved, including the children. His court appearance was extremely stressful, and he began to question his own competence, particularly when evidence was introduced that his patient had been physically abusive to her daughter.

Case Example 3

Mark, a 16-year-old convicted (as an adult) of attempted murder, was referred for evaluation after telling the prison chaplain that he wished to kill himself. Mark had just been sentenced to a period of punitive segregation (solitary confinement) for threatening a corrections officer. While escorting Mark to the medical clinic for evaluation, the corrections officer joked in the waiting room that Mark would be "doing us all a favor" had he actually killed himself. The nurse and psychiatrist, Dr. Roberts, laughed along with him. Dr. Roberts examined Mark and decided that he was malingering in order to avoid the period of segregation and deemed him "not suicidal." The following night, corrections officers found Mark hanging by a bedsheet in his cell. He was resuscitated and rushed to the local hospital where he was admitted to the intensive care unit; he remained intubated for 4 days.

DEFINITION OF VICARIOUS TRAUMATIZATION

Vicarious traumatization refers to the experience of psychological trauma as a result of seeing or hearing about the traumatic experiences of others. Review of the literature, which is derived more from studies of the effects of witnessed trauma on emergency and other personnel, reveals that the issue of psychological trauma in clinicians, in general, and in forensic clinicians, in particular, has received scant attention.

Most clinicians involved in forensic work would not consider themselves to be particularly at risk. Patients are traumatized, not clinicians. The professional role means we can "handle" the work. We do not wish to upset our friends and families with the horrors encountered in the course of our work. As a result, most forensic practitioners lack an appropriate context in which they can explore their reactions to the stories of violence and cruelty encountered in their work. In the past, formal supervision provided a context in which individual reactions to the work could be processed. With the passing of psychoanalytically based forms of treatment, formal supervision and analysis of countertransference are no longer in vogue. Problems are ignored, and the consequences of doing so are often a surprise. They may include, but are not limited to, overinvolvement with a victim or failure of empathy for a perpetrator. Professional consequences can include poor work performance, ethical violations, and even legal sanction. Over time, faced with chronic trauma, the forensic professional is vulnerable to developing the symptoms of burnout.

RISK FACTORS FOR VICARIOUS TRAUMATIZATION

Working With the Perpetrators

Working with the perpetrators of violent crimes, whether in a forensic or correctional setting, involves, at times, hearing firsthand accounts of horrific events. Whether it is the account of a killing during a drug deal by an inner-city adolescent or of the rape of a 12-year-old girl, hearing the stories, seeing the crime scene evidence, reviewing the autopsy reports, and listening perhaps to the victim's screams on a 911 tape can evoke powerful visceral responses in the clinician, for which he or she may not be fully prepared. There is a need, as always, to balance the inner response with the external demands imposed by the professional role. The sadistic patient or examinee may graphically recount details precisely designed to elicit a painful response in the clinician or evaluator. Surprise can intensify the response. A clinician may feel physically threatened or frightened. Disgust and anger can feel overwhelming at times, as the clinician identifies with the victim or victims.

All violence and abuse share the characteristic of being a massive failure of empathy. Anger and withdrawal are common responses in clinicians working with violent patients or in the course of forensic evaluations. Group failure of empathy may occur in clinicians working in corrections. In response to, or in anticipation of the difficulties of encountering the perpetrators of violence, some clinicians will avoid them. There is an unwillingness to see perpetrators as sick. In Case Example 3, an adolescent who was recently incarcerated with adult prisoners, with symptoms of major depression and epidemiologically at high risk for suicide, was deemed well. His sharing of suicidal thoughts with the pastor was attributed to

his desire to avoid solitary confinement. As is often the case, the clinicians joined with the corrections officers in distancing from the patient, expressing their anger at the inmates in the form of aggressive humor, and perpetrating, themselves, a considerable failure of empathy.

Failure of empathy in clinicians in forensic settings can include premature closure regarding diagnoses of malingering or psychopathy, as when, for example, in sex offender or domestic violence group therapy, the failure of offenders to develop "appropriate" victim empathy is attributed to sociopathy, without having addressed the perpetrators' own "victim" issues.

When a forensic clinician is retained by the prosecution in a criminal case, responses to working with perpetrators can lead to loss of neutrality and bias. Seeking revenge in the courtroom, a forensic evaluator may fail to consider all data in assessments. Clinicians may sometimes deal with the inevitably painful feelings that occur in response to accounts and images of horrific acts through a kind of counterphobic exhibitionism from the witness stand. Anger at the alleged perpetrator can lead to premature closure regarding motive and mitigation as well as diagnosis.

Responses to working with perpetrators can also lead to an overemphasis of some data at the expense of other data. Such responses put clinicians at risk of seeing the perpetrator as a victim of the "system." They may overinterpret reports of early trauma or accounts of psychopathology. Seeing the alleged perpetrator as a victim, the defense expert may find himself or herself interpreting the behavior of the other side as vengeful. There can be premature closure regarding responsibility and capacity for choice. The temptation is to simply accept the defendant's account of events. Clinicians may find themselves unwilling to review the forensic material in detail. Analysis of the data is limited to the subjective accounts provided by the defendant. Analysis of the actual behavior is avoided.

Working With the Victims

Encountering the images of abuse and violence in the narratives of victims can elicit powerful responses in clinicians and those involved with forensic evaluations. When clinicians fail to process these feelings, problems can arise as was seen with Dr. Berry (Case Example 1), who found herself thinking about her patient's accounts of torture at odd times. She would become acutely distressed at images that reminded her of what had happened to him. As her symptoms worsened, she began to drink heavily to obtain some relief. When her supervisor cautioned her regarding identification with the victim, she felt strongly that a neutral stance in treatment would somehow represent a morally inadequate response to the issue of torture. She felt guilty about "not doing more" and came to believe that neither her peers nor her teachers "really understood." She stopped speaking about her own feelings, and focused exclusively on medication issues, in sessions with her supervisor. Her supervised sessions ceased to reflect what was happening, not only in the countertransference but in the treatment. Her sense of isolation increased when the patient was threatened with deportation to the country and the authorities from whence he had escaped. She interpreted her own increasing depression as an appropriate response to events. She did not seek treatment.

Mr. Bell (Case Example 2) spent much of his time working with the victims of domestic abuse. When his patient asked him to testify on her behalf at the custody hearing, he gladly said yes, even though he had not performed a custody evaluation, per se. An experienced clinician, he believed that issues regarding clinical limit setting, rescue fantasies, and overidentification were behind him. Rationalizing his decisions in terms of victim advocacy, he failed to set limits and violated the boundaries of his work.

Working With Families and Children

For many clinicians, the performance of custody evaluations for the courts is one of the most stressful tasks faced in forensic practice. The stakes are high when one parent accuses the other of abusing the children in some way. Parents may try to enroll the evaluator in their individual cause and can become angry when things do not go their way. Threats of physical harm are not uncommon. Accounts of spousal or child abuse are distressing. Retaining a neutral stance and continuing to work (avoiding pessimism) within the limits of one's expertise (avoiding grandiosity) can be challenging.

When asked by the court to assess a child in regard to alleged sexual abuse, one pitfall is confusing clinical objectivity and neutrality with moral ambiguity. Years ago, children were simply not believed when they reported that they were being sexually abused by an adult. The reality constructed by society was that this simply did not happen and that children had fantasies about having sex with adults, which they had trouble distinguishing from reality. Today, few clinicians hold those views. Epidemiological research and clinical research on sex offenders and victims have shown that the sexual abuse of children is all too common. The shift in perspective also came about as a result of political and social action, particularly by feminists, aimed at protecting chil-

dren and educating the public. In both clinical and forensic work, the merging of ideology with clinical theory can lead to loss of objectivity and neutrality.

The apparent loss of objectivity seems to be reflected in the research also. Research into memory in children by some authors has focused on how children can be lead, by adults, to report and elaborate on events that never occurred. There is a paucity of experiments, however, looking at how children can be lead, at the insistence of the adults in their lives, to forget and deny events that did occur. The stakes are high, and group data, in any case, can only be a guide in assessing an individual child. The forensic clinician is left alone, in the end, to deal with what can be horrific material.

Individual Risk Factors: Temperament, Personal History, and Adaptation

The outcome for any individual exposed to a traumatic event is determined by a complex interaction of factors: those derived from the trauma itself, such as contextual and environmental factors, as well as group and individual responses. Individual temperament, a past history of psychological trauma or PTSD, self-esteem, and individual coping styles are important in considering an individual's risk for vicarious traumatization.

Temperamental factors associated with increased risk for psychological symptoms following exposure to traumatic stimuli include a negative depressive or avoidant style, hostility, psychological or cognitive rigidity, and mood instability. Flexibility and mood stability and rhythmicity, as well as a positive or optimistic style, are associated with diminished risk.

Temperamental variables exhibit a nonlinear relationship to coping and outcome. For example, an individual with a strong tendency toward sensation seeking will be able to experience events that are often traumatizing for others in a positive way—as challenging and exciting. Taken too far, these individuals may have difficulty dealing with less stimulating activities and may become "addicted" to the excitement. Likewise, individuals who respond to stressors by increasing their activity level will do well in emergency situations; however, responding in this way may interfere with their functioning in other circumstances. An excessive increase in activity level can lead to impulsive and possibly impaired decision making.

Temperament is only one factor to consider in predicting a response to stressful or traumatic life events. An individual's coping style can also affect outcome. Maladaptive coping styles, such as avoidance, isolation, and alcohol and drug abuse, worsen the situation over time. Adaptive coping styles, such as affiliation, humor, altruism, self-nurturing, and the search for meaning, enhance one's ability to manage stress and grow from the experience.

Temperament is related to the ability of an individual to maintain a sense of self-efficacy in the face of overwhelming aversive stimulation. An internal locus of control, a tendency to interpret life events in a positive way, cognitive flexibility, and social extroversion would allow an individual to maintain a sense of self-efficacy even when exposed to chronic or repeated psychological trauma. Traits like avoidance, a tendency to interpret life events in a negative way, and an external locus of control would be associated with a sense of personal impotence and with a negative outcome.

The impact of differing temperamental styles in response to overwhelming aversive stimulation is modulated, always, by contextual variables. It is not the style or the exposure that determines outcome, but the appropriateness of the response to the stimulus at any given time that is significant. For example, the use of dissociation by children exposed to abuse by parents on whom they depend for survival, or by adult victims of sociopolitical torture, is adaptive when the abuse is ongoing. Later on, however, when the coping mechanisms persist and are no longer related to environmental stimuli, they become the symptoms we treat.

Previous exposure to traumatic events or stimuli is a well-documented risk factor for the experience of psychological distress following reexposure to traumatic situations. People who have been traumatized tend to dissociate, and people who dissociate tend to be at increased risk of developing symptoms following reexposure to traumatic situations. Again, it is not the tendency to dissociate that leads to the increased vulnerability, according to this review, rather, people who dissociate and who have been previously traumatized may be more at risk for feeling out of control in association with a traumatic event. Even this is not a simple relationship however. Not all individuals with a tendency to dissociate have a history of abuse or psychological trauma. About 5% of the population is characterized as highly hypnotizable and therefore prone to dissociate.

Other studies identify a history of depression or anxiety disorder and concurrent stressful life events as risk factors for the development of symptoms following exposure to psychological trauma.

A recurring theme in the accounts of individuals who become symptomatic following exposure to a traumatizing event is that of frustrated helplessness. Repeated exposure to traumatizing stimuli can induce a state analogous to that of the learned helplessness paradigm. In animals, this paradigm is used to induce a state that is a model for human depression. Animals are exposed repeatedly to a traumatizing stimulus. The animal is unable to do anything that would stop the painful or aversive stimulus, and the stimulus cannot be avoided or escaped. After a time the animals stop trying. The effect is abolished when the animal is able to control the stimulus in any way. This paradigm has been used to understand the behavior of people exposed to chronic or repeated psychological trauma, such as victims of domestic abuse. An individual's ability to maintain a sense of personal effectiveness in the face of psychological trauma will strongly influence the psychological outcome.

Traumatic events elicit responses in an individual's social group. A dynamic relationship exists between an individual's response to a given stressor, temperament and past history, and the response of the group to the exposure. An individual's ability to cope with psychological trauma can be supported by social factors within the group, such as training, leadership, the availability of support, and group rituals for dealing with the trauma.

Professional Role and Professional Identity

Forensic assessments differ in purpose from clinical evaluations, as has been noted in Chapters 3, "Forensic Ethics," and 4, "Introduction to Forensic Evaluations." The results of forensic assessments can be legally or financially harmful to people, such as when we assess an individual's mental state at the time of a crime or when we evaluate the extent to which a person is or is not actually disabled. Ethically, we must strive for objectivity.

Balancing our internal response to intense and often horrific material with the need to maintain a professional demeanor externally is a common challenge in forensic work. People expect professionals to be calm and neutral and to express little emotion. We expect it of ourselves. Indeed, this may be desirable in the short term, for example, on the witness stand or during an interview. The problems begin when we expect ourselves to be "professional" all the time.

In forensics, unlike in clinical work, our colleagues are not interested in debriefing after a difficult interview. The context of the work is not supportive. For example, one can spend hours and hours on the witness stand, enduring prolonged, emotionally charged cross-examination. After stepping down from the stand, emotionally drained, the forensic expert is alone. There is no one from whom we can seek support. If we carry the "professional" attitude home, we will not seek support in our personal lives either. We do not wish to horrify our friends and families with the details of our work. Most forensic professionals do not seek treatment or supervision. Isolation and lack of support in the context of psychosocial stress are risk factors for depression and traumatic symptoms.

INDIVIDUAL RESPONSES TO VICARIOUS TRAUMATIZATION

Perception and Cognition

When clinicians are exposed to horrific accounts of violence and terror, a range of responses are possible. Visual images may be elicited, with or without an associated affect. External images may trigger recollections of the traumatic material. Elements of the narrative may recur, with varying frequency and intensity.

The clinician will have associations in response to the stimuli. Visual images from the past and memories of past trauma can recur. Reflections on one's own family and one's own responses to similar stories in the past can be elicited. The social worker from Case Example 2 recalled how when he heard a patient begin an account of domestic violence, he could almost finish the story himself. He already knew what would come next. The familiarity fed a sense of personal competence. The physical abuse of the child was not part of the scenario. When victims become perpetrators and perpetrators have been victims, stereotypes break down and challenge the clinician's preconceived notions.

The psychiatrist and nurse working with the depressed adolescent in Case Example 3 were horrified when they first began to work at the prison. They learned that a prison environment is harsh, that the noise can be overwhelming, and that there is marked resistance to change in the system. The focus is on security. Clinicians who try to perform effective clinical work sometimes describe a sense of frustration. Allying with the corrections officers' perspective allows clinicians to avoid the painful awareness that there is little they can do for an adolescent experiencing major depression who is sentenced to an adult male prison and even allows them to avoid seeing the inmate's depressed affect. They attribute the sleep disturbance to the noise and his reported wishes to die to escape the horror of his reality as manipulation, an attempt to escape the consequences of his actions.

Affect and Mood

The affective states induced in response to traumatic stimuli range from anger to fear to numbing. The affec-

tive response shapes and colors the associations stimulated, as well as their interpretation, in response to a given stimulus. As Beck showed for depression, the cognitive distortions related to the depression tend to induce a depressed response. The same may occur with fear, anger, or helplessness. Affect shapes perception, thought, and ultimately behavior. The quality of associations will be determined by the affect experienced. As forensic professionals go through the process of evaluating individuals, their conclusions will, in the end, be commensurate with their affect. A hypothesis-testing approach, interviews with collaterals, and objective testing are ways in which the distortions induced by affect can be alleviated, whether the clinician is suffering the effects of vicarious traumatization or is simply responding in a manner determined by his or her own past experiences and prejudices.

Meaning and Behavior

Whether responding with a sense of frustrated helplessness, fear, guilt, or anger, the forensic clinician can be led to question the meaning of what he or she is doing, and at times, his or her own competence. Allying with polarized groups on an issue, the sense of isolation and helplessness is abated at first. There is a clear sense of right and wrong, a sense of familiarity with the territory. Trauma intensifies group dynamics. External boundaries become the line between *them* and *us*. There is little tolerance for complexity and ambiguity. Individuals who challenge the group defenses are often scapegoated. The social worker described in Case Example 2 had sought the support of like-minded professionals in response to the trauma of working with the victims of domestic violence. For him, as for many of his colleagues, clinical and forensic data had political meaning. He saw his patient not as an individual but as representative of a group that was victimized and abused by representatives of another group. He understood, intellectually, the distinction between clinical work with a mother and a custody evaluation for the courts. Yet he decided to testify anyway. On the witness stand, his bias was clear. Confronted with material he might have uncovered had he performed a full assessment, he questioned his own competence and was traumatized anew.

Dr. Berry (Case Example 1) began to avoid references to and reminders of torture, and her unfortunate patient, after a brief initial attempt to share her concerns with her supervisor. She stopped watching television because reminders of her patient's suffering would trigger hours of painful preoccupation. She withdrew from people she felt did not understand. She became preoccupied by the issues raised by the experiences of her patient. That there was a possibility that he might be returned to the country where he had been tortured increased her sense of urgency. She lost interest in anything that did not relate to the problem of torture and felt guilty that she could not do more. She questioned her career choice. Her patient's situation began to improve; he was no longer under threat of deportation. His symptoms began to abate because the medication was working and because he was processing his experience through treatment. But by now, Dr. Barry had begun to drink to excess. She no longer felt connected in her residency program. She joined a human rights organization, and at their meetings, she would hear accounts of torture, not unlike those of her patient, over and over. She was no longer able to let go.

PROFESSIONAL AND PEER RESPONSES TO VICARIOUS TRAUMATIZATION

Group Responses to Psychological Trauma

The availability of social support can mitigate the effects of stress from overwhelming or traumatizing events. Isolation renders individuals more vulnerable to the effects of stress.

People tend to affiliate themselves with like-minded groups. People who respond to psychologically traumatizing material by identification with the victim will seek support from groups that are supportive of victims, while those who tend to identify with the aggressor will seek support from groups with a similar emphasis. An example of this kind of polarization has been seen recently in the so-called false memory debate. Groups on one side emphasized the victim's need for support in recalling traumatic or painful material in therapy, while other groups emphasized the influence of the therapist on such recollections, and the detrimental effects such recollections have on family relationships. The latter groups may emphasize the need for proof, often considerably beyond a reasonable doubt, before complaints of abuse are believed. The groups that are more supportive of victims may consider requests for objective assessment or clinical neutrality to represent nothing less than the moral sanction of violence, cruelty, or abuse. Data may be oversimplified and overinterpreted. Hypotheses go untested and alternatives go unexplored.

Mental health professionals have always had to deal with stories of pain, loss, and trauma. Group defenses can include denial, intellectualization, and isolation of affect. Clinicians do not suffer, patients do. An individual clinician who complains openly of psychological symptoms in relation to psychological trauma may threaten group defenses. In order to maintain homeostasis, these individuals may be isolated and scapegoated. Clinicians may be reluctant to disclose their own reactions to traumatic stimuli in order to avoid negative appraisal by peers or supervisors. In a way, Dr. Berry and her supervisors colluded in the denial of her problems. Questions regarding her emotional response to dealing with horrific accounts of torture in her work were left without answers. In resisting dealing with painful material, both Dr. Berry and her supervisors invoked concerns that supervision should not become therapy and focused on medication strategies in the treatment of PTSD, to the exclusion of all the other issues emerging in the therapy.

Vicarious Traumatization as Countertransference— Supervision and Education

In 1910, Freud introduced the concept of countertransference to psychiatry in reference to the patient's influence on the therapist's unconscious feelings. Today, *countertransference* can be defined as responses to the patient that are based on the therapist's past rather than the patient's issues, or more broadly, almost any response the therapist has to the events described by the patient. Countertransference can be used as a useful source of clinical data that can be understood and used in a manner profoundly helpful to patients. Nonetheless, as discussed in the clinical literature, the term often conveys a critical valence, implying that the clinician has somehow erred in having these responses in the first place. That a clinician should have any feelings at all, is indeed, counter to the expectations of the professional stereotype. In medical school, psychiatrists learn that individuals who express feelings of distress are, in some way, weaker than their colleagues. They have to "tough it out." The experience of psychological trauma was even cited in one article as being good, because it helped doctors develop compassion. In former times, terms like *character building* were used to describe the beneficial effects of overwork in stressful and sometimes traumatizing situations.

Education regarding dealing with one's own feelings when dealing with a patient's violence, trauma, or loss is meager at best. In addressing countertransference, there is an emphasis on the intellectual understanding of problems. Little attention is paid to feelings.

Avoiding Pitfalls

Maladaptive attempts to deal with the stress of forensic work include social isolation, which can result from spending too much time on the work, withdrawal from pleasurable activities (because there is so much to be done), eating too much or too little, not sleeping enough or chronic fatigue, avoidance, and the inability to shift to less dramatic, if important, details in life such as paying bills, returning phone calls, and so on. Inappropriate use of alcohol often begins slowly and worsens over time. Should the symptoms of psychological trauma emerge, early recognition and intervention are essential. Formal and informal consultation with colleagues avoids intellectual isolation and helps one gain perspective not only on the case but also on one's own countertransference.

Seeking Support

Clinicians who work in correctional or forensic settings are often not at liberty to share with others material related to cases they encounter in their work. Yet the work is stressful. Support from colleagues is helpful. The Internet provides a means by which they can stay in contact with other professionals in the area. Bulletin boards offer the opportunity of seeking advice in an anonymous way from others who work in the field. Joining local professional societies is helpful also. Psychotherapy provides a more formal setting in which one can explore one's feelings in a safe way. Consultation with a psychiatrist is essential should symptoms become severe enough to warrant treatment with medication.

Although one may not be able to share the facts of cases with friends and family, maintaining relationships outside the work is also essential. Allowing oneself to be cared for by family and friends helps restore one's optimism and perspective.

Sports not only allows one to get exercise but participation can help restore a sense of self-efficacy that is battered by working in the darker spheres of life. Crafts can have a similar effect, and handiwork can be especially relaxing. Encountering beauty in art, music, literature, or other endeavors can provide a welcome relief when faced with the daily horrors of forensic work.

Supervision

Experienced clinicians rarely consider themselves to be in need of supervisory sessions. Many clinicians never learned to use supervisory sessions effectively. During training, because of the inevitable confusion between evaluation and supervision, many clinicians never experienced supervision to be the safe, supportive procedure it was originally meant to be. Engaging the services of another clinician for the purposes of formal supervision can be invaluable. Sessions in which the material is

reviewed as the source of the countertransference reactions can greatly aid in the development and maintenance of a neutral stance and an objective approach. Such sessions are confidential, privileged, and supportive. By paying for the service, instead of having to endure it as a requirement, the clinician retains control of the process.

The Search for Meaning

Death, loss, aloneness, freedom, and the search for meaning, justice, and truth—all are existential or spiritual issues at heart. Whether in psychotherapy or in the course of spiritual or religious practice, the search for the meaning of our experiences helps us maintain perspective. Spiritual and religious practice can be helpful in alleviating stress. Understanding the limits of one's power and responsibility can help ease our concerns. Belief in something greater than ourselves provides solace. We are asked, in forensic work, to bear witness to the actions and intentions of others. Keeping it simple and resisting the temptation to affect the outcome of the proceedings, to "do something," will improve the quality of our work, alleviate some of the psychological pressures of forensic work, and help us contribute to the overall process in a more constructive way.

CASE EXAMPLE EPILOGUES

Case Example 1

Dr. Berry resigned from the department of psychiatry and went to work for a human rights organization. She continued to treat her patient, who was allowed to stay in the country and who ultimately recovered from his PTSD.

Case Example 2

Mr. Bell confronted his patient, who admitted to having severely physically abused her 5-year-old daughter from the time she was an infant. The father was awarded custody of the child. Mr. Bell sought supervision, and, having worked through the crisis provoked by his courtroom experience, he began to explore his patient's abusive behavior.

Case Example 3

Mark recovered with no neurological sequelae. He returned to prison where he was treated by Dr. Roberts with an antidepressant and therapy. Shaken by the experience, Dr. Roberts began to address the use of gallows humor among staff.

ACTION GUIDELINES

Preparation

The ability to control aspects of any painful or noxious stimulus reduces its intensity and impact. By knowing in advance the kind of material that will have to be addressed, and the potentially difficult issues raised, one is less likely to be taken by surprise in an interview with an individual with a horrific tale to tell, whether for the first time or in the course of a time-limited evaluation. Allowing oneself to be desensitized by repeated, if limited, exposure to difficult material can be helpful and can increase one's sense of self-efficacy. Ensuring that support is available, as needed, will also be helpful.

Managing Stress

Concomitant life stresses increase the likelihood that clinicians working with traumatizing material in their work will experience psychological distress. Clinicians are often poor judges of their own capacity for stress. Motivated by ambition, greed, or myriad other issues, we agree to take on challenging cases regardless of the status of our personal lives. Clinicians forget how to take care of themselves in terms of food, sleep, and exercise. Recognizing when one is stressed and taking appropriate action are essential. Awareness of one's boundaries and one's limits and maintaining a reasonable frame in which one works can protect the clinician from becoming overextended.

SUGGESTED READINGS

Beck AT, Rush AJ, et al: Cognitive Therapy of Depression. New York, Guilford, 1979

Gershuny BS, Thayer JF: Relations among psychological trauma, dissociative phenomena and trauma-related stress: a review and integration (abstract). Mich Med 95(2):20, 1996

Gunther MS: Countertransference issues in staff caregivers who work to rehabilitate catastrophic injury survivors. Am J Psychother 48(2):208–220, 1994

Harvey MR: An ecological view of psychological trauma and trauma recovery. Clin Psychol Rev 19(5):631–657, 1999

Hayes JA, Gelsc CJ, Van Wagoner SL, et al: Managing countertransference. Psychol Rep 69(l):139–148, 1991

Schetky DH, Coldbach E: Countertransference on the witness stand. Bulletin of the American Academy of Psychiatry and Law 10:15–21, 1982

Schetky DH, Devoe L: Countertransference issues in forensic child psychiatry, in Clinical Handbook of Child Psychiatry and the Law. Edited by Schetky DH, Benedek EP. Brunner Mazel, 1992, pp 230–245

Sims A, Sims D: The phenomenology of post traumatic stress disorder: a symptomatic study of 70 victims of psychological trauma. Br J Psychiatry 167(6):812–817, 1995

Spiegel D, Hunt T, Dondershine HE: Dissociation and hypnotizability in post traumatic stress disorder. Am J Psychiatry 145:301–305, 1988

Thomas Blair D, Ramones VA: Understanding vicarious traumatization. Journal of Psychosocial Nursing 34(11):24–30, 1996

PART II

Child Custody

Dr. Herman provides a foundation for approaching child custody disputes and discusses current social dilemmas that pose ethical and clinical questions for the forensic examiner in Chapter 8. In Chapter 9, Dr. Barnum provides an extensive framework for assessing parenting capacity and considering how parents' skills mesh with the developmental needs of their children. He also discusses specific problems that arise in various mental disorders and their impact on parenting.

In Chapter 10, Drs. Wasserman, Rosenfeld, and Nickman take us into the world of the foster child and discuss how the foster care system affects the foster child's development and mental and emotional well-being. They discuss the advantages and disadvantages of foster care and provide useful information on how the system operates. Visitation with parents and related issues are also discussed. When parental reunification is not possible, there is currently much effort being put

forth toward getting children placed in adoptive homes. Dr. Schetky discusses the legal requirements for termination of parental rights, weighing whether it is in the best interests of the child, and considers alternatives to absolute termination of parental rights in Chapter 11.

Given the scarcity of healthy Caucasian newborns available for adoption in the United States, we have seen a rise in the number of adoptions of children from abroad as well as transracial adoptions. Drs. Norris and Ferguson provide a balanced view of the issues that arise in these types of adoptions and offer guidelines for the forensic examiner who becomes involved in these cases in the last chapter in Part II.

Together, these chapters speak to the ever-changing world of child custody and the need to operate within a clear framework regarding one's role, ethical tenets, and the law.

CHAPTER 8

Child Custody Evaluations

Stephen P. Herman, M.D.

Case Example 1

Elizabeth Resnick and Harvey Cramer never married but were living together when Elizabeth became pregnant. Soon after the birth of their son, Hal, their relationship deteriorated. Even though she was angry and disappointed, Elizabeth agreed to a coparenting plan with Harvey. She would have Hal for at least 3 months, with his father coming over whenever he liked. After 3 months, the infant would live with his father, with his mother visiting regularly. This plan would continue, the parents agreed, until Hal went to nursery school, at age 3. Then, the couple agreed, they would consult a child mental health expert for advice.

Things did not work out the way they expected. It took Harvey 10 months before he was able to settle into a home of his own. There were periods of time—sometimes 2 weeks in length—when he would not see his son at all. When he finally arrived at Elizabeth's home to take his son, she informed him she had gone to family court and had been given temporary custody of Hal. Harvey was escorted off the property by the police.

Several months later, a family court judge appointed Dr. Smithson to perform a custody evaluation and to make recommendations regarding the best interests of the child, who was now 2 years old.

Case Example 2

Marilyn and Bruce Greene were divorcing and battling over custody of their 7-year-old daughter, Hallie. They had originally fashioned an out-of-court settlement with Marilyn getting sole custody and Bruce having extensive visitation with his daughter. Then, unexpectedly, Marilyn received an extraordinary offer of employment in her field of meteorology—in a city 1,000 miles away. When he learned of his wife's plans to move, Mr. Greene initiated a lawsuit seeking sole custody of Hallie. Dr. Wellington, a forensic child and adolescent psychiatrist, was appointed by the court "to conduct a full evaluation as to the best interests of the minor child, Hallie Greene, specifically as they relate to custody and visitation and to prepare a report for the court with any and all pertinent recommendations."

Case Example 3

A mother of seven children, receiving state assistance and involved in an abusive relationship with the father of six of the children, was addicted to crack cocaine. Over a period of 8 months, she purposely starved and physically abused her youngest child, 3-year-old Cathy. Eventually, Cathy was found dead in her crib, and her mother pleaded guilty to homicide. The maternal grandmother petitioned the city to become the kinship foster mother for the surviving six children, ranging in age from 4 to 15 years.

The city's child protective services agency was against placement with the grandmother. It believed that the grandmother had known about the starvation of the deceased child but had done nothing about it. She was never charged. The grandmother visited the children regularly. They repeatedly expressed their unanimous desire to live with their grandmother, with whom they had been involved since each of them had been born.

The family court appointed Dr. Baird to perform an impartial evaluation in order to recommend a placement plan in the best interests of the children.

LEGAL ISSUES

Child Custody

Evolution of Judicial Presumptions

Child custody disputes have always reflected societal views of the family and the specialized roles of mothers and fathers (Derdeyn 1976). As noted in Chapter 1, "History of Child and Adolescent Forensic Psychiatry," the principles governing child custody decisions have undergone many changes and have gradually shifted from being parent-centered to child-centered. Courts now examine custody disputes on a more individualized basis in order to determine the needs of each child. This best interests presumption is the guiding principle in deciding custody disputes (Weithorn 1987). All states adhere to this presumption, explicated in the 1966 landmark case from Iowa, *Painter v. Bannister*. The clinician should be aware of the exact wording of local statutes governing custody.

Types of Custody Arrangements

Custody disputes can arise when divorcing parents are not able to agree on residential and parenting arrangements for their children or when one parent uses the issue as a wedge against an unfavorable divorce outcome. Regardless of parental motivation, the types of custody are usually sole or joint. In sole custody, one parent has the legal authorization to make all major decisions regarding the growth and development of the child. The non-custodial parent's rights are not terminated but major decision-making powers are. (Sometimes, however, a termination of parental rights case may occur in connection with an ongoing custody or child placement case. In 1982, the U.S. Supreme Court held in the landmark case *Santosky v. Kramer* that in such cases of termination, the constitutionally required burden of proof shall be clear and convincing evidence.)

In a joint custody arrangement, the precise definition depends on what the parties work out. It does not automatically mean that a child lives with each parent half of the time. It does mean, however, that both parents have the legal right and responsibility to share in their child's growth and development (Tibbits-Kleber et al. 1987). Joint custody, heralded by some as a panacea for the ills of custody disputes, can be successful in certain circumstances, if both parents are able to set aside their anger and frustration with each other, tolerate each other's differing parenting styles, and communicate frequently with relative comfort (Steinman 1981, 1985). However, such a postdivorce situation is unusual for many parents and might be impossible for most. What seems to be important psychologically for children of divorce is the ongoing relationship between the parents and between the parents and the children, rather than the legal custody arrangement (Atwell et al. 1984; Derdeyn and Scott 1984; Pruett and Hoganbruen 1998; Wallerstein and Johnston 1990). In addition, recent research findings suggest that the problems seen in children of divorce may, in fact, primarily relate to the extent of the troubled marriages of their parents *prior* to the divorce, rather than the divorce itself (Kelly 2000). Such children may have serious psychological problems following their parents' divorce because of high levels of conflict, including domestic violence and verbal abuse, while the family was still "intact."

Visitation

Custody disputes often include determinations about visitation. Sometimes, in fact, the expert witness is evaluating a visitation dispute, rather than an argument over custody (Benedek and Schetky 1985). Disorders of visitation arise when parents disagree about implementing a court-ordered visitation arrangement, when parents accuse each other of sabotaging a visitation schedule, when parents are unable to formulate a workable visitation arrangement, or when one parent maintains that the child is reluctant to visit the other parent (Levy 1982). It has been argued that the sole custodial parent should control visitation arrangements in the interests of reducing the child's anxiety and avoiding further court interference in this family issue (Goldstein et al. 1973). However, courts do become involved in visitation disputes that are part of (or separate from) a custody dispute.

Visitation crises during or after divorce may occur when children are used as "messengers" by a parent, when one parent begins a new relationship, when a parent radically changes a lifestyle, when there is resentment over money, or when one or both parents exhibit significant psychopathology. Visitation problems may be unlikely when both parents easily agree on which parent ought to be the custodial parent, when there are few disputes over parenting, and when parents work hard with attorneys and mental health professionals to minimize conflict (Hodges 1986).

Two areas of controversy surrounding visitation problems include allegations of sexual abuse and visitation schedules when infants are involved. The evaluation of sexual abuse allegations will be discussed elsewhere in this volume; however, there is a perception that they have increased in the last decade and have become a wedge designed to reduce parental access during or following a divorce. Yet it is probable that only a small proportion of contested custody and visitation cases involve sexual abuse allegations (Thoennes and Tjaden 1990). Still, visitation is often suspended entirely with the accused parent until he or she is exonerated. This could last over a year.

When infants are involved, courts may rely heavily on the recommendations of mental health professionals.

However, there are virtually no clear-cut guidelines in the behavioral sciences literature to guide clinicians in their recommendations to the court. Although a custodial parent may feel otherwise, there are no data supporting the notion that visitation involving infants, toddlers, or preschoolers is in and of itself harmful to the child or need be severely restricted. Each case will have to be evaluated on its own merits, because the issue of infant overnight visitation remains controversial (Levy 1998). Obviously, the following factors must be taken into account: parental conflict, parental inadequacy or irresponsibility, significant geographic distance between parents, severe mental illness in a parent, and an abusing parent.

Mediation

Like joint custody, mediation has been heralded by some as an important alternative to the adversarial system. By the 1980s, as most states adopted no-fault divorce laws, mediation's popularity grew. In several states, including California, Maine, and New Mexico, mediation is mandated by the court before custody litigation begins. Maryland courts have also adopted this process, except in cases in which a good-faith allegation of sexual or physical abuse has been made. Connecticut requires all custody disputes to go through a pretrial mediation lasting one full day, held at the same courthouse where the actual trial would be held if the mediation is not successful in settling the case. The mediators are two experienced practitioners—a matrimonial lawyer and a mental health professional—of opposite sex. The success rate of these one-day "marathon" sessions in settling the custody dispute is over 50% (B. Carey, Middletown, CT, Superior Court, personal communication, June 6, 2001). Mediation programs may differ throughout the country in terms of the professional backgrounds of the mediators, the number of sessions, the inclusion or exclusion of children's direct participation in the process, and the presence or absence of lawyers, members of the clergy, accountants, or other related professionals. Thus there is no single, clear-cut definition of mediation when applied to resolving custody disputes (Miller and Veltkamp 1987).

Proponents cite advantages of mediation: parents avoid litigation and the necessity for a court to direct their behavior; the process is more personalized, with more attention directed to the unique characteristics of the family; parents take an active role in deciding their family's fate; and there is greater likelihood of long-term compliance.

In one study, nearly a decade after custody mediation, noncustodial parents reported more frequent current contact with their children and greater involvement in current decisions about them. Parents who had used mediation reported more frequent communication about the children since resolution of the dispute (Dillon and Emery 1996).

Critics of mediation argue: there is too wide a variety of backgrounds and skills in mediators; there are no standards for what constitutes adequate mediation in custody disputes; failed mediation can lead to even more acrimony once the parties enter the judicial system; and mediation may lead to an imbalance of power that could favor men, who seem to mediate differently from women. It is thought by some that in these situations, a man's verbalizations relate more to gaining power and the upper hand, whereas a woman's may be more about feelings and compromise.

A 1-year follow-up study of parents who used mediation reported differences in levels of satisfaction between fathers and mothers. In this study, fathers involved in mediation were substantially more satisfied and were in greater compliance with child support orders than were fathers who had not used mediation. However, mothers appeared to be less satisfied (Emery et al. 1994).

Mediation may work if couples are motivated to be child-centered in their custody negotiations and both parents are able to trust and work with the mediator or comediators. During or following the custody evaluation performed by the court-appointed expert, the process may evolve into mediation or may lead to the parents entering mediation with someone else. In this way the custody evaluation may serve a therapeutic purpose and may help the parents concentrate their energies toward a settlement and away from further litigation.

Special Issues

Child custody evaluations are frequently complicated by special issues presenting additional challenges to the expert witness (Herman 1990). Many of these issues reflect current social dilemmas and raise ethical as well as clinical questions. These include homosexual parenting and the impact of AIDS (Allen and Burrell 1996; Bozett 1987; Kleber et al. 1986; Mason 1998); grandparents' and stepparents' rights (Stanton 1998); mentally ill parents and parental kidnapping (Long et al. 1991; Schetky and Haller 1983); allegations of sexual, physical, and spousal abuse (Green 1986; Lieberman and Van Horn 1998); controversies arising from advances in reproductive technology, such as surrogate parenting, oocyte donation, artificial insemination, and in vitro fertilization (Kermani 1992); and issues related to parental relocation. The evaluating mental health professional faces the dual responsibilities of performing a competent and fair clinical evaluation and communicating to the court how the special issue affects the particular family.

Homosexual parents. The expert evaluating a custody dispute in which one parent is homosexual will need to review the current literature on children of homosexuals in order to best advise the court. This highly emotional topic is handled quite differently in legal jurisdictions across the United States. Some states have equated homosexuality with parental unfitness. New Hampshire law bars homosexuals from serving as foster or adoptive parents (*Opinion of the Justices* 1987). In Missouri, the court of appeals denied custody to a lesbian mother and then restricted visitation on the basis of the mother's sexual orientation (*S.E.G. v. R.A.G.* 1987). But in New York State, for example, a lesbian couple sought and were granted legal recognition of their status as parents of a 6-year-old boy, in what was the first legal recognition of lesbian coparenting in the state (*In the Matter of the Adoption of a Child Whose First Name Is Evan* 1992).

Studies on homosexual parenting appear to suggest no significant differences in the psychological development and gender identity of their children, as compared with families with heterosexual parents. In one study of children conceived via donor insemination and raised by either heterosexual or homosexual parents, ongoing adjustment was unrelated to their parents' sexual orientation (Chan et al. 1998). A meta-analysis of research findings has failed to identify differences between heterosexual and homosexual parents regarding parenting styles, emotional adjustment, and sexual orientation of children (Allen and Burrell 1996). Less is known about the families of gay fathers, although studies suggest they are as nurturing and supportive of their children as are heterosexual fathers. Children of gay fathers, however, may be distressed at some point in their development about their father's homosexuality (Bozett 1987).

Parental kidnapping. The expert should know about the impact on the child of parental kidnapping, if that has occurred (Cole and Bradford 1992). Schetky and Haller (1983) have noted the agonizing conflicts undergone by children kidnapped by their disturbed and/or desperate parents caught up in custody litigation as well as legal attempts to deal with this issue. The expert evaluating such a case should be familiar with state and national laws that apply, along with the 1980 Hague Convention on the Civil Aspects of International Child Abduction, to which the United States is a signatory.

Grandparents' rights and other third-party rights. The expert should be aware of the legal and clinical ramifications of grandparents, stepparents, and other third parties seeking visitation rights or custody (Stanton 1998). State laws vary in their permissiveness regarding such visitation and custody. In June 2000, in what is certain to be a landmark ruling, the U.S. Supreme Court held in *Troxel v. Granville* that a Washington state law was applied unconstitutionally as it related to visitation in a particular family's case. The law allowed "any person" to petition for visitation rights "at any time." The law had authorized state superior courts to grant such rights whenever it was deemed to be in the child's best interest.

In a decision delivered by Justice O'Connor and joined by the Chief Justice and Justices Ginsburg and Breyer, along with Justices Souter and Thomas concurring in separate statements, the Court discussed the protection afforded by the Fourteenth Amendment against any state depriving "any person of life, liberty, or property, without due process of law." The court held: "The liberty interest at issue in this case—the interest of parents in the care, custody, and control of their children—is perhaps the oldest of the fundamental liberty interests recognized by this Court." Justice O'Connor criticized Washington State's "breathtakingly broad" statute, which would disregard a fit custodial parent's decisions regarding visitation and would instead substitute the determination of a judge. The Court did not, however, declare state laws allowing for grandparent visitation (in all 50 states) to be unconstitutional. Justice O'Connor wrote: "We do not, and need not, define today the precise scope of the parental due process right in the visitation context."

Reproductive technology. In areas on the very frontier of reproductive technology, mental health professionals and legal experts alike will struggle and agonize over profoundly complex questions. Here, all too often, social practices and medical decision making outstrip statutes and coherent and predictable case law.

Relocation cases. A common special issue arising with greater frequency since the end of the twentieth century is the issue of parental relocation. This additional factor is an outgrowth of three demographic phenomena: our nation's high divorce rate, corporate downsizing, and our increasingly mobile society. Typically, a parent seeking custody also wishes to move out of the local area because of an important employment opportunity. In a landmark case in New York State, that state's highest court, the New York Court of Appeals, addressed this issue (*Tropea v. Tropea* 1996). The court adopted a best interests approach in its decision: "[E]ach relocation request must be considered on its own merits with due consideration of all the relevant facts and circumstances and with predominant emphasis being placed on what outcome is most likely to serve the best interests of the child" (*Tropea v. Tropea* 1996).

In such relocation cases, the expert must examine a number of factors, such as how the particular child would most likely cope with the loss of regular contact with the parent left behind, the psychological impact of cutting ties with the home community and establishing new ones elsewhere, whether the custodial parent would facilitate reasonable opportunities for the child to visit with the other parent, and the parent's motivation for wanting to move away (Herman 1999).

Parents with criminal convictions. Another complicating issue involves a foster or pre-adoptive parent found to have a criminal conviction. The expert psychiatrist may be asked to evaluate the relevancy of such a conviction on parenting and the best interests of the child. A new law in New York State mandated that the discovery of a prior criminal conviction in a foster parent is grounds for immediate removal of foster children—no matter how long they have lived in the home or how appropriate the placement has been (NY Social Services Law 1999). This law has been found unconstitutional in several New York courts.

Whatever the special issue might be, the evaluating clinician considers that issue in terms of how it affects the child and the parent-child relationship. The question then becomes not that a parent has a history of psychiatric illness, for example, but rather, what is the impact of the illness on this particular child and the relationship with the child? In this way, the expert can put an issue in proper perspective and possibly defuse what might otherwise be a false issue serving one side's legal strategy.

Role of the Expert Witness

Because custody disputes are complicated processes, the court-appointed mental health expert has an important role to play. Various professional organizations have published guidelines and practice parameters that assist clinicians and help to promote and maintain standards of care (American Academy of Child and Adolescent Psychiatry 1997; American Association of Family and Conciliation Courts 1994; American Psychiatric Association 1988; American Psychological Association 1994). Studies bear out that judges *are* influenced in their decisions by clinical evaluations (Ash and Guyer 1984). Jurists rely on the expertise of psychiatrists, psychologists, and clinical social workers when deciding custody and visitation cases. Through the written report and testimony, the mental health professional provides important information to the judge. The expert witness may also assist the

families by helping to make the clinical evaluation therapeutic. As the one who tries to elucidate the best interests of the child, the expert may be the first professional who is able to get the disputing parents on a more child-centered track. Sometimes, the child custody evaluation evolves into mediation or even arbitration, when both parents have come to trust the clinician and are motivated to reach an agreement themselves.

THE CLINICAL EVALUATION AND WRITTEN REPORT

Becoming Involved

Therapists desiring to perform child custody evaluations may want to notify local courts (including judges and their law secretaries and court clinics), attorneys, mental health colleagues, and agencies that may provide this service. Neophytes should make contact with an experienced colleague who can act as a mentor. Newcomers to this work should also read about their state's legislative and judicial history of handling child custody and visitation disputes. Those interested in this and other types of forensic work should consider an approved fellowship in forensic psychiatry, now required for those desiring the American Board of Psychiatry and Neurology Certification in Forensic Psychiatry.

The initial referral call may come from the judge's law secretary, from an attorney, the guardian *ad litem*, or from a parent. The expert should know precisely what questions the judge is asking and whether, in fact, they can be properly answered. Sometimes, judges have unrealistic expectations of what a psychiatrist can do. It is important to have the court issue a written order appointing the expert as the court's witness. In this way, the mental health professional is usually protected from liability under the umbrella of judicial immunity (Curran 1985).

The expert should inform lawyers and parents alike that he or she will perform a custody evaluation *only* if both sides agree that the expert will do an impartial evaluation. Experts should avoid one-sided custody and/or visitation evaluations, seeing only a part of the family. Judges and lawyers alike view such experts as "hired guns," whose credibility and objectivity become suspect. Mental health professionals should strive to avoid doing one-sided and incomplete evaluations. Occasionally, this rule may have to be modified, if, for example, one party fails to cooperate sufficiently or cannot be located. Such a situation should be explained in full in the report.

Prior to the evaluation, the expert should explain the fee and request full payment. In private custody cases, payment is usually shared by both sides. Sometimes the judge will order each party to pay a percentage of the fee based on their financial situation at the time. Government and/or social welfare agencies may have their own billing practices that apply to experts.

Interviewing Parents

The expert can offer both parents the opportunity to meet together with him or her for the first session. Sometimes, one or both parents decline this suggestion, saying that such a meeting would be too painful and upsetting. The clinician should explain that refusing this initial joint meeting in no way puts the objecting parent in a bad light, as far as the expert is concerned. But if such an opportunity is taken by both parents, the clinician has the opportunity to observe their interaction and explore in a preliminary way whether or not there is any chance of a settlement. At the very least, the clinician can use the session to explain how the evaluation will be conducted and can assess the current level of animosity or cooperation between the litigating parties.

Prior to the start of the session, the clinician should explain to parents or any other party being interviewed that because of the forensic nature of this evaluation, they must waive their rights of confidentiality and privilege. The expert might have interviewees sign such a waiver. In every case, the expert should document in the record that such an explanation has been given and agreement has been obtained.

Each parent should be seen several times alone in sessions of 45 to 60 minutes. In the first session, the expert gives the parent a chance to speak about the background of the case, the marital problems, and his or her desires regarding the arrangements for the child or children. In subsequent sessions, the clinician asks about the history of the parent-child relationship and seeks to know how well each party knows the child, what the child's special needs might be, and the party's plans for that particular child (American Academy of Child and Adolescent Psychiatry 1997).

Many parents or other caregivers use these sessions for severe criticism of the opposing party and to "prove" to the expert that only he or she is truly "fit" to parent the child. The expert can allow this to a point, noting what each party chooses to criticize in the other, but should eventually limit these critiques in order to move on to other subjects.

In addition, the forensic expert must remember he or she is not a detective or human polygraph. He or she is not the trier of fact; the judge fulfills that role. The object of these sessions with the parents or other caregivers is to learn about their relationships with the child or children—not to conclude who is telling the truth and who is lying. Litigating parties will repeatedly try to convince the clinician of one thing or another and will sometimes bring in "evidence" to support their case. The clinician should remind each party what his or her proper function is to be. Frequently a party will bring in a videotape or audiotape, a "found" diary or other journal, telephone bills, or receipts. The party might ask the expert to listen or watch a tape. In general, it is wise to decline such a request unless both sides are in agreement that the expert do so. Watching a video or listening to a recording (perhaps made surreptitiously by one side) puts the psychiatrist in a difficult and uncomfortable position and threatens the impartiality of the evaluation. In some states, surreptitious recordings may be illegal.

The evaluation of the caregivers should also include inquiring about their own family backgrounds and educational, social, work, medical, and mental health histories.

The evaluation for custody is *not* a formal psychiatric examination. The primary object is not to arrive at psychiatric diagnoses but rather to assess parenting ability, the parent-child relationship, and, ultimately, the best interests of the child. If a parent or caregiver is given a psychiatric diagnosis, the expert must include the mental status examination, defend the diagnosis and, most importantly, put that diagnosis in the context of how it does or does not affect parenting.

Interviewing Children

Prior to the first interview with the child, which should occur early in the evaluation process, one or both parties may try to involve the expert in a controversy over which parent brings the child to the session. If just two sessions are planned alone with the child, then each parent can take a turn. Otherwise, the parties will attempt to involve the clinician in this dispute within a dispute. The expert should refrain and can suggest that the parents not struggle over this question. Each party may feel the child will be influenced by the transporting adult. The therapist should point out that in many cases the child already is influenced by the adults and this will be factored in during the evaluation. Each party may also ask the expert how to prepare the child for the interviews. The expert can turn the question around and ask the adult what he or she deems appropriate to say to the child. That party's response may give additional information about how he or she relates to the child and understands the child's developmental level. Adults can and should be honest with the child about the purpose of the evaluation. Even a 3-year-old knows that her parents are fighting about where she will live. It creates more anxiety and confusion for the child to say, "You're going to meet a nice man who likes to talk to kids."

Although the litigating parties are seen at least once each at the start, the child or children should be seen as early into the process as possible. Although custody disputes are supposed to be about children, the clinician may find himself caught up in the struggle between the litigating parties and delayed in actually meeting the child. Children as young as 3 years or even slightly younger can be seen alone, assuming they are able to separate from the caregiver who brought them.

Therapists conduct the interview with the child as they would any evaluative session. They try to develop a comfortable, anxiety-free relationship early on, through the use of drawing, building toys, a board game or electronic game, or any other toy. A dollhouse may be especially evocative of play with domestic themes and symbols. The experts are interested in how the child perceives the family conflict and what he or she thinks might happen. The expert can explain to a child of 4 years what a judge is and how the doctor is meeting with the family to help the judge figure out where the child is going to live.

It is not necessary—and may, in fact, be detrimental—to ask a child his or her parental preference. Such a question often puts added pressure on a child already dealing with enough. A child who volunteers such information, however, may do so for a number of reasons. Perhaps he was coached by an adult. Or perhaps the child has a legitimate reason that he can explain and support. The child's preference, when volunteered, should be noted and considered as part of the data collected. More weight is usually given to preferences expressed by preteens than those of 4- or 5-year-olds. The expert considers the developmental context, whether there is evidence of coaching or coercion, and the child's stated reasons for the preference. When siblings are involved, they should be seen first together and then in separate sessions. A child may be more inclined to speak about the home situation or her own concerns when supported by the presence of a brother or sister.

Interviewing Adult and Child

It is important to have one or two interviews with each party and the child or children. The joint session can be unstructured and should occur in most cases after the child has already had a session in the office. Thus, he or she will have become familiar with the office, the furniture, games, toys, and so forth, and can choose to direct the play and/or discussion with the adult. The evaluator does not have to be an active participant in this session but instead can observe and record the child-adult interactions. The expert should factor in adult anxiety at seemingly being "graded" during the interview and should stress that this is a time for adult and child to be together in any manner they wish. The therapist observes the interaction, the ease with which adult and child relate to each other, how they play together, what they say to each other, and their levels of anxiety, conflict, and comfort.

The therapist might want to conduct this session in the adult's home. A home visit—even though it is planned and, therefore, not a surprise drop-in—nevertheless affords a view of the family in its own surroundings. There may be much material gained in such a visit that would otherwise be missed if the evaluations are conducted solely at the office.

Interviewing Others

Occasionally, the expert may wish to interview others who play an important role in the proceedings. For example, a divorcing father or mother may be already living with the person he or she intends to marry. Such a potential stepparent should be interviewed in person. Sometimes a nanny, babysitter, grandparent, or other adult who knows the child well may provide useful information. The clinician may see fit to conduct telephone interviews with therapists involved with the adults or the child, schoolteachers, or other professionals, such as medical doctors, tutors, or speech therapists. The expert should seek the agreement of both parents before involving others in the custody evaluation.

The Written Report

The expert communicates to the judge, a family services court clinic, or the attorneys through the very important written report. This report should be succinct, in plain language without unexplained psychiatric jargon, long enough to be complete, but short enough to maintain the professional interest of those non–mental health professionals who read it. The report can be written in letter form, addressed to the judge, the clerk of the court, or other appropriate individuals, depending on the locale. The expert should know in advance the primary recipient.

Psychiatric diagnoses are usually not necessary; this evaluation is about parenting. The report should be written with the expectation that at some point the parent or other caregiving adult might read it. Read and reread the report before submission. It is a permanent record of the expert's work and a reflection of the level of professional competence.

Testimony

A complete and comprehensive written report, accurately reflecting the clinical interviews, with conclusions amply supported by the data that are presented, stands on its own and can help lead to a settlement. Sometimes, though, the expert will be required to testify in court about the report. The expert may be called by the side apparently favored in the report, by the other side, or by both. For further guidance on testifying, the reader is referred to Chapter 5, "Testifying: The Expert Witness in Court."

PITFALLS

Accepting Cases

Avoid unilateral evaluations. An expert may be under intense pressure from an attorney to evaluate a child and one caregiving adult—the attorney's client. The attorney may state that the expert will not be asked to offer an opinion as to custody—just to evaluate and comment (favorably) on the adult-child relationship. The expert should avoid such one-sided participation, as mentioned earlier. Such a limited evaluation puts added stress on the child and often subjects him or her to yet another evaluation for the other side. Conducting a unilateral evaluation does little to enhance the professional reputation of the expert. It is just not possible to compare and assess two parents if only one has been seen.

Avoid wearing two hats. The treating therapist should not assume the additional (and highly contradictory) role of forensic expert. Nor should the court-appointed impartial expert become involved in treatment or even in giving occasional advice.

Avoid conflicts of interest. Forensic experts should assiduously avoid situations suggestive of a conflict of interest or any instances in which their impartiality could be challenged.

Evaluation

Parents or other caregivers often feel they have not had enough time to explain their side to the expert. It is important to give them an opportunity to be heard and not be unduly strict about limiting their time. On the

other hand, the clinician should explain that the evaluation cannot be prolonged indefinitely. The expert should not refuse to read documents prepared by or on behalf of one side, even if he or she feels they will have little relevance. It is important for adults to feel they have been heard with respect and are being evaluated by an impartial expert. To reiterate, the expert should avoid trying to decide when someone is lying and should not confuse his or her role with that of the judge.

Report

A major pitfall in preparing the written report is failure to have the conclusions follow from the data presented (Herman and Levy 1989). The reader should appreciate a flow in the material and a cogent and credible formulation at the end. The conclusions and recommendations should emerge in a rational way and should not take the reader by surprise. The report should contain enough process from the interviews so that the judge can appreciate that the expert did solicit and analyze enough information.

Testimony

A common pitfall in testifying is not being properly prepared for court. The expert should carefully review the written report and contemporaneous process notes prior to testimony. It is advisable for the court-appointed expert to refrain from meeting with attorneys prior to testimony. Unilateral meetings—even with the "friendly" attorney—reduce the expert's stature as impartial. Although experts are usually permitted to review their reports and other notes when on the witness stand, they ought to be prepared and should convey the impression of having put considerable time and thought into the testimony.

CASE EXAMPLE EPILOGUES

Case Example I

Dr. Smithson interviewed Elizabeth and Harvey together once and separately five times each. He also saw each of the parents with Hal. Harvey accused Elizabeth of "duplicity" by obtaining an ex parte order of temporary custody. He said he had great difficulty finding a home and had to go out of town for business. It was his business, he emphasized to the doctor, that provided the child support for Hal. He also told Dr. Smithson that Elizabeth had used cocaine and marijuana regularly before the pregnancy.

Elizabeth questioned Harvey's ability to care for their child. She also reported that Harvey had pushed her down in anger on the day he attempted to take his son. She admitted to using cocaine and marijuana but insisted that she had stopped 4 years before she became pregnant with Hal. Both parents agreed that joint custody was no longer a possibility for them. Elizabeth did say she saw nothing wrong with Hal spending an overnight with his father every other week, and she knew Hal enjoyed being with his father.

Dr. Smithson observed both parents acting lovingly and appropriately in their sessions with Hal. The child psychiatrist did notice Harvey being more physical with his son; Elizabeth's style with the infant was calmer and even sedate at times.

The forensic expert recommended that custody be awarded to the mother, opining that Hal's routine and comfortable, predictable, and stable arrangement with his mother ought to be maintained. He recommended that the father have Hal with him one overnight every other weekend, to be gradually increased to two overnights on alternate weekends. He could also have his son for 2 hours for a midweek dinner, if he wished. The written report helped settle the case; there was no trial, and each party entered into a written stipulation agreeing to Dr. Smithson's recommendations.

Case Example 2

Dr. Wellington did her usual child custody and visitation evaluation of the Greene family. After all of the clinical interviews, including telephone contact with therapists for each parent and with Hallie's teacher and three sessions alone with Hallie, the child psychiatrist was stumped. She found both parents to be quite fit and eminently qualified and capable to take primary care of their daughter. The doctor found Hallie's sessions quite compelling. Although she was only 7 years old, she was quite bright and articulate. She talked about feeling caught in the middle, of loving and being attached to both of her parents, of the positives and negatives about the potential move 1,000 miles away from her father, and about how much she would miss her father.

Dr. Wellington found that she was unable to recommend one parent over the other. She decided that she could best assist the court by elucidating each parent's strengths and the nature of each parent's attachment to Hallie. She discussed her analysis of the mother's motivation for the move. Most importantly, she conveyed to the court the emotional state of the minor child and described in detail the nature of Hallie's attachments to her mother and her father. She concluded that the ultimate decision would have to be the court's; the best she could do as a forensic clinician was to help the court understand the emotional needs of the child.

Case Example 3

Because Dr. Baird had been appointed by the court, he had access to many documents as well as the family itself. Along with interviewing the grandmother sev-

eral times, each of the children—alone and all with the grandmother—the mother, who was incarcerated, and other family members who might assist the grandmother in caring for the six surviving children, the child psychiatrist reviewed the entire foster agency case record, including every progress note written about the children, their placement, and their visits with their grandmother. He also reviewed protective services documents in opposition to the placement, along with other interim psychiatric and psychological evaluations of the children and their grandmother.

Dr. Baird concluded that the children's best interests would be served by allowing them to live with their grandmother. All of them had expressed this desire. Dr. Baird wrote—and later testified—that such a permanent placement would give the children the message that there was much good in their family to provide balance against the evil committed by their mother. Living with their grandmother, they would be better able to begin the long process of healing within the loving environment of their family.

The family court judge, twice having denied the grandmother's petitions to care for her grandchildren, after hearing what she referred to as "Dr. Baird's compelling and most sensible testimony—a reflection of a most complete and comprehensive clinical evaluation," finally authorized the placement with the grandmother.

ACTION GUIDELINES

A. Getting involved
  1. Agree to be a court-appointed expert only, or someone agreed to by both sides.
  2. Make sure the questions posed by the court are understood and appropriate for someone of your profession to answer.
  3. Make fee requirements clear and whenever possible request full payment at the start of the evaluation.

B. Doing the evaluation
  1. Explain to all parties how the evaluation will be conducted and be sure to get waivers of rights of confidentiality and privilege.
  2. Consider the evaluation a profile of parenting—not a psychiatric examination.
  3. Be sure all relevant people are interviewed and for adequate time.

C. Writing the report
  1. Remember that the report is a *communication* with a non–mental health professional; it should be written clearly and should be free of undefined jargon or arcane terminology.

2. Clearly list who was seen, when, and for how long. Include all important data from the interviews, along with direct quotes.

3. Be sure conclusions and recommendations flow naturally and logically from the data that are presented.

4. Proofread carefully!

REFERENCES

Allen M, Burrell N: Comparing the impact of homosexual and heterosexual parents on children: meta-analysis of existing research. J Homosex 32:19–35, 1996

American Academy of Child and Adolescent Psychiatry (Herman SP, principal author): Practice parameters for child custody evaluation. J Am Acad Child Adolesc Psychiatry 36 (suppl):57S–68S, 1997

American Association of Family and Conciliation Courts: Model Standards of Practice for Child Custody Evaluation. Madison, WI, American Association of Family and Conciliation Courts, 1994

American Psychiatric Association: Child Custody Consultation: Report of the Task Force on Clinical Assessment in Child Custody. Washington, DC, American Psychiatric Association, 1988

American Psychological Association: Guidelines for child custody evaluations in divorce proceedings. Am Psychol 49:677–680, 1994

Ash P, Guyer M: Court implementation of mental health professionals' recommendations in contested child custody and visitation cases. Bulletin of the American Academy of Psychiatry and the Law 12:137–147, 1984

Atwell A, Moore U, Nielsen E, et al: Effects of joint custody on children. Bulletin of the American Academy of Psychiatry and the Law 2:149–157, 1984

Benedek E, Schetky D: Custody and visitation: problems and perspectives. Psychiatr Clin North Am 8:857–873, 1985

Bozett F (ed): Gay and Lesbian Parents. New York, Praeger, 1987

Chan R, Raboy B, Patterson C: Psychosocial adjustment among children conceived via donor insemination by lesbian and heterosexual mothers. Child Dev 69:443–457, 1998

Cole W, Bradford J: Abduction during custody and access disputes. Can J Psychiatry 37:264–266, 1992

Curran W: The vulnerability of court-appointed impartial experts in child-custody cases. N Engl J Med 312:1168–1170, 1985

Derdeyn A: Child custody contests in historical perspective. Am J Psychiatry 133:1369–1376, 1976

Derdeyn A, Scott E: Joint custody: a critical analysis and appraisal. Am J Orthopsychiatry 54:199–209, 1984

Dillon P, Emery R: Divorce mediation and resolution of child custody disputes: long-term effects. Am J Orthopsychiatry 66:131–140, 1996

Emery R, Matthews S, Kitzmann K: Child custody mediation and litigation: parents' satisfaction and functioning one year after settlement. J Consult Clin Psychol 62:124–129, 1994

Goldstein J, Solnit A, Freud A: Beyond the Best Interests of the Child. New York, Free Press, 1973

Green A: True and false allegations of sexual abuse in child custody disputes. Journal of the American Academy of Child Psychiatry 25:449–456, 1986

Herman S: Special issues in child custody disputes. J Am Acad Child Adolesc Psychiatry 29:969–974, 1990

Herman S: Child custody evaluations and the need for standards of care and peer review. Journal of the Center for Children and the Courts I:139–150, 1999

Herman S, Levy A: Does peer review have a place in child custody evaluation? Children Today 18:15–18, 1989

Hodges W: Interventions for Children of Divorce. New York, Wiley, 1986

In the Matter of the Adoption of a Child Whose First Name Is Evan, 583 NYS2d 997 (NY Surr 1992)

Kelly J: Children's adjustment in conflicted marriage and divorce: a decade review of research. J Am Acad Child Adolesc Psychiatry 39:963–973, 2000

Kermani E: Issues of child custody and our moral values in the era of new medical technology. J Am Acad Child Adolesc Psychiatry 31:533–538, 1992

Kleber D, Howell R, Tibbits-Kleber Λ: The impact of parental homosexuality in child custody cases: a review of the literature. Bulletin of the American Academy of Psychiatry and the Law 14:81–87, 1986

Levy A: Disorders of visitation in child custody cases. Psychiatry and Law, Winter, 1982, pp 471–489

Levy R (ed): Visitation with infants, in Legal and Mental Health Perspectives on Child Custody Laws: A Deskbook for Judges. Danvers, MA, Westlaw, 1998, pp 15.1–15.5

Lieberman A, Van Horn P: Attachment, trauma, and domestic violence: implications for child custody. Child Adolesc Psychiatr Clin N Am 7:423–443, 1998

Long N, Forehand R, Zogg C: Preventing parental child abduction: analysis of a national project. Clin Pediatr (Phila) 30:549–554, 1991

Mason S: Custody planning with HIV-affected families: considerations for child welfare workers. Child Welfare 77:161–177, 1998

Miller T, Veltkamp L: Disputed child custody: strategies and issues in mediation. Bulletin of the American Academy of Psychiatry and the Law 15:45–56, 1987

NY Social Services Law § 378-a(2), 1999

Opinion of the Justices, No 87–080, NH S Ct (1987)

Painter v Bannister 258 Iowa 1390, NW2d 152 (1966)

Pruett M, Hoganbruen K: Joint custody and shared parenting: research and interventions. Child Adolesc Psychiatry Clin N Am 7:273–294, 1998

Santosky v Kramer 455 US 745, 102 S Ct 1388 (1982)

Schetky D, Haller L: Parental kidnapping. Journal of the American Academy of Child Psychiatry 22:279–285, 1983

S.E.G. v R.A.G., 735 SW2d 164, MO App ED (1987)

Stanton A: Grandparents' visitation rights and custody. Child Adolesc Psychiatr Clin N Am 7:409–422, 1998

Steinman S: The experience of children in a joint-custody arrangement: a report of a study. Am J Orthopsychiatry 51:403–414, 1981

Steinman S: A study of parents who sought joint custody following divorce: who reaches agreement and sustains joint custody and who returns to court. Journal of the American Academy of Child Psychiatry 24:554–562, 1985

Thoennes N, Tjaden P: The extent, nature, and validity of sexual abuse allegations in custody/visitation disputes. Child Abuse Negl 14:151–163, 1990

Tibbits-Kleber A, Howell R, Kleber D: Joint custody: a comprehensive review. Bulletin of the American Academy of Psychiatry and the Law 15:27–43, 1987

Tropea v Tropea, 642 NY S2d 575 (Ct App 1996)

Troxel v Granville, 530 US 57, 120 SCt 2054, US Wash (2000)

Wallerstein J, Johnston J: Children of divorce: recent findings regarding long-term effects and recent studies of joint and sole custody. Pediatr Rev 11:197–204, 1990

Weithorn L (ed): Psychology and Child Custody Determinations. Lincoln, NE, University of Nebraska Press, 1987

CHAPTER 9

Parenting Assessment in Cases of Neglect and Abuse

Richard Barnum, M.D.

Case Example 1

Ms. Alvarez, a recent immigrant from Central America, brought her infant child to a hospital emergency room, concerned that the child was sick. Hospital staff noticed that Ms. Alvarez was dirty, seemed vague and distracted, and was reluctant to answer questions. They made a report to the child protection agency. The agency's investigation noted that Ms. Alvarez was socially isolated and continued to resist service involvement and raised questions regarding possible substance abuse. The agency brought a petition to have the child removed from Ms. Alvarez because of neglect.

Case Example 2

Mr. Brown was a middle-age single man who was raising three children in conditions of poverty and social disadvantage. Because of poor school attendance and hygiene concerns on behalf of all three children, the child protection agency became involved with the family. Over a period of some months, the agency's efforts to establish a relationship with Mr. Brown met with increasing resistance, and the agency petitioned the court for custody of the children. The children were placed in short-term foster care but showed increasing signs of anxiety and depression. The court referred the case for clinical evaluation of Mr. Brown's parenting abilities.

Case Example 3

Ms. Green was a 35-year-old woman with a history of victimization by domestic violence with depression, substance abuse, and chaotic family functioning. Her two older children were removed from her custody, and her parental rights were terminated. She became

successfully involved in services for battered women and was substance-free when she had a third child, but she remained homeless. When she failed to follow the rules of her homeless shelter and was expelled, custody of her infant child was awarded to the child protection agency; the child remained in foster care for 3 years because of the court's concerns about Ms. Green's history and her continuing homelessness.

LEGAL ISSUES

Key legal issues in the assessment of parental capacity include the context and questions posed, the legal standards of parental capacity, and the consultant's role.

Questions and Context

Sometimes questions about parental capacity are clearly posed and explicit; often they are implicit and difficult to articulate. They arise in a broad range of legal contexts, including juvenile delinquency, status offenses, marital separation and divorce, guardianship and adoption, and both civil and criminal proceedings arising from allegations of child abuse and neglect. Even within the realm of child abuse and neglect, legal contexts can vary widely. Criminal prosecution of abuse and neglect may raise questions about parents' criminal responsibility or competence to stand trial (which may relate to issues of parental functioning), and sentencing decisions in criminal cases may take parental functioning into account.

Civil proceedings vary in their formality and stakes depending on the seriousness of the allegations and the stage of the case. Newer and less serious allegations may tend to focus more on questions of temporary custody and service planning (Kamerman and Kahn 1989), whereas more serious allegations (or cases where efforts at providing services to parents have failed) may focus on the higher-stake issue of terminating parental rights permanently (see Chapter 11, "Termination of Parental Rights," and Quinn and Nye 1992). With each of these differing areas of focus, the relevant issues in parental functioning may vary, as will the legal standards for deciding the matter.

Legal Standards

Even within legal contexts in which the focus is squarely on characterizing parents' capacities to provide for their children, the breadth and vagueness of the concept of *parental capacity* present serious challenges for forensic consultation in this area. Parental behavior and characteristics have been the subject of considerable empirical research. This research certainly suggests some basic characteristics of parents that may be associated with various kinds of risks for children and others that may be less clearly associated with good outcomes (National Research Council 1993). Though most mental health professionals have strongly held beliefs about what features in a parent promote success in children, and what features may tend to be harmful, they differ from one another on questions of which features tend most to be helpful or harmful and in what combinations, in what ways, for what kinds of children, at what ages, and in what sorts of circumstances. There is no standard clinical consensus as to what the essential features of parenting are, let alone on how to characterize or measure those features.

Consultant's Role

As detailed in Chapter 4, "Introduction to Forensic Evaluations," clinicians undertaking forensic evaluations need to be as clear as possible regarding the specific role they are asked to take and the question(s) they are asked to answer. Clinicians involving themselves in child abuse and neglect cases may have some appropriate role in addressing the credibility of an alleged child victim, but they need to appreciate that the legal system has complex nonclinical means of determining the facts of a case. Though the consultant should avoid serving as a fact finder, it is critical for the evaluator of parental capacity to understand the specific allegations of abuse or neglect as clearly as possible in order to appreciate the significance of the parent's alleged behavior for parental capacity.

Although nonclinical means are the ultimate basis for the finding of facts regarding events of abuse or neglect, the key legal findings in many child abuse and neglect cases will not rest solely (or even significantly, in some cases) on a determination of what a parent did or did not do in a specific allegation of abuse or neglect. In many cases, the issue will have come to legal attention because of a relatively minor instance of abuse or neglect or even because of an instance in which a child was at risk without any true abuse or neglect occurring at all. In such cases, and in some involving more salient abuse and neglect, the legal determinations of child custody and of parental rights rest not on findings of fact about specific events but instead on legal findings regarding more vague civil issues, such as a parent's ability to provide proper care and custody or a prognosis for improvement or deterioration for a parent with a mental disorder. In such cases the forensic clinician's opinions regarding the facts of an alleged event of abuse or neglect will properly be of little importance legally, but the clinical opinions regarding the basic issues of parental capacity and prognosis will be central to the adjudication and disposition of the civil matter.

Clinical interviewing of parents needs to include careful attention to the purpose to which evaluation results will be put. It is especially important to be clear as to whether specific admissions of child mistreatment made by parents to a clinical consultant can be used as evidence in criminal adjudication. Because one of the issues in civil proceedings stemming from child abuse will be the risk of mistreatment recurring, a parent's ability to acknowledge the mistreatment, and to engage in a specific plan to reduce the risk of recurrence, can be a critical element of the consultation. If the parent faces subsequent criminal liability for any admission made in the clinical consultation, the parent may be inhibited from making such an admission. In that case, the consultant will be hard pressed to know whether the parent's denial is a means of avoiding prosecution or whether it represents a more malignant form of psychological avoidance of responsibility, with a potentially more negative prognosis (Barnum 1990b). It is usually important that the consultant, the referring client (court, agency, or lawyer), the parent, and the parent's counsel all be clear on what protections, if any, a parent may expect from criminal liability based on admissions in a clinical evaluation.

The consultant needs to be sure that the parent understands that the results of the interview may be used to counter the parent's interests. In addition, however, ideally the consultant will help the parent to be comfortable enough in the interview process that the parent can communicate valid information about his or her history and state of mind, and the consultant will notice and document indications of caution or guardedness in the parent that might undermine the validity of the information the parent provides.

CLINICAL ISSUES

Because the realm of parental capacity is so broad and because it is not possible to observe directly more than a small fraction of relevant parental behavior, it is necessary to find surrogate variables to stand in for direct observation. Articulating the issues to select for examination in an assessment of parental capacity thus requires a theory of parenting. As suggested above, the field lacks consensus on a basic theoretical understanding of parental capacity. What follows, therefore, is a suggested theoretical framework for understanding parenting. This framework is offered as a basis for articulating surrogate variables for observing, organizing information, and linking observations to predictions of broader functioning as a parent.

Theoretical Conceptions of Parental Capacity

As in any other forensic assessment, the evaluation of parental capacity requires a preliminary articulation of the specific functions at issue. The organizing theory offered here avers that parenting involves two distinct basic functions; these can be thought of simply as care and protection. Care is a broad term referring to the complex processes of socialization, the essential teaching function of parents that promotes appropriate growth and development in a variety of psychological realms. Protection refers to the provision of a safe and supportive boundary between the child and the outside physical and social worlds.

Socialization

A parent's responsibility is to teach children, to enable them to become well-adapted members of society. Socialization involves concurrent teaching in multiple realms, involving three basic kinds of learning: cognitive, behavioral, and emotional (Levinger 1971).

Cognitive development and skill building. Parents support cognitive development in two basic ways. They impart knowledge, and they foster the development of various skills. The specific areas of knowledge and skills vary greatly with the child's stage of development and with cultural background. Methods of supporting cognitive development also vary with the child's development and with the parents' interests and style. Among the most important areas of cognitive development are language functioning, self-care skills, school and vocational functioning, and social skills. Parents promote these areas of development through explicit teaching and through promoting practice and autonomous performance.

Supervision and discipline. Behavioral learning is an important basis for the development of overall personal discipline. Parents have a fundamental responsibility to promote good habits in a wide variety of areas, not only by teaching them but also by shaping and enforcing them with appropriate patterns of supervision, reward, and punishment. The specific habits to be taught may vary considerably with culture and values, as may the specific techniques by which reward and punishment are applied. But some consistent principles of behavioral learning do inform good parental practice in this area generally. These principles begin with the importance of parents maintaining awareness of their children's behavior through adequate supervision. No plan of discipline can be effective if it does not rest on accurate vision of what a child is doing; without this vision, responses to behavior will be essentially random.

Parents who are able to provide adequate supervision can consistently and reliably respond to desired behavior in the child with positive sanctions, and to undesired behavior with negative or aversive sanctions (Patterson and Stouthamer-Loeber 1984; Patterson et al. 1989). Explicit positive rewards of moderate intensity, offered intermittently, are probably most effective in shaping specific behaviors consistent with positive emotional functioning. However, some aversive sanctions are also usually necessary to extinguish specific undesired behaviors (Snyder and Patterson 1986). Mild aversive sanctions, such as withdrawal of approval, explicit expression of disapproval, time out, and restrictions, are usually sufficient and effective, especially if applied reliably. Parents who choose to use various forms of physical punishment as aversive sanctions are expected to ensure that such punishment is mild enough not to be physically harmful, consistent enough in its application to be effective, and careful and infrequent enough to avoid generating compelling adverse emotional effects (Barnum 1990a).

Emotional support, nurturance, and direction. Elements of parental behavior that foster positive emotional development and functioning have always been the subject of exploration and debate. It is probably beyond the current reach of child psychology and psychiatry to articulate definitive active ingredients in parenting for promoting emotional growth, given the variety of parent-child inter-actions at various stages of development and the uncer-tainties regarding the relative impact of these interactions and other genetic and environmental influences on emotional development. However, it is reasonable to suggest that a parent's own general emotional coping has some impact on that of a child, both directly (through the process of learning by identification) and indirectly (through its impact on the general tone of emotional comfort and security in the family).

Parental emotional coping that is dominated by anger and conflict can be expected to contribute to anxiety and to a greater propensity for aggressiveness in a child (Farrington and Hawkins 1991; Loeber and Dishion 1983). Overly critical or rejecting parental behavior may contribute to poor self-esteem, low confidence, and anger (Goodman et al. 1994). Overly nurturant and protective parental behavior may foster a sense of insecurity and undermine a child's feelings of confident autonomy and independent competence. Parental styles of emotional communication marked by either high levels of conflict or by distance and withdrawal probably teach less effective emotional coping than do more moderate styles of direct but respectful emotional interchange.

Advocacy and Protection

Besides affording children the variety of cognitive, behavioral, and emotional teaching that promotes positive socialization, parents also need to protect their children from various dangers and to advocate for their child's interests with the world at large.

Safety.   Routine expectations of parents include that they will make reasonable efforts to keep their children safe from foreseeable physical harm. Parents are also expected not to harm their children and to keep others from harming their children as well. Foreseeable harms that parents are generally expected to try to prevent include physical injury and some infectious diseases and nutritional insufficiencies, and foreseeable harms may also include emotional injuries caused by exposure to experiences such as domestic violence, sexual abuse, and other emotional maltreatment (Jaffe et al. 1990).

Supportive interface with the world.   In addition to providing for a child's basic safety, a parent's protective responsibility also includes furthering the child's interests in the world at large. Parents are expected to provide for appropriate medical care and to ensure their children's attendance at school. Parents are expected to have some understanding of their children's individual needs and to make reasonable efforts to provide for these needs, within the limits of individual circumstances. If a child has a mental or physical disability, a parent is generally expected to recognize and understand the disability and provide help and accommodation for it.

Obviously there can be great variation in what is expected of parents depending on individual circumstances. Though in most circumstances a parent would probably be found neglectful for not noticing or providing for appropriate treatment for a child's broken leg, the extent of a parent's obligation to seek and authorize medical treatments for conditions such as acne or depression is likely to be more ambiguous. A parent's consistent refusal to allow a child to attend school, requiring instead that the child remain at home to care for younger siblings and to work in the family business, will ordinarily be seen as different from a parent's refusal to authorize a particular plan for special education, with which the parent may not agree. In such conditions, legal judgments may vary and will likely take a variety of indicators of parental capacity into account in reaching a determination of neglect or abuse.

Developmental Issues

In understanding the variety of specific parental characteristics that make up overall parental capacity, it is important to consider the variations in children's needs across the range of development. Parental characteristics that support good care of an infant may not be as positive in dealing with an older child, and problems in caring for an infant may not predict similar difficulties in meeting the needs of a school-age child (Cicchetti and Toth 1995). Table 9–1 summarizes the specific parental tasks for each area of parenting at different developmental stages.

Parental Strengths

In meeting the developmental needs of children for advocacy, protection, and socialization, some specific strengths are especially important.

Cognitive Capacities

Parents need to have some knowledge of basic child development and health and sufficient knowledge of the world to be able to keep the child safe and to provide for the basic needs of the family (Dowdney and Skuse 1993; Feldman 1986). The parent needs to know when to seek help and where to turn for it and to have at least some basic problem-solving ability.

TABLE 9–1. Parental tasks at stages of child development

	Infancy	Toddlerhood	School age	Adolescence
Safety	Provide food, shelter, and warmth; safety from physical harm; routine medical care.	Prevent poisoning, burns, falls, or other accidents.	Teach autonomous safety skills and habits.	Support continuing safe practices, with less supervision in response to good habits.
Understanding and advocacy	Recognize developmental progress; deal with medical and other providers.	Continue to note development; deal with medical, day care, other parents.	Recognize child's function in various settings; deal with teachers and other professionals for services.	Communicate with child and others; promote appropriate education and other services.
Cognitive support	Talk and read with baby; provide other appropriate stimulation.	Read and provide other stimulation; support arts, crafts, sports, chores, and natural curiosity.	Support school functioning; provide direct support for learning, with homework.	Support range of alternatives for education and vocational training.
Discipline	Establish regular routines for sleeping, eating, and other activities.	Supervise child's behavior; begin active provision of consistent rewards and punishments; foster good habits.	Supervise the child's activities outside of home; provide punishment for conduct problems and restrict access to antisocial peers. Foster work habits.	Provide appropriate supervisory attention without being overly intrusive; provide realistic sanctions; support autonomy.
Emotional support	Ensure secure attachment and early relatedness; respond to signs of distress and support infant's tolerance of distress.	Enable confident and safe exploration, with return for parental support. Allow opposition without struggle, maintaining control and safety.	Support peers and independence; add self-esteem through genuine success in forming skills and friendships; provide stable support, help, and problem solving.	Have stable expectations and provide support; note signs of distress and provide reliable communication; foster emotional growth, accepting greater maturity and relating as a peer in response.

Reliability and Organization

Parents need to be organized enough in their own functioning to be able to provide reliable structures for the child's functioning, to enable the child to take part consistently in activities outside the family (especially including school), and to provide the child with a sense of security and support for the child's own developing capacity for structure. The parent's overall personality functioning should be such that a child would learn responsibility by identifying with the parent.

Social Supports

A parent's membership in a social network is an important characteristic for success in raising children (Wolfe et al. 1995). Connection with others in a community—whether defined by neighborhood, school or church attendance, or some other affiliation—helps parents to know about both problems and resources within the community that may affect the child. Having a network of connections with others provides parents with emotional support for dealing with the stresses of parenting;

knowledge, perspective, and direction regarding specific problems that may arise; and some flexibility in sharing responsibilities for child care, supervision, transportation, and other specific tasks. These connections also help to foster children's social development directly, by bringing them into contact with a variety of other families, providing them perspective and an opportunity to develop broader relationships and supports for themselves.

Warmth and Caring

A parent who feels warmly toward a child, who has some empathy for the child's experience, who is happy to have responsibility for the child and is proud of the child, will likely be more motivated and successful in providing for the child than one who is not. Furthermore, a parent's overall emotional functioning makes a critical contribution to the child's development, through identification and through the establishment of an overall emotional tone in the family environment. Emotional stability, enthusiasm, optimism, generosity, engagement with others, and skill in coping with stress, frustration, conflict, and loss without becoming emotionally overwhelmed are all parental traits that can contribute to a child's emotional development.

Parental Deficits

Just as various positive traits contribute to success in parenting, a number of psychological problems in parents can contribute to impairments in abilities to meet parental responsibilities. In appreciating the impact of these problems, it is especially important in a forensic assessment to be as explicit as possible in linking the psychological impairment to the specific functional deficits in parenting that result from it.

Mental Retardation

Mental retardation can be associated with a variety of parenting problems, depending in part on the severity of the overall cognitive deficit and in part on the extent of other co-occurring psychological problems. Chapter 32, "Legal Aspects of Mental Retardation," provides a detailed account of the impact of mental retardation on parenting.

Depression

Parents with depression face particular risks, stemming primarily from the overall reductions in energy, emotional investment, motivation, attention, and cognitive acuity that depression may bring. They may fail to provide adequate cognitive stimulation and support, either as a result of dulling of their own cognition or from reduced motivation. Preoccupation or anergia and inattention can result in inadequate consistency of behavioral supervision; this may put a child at risk for unsafe behavior and may contribute to inconsistent and ineffective discipline (Wahler 1980). Discipline may be further impaired by a depressed parent's irritability, anger, and negative attributional style, contributing to an overall tendency for angry blaming of children for misbehavior and for overly harsh or abusive punishment (Webster-Stratton and Hammond 1988; Zuravin 1989). Depressed parents can fail to promote normal attachments in infants, owing to their own emotional withdrawal and lack of interest (Beardslee and Wheelock 1994; Field et al. 1990; Teti et al. 1995), and can contribute to the development of an anxious and depressed emotional orientation in older children as a result of identification as well as the child's defensive responses to the parent's emotional inconsistency (Weissman et al. 1984).

Substance Abuse

Substance abuse can have a compelling negative impact on parental responsibility (Regan et al. 1987). Opiate addiction puts parents at risk for antisocial behavior to support the acquisition of drugs and contributes to direct pharmacological impairment in energy, attention, engagement, and motivation. The resulting impact on child development can be similar to that of depression (Mayer and Black 1977). Heavy use of cocaine (especially free-based cocaine) generates serious emotional and behavioral instability, with an increased risk for violence and for sexually abusive behavior (Famularo et al. 1992; Hawley et al. 1995). Alcoholism can have a wide variety of manifestations and tends to affect parenting negatively in various ways, depending especially on the chronicity of the intoxication, on the degree and type of the resulting behavioral disinhibition, emotional withdrawal, and failure of judgment, and on the social and occupational consequences of the drinking (Reich et al. 1988; West and Prinz 1987).

History of Abuse

A parent's own history of suffering abuse or neglect in childhood can have some negative effects on parenting (Egeland et al. 1988; Rutter 1989). These effects may stem from general manifestations of personality disorder, resulting in part from a childhood history of maltreatment (Bryer et al. 1987; Herman et al. 1989). Such traits as general emotional instability, guardedness, defensive self-involvement, anger, irritability, and blaming may be expected to have the same kinds of impacts on parenting that these problems do when they appear as symptoms of a more acute mental disorder. A parent's own history of abuse can also affect parental responsibility in more specific ways, however. It may lead to a parent resenting the child's dependency or feeling entitled to behave badly or to expect indulgence from the child (Main and Goldwyn 1984). It may contribute to feelings of anxiety, doubt, or guilt, which may in turn undermine the parent's confidence in setting limits and in conveying broader expectations and values to the child. A history of sexual abuse may be associated with a parent being either especially preoccupied with, or avoidant of, the possibility that a child may be experiencing sexual abuse (Famularo et al. 1994).

Course and Context

In assessing the impact of a mental disorder or substance abuse on parenting, it is important to recognize the specific pattern of parental symptoms and the course of the illness. A parent with a chronic psychotic illness in which the child becomes involved in the parent's paranoid delusions presents an enduring risk both to the child's safety (if the parent is prone to act preemptively against delusional enemies) and to the child's overall emotional development (if the child is constantly blamed or otherwise mistreated). On the other hand, a parent with intermittent episodes of hypomania, delusions, or depression who functions well most of the time is likely to have a different and generally less negative impact on a child's overall development. A parent who has occasional binges of freebasing cocaine during which he becomes violent, hypersexual, and disinhibited may place a child at considerably more acute risk for serious harm than a parent who gets drunk every evening after the child goes to bed.

The significance of a disorder for parenting function also depends critically on the overall social network of the family. The effect of even a serious mental illness in a parent will be far less in a family in which the other parent has a strong relationship with the children than it will for an isolated single parent (Emery 1982). The "buffering" of impaired functioning in one parent can be achieved by another parent, by grandparents or other extended family members, and even by responsible older siblings (on behalf of younger ones). Successful buffering includes protecting the children from specific potential harm that may result from the impaired parent's disorder, as well as providing active socializing support. It also includes helping the children to understand the nature of the other parent's difficulty so that they are not made anxious or guilty by it.

Techniques for Assessment of Specific Parenting Capacities

As with any other forensic evaluation, the most challenging elements in the assessment of parental capacity concern the foregoing articulation of the specific functions in question. Once the forensic clinician has a sound grasp of the functional elements of parenting, the gathering of relevant clinical data is directed by that understanding. As in any other forensic evaluation, data gathering techniques are both clinical and investigative.

Interviewing Parents

The consultant's interviews with the parent need to include a thorough clinical history and mental status examination to provide a sound basis for an overall clinical assessment. Beyond articulating clinical history and diagnosis, interviews need to focus specifically on the variety of functional strengths and weaknesses that are relevant to parenting and to link specific weaknesses (if possible) to specific disorders. Clinical assessment needs to consider the prognosis (with and without treatment) of whatever disorders contribute to functional deficits and include in this consideration an exploration of the

parent's own understanding of the disorder, its impact, and its treatment.

A variety of specific areas in the parent's experience can be important to explore in taking a clinical history for a parenting assessment.

History of child abuse.   It is important to explore the parent's possible exposure to abuse or neglect in her own childhood. If there was such exposure, the interview needs to examine how she responded to it at the time, how it affected her subsequent development, and what lingering impact it may still have in symptoms of anxiety, depression, emotional instability, guardedness and isolation, or dissociation. A parent who experienced abuse in childhood that was recognized and that led to protective intervention and psychological treatment may have experienced limited negative emotional consequences. In contrast, a parent who experienced similar abuse but who did not get help and continued to suffer more lasting abuse, or simply contained a more limited abuse experience in isolation, may have experienced more compelling and lasting emotional consequences of the abuse.

Substance abuse and mental disorder.   It is essential that the clinical evaluation of parents includes careful and thorough attention to questions of substance abuse and mental disorder. Substance abuse disorders are the most significant contributing factor to serious child abuse and neglect (Murphy et al. 1991). Mood disorders are also prevalent among parents who maltreat their children, and other mental disorders can contribute to specific parental failures as noted above.

Recent and current relationships.   The parent's relationships within his or her own family of origin can be an important source of support or of ongoing disruption in emotional functioning. It can be important to explore relationships with both parents and with siblings, since in many cases there may be discord or isolation in some relationships but warmth and support in others. The parent's network of friends and neighbors can be especially important. When these relationships are extensive and positive, they can have great value in providing both emotional and practical support in dealing with children. When they are conflicted, suspicious, or distant, they may offer little in terms of practical or emotional help and may contribute to a parent's overall stress and difficulty coping.

The parent's relationships within the nuclear family are probably of greatest significance to parenting function. The sharing of responsibility for raising children is always a serious challenge to any spousal relationship. Partners bring different basic expectations about children and parenthood to their relationship, and these may only emerge in the course of having children and dealing with them. A comfortable spousal relationship, with trust and good communication, can enable parents to resolve conflicts about children in a calm and creative manner, improving their overall ability to understand and respond appropriately to their children's needs.

The consultant should explore with each parent the history of the relationship with the other parent, including their meeting and attraction to one another, the growth of their involvement with one another, and how they have dealt with conflict. The exploration should attend particularly to how they each have dealt with any differences regarding the children, and to how these differences have led either to increased conflict or to improved understanding and mutual support. If either parent has problems with mental disorder or substance abuse, then the other parent's buffering of the impact of these problems on the children is especially important to explore.

Exploration of the parenting experience.   Because the clinician will have limited opportunity to observe the parent's overall dealings with the child over time and in a variety of contexts, it is important in the interview context to try to learn as much as possible directly from the parent about her own specific functioning as a parent. This exploration is structured around a basic history of the child's development and functioning.

The parent's experience of the child's conception can have an impact on the parent's overall feeling about the child. If the child was unwanted, the parent may be more prone to relate poorly to the child; if the child was conceived by rape, the parent may face special challenges in establishing an emotional connection. At the other extreme, some parents of children conceived as a result of extraordinary efforts may experience high levels of stress around the conception and pregnancy, may have trouble relaxing with the child, and may set especially high expectations for the child, leading to ultimate frustration and conflict (Rojo-Moreno et al. 1996).

The nature of the parent's initial attachment to the child may have an impact on the development of an enduring sense of closeness with the child (Kumar 1997; Minde 1986). Exploration of the parent's account of the infant period focuses on the parent's adjustment to having a new baby, including such challenges as getting enough sleep, establishing the child's schedule, helping older siblings to adjust to the baby, and coming to appreciate the infant's temperament. It is valuable to question parents about how they have coped with stresses, such as

a fussy or colicky baby, the child's medical problems, and the parent's own mood changes, and to ask for an account of the process of getting to know, understand, and relate to the baby as an individual.

In asking about toddler development, it is important to consider the parent's recognition of basic progress in motor and language development. Insight into parental discipline comes from the parent's account of how he or she has established regular behavioral routines with the toddler, taught the child about safety, and responded to the child's discovery of saying no and temper tantrums. A parent's sensitivity to and response to the toddler's insatiable curiosity can provide some indication of his or her support for the child's cognitive development.

Examination of the parent's experience with the school-age child focuses especially on support for school and social functioning and on the growth of independent responsibility in managing those tasks and chores at home. Questioning the parent about the child's interests and friends can provide information about the parent's continuing awareness of the child's activities and about the degree of breadth and sensitivity in the communication between parent and child. Similar themes inform the parent interview regarding the adolescent, but with more focus on the parent's means of developing an appropriate balance of independence with disciplinary supervision, and on the parent's recognition and adjustment to indicators of the adolescent's developing genuine independence.

Regardless of the child's age, some specific issues are always worth exploring when interviewing parents. The consultant needs to ask the parent about his or her understanding of the child's progress in reaching developmental expectations and about any special needs the child may have. How clearly and accurately does the parent understand the nature of any problems, and what is his or her plan for responding to them? If services for developmental delay, learning disability, mental disorder, or medical problems are in place, how does the parent experience and use those services?

It is always instructive to ask parents about their approach to discipline. What theoretical basis do they have for discipline, what specific practices do they use to shape the child's behavior, and what expectations of the child inform these practices? Where did the parents learn this approach to discipline, and what is their sense of how well it actually works?

A useful approach to filling in details about parenting function is to ask the parent to describe some daily routines in as much detail as possible. For example, on a school day, when and how does the child get up, get dressed, have breakfast, and get to school? What is the parent's specific role in those activities? What is the specific routine for after school, dinnertime, evening, and bedtime? How are weekends different? What other variations seem to make a difference? When does the child get together with friends and extended family, and how is the routine adjusted to those relationships? Asking the parent to describe both favorite and difficult times with the child can sometimes shed important light on the emotional quality of the relationship with the child. A mother whose favorite times with the child are when the child comforts her when she is upset probably has a different overall emotional relationship from one whose favorite time involves the child posing questions about his experiences at school or with friends, which lead to them talking at length about the child's concerns.

Finally, parent interviewing should always include specific attention to how the parent shares responsibility for parenting with others. How do the other parent, extended family members, friends, child care providers, and others contribute to the parent's ability to provide for the child? Are they helpful and supportive or critical and undermining? What specific help do they provide and with what reliability? What problems (if any) characterize their relationships with the parent?

Interviewing Children

Ideally, thorough assessment of parent capacity will include directly interviewing the children involved. The child's individual characteristics can be important to an appreciation of how the parent needs to deal with the child, and the child's perspective on the relationship with the parent will usually add to the understanding of that relationship. The consultant should attend to the following concerns in child interviews.

Thorough history and mental status examination. As with the parent, interviewing the child should include a thorough history and mental status examination. It is critical to determine what particular individual characteristics in the child the parent needs to understand and respond to. A child with a mental or developmental disorder will present special challenges to the parent, in both advocacy for treatment and special education and socialization. In order to appreciate the nature and depth of those challenges, the assessment of the child needs to note the child's overall cognitive and emotional functioning and any special concerns regarding discipline that may arise, such as with an impulse control problem or a disruptive behavior disorder.

Children who have experienced trauma present additional challenges to the assessment process. Beyond the issues of the specific nature of abuse or neglect a child may have experienced (which will be addressed below), the assessment needs to understand the child's emotional response to the trauma in order to appreciate what parental response will be most important for the child's recovery. If the child has suffered abuse or neglect by the parent in question, the assessment needs to take a careful account of the child's emotional reaction to this abuse. The child may experience continuing high levels of anxiety about the parent, which may be exacerbated simply by being in the parent's presence. Alternatively, the child may experience a strong traumatic attachment to the parent or a sense of having to care for the parent to compensate for the parent's problems. These different emotional responses would call for different responses from a parent to promote the child's well-being.

Fact explorations.   Sometimes the assessment of parental capacity needs to include clinical interviewing of the child in an attempt to clarify the basic fact questions about what sort of abuse or neglect the child may have experienced, and by whom. The technical issues in interviewing children for fact questions are covered in Chapters 14, "Reliability and Suggestibility of Children's Statements," and 15, "Interviewing Children for Suspected Sexual Abuse." Key elements include establishing a supportive but objective relationship; encouraging the child to communicate without a sense of pressure; avoiding specific leading questions; asking open questions, which encourage the child to describe his experience in his own terms; asking clarifying questions; and asking more specific questions if needed, recognizing that the more specific and leading the questions, the less reliable the child's account will be, both legally and clinically.

Specific issues regarding parental functioning. In addition to specific fact questions concerning the child's abuse history, the interview of the child can address other aspects of the child's relationship with the parent that may be relevant to parental functioning. The consultant can ask the child general questions similar to those asked of the parent, regarding favorite events, special times, problems in the relationship with the parent, and daily routines, as a way to gain general information on the quality of the parent-child relationship. Appropriate questions concerning discipline include asking the child about what rules apply in the family and what specific rewards and punishments (if any) apply to various behaviors. The child can also provide information about the parent's role in helping with schoolwork, with daily tasks, and with other cognitive learning.

Medical and Psychological Tests

Medical.   In cases in which clinical assessment suggests that medical or neurological problems may be contributing to parent incapacity, it may be helpful to undertake specific testing to clarify the diagnostic issues. Tests of blood cell counts, thyroid and adrenal function, and other metabolic functions can contribute to the recognition of functional deficits in parental energy and emotional regulation that may be quite treatable. In rare cases a parent's deterioration in functioning may result from organic brain pathology requiring neurological assessment with special imaging techniques. As with other test results, the results of all such tests need to be made relevant to the specific functioning of the parent; abnormalities should not be understood as significant in themselves without such interpretation.

Psychological.   The uses of psychological testing in forensic assessment are covered extensively in Chapter 6, "Psychological Testing in Child and Adolescent Forensic Evaluations." In assessing parent capacity, it is most important to appreciate the empirical validity of various tests and to ensure that test results are relevant to specific areas of functional strength or deficit. Tests of personality functioning may be especially helpful when a parent is not forthcoming in interviews, but results need to be interpreted cautiously.

Behavioral Observations

The final source of direct clinical assessment of parental capacity is direct behavioral observation of the parent engaged in specific activities in situ.

Home visits.   A visit to the parent's home can provide important information about elements of functioning that may not be otherwise available. Visits provide a more immediate sense of the parent's neighborhood than the consultant might otherwise have and more direct current impressions of the parent's housekeeping capacities than are available from a protective services investigation. How the home is configured may provide some indications of the parent's style and priorities: whether a parent has made provisions for privacy in a crowded space provides some information as to the parent's respect for intergenerational boundaries; whether a child has a quiet space available to do schoolwork tells something about a parent's concern for the child's learning. The specific pictures of family members and others on display in a home can tell something about whom the parents care about.

Parent-parent interactions.   When parents live together or otherwise interact significantly with one another around the child, it is important for the assessment to include some direct observation of their interaction with one another. Such observation may be part of ordinary conjoint clinical interviewing, but if the interviewer is too structured or directive in the interview process, then spontaneous interaction between the parents will not be observed. The consultant should be especially interested in what specific attitudes about the child each parent conveys, how each contributes to the conversation with one another, how conflict between them emerges, and whether the parents explore and resolve conflict constructively, ignore it, or build it into more substantial strife. The consultant should be cautious about encouraging conjoint interviewing or other direct observation of parent-parent interaction in situations involving interparental violence (Lerman 1984).

Parent-child interactions.   Direct observation of interaction between the child and the parent can happen in an informal home visit. If the child is in foster care or other out-of-home placement, it can happen at a scheduled parent-child visit.

The consultant should notice as carefully as possible the specific interaction between parent and child. It is more useful in articulating parental functioning to describe how the parent initiates various interchanges and how the parent responds to various behaviors in the child than simply to characterize the interaction as "good" or "warm" or "distant." How do parent and child use the visiting time together? How does the parent structure the time, if at all? How well does the parent notice and respond to cues in the child of the child's feelings and desires?

In attending to the quality of the emotional interaction between parent and child, the consultant should notice how the child and parent initially greet one another and how the interaction develops from there. When a child is initially anxious or cautious about opening up with a parent, the parent may feel hurt and respond in a defensive manner, inhibiting further closeness, or the parent may try to overwhelm the child with exuberant enthusiasm. Sometimes either of these extremes will lead to an overall interaction of consistently poor quality, but sometimes a different initiative by parent or child will succeed in breaking through; it can be helpful in planning further services for the family to notice what seems to work well and what does not in the repertoire of interactions.

It is important to note how well the parent supervises the child. Does the parent simply allow the child to do what the child wants, or does the parent direct the child's activities? Does the parent ensure that the child's behavior is safe, or does the parent seem to miss potentially risky situations, such as infants or toddlers mouthing small objects or climbing on chairs and tables? Does the parent take initiative to teach the child safe and proper behavior? Does the parent use appropriate praise and punishment (such as speaking sharply or giving a brief period of time-out) in response to a child's obvious misbehavior? Noticing and recording such observations can be very important in characterizing interaction generally and, potentially, in documenting changes in interaction that may have developed in response to services (Barnum 1987; Loar 1998).

Parent-professional interactions. It can also be helpful to observe and document interactions between parents and other professionals. Sometimes direct observation of interaction between a parent and an attorney is important in addressing the question of the parent's competence to collaborate with counsel in litigation. Sometimes observation of interaction between a parent and an agency caseworker can help in recognizing deficits in communication, which may be exacerbating their antagonism toward one another.

Investigating Records

The forensic clinician routinely needs to seek a variety of records to provide information about specific allegations of abuse or neglect, and about a parent's overall functioning. Records of the parent's involvement with the court and with a child protection agency, of police and probation contacts, and of a parent's clinical service contacts and clinical records of a child's treatment (including medical care) may yield important information. If a parent is reluctant to authorize release of confidential records, sometimes a court can order their release, if the provider is known, but rules regarding such authority vary depending on the location and on the type of case. If a parent is guarded about this information and succeeds in keeping a past or ongoing treatment involvement secret, it can become a challenge even to learn of it, let alone to obtain a record of it. The evaluator needs to be attentive to clues about a parent's clinical involvements that may be embedded in other available records, to pursue such clues with the parent directly, and to ask for help from the court or referring agency in seeking authority to obtain records from a variety of sources, even if it may not be certain that such records exist. The child's records of medical care, day care, and school functioning can provide important information about the child's functioning, the child's relationship with the parent, and the parent's advocacy abilities on behalf of the child.

Investigative Interviews

In addition to reviewing records, it is often helpful to interview collateral sources to gain important historical information. Commonly, relevant sources include extended family members, foster parents, teachers, agency workers, and other clinical service providers. It can sometimes be helpful to interview neighbors, employers, and other individuals who may have had important contacts with the family, especially if the usual primary investigation services of the court or child protection agency have not included these sources in their initial gathering of information.

The Report

The consultant may be expected to write a report to the referral source at the conclusion of the clinical assessment, detailing findings and providing opinions and recommendations.

General Clinical Data

In presenting the basic clinical history, mental status, and test results (as outlined in Chapter 4, "Introduction to Forensic Evaluations"), the writer should identify the salient clinical observations and document them explicitly, avoiding jargon in favor of ordinary language and clear description.

Specific Data on Parenting Function

A subsequent data section provides the clinical data of most specific relevance to the evaluation. It includes information from others' observations and reports, from parent and child interviews and observations, and from specialized tests, all focused on the specific areas of parental functioning.

A subsection on understanding and advocacy will include the parent's account of how she understands her child's development generally, including, especially, her recognition and understanding of any special characteristics or needs the child may have. It will include an account of how the parent has responded to these needs, from both the parent and from other sources, including her successes and difficulties in relationships with providers of services. The subsection on protection will address specific concerns about the child's safety, including information from the parent and others regarding the parent's recognition of risks in the child's environment and the actions she has (or has not) taken to manage those risks.

The subsections on socialization will include the parent's account (and others') of his support for the child's cognitive development, through appropriate stimulation and teaching at home and through support of the child's school and vocational experiences, as well as accounts of the parent's disciplinary theories and practices. They will include descriptions from the parent and others of the wide range of emotional interactions between parent and child affecting the child's attachment, self-esteem, emotional regulation, social skills, and empathy for others, including accounts of the parent's own emotional functioning that may be relevant to the child's learning in these areas through identification.

Organizing Opinions

The simplest way to offer opinion statements is to solicit clear questions at the time of the referral and to answer them as explicitly as possible. However, child abuse cases tend to be quite complex, and referral questions are not always formulated with sufficient care and attention to the variety of issues in the case. Therefore, it can be helpful to have in mind a detailed vision of what opinions are most often important in child abuse cases, of how they relate to one another, and of how they each specifically inform and are informed by the assessment of parent capacity (Barnum 1997).

Summary of clinical assessment. The first kind of relevant opinion concerns the general diagnostic assessment of the parent. It is often helpful to begin the opinion section of the overall report with a very brief summary of only the salient points of the parent's clinical history, followed by diagnostic opinions regarding the parent's specific areas of clinical disorder, if any. At this point in the report, the clinical diagnostic opinions can stand alone as background, without immediate linkage to the issue of parent capacity; this linkage is addressed in the subsequent opinion sections described below.

The four H's. Each child abuse case tends to raise four discrete questions, either implicitly or explicitly. These are easily remembered as *the four H's:* What happened? What harm did it cause? What help can the parent provide? What hope is there for the future? Most often only one or two of these questions are raised explicitly in the referral for assessment; when the referral is for parenting assessment, the explicit question raised is the third H, that is, what is the parent's current capacity to provide appropriate care for the child? Even when the referral question is explicit and limited to assessment of parent capacity, it is valuable for the consultant to attend routinely to each of the four questions, because how one understands the parent's capacity can be critically affected by how one understands the facts of the case and

the child's condition (the first two H's). Furthermore, in many child abuse cases the assessment of parental capacity is most useful when it includes consideration of prognostic issues and treatment recommendations (the fourth H).

1. What happened? This question concerns the facts of the alleged abuse and neglect. In many cases there may be little or no dispute as to what actually happened to bring the case to the attention of an agency or court. In some cases, however, there may be very serious dispute as to whether there was any abuse or neglect at all, and if there was, by whom. Cases of alleged sexual abuse of young children, of some physical abuse, and of disputes regarding parental overinvolvement in a child's medical or psychiatric care (Meadow 1982) are all situations in which the most critical issue in the case tends to be who did what to whom.

The consultant may be entirely unable to answer this question, because adequate information is not available, because evidence is in dispute and the consultant is not a fact finder, or simply because the scope of the requested evaluation does not include the sort of investigation that would be required to develop adequate information to determine what happened. But it is always helpful for the consultant addressing parental capacity to pay some heed to what is known about what happened to the child as background to any opinion regarding parental capacity, because disputes or uncertainty as to the parent's involvement in the original instance of abuse or neglect may be absolutely critical to appreciating the parent's current capacity. If the parent did abuse the child, then it is reasonable to demand that some elements in the parent's functioning change; however, this demand may not be so reasonable if the facts of the abuse are unclear.

2. What harm did it cause? This question concerns the harm done to the child by the alleged abuse or neglect. Even if it is clear that a child has suffered from abuse or neglect, there can be quite substantial variation among children in how seriously they are damaged by it (Rutter 1983). The extent and nature of emotional injury suffered by the child can be a critical factor in determining the parent's capacity to care for the child, as it will likely affect the child's overall condition and special needs, and thus, the particular skills required of the parent in caring for the child. In the case of a child with multiple problems that may have preexisted the abuse, the issue is complicated by the problem of determining how much of the child's difficulty could have been expected to develop spontaneously without the abuse, and how much of it may stem more or less directly from the abuse itself.

3. What help can the parent provide? This opinion statement is the focus of the assessment of parental capacity: What is the parent's current ability to provide adequate care for the child? Obviously this opinion cannot be stated as a simple overall approval or disapproval of the parent's capacity for two reasons: First, the issue of whether the parent's capacity is ultimately good enough is a value question that is beyond the consultant's expertise, as detailed further below. Second, as the analysis of parental functioning provided here explains, parental capacity is not a unitary concept but instead involves a variety of different functions, which may vary quite independently of one another.

The appropriate expression of opinion in this section on parental capacity involves summarizing the salient findings from the previous sections describing specific parental functions and then offering opinions regarding the nature and extent of particular strengths or weaknesses that these findings indicate. It is then appropriate to address the issue of whether this specific constellation of strengths and weaknesses would put a child (in that parent's care) at risk of further abuse or neglect. The consultant should be as explicit as possible in characterizing the particular type of apparent risk (such as physical abuse, neglect, emotional harm, or sexual abuse) and how it might be expected to arise in specific relation to the articulated parental deficits. Ideally, the consultant can also be explicit in characterizing the level of risk, the specific precipitating factors that would tend to activate the risk, and the degree of certainty with which the consultant's opinion is held.

4. What hope is there for the future? (prognosis and clinical recommendations) This final opinion statement concerns the parent's prognosis for improvement. Articulating treatment needs and expectations is critical for service planning, and opinions as to a parent's prognosis for relapse or other future deterioration can be a relevant issue in determining current fitness (Barnum et al. 1998). Opinions in this section should draw on the summary of the parent's clinical condition and on the opinions regarding specific functional deficits and risk situations in the previous section. To the extent that parenting deficits and risks are linked to a specific disorder in the parent for which treatment might be effective in improving function and reducing risk, it is of critical importance to articulate that linkage and to offer frank prognostic opinions regarding the extent to which treatment may realistically be expected to make a difference (Rogers and Webster 1989). In reaching this opinion the consultant should attend to 1) what is known empirically about the likely success of specific treatments for the parent's

particular disorders, 2) the parent's history of past treatment involvement, noting both successes and failures, 3) the parent's current recognition of the disorder and motivation for treatment (including consideration of any changes in these states from the past), and 4) issues of realistic access to adequate treatment, including availability of appropriate treatment, funding, transportation, and language and cultural matching. If the parent's disorder is not likely to respond to treatment, the consultant should note this and explain why. If the nature of the parent's deficit is not closely linked to a clinical disorder but instead reflects educational disadvantage (such as a lack of knowledge of ordinary child development or medical problems) or social problems (such as homelessness, poverty, or domestic violence victimization), the consultant should articulate this point and may offer suggestions about other services that may be appropriate and helpful.

PITFALLS

Dealing With Ambiguous Facts

As in any forensic evaluation, the facts on which the parenting evaluation rests are critical to its validity. Ambiguous or disputed facts usually concern the question of what abuse or neglect actually took place, uncertain details of clinical history, and varying third-party impressions of the parent's functioning. The consultant should take care to consider all the available information and may offer an opinion as to how it is most reasonable to understand inconsistencies in clinical data. However, the consultant should generally avoid explicit fact-finding unless he or she is specifically authorized by the referral source to reach and offer opinions on facts.

Staying Within Expertise

It is essential that the consultant understand that the overall issues addressed by courts and protective services agencies are broader than issues of diagnostic assessment, treatment, and prognosis. Issues of balancing children's and parents' rights, determining the relative moral and social value of one approach to parenting compared with another, and deciding what level and what type of risk to children may or may not be acceptable are basic issues of law and social policy, which are outside the expertise of the consultant. The consultant should avoid expressing personal opinion on these issues of social policy in a form that may be mistaken for an expert opinion (Melton et al. 1987).

Articulating Recommendations as Clinical Prognoses

In making recommendations, the consultant needs to be aware of the competing interests in the case and of the basic questions of social policy and value at stake. The consultant may undermine his or her own credibility as an expert by appearing to reach beyond appropriate clinical opinions to offer global recommendations for resolving a case. The consultant may be more successful in staying within the role of expert by offering opinions in the form of prognostic statements regarding likely outcomes of different actions rather than in the form of global recommendations. For example, it may be more successful to say, "Given this parent's specific strengths and weakness as described here, and his favorable prognosis for treatment, the risk of long-term harm to this infant will likely be greater if the child remains in foster care than if he is returned to the parent," than to offer the blanket recommendation, "This child should be returned to the parent."

Specific Legal Questions

Finally, ideally the consultant should be aware of the local laws and regulations governing child abuse and neglect matters and should try to determine at the time of referral whether there are specific legal findings at issue. Potential findings include determinations of parental fitness according to specific factors that may be articulated by statute or case law or of what treatment services might constitute "reasonable efforts" to make in trying to return a child to a parent's custody (McCarthy et al. 1999). When such specific issues are at stake, the consultant is far more useful (and may have a much less complicated assessment to perform) if those issues are made clear at the start and if the assessment focuses on addressing them.

CASE EXAMPLE EPILOGUES

Case Example 1

The court temporarily awarded custody of the child to the agency but referred the case for clinical evaluation to a bilingual psychiatrist from Central America. The psychiatrist enabled Ms. Alvarez to recount her traumatic experiences of immigration and her symptoms of postpartum depression and helped her to engage in treatment supported by the agency. Her condition improved substantially with the help of treatment and encouragement for her developing

social supports, with specific improvements in energy, warmth, and relatedness with the baby observed at visits. The child was returned to her care after 3 months.

Case Example 2

Clinical evaluation of Mr. Brown found a history of neglect by his family in childhood and experiences of abuse when he was in foster care; mild mental retardation along with a somewhat guarded interactional style, but no other clear psychopathology, and close and caring relationships with each of the three children. Observation of Mr. Brown's interaction with the agency caseworker noted the worker's rapid, brusque manner and the elaboration of complex tasks in the service plan, which Mr. Brown did not understand. Articulation of Mr. Brown's cognition and background along with specific recommendations for communicating in a simpler and more supportive style led to some improvement in the relationship between Mr. Brown and the agency, and marginal improvements in service compliance. The clinician could not make an ultimate recommendation as to custody but was able to articulate expectations regarding the children's likely progress 1) if they remained in foster care or 2) if they returned to Mr. Brown. The court took those expectations into account in its ruling on custody.

Case Example 3

Ms. Green maintained visiting contact with her child, but the child showed increasing anxiety at visiting times, withdrew from her mother, and showed more anxiety and regressed dependence with her foster mother, who hoped to adopt her. Careful evaluation of parental functioning showed that Ms. Green related well with her child at visits, but also found her continuing to be vulnerable to emotional disorganization. The consultant noted that her child had developed a strong bond with the foster mother, and averred that Ms. Green would not be able to respond successfully to the emotional harm her child would experience if separated from the foster mother. The legal standard in the case allowed the court to find Ms. Green unfit on this basis, and her child was adopted by the foster mother.

ACTION GUIDELINES

A. Establish the context and question(s).

1. Identify referral source; clarify and negotiate referral question(s).
2. Establish the expected database for the clinical evaluation.
3. Understand the legal issues and standard(s).

B. Conduct the evaluation.

 1. Obtain existing records.
 2. Meet with parent(s):
    a. Establish expectations about confidentiality, dissemination, and legal use.
    b. Establish comfortable and valid communication.
 3. Obtain additional records.
 4. Meet with children and others, if indicated.
 5. Arrange for specialized testing, if indicated.
 6. Observe visits and home when possible.

C. Report findings, opinions, and recommendations.

 1. Gather documents, notes, tapes, and other sources.
 2. Write up clinical and forensic data sections.
 3. Review what you have written, and write a clinical summary.
 4. Write opinions:
    a. Answer referral question(s).
    b. Address the 4 H's.
    c. Avoid fact-finding and nonclinical recommendations when possible.

REFERENCES

Barnum R: Understanding controversies in visitation. J Am Acad Child Adolesc Psychiatry 26:788–792, 1987

Barnum R: Managing risk and confidentiality in clinical encounters with children and families, in Confidentiality and the Duty to Protect: Foreseeable Harm in the Practice of Psychiatry. Edited by Beck J. Washington, DC, American Psychiatric Press, 1990a, pp 77–105

Barnum R: Self incrimination and denial in the juvenile transfer evaluation. Bulletin of the American Academy of Psychiatry and the Law 18:413–428, 1990b

Barnum R: A suggested framework for forensic consultation in cases of child abuse and neglect. Journal of the American Academy of Psychiatry and the Law 25:581–594, 1997

Barnum R, Kinscherff R, Ayoub C, et al: Implications of changes in child abuse laws for forensic mental health consultation to courts, in Guardian ad Litem Practice in Probate and Juvenile Courts: An Interdisciplinary Approach. Boston, MA, Suffolk University Law School, 1998, pp 417–426

Beardslee WR, Wheelock I: Children of parents with affective disorders: empirical findings and clinical implications, in Handbook of Depression in Children and Adolescents. Edited by Reynolds WM, Johnston HF. New York, Plenum, 1994, pp 463–479

Bryer JB, Nelson BA, Miller JB: Childhood sexual and physical abuse as factors in adult psychiatric illness. Am J Psychiatry 144:1426–1430, 1987

Cicchetti D, Toth SL: A developmental psychopathology perspective on child abuse and neglect. J Am Acad Child Adolesc Psychiatry 34:541–565, 1995

Dowdney L, Skuse D: Parenting provided by adults with mental retardation. J Child Psychol Psychiatry 34:25–47, 1993

Egeland B, Jacobvitz D, Sroufe LA: Breaking the cycle of abuse. Child Dev 59:1080–1088, 1988

Emery RE: Interparental conflict and the children of discord and divorce. Psychol Bull 92:310–330, 1982

Famularo R, Kinscherff R, Fenton T: Parental substance abuse and the nature of child maltreatment. Child Abuse Negl 16:475–483, 1992

Famularo R, Fenton T, Kinscherff R, et al: Maternal and child post-traumatic stress disorder in cases of child maltreatment. Child Abuse Negl 18:27–36, 1994

Farrington DP, Hawkins JD: Predicting participation, early onset and later persistence in officially recorded offending. Criminal Behavior and Mental Health 1:1–33, 1991

Feldman MA: Research on parenting by mentally retarded persons. Psychiatr Clin North Am 9:777–796, 1986

Field T, Healy B, Goldstein S, et al: Behavior-state matching and synchrony in mother-infant interactions of nondepressed versus depressed dyads. Dev Psychol 26:7–14, 1990

Goodman SH, Adamson LB, Riniti J, et al: Mothers' expressed attitudes: associations with maternal depression and children's self-esteem and psychopathology. J Am Acad Child Adolesc Psychiatry 33:1265–1274, 1994

Hawley TL, Halle TG, Drasin RE, et al: Children of addicted mothers: effects of the crack epidemic on the caregiving environment and the development of preschoolers. Am J Orthopsychiatry 65:364–379, 1995

Herman JL, Perry JC, van der Kolk BA: Childhood trauma in borderline personality disorder. Am J Psychiatry 146:490–495, 1989

Jaffe PG, Wolfe DA, Wilson SK: Children of Battered Women. Newbury Park, CA, Sage, 1990

Kamerman S, Kahn A: Social Services for Children, Youth and Families in the United States. Greenwich, CT, Annie B. Casey Foundation, 1989

Kumar RC: "Anybody's child": severe disorders of mother-to-infant bonding. Br J Psychiatry 171:175–181, 1997

Lerman LG: Mediation of wife abuse cases: the adverse impact of informal dispute resolution on women. Harvard Women's Law Journal 1:57–113, 1984

Levinger J: Patterns of parenthood as theories of learning, in Families in Transition. Edited by Skolnick A, Skolnick J. Boston, MA, Little, Brown, 1971, pp 342–346

Loar L: Making visits work. Child Welfare 77:41–58, 1998

Loeber R, Dishion RJ: Early predictors of male delinquency: a review. Psychol Bull 94:68–99, 1983

Main M, Goldwyn R: Predicting rejecting of her infant from mother's representation of her own experience: implications for the abused-abusing intergenerational cycle. Child Abuse Negl 8:203–217, 1984

Mayer J, Black R: Child abuse and neglect in families with an alcohol- or opiate-addicted parent. Child Abuse Negl 1:85–98, 1977

McCarthy J, Myers J, Jackson V: The Adoption and Safe Families Act: Exploring the Opportunity for Collaboration Between Child Mental Health and Child Welfare Service Systems. Washington, DC, National Technical Assistance Center for Children's Mental Health, Georgetown University, 1999

Meadow R: Munchausen syndrome by proxy. Arch Dis Child 57:92–98, 1982

Melton GB, Petrila J, Poythress NG, et al: Psychological Evaluations for the Courts. New York, Guilford, 1987

Minde K: Bonding and attachment: its relevance for the present-day clinician. Dev Med Child Neurol 28:803–806, 1986

Murphy JM, Jellinek M, Quinn D, et al: Substance abuse and serious child maltreatment: prevalence, risk, and outcome in a court sample. Child Abuse Negl 15:197–211, 1991

National Research Council Panel on Research on Child Abuse and Neglect: Understanding Child Abuse and Neglect. Washington, DC, National Academy Press, 1993

Patterson GR, Stouthamer-Loeber M: The correlation of family management practices and delinquency. Child Dev 55(4):1299–1307, 1984

Patterson GR, DeBaryshe BD, Ramsey EA: A developmental perspective on antisocial behavior (Special Issue: Children and Their Development: Knowledge Base, Research Agenda, and Social Policy Application). Am Psychol 44(2):329–335, 1989

Quinn KM, Nye SG: Termination of parental rights, in Handbook of Psychiatric Practice in the Juvenile Court. Edited by Kalogerakis MG. Washington, DC, American Psychiatric Press, 1992

Regan DO, Erlich SM, Finnegan LP: Infants of drug addicts: at risk for child abuse, neglect, and placement in foster care. Journal of Neurotoxicology and Teratology 9:315–319, 1987

Reich W, Earls F, Powell J: A comparison of the home and social environments of children of alcoholic and non-alcoholic parents. British Journal of Addiction 83:831–839, 1988

Rogers R, Webster CD: Assessing treatability in mentally disordered offenders. Law Hum Behav 13:19–29, 1989

Rojo-Moreno J, Valdemoro C, Garcia-Merita ML, et al: Analysis of the attitudes and emotional processes in couples undergoing artificial insemination by donor. Hum Reprod 11:294–299, 1996

Rutter M: Stress, coping, and development: some issues and some questions, in Stress, Coping and Development in Children. Edited by Garmezy N, Rutter M. New York, McGraw-Hill, 1983, pp 1–41

Rutter M: Intergenerational continuities and discontinuities in serious parenting difficulties, in Child Maltreatment. Edited by Cicchetti D, Carlson V. New York, Cambridge University Press, 1989, pp 317–348

Snyder J, Patterson GR: The effects of consequences on patterns of social interaction: a quasi-experimental approach to reinforcement in natural interaction. Child Dev 57(5):1257–1268, 1986

Teti DM, Gelfand DM, Messinger DS, et al: Maternal depression and the quality of early attachment: an examination of infants, preschoolers, and their mothers. Dev Psychol 31:364–376, 1995

Wahler RG: The multiply entrapped parent: obstacles to change in parent-child problems. Advances in Family Intervention, Assessment, and Theory 1:29–52, 1980

Webster-Stratton C, Hammond M: Maternal depression and its relationship to life stress, perceptions of child behavior problems, parenting behavior, and child conduct problems. J Abnorm Child Psychol 16:299–315, 1988

Weissman M, Prusoff B, Gammon G, et al: Psychopathology in the children (ages 6–18) of depressed and normal parents. J Am Acad Child Adolesc Psychiatry 23:78–84, 1984

West MO, Prinz RJ: Parental alcoholism and childhood psychopathology. Psychol Bull 102:204–218, 1987

Wolfe D, Reppucci ND, Hart S: Child abuse prevention: knowledge and priorities. J Clin Child Psychol 24(suppl):5–22, 1995

Zuravin SJ: Severity of maternal depression and three types of mother-to-child aggression. Am J Orthopsychiatry 59:377–389, 1989

CHAPTER 10

Foster Care and Adoption

Saul Wasserman, M.D.
Alvin Rosenfeld, M.D.
Steven Nickman, M.D.

Case Example 1

Roberto, a 13-year-old foster child who had regular visits with his biological mother, had a tenuous adaptation in his foster home. The foster parents noticed that the child's behavior and attitude seemed worse after each visit, with more talk about "getting high" and more resistance to the foster parent's authority. For that reason, they asked that visits with the biological parent be limited. The court asked for a forensic consultation.

Case Example 2

A clinician is asked by the court to "evaluate the needs" of Tran, an extremely hyperactive and anxious 6-year-old who, because of extensive physical abuse, was recently placed in a foster home.

Information about the child's family history and development is sketchy. Developmental assessment reveals that the child is 6 months to a year behind, with scattered abilities and deficiencies. Play and drawing reveal a preoccupation with themes of aggression, violence, and loss. The child meets the criteria for an attentional disorder, as well as an adjustment disorder with anxiety, and probably a posttraumatic stress disorder.

The biological mother refuses to participate in the consultation. In a phone call she says that the child has no problem that wouldn't be solved by being returned to her. She strongly opposes medication for her son and said she will sue the psychiatrist if he gives the child Ritalin because she was sure it "would stunt his growth."

LEGAL ISSUES

Entering Foster Care

Today, becoming a foster child usually begins with an allegation of abuse or neglect that triggers an investigation to determine whether the accusation is valid. Even if it is not, the process distresses the family substantially. If the abused child is considered to be in significant danger, child welfare professionals, often in consultation with a clinician, must assess the family's capacity to prevent future mistreatment. If they feel the child cannot be protected in the home, they submit a report to the court. When a child is to be placed in a foster home for more than immediate protection, a judge must sift through contradictory data and competing arguments—assessing the potential benefits and harms that occur when a child is removed from her or his biological parents' care—and must ultimately decide the family's fate.

Agency Response

Being accused of child abuse or neglect is a highly personal, distressing event in any individual's life that deserves careful investigation. Yet in most localities the system is not set up that way. Usually overworked and underfunded, child protective agencies are high-volume operations. Referrals range from life-threatening situations to trivial reports made by uncertain, anxious, mandated reporters. With so many cases and so much at stake, agencies must concentrate their efforts on seemingly severe cases. Generally speaking, the more immediate the situation, the more serious the danger to the child, and the more reliable the reporter, the higher the likelihood that the report will receive immediate attention. Most other reports are simply filed, with little or no action taken.

Investigation may be difficult because families give widely fluctuating degrees of cooperation to the investigative process. Few take kindly to a social worker appearing at the door, implicitly threatening to take away their child. Mistreating a child is a crime, and the police are frequently involved. Families being investigated often see the child welfare worker as a punitive, accusatory agent of social control. Furthermore, many workers' training is spotty: the field investigator charged with a very serious statutory responsibility that requires interviewing skills, considerable knowledge, and the ability to make subtle distinctions and difficult judgments may not even have a bachelor's degree.

Gathering information in these tense situations is hard, time-consuming, and may require tenacity. The simplest task may be complicated. For instance, in some localities just accessing internal agency records may be difficult. Families move frequently, change their names, and their records can be scattered across several jurisdictions. Assembling school, police, and physician reports, interviewing relatives, teachers, and such all takes time, sophistication, and effort, which may not be available in a particular case. Relying on children for valid information is also fraught with difficulty as discussed in Chapters 14, "Reliability and Suggestibility of Children's Statements," and 15, "Interviewing Children for Suspected Sexual Abuse."

If the investigating social worker fears that the child cannot be protected with voluntary services, the child is likely to be removed from the home, at least temporarily, and placed with relatives or a temporary foster family or in a children's shelter. The matter is then forwarded to the court for a formal hearing.

Emergency Placements

A child can be removed from a home by a social worker or by the police based on "reasonable cause" to believe a child is abused or neglected. When a child is removed from a family on an emergency basis, the agency must follow a relatively strict timeline. Some form of probable cause hearing, which provides preliminary court oversight, must be held quickly, usually within a few days of removal. Parents have a right to counsel and often try to persuade the hearing officer that the child should be returned home immediately. In practice this rarely happens before a fuller hearing, usually called an *adjudication hearing*, which occurs later and in which the court must decide whether the state should establish temporary custody over the child. The legal standard for removal is "clear and convincing evidence." If the child is adjudicated "a dependent of the court," a dispositional hearing is held to decide where the child should be placed.

Balancing Rights of Children and Parents

In passing child abuse and neglect laws, the state assumed responsibility to protect children from serious mistreatment. The child's right to physical safety and parental care must be balanced with the parent's right to be free of state intrusion. By mandating increasingly formal judicial review as the government intrudes more deeply into the family's situation, the process aims to give workers the flexibility to protect children while simultaneously protecting parents' rights.

Reunification Plans

If the child is in foster care involuntarily, the agency must make "reasonable efforts" to help the parents remedy whatever issues led to mistreatment and placement. This *reunification plan* might include substance abuse treatment for the parent, social services to prevent homelessness, mental health treatment, parent education through parenting classes, or some sort of training in anger management. Some responsible experts argue that more needs to be done to empower biological families; others insist that "reasonable efforts" have become extraordinary (Washington Social Legislation Bulletin 1996).

Hearing at 6 Months

When a child is removed from a biological parent's care, the court provides ongoing oversight. Typically, a court hearing, held 6 months after removal, reevaluates the situation. If the biological parent demonstrates an improved capability to parent, the judge may return the child and close the case. Conversely, if the parent has not complied with the plan, the child may remain in foster care for another 6 months. If within 12 months the parent has still not complied with the reunification plan to the court's satisfaction, the agency begins permanency planning. In extreme circumstances, or for some young children, this process may be accelerated. Recent federal law emphasizes the need for children to be in permanent settings after 18 months in the state's care. So when a parent is not likely to improve, their rights are legally terminated, freeing the child for adoption.

The state prefers that parents rehabilitate themselves, but it recognizes the need to provide permanency in the child's life, both because the child needs it developmentally and because state rehabilitative resources are limited. Although there are conceptual criticisms of the child protective services and welfare systems, their difficulties are more in practice than with their theoretical designs.

Judge's Dilemma

A child who lives in an abusive or neglectful home risks suffering physical and/or psychological injury that will have long-term negative sequelae. But the United States has a basic principle that families deserve privacy in all but exceptional circumstances. Furthermore, by our nature as primates, children and parents are emotionally attached, even if this attachment demands considerable distortion for the child to fit into a pathological family. In most cases, breaking this attachment causes severe distress and potential long-term psychological injury.

In effect, the judge reviewing a particular case frequently has to choose between two unappealing alternatives and has to select the less detrimental one (Wasserman and Rosenfeld 1985). The first is leaving the child in a home in which he or she is being mistreated. The second is placing the child in an overburdened system that may not respond to the child's specific needs. In fact, a seriously abused or neglected child placed in foster care is likely to grow up in a safer, more hospitable environment. Removing the child, or even threatening removal, may serve as a wake-up call to a parent(s) to make a significant change in lifestyle. Sometimes placing the child frees parents from the daily responsibilities of parenting and allows them the time and energy to focus on making needed changes. Yet foster care has significant negatives. Besides the distress associated with breaking the parent-child bond, the foster system may also not offer the child very good alternatives (Rosenfeld et al. 1998). We will briefly review the history of American foster care to understand why this is.

CHILDREN IN FOSTER CARE

Changing Face of Foster Care

The American foster care system has about 500,000 children and adolescents living in it. Foster care had originally been provided through private charities founded by or working with religious groups. In the late nineteenth century, governmental agencies began to assume responsibility for children who could not live with their parents. In 1909, the first White House Conference on Children codified this system, which served the country until the 1960s. At that first conference, and during each succeeding generation, a debate raged about whether it is best to try to provide services that solidify a shaky home or place the child in a more "wholesome" situation.

After Kempe and colleagues' 1962 article, "The Battered Child Syndrome," legislation was enacted that mandated reporting child abuse. Child welfare agencies were empowered to forcibly remove children from abusive homes. The placement of choice, primarily because no better one seemed available, was foster care; a system designed 100 years earlier for voluntary placements. It was unprepared for the influx of large numbers of abused and neglected children. Inadvertently, foster care became an involuntary system (Rosenfeld et al. 1998). The children entering care differed from the traditional foster care population; often they had experienced much more early deprivation and abuse and were less securely attached, or attached in more pathological ways than in the past. Both the volume and severity of the children's pathology rapidly overwhelmed the system. Furthermore, over time children were staying in care longer. Average stays were approximately 5 years (Fanshel 1978).

Sound research suggested that long stays without a permanent commitment were detrimental to children's healthy development. During World War II, Anna Freud (Freud and Burlingham 1944) and others had observed that children separated from their families could be damaged emotionally, even when placement made them safer physically. After the war, Bowlby (1966), Spitz (1945), and others published well-done empirical research that documented how important good attachment was for normal development. A foster system that cared for infants impersonally, in large institutions, and that moved children around frequently seemed likely to interfere with the bonding process and psychological health.

In 1980, to stop children from moving from one foster home to another, the federal government enacted legislation to promote permanent placements (Fialkov 1988). Public Law 96-272 emphasized stabilizing biological families. It mandated "reasonable efforts" be made to help the biological family improve so that a child would not need to be removed or could safely return home. But if the family made insufficient progress after a year, the social worker needed to start making alternative plans to give the foster child a stable, long-term living situation. After 18 months of foster care, a social worker could petition the court to terminate parental rights, freeing the child for adoption or guardianship status.

Initially this effort seemed successful. From 1977 to 1982, the foster care population declined from 502,000 to 243,000 (Fein 1991). Experts felt that foster care for all but a relatively small number of children would soon be a thing of the past. In the 1980s, preventive services were cut back. Few were perceptive enough to realize that Reagan-era social policy combined with the then-growing explosion in substance abuse (including crack cocaine), homelessness, and HIV would lead to an increased need for placements. The population in foster care soared in the late 1980s. By 1993, the foster care population had almost doubled. The system was again badly overloaded.

Problems of Foster Children

Numerous studies have documented that a high percentage of children currently in care have significant physical and/or psychological difficulties (Dale et al. 1999; Halfon et al. 1992, 1995; Pilowsky 1995; Simms 1989). In Simms's study, 60% of the children had developmental delays, 35% had a chronic medical problem, 15% had a birth defect, 15% were of a short stature (suggestive of physical growth delays), 12% had no routine health care, 34% were not properly immunized, and 32% continued to have unmet health needs after placement. Study after study has documented that the foster care population is a very damaged group. In addition to being far more likely to have chronic medical conditions, children in foster care weigh significantly less, are significantly shorter than the general population, require a significant amount of medical subspecialty care, have a high incidence of developmental delays, have major deficits in adaptive behavior, and have a high number of behavioral problems (Hochstadt et al. 1987).

The situation for infants is of particular concern. Despite good evidence that infants and young children are uniquely vulnerable to the medical and psychosocial hazards of institutional care, such as increased risk of serious infectious illness and delayed language development (Frank et al. 1996), infants and very young children still spend extended periods of time in shelters.

Although the child welfare system tries to abide by the principle that poverty alone should not be a reason for a child to be removed from a family, in practice the overwhelming number of child welfare families are poor. A national study (Lindsey 1991) found that parents' inadequate income, *not how severely the child had been abused*, best predicted whether a child is placed in foster care rather than the family receiving supportive services.

Kinship Care

When the foster care population increased dramatically in the late 1980s, skilled homes were scarce so children were placed with biological relatives who became their legal foster parents. *Kinship care* became a legal alternative that grew dramatically more prevalent when several courts ruled that if a child's relatives fostered the child, they were entitled to receive the same financial benefits as unrelated foster families. The number of children in such placements mushroomed. By 1991, over 40% of foster homes in New York City were kinship foster homes (Child Welfare League of America 1994).

Kinship care has some obvious benefits, such as the likelihood of cultural and geographic proximity, blood ties, the option of greater personal involvement by the foster parent, the possibility that the biological parent will be more accepting of the placement, and the hope that the child can build on an preexisting personal relationship with the related foster parent.

At the same time, kinship care can have its own set of difficulties. Children in kinship care still show a significant incidence of mental health problems (Dubowitz et al. 1993). Grandparents are frequently elderly and have their own health problems. Sometimes biological parents and fostering relatives have ongoing conflicts. Often fostering grandparents have their own goals, such as the hope that the responsibility of child rearing may contribute to a biological parent's rehabilitation. Some argue that the grandparents who raised the dysfunctional parent are likely to be deficient as parents to the next generation. Unfortunately, as kinship care became the preferred form of fostering, child welfare agencies sometimes sought out relatives whether or not they had an emotional tie to, or even personal familiarity with, the child. In actual practice, kinship homes are less thoroughly monitored and supervised than conventional foster homes, which can diminish the extent to which they protect and nurture children.

Advantages and Disadvantages of Foster Care

Parenting foster children is not easy. Foster children have a threefold greater risk of maltreatment in their foster home in comparison to the general population and a sevenfold increase in risk for physical abuse (Benedict et al. 1994). Yet in spite of the problems, fairly good empirical evidence indicates that foster care, overall, convenes some benefits (Fanshel 1978; Fein 1991; Wald et al. 1988). Children entering foster care are often small for their age yet show gains in growth in the first year of care that do not appear to be simply nutritionally related (Wyatt et al. 1997). The delinquency rate for children in foster care is roughly similar to a group of maltreated children who were not removed (Runyan and Gould

1985). A study of the long-term outcome of children who had spent at least 5 years in foster care and are now grown up found that 56% of the children were considered well integrated socially, 12% had an average integration, 20% were considered partially integrated, and 10% were in situations of failure. Multiple family disturbances and repeated traumatic experiences in childhood increased risk (Dumaret et al. 1997).

For many years, family preservation has been advocated partly out of the belief that no one cares as much as the child's own parents. Proponents argue that leaving a child in the home and offering intensive remedial services is a far better alternative than foster care, but this has yet to be proven empirically. Some research indicates that leaving the child in the home with intensive family preservation services is not always the best solution. Eight of 10 studies of such services show no reduction in out-of-home placement for children at risk (Heneghan et al. 1996). Furthermore, it has been argued that when children are in need of a permanent substitute family, such adoptive placements are much more successful when they occur as early in the child's life as possible.

Adolescents in Need of Placement

The law distinguishes between children who are abused or neglected and older children, usually teenagers, who are in conflict with their parents. This adolescent population may be called *beyond control, chronic runaway*, or *PINS*—person in need of supervision. Most observers agree that the foster care system, which is focused around at-risk *children* who are usually dependent and thus submissive to adult authority, does not work well with rebellious, oppositional teenagers. In the last 20 years, services for this population, whose needs lie between child welfare, juvenile justice, and mental health, have been cut back markedly despite the sense that programs designed for this group may be effective and valuable. In a family-centered diagnostic assessment program for PINS, placement in short-term foster homes combined with outreach efforts to engage families in counseling led to a sharp reduction in the number of youths needing institutional placement (Kagan et al. 1987).

Children in Foster Care

Child's Experience of Removal

The removal process, which has been likened to emergency surgery (Rosenfeld et al. 1998), is usually quite disruptive for the child. Most children coming into care are removed from their homes suddenly and are confused and frightened. The child may have no opportunity to even take treasured possessions, such as a pillow, a stuffed bear, and photographs of loved ones, into care. The social worker may not make time to explain the process and allay the child's fears. For a child who cannot move immediately into a familiar and loving relative's care, coming into care means being forced to live with strangers, hopefully ones who are sympathetic to the child and have a nurturing, organized home. The child may find himself in a new school and may have very limited contact with parents. Less fortunate children are placed in children's shelters, some of which are homelike but which are more likely to be institutional. Older children, many of whom have spent long periods of time in shelters, may harshly introduce younger children into street life.

Physical and Medical Needs

Foster children frequently have not had basic medical and dental care. Immunization records may be incomplete and vaccinations nonexistent; growth charts and critical medical information, such as drug sensitivities, may be unavailable. If a child moves from one foster home to a new foster home, medical records may not follow. In response, some localities have pioneered medical passports, which move with the child and carry information that is available to new foster parents and physicians.

Because a foster child's medical bills are typically paid through Medicaid, which has low reimbursement rates and onerous practices, competent physicians may be unwilling to treat these children. For this reason, some regions have established special clinics where foster children have ongoing relationships with a treatment team.

Educational Issues

Many foster children have attended school erratically and performed marginally. Placement in a foster home may give children a parenting figure who makes sure that she attends school daily, is well fed, and is ready to learn. Some children have neurological and/or psychiatric problems that contribute to their learning difficulties. Often, mistreating parents have not been willing or able to cooperate with the school to evaluate these needs. Clinicians who are already used to working cooperatively with teachers and parents can help foster parents, social workers, and teachers develop a good educational plan for the child. This is especially important in situations in which children present with a mixed pattern of cognitive, developmental, and emotional difficulties.

Emotional Issues

Given the amount of stress foster children have had and are experiencing, they may temporarily regress. Their personal issues are compounded by the reality that they, by definition, have not come from normal homes. Thus, the stresses each child experiences, and the way in which each reacts to care, are influenced by his or her previous experience (Rosenfeld and Wasserman 1990). Some may become withdrawn, enuretic, and depressed; others may become irritable, explosive, or aggressive. A neglected child used to considerable freedom may find the rules, restrictions, and supervision typical of foster homes too confining. A child from a violent home who has learned to be aggressive for self-protection may quickly employ that strategy to protect personal possessions and space. Children who have grown up as caretakers will worry about their parents' and siblings' well-being. Many children become discouraged and depressed. A few will act out sexually; some threaten suicide (perhaps repeating threats they have heard their parents make), and occasionally, out of desperation and hopelessness, a child will make a serious suicide attempt. More typically though, older ones will run away when pressures mount.

Most foster children will not receive psychotherapy; in fact, the foster homes are conceptualized as the agent of healing. Foster infants and young children may present with a variety of eating, sleeping, mood dyscontrol, and behavioral problems that foster parents are expected to manage. For that reason, several authors have advocated intensive early intervention for infants placed in foster care (Ruff et al. 1990; Zeanah and Larrieu 1998). Foster parents, the main resource to help the child deal with the most pressing emotional issues, vary widely in their ability to understand children's emotional needs and to develop specific, constructive strategies. Most states do not provide much ongoing training or support for foster parents, who need unusual inner and educational resources to deal with difficult children. Some foster parents can be remarkably effective with a highly disturbed child; other foster parents may quickly want to be rid of the problem. Some locales have developed creative ways to help foster parents deal with emotionally troubled children. A common strategy is the use of *therapeutic foster homes*.

Therapeutic foster home care may provide extensive consultation to foster parents, either on a case-by-case basis or through some form of foster parent group. Extra resources such as respite care, family therapy, funds for enrichment programs or staffing, on-call backup to help deal with difficult situations, and in-home support may also be available (Reddy and Pfeiffer 1997; Rosenfeld et al. 1997). Although data are limited and the programs follow different models, this approach is promising.

The Role of Foster Parents

People become foster parents for a variety of reasons. Some are drafted into the role to assist family members in serious trouble; others are motivated by altruistic concerns. Some become foster parents to compensate for their inability to bear biological children and hope that fostering will lead to adoption. A few do it for the money. Just a few decades ago, foster parents were routinely advised not to form a strong attachment to their foster child because the child would eventually return to the biological parents. Even today, foster parents have legitimate reasons to be tentative in their attachment and commitment to the child. On one hand, foster parents have to build a relationship with a child who may stay for only a short time. They must be sensitive to the child's emotional needs and respectful of the child's relationship with the biological parent, without feeling competitive or critical. This is no easy task. Foster parents are treated like the foster care system: Great expectations are placed on them, yet, usually, far too few resources are provided for them to do the job very well.

In the past, many child welfare agencies had a policy of deliberately not giving family foster agencies or foster parents any information about the biological parent, which seems counterproductive. More frequently, today's foster parent is expected to "partner" with the biological parent, not always an easy task. Some foster parents have great difficulty partnering with an abusive, drug-addicted, sometimes violent parent. Others find that their fantasies about the biological parent's awfulness are unfounded, and they feel a sense of identification or kinship with the birth parent.

Visitation With Biological Parents

During the time when biological parents are supposedly working to improve functioning, they are allowed contact with the child, unless a good reason exists to prohibit visitation. This helps preserve the parent-child relationship. Children whose parents have abandoned them often suffer severe psychological scars. Yet visitation can be problematic. For some parents, economic practicalities or lack of transportation may make regular visits hard. Others find visitation painful; it forces them to face personal inadequacies. Some make promises that they cannot fulfill and regularly disappoint their child or do not even show up for a visit. Other parents are too drunk, disturbed, impulsive, or delusional to comply with basic visitation rules. Even under the best circumstances, visitation stirs up psychological issues about the separation; foster parents may see evidence of increased anxiety, such as sleep disturbances, before the visit and anger and sadness afterward.

Consistent parental visitation is the single most powerful predictor that the child ultimately will return to the biological parents' care (Lawder et al. 1986). Foster children whose biological parents visit them regularly exhibit fewer externalizing and internalizing behavior problems (Cantos et al. 1997). Whether this indicates a stronger attachment before removal, and thus a better prognosis, is unclear. A biological parent who visits regularly certainly can help a child maintain a hopeful attitude about reunification and avoid a sense of total abandonment. Visitation may also serve as a source of hope for the biological parent and help reinforce a commitment to a treatment program. Yet under other circumstances, such as the parent who is very unreliable, overpromises, or acts in a way that undercuts the foster parent, visitation may make the child's situation much worse.

Children may regress in connection with parental visits. In those circumstances, clinicians need to assess the child's capacity to handle these visits and to develop a strategy that best suits the child's unique needs. Sometimes the agency needs to go to court to prohibit visitation because it is too disruptive to the child's well-being. It is important to distinguish between regression in response to sadness at leaving an important attachment and regression as a response to previous trauma.

Return Home

In one study, over half of children in foster care returned to their biological parents. Of children who went to what was intended to be a permanent placement, 78% were still there 12 to 18 months later. Most children in permanent placements were functioning well (Fein and Maluccio 1984). A child's return to the biological parents' home does not guarantee that problems have been resolved. Actually, the child's preplacement behavioral and emotional problems may have worsened. The child may be more cynical about parental authority; occasionally a child manipulatively threatens to go back into care to control the parent. For children who first experienced stable and competent parenting in the foster home, returning may force them to painfully acknowledge that the birth parent is woefully inadequate and that life in a foster home really is better. Some children will deny recurring abuse, preferring to live in the abusive home than to return to foster care.

Most states allow some time to elapse with the child back in the biological home before formally dismissing

court control. Some birth parents may shift into "family maintenance" status and receive voluntary services. Although some parents recognize the necessity for the court to have intervened, others see themselves as having been unfairly treated and want little to do with the system once dependency is dismissed.

CLINICAL EVALUATION OF THE FOSTER CHILD

Problems of Evaluation

Child clinicians frequently consult on children in foster homes, either to assess the child's possible treatment needs, to develop strategies to better control a child's behavior, or to make recommendations about parental reunification. In assessing such highly stressed children, it is hard to sort out how much of the child's difficulty emerges from the environmental pressures operating at the time and how much reflects more inherent biological and psychological tendencies.

As noted, foster children have parents with a high incidence of substance abuse and diagnosed and undiagnosed mental illness. So they have a higher-than-average genetic loading for mood, thought, and attentional disorders, combined with being enormously stressed psychologically. Time's passage and foster parents' patience and understanding may help a child reintegrate psychologically, or at least adapt better, to the new setting.

Therapeutic Treatment of Foster Children

Numerous articles provide detailed discussions of treatment issues (Fraiberg 1962; Hughes 1998; Pilowsky 1995; Rosenfeld and Wasserman 1990; Rosenfeld et al. 1997; Steinhauer 1991). Almost all clinicians emphasize the attachment problems that foster children have, although how to best approach that issue depends on the specific clinical situation and treatment goals.

ISSUES RELATED TO ADOPTION

The Child's Attachment Status

By the term *attachment status* we mean the child's capacity to establish a bonded, meaningful relationship with the adoptive parent. This may be crucial subsequently. Sometimes clinicians are asked to assess this issue to determine whether parental rights should be terminated and a child freed for adoption. To assess attachment status, the clinician needs to know about the relationships the child has had, and has, with the biological parents, caretaker relatives, and previous foster parents. It is helpful to know if the child has ever had a secure attachment with anyone and to what extent the child remembers and thinks about the past caretakers. Even if good information is available (and usually it is not), this type of assessment is imprecise and difficult.

Foster care and adoption are closely linked. Many foster children get adopted, either in the same or different homes. Furthermore, both groups live and grow up with parents who are not their biological parents. Clearly the two groups include a very wide range of children, from those adopted in infancy who may develop few if any difficulties to neglected, traumatized children who go through a succession of foster homes and suffer progressive deterioration in their capacity to attach and trust.

Nickman (1999) has written an extensive review of issues related to adoption. To some degree all adopted and foster children may suffer three types of loss: loss of caretaker continuity, familiar environment, or attachment capacity (overt loss); loss of the inner certainty of belonging, having a clear-cut identity, and being wanted (covert loss); and vulnerable self-esteem by virtue of stigmatizing life experiences (status loss) (Nickman 1985).

Children Adopted From Abroad After Infancy

These children may have spent long periods in relatively impersonal environments such as group homes or institutions. Some have suffered multiple overt losses, including loss of their linguistic environment, and later, loss of their original language and culture. In addition, because they may have impaired attachment capacity and significant learning disabilities (Gindis 1998) or are seriously at risk for these problems, these adoptions are disrupted more frequently than those from domestic foster care. Nevertheless, many of these children do exceedingly well in adoptive homes. Mental health professionals dealing with these families need to recognize overt, covert, and status losses, simultaneously making sure that the children's cognitive capacities are adequately assessed and that parents attend to their children's educational and medical needs.

Managing Previous Relationships

The child's relationship and contact with the birth parents and relatives, and occasionally previous long-term foster parents, can be important for adopted children. Clinicians may be asked for guidance when adoptive par-

ents are puzzled about whether these contacts are valuable or destructive to the child. Clarification of this question is important. Intervention may be needed, and may involve the birth parent, to improve contacts or occasionally to end them. These decisions need to be made on the basis of each child's unique situation.

Psychotherapy often helps these families; they may benefit if the same therapist sees both child and parents in a flexible arrangement, at times separately and at times in conjoint meetings. Children dealing with these relationship issues often have externalizing behavioral problems, and the family needs ways to deal with them (Delaney and Kunstal 1993; Keck and Kupecky 1995).

SUMMARY

Foster care is a complex combination of a framework of laws and governmental policy based on a concern for the physical and psychological needs of children and families. It reflects a high humanitarian ideal and a reality that falls far short of that ideal. Our task as clinicians is to use our clinical expertise and wisdom to assist the child, the family, the social worker, and the judge as they try to meet their responsibilities within this framework and to make a far-less-than-optimal situation better.

PITFALLS

Clinician-Related Issues

Biases

Issues related to race, class, and culture abound in the foster system. The clinician may be asked to evaluate children from a multitude of ethnic groups with widely divergent views about the relationships between parents and children, schools, and government. Cultural sensitivity is important. But respect for cultural differences ought not be used to justify what would be considered poor parenting in any culture.

At times, parents, children, and social workers may be adversaries; the clinician must not overidentify with any particular viewpoint. An honest and reality-based assessment of parental and system capabilities ultimately serves everyone's interests best.

Emotional Demands and Pressures

Child protection work involves extremely distressing situations, and the work is emotionally demanding. Our personal reactions to cruelty can either lead us to deny such situations or lead us to respond angrily, ultimately harming children and their families. The ongoing pressures and responsibilities can lead to cynicism, fatalism, and apathy.

Power Relationships

The clinician typically serves as a consultant in child protection issues. Most day-to-day decisions are made by social workers, some of whom may have ambivalent feelings about working with professionals with more education and income. Many will welcome the clinician's expertise and value the contribution; some will be antagonistic and defensive.

Information Issues

Information may not be available, or it may be prohibitively expensive and time-consuming to obtain. Parents frequently lie or omit important information; occasionally, social workers may deliberately omit information or falsify records to protect themselves. Therapists with weak forensic training or poor boundaries may draw unwarranted conclusions from limited evidence.

In some situations, children may have voluminous charts that are poorly organized, making it hard to pick out key items. Quarterly reports may track clothing inventories but provide little information about the status of the child's relationship with the foster parent or academic progress. Social workers may be reluctant to allow access to agency records for a variety of reasons. Photocopies of handwritten notes may be illegible.

System Issues

Working with governmental agencies can be frustrating because of their bureaucratic complexity. Decision making at times can be very slow and at times appear arbitrary. Resources may be quite limited. Agency priorities may change erratically based on current political sentiment or budget.

As children move into care, their cases typically move from emergency response workers to evaluators to foster home supervisors. Each new worker must become familiar with the case, make decisions, and implement those decisions. For the child who is "the case," this means dealing with a confusing array of people who may each have different views, approaches, and skills. Tensions can develop between the consultant who is working on behalf of the needs of a particular child and workers who have differing agendas or are responding to other agency needs.

Court Issues

As in all forensic work, the clinician must operate within a preexisting format and rules for decision making and conflict resolution. Failure to understand and respect these rules can lead to catastrophic consequences. Within his or her area of expertise, a clinician can make a valuable contribution to the court process, but the clinician must be careful not to either overstate expertise or draw conclusions beyond the evidence. The legal system functions (or at least tries to function) on the basis of facts and is a highly formalized form of conflict in which every statement may be carefully scrutinized and challenged. Emotionally based statements or opinions disguised as fact may interfere with the process.

CASE EXAMPLE EPILOGUES

Case Example 1

A relative of the child told the clinician that the birth mother, who had serious drug, alcohol, and psychiatric problems, was giving the boy alcohol to drink and marijuana to smoke during visits. The boy confirmed this, adding that the mother had instructed him not to tell anyone. When the issue surfaced, the mother said the child was lying and was just trying to get her arrested. The boy was furious with his mother, the clinician, and the foster parent. He felt betrayed and didn't know whom to trust. He immediately got into trouble for fighting at school and vandalism. He ran away from the foster home, spent several weeks homeless, and subsequently was placed in a juvenile detention facility.

Although the boy was told that the forensic consultation was not confidential at the start of the evaluation, the boy's anger at adult authority figures was far stronger than his ability to understand the legal distinctions in the situation.

After a few months he calmed down and went to live with an uncle. He has done well since.

Case Example 2

The clinician thought that the child suffered from anxiety difficulties as well as attention-deficit/hyperactivity disorder. She recommended to the court that the child receive stimulant medication for the attentional disorder and psychotherapy to help the child overcome his fears, as well as extra support at school. The court signed the consent for medication on behalf of the child. The child responded quite well to the medication with a marked decrease in hyperactivity and improved ability to focus on schoolwork. In time the child moved up to grade level. The therapy work progressed slowly, with the child only gradually mastering his anxieties. During this period his mother disappeared for several months. The social worker made plans for the foster parent to assume long-term guardianship.

ACTION GUIDELINES

Know and Respect the Law

The foster care system operates according to rules defined by law. Sometimes these rules are contrary to our clinical judgment or wishes, but they are paramount, so clinicians have to understand the rules, respect the framework they provide, and abide by them.

Know and Understand How the System Works

To move cases along in a way that best serves the interests of children and their families, clinicians need to understand how the system works. Utopian or unrealistic recommendations may lead to unnecessary, destructive delays and to families getting less than they might. Realistic opinions about the system and parents' capabilities help the judge make better decisions.

Participate in Multidisciplinary Learning

The research literature on foster care may appear in journals of social work, psychology, psychiatry, child abuse, education, and pediatrics. Little of it is well done or data based. But all of these disciplines contribute a perspective and clinical wisdom to the field; colleagues with expertise in each of these areas often provide a valuable way of sharing ideas, creative solutions, and insights. Participation in multidisciplinary consultation teams or death review teams can help broaden an appreciation of how to prevent the terrible.

Try to Maintain a Balanced Perspective

Although the foster care system deals with many painful situations, it represents a major effort to see that children and their families are treated humanely. As imperfect as the system is, the collaboration of many dedicated people does often make a difference in children's lives. To be most effective on a long-term basis, clinicians need to maintain good morale without too much cynicism in a world of great imperfection.

Educate the Public and Government Leaders

All too often, understanding of the foster care system is based on media cameos focused on catastrophic events.

This can lead to poorly thought out changes in policy. Realistic and accurate information about the strengths and weaknesses of the system is a prerequisite to more intelligent planning and improvement.

REFERENCES

Benedict MI, Zuravin S, Brandt D, et al: Types and frequency of child maltreatment by family foster care providers in an urban population. Child Abuse Negl 18(7):577–585, 1994

Bowlby J: Maternal Care and Mental Health. New York, Schocken, 1966

Cantos AL, Gries LT, Slis V: Behavioral correlates of parental visiting during family foster care. Child Welfare 76(2):309–329, 1997

Child Welfare League of America: Kinship Care: A Natural Bridge. Washington, DC, Child Welfare League of America, 1994

Dale JR, Kendall JC, Humber KI, et al: Screening young foster children for posttraumatic stress disorder and responding to their needs for treatment. American Professional Society on the Abuse of Children Advisor 12(2):6–9, 1999

Delaney R, Kunstal F: Troubled transplants: unconventional strategies for helping disturbed foster and adopted children. Portland, ME, National Child Welfare Resource Center for Management and Administration, Edmund S. Muskie School of Public Service, University of Southern Maine, 1993

Dubowitz H, Zuravin S, Starr RH Jr, et al: Behavior problems of children in kinship care. J Dev Behav Pediatr 14(6):386–393, 1993

Dumaret AC, Coppell-Batsch M, Couraud S: Adult outcome of children reared for long-term periods in foster families. Child Abuse Negl 21(10):911–927, 1997

Fanshel D, Shinn EB: Children in Foster Care. New York, Columbia University Press, 1978

Fein E: The elusive search for certainty in child welfare. Am J Orthopsychiatry 61:576–577, 1991

Fein E, Maluccio AN: Children leaving foster care: outcomes of permanency planning. Child Abuse Negl 8(4):425–431, 1984

Fialkov MJ: Fostering permanency of children in out-of-home care: psycho-legal aspects. Bulletin of the American Academy of Psychiatry and the Law 16(4):343–357, 1988

Fraiberg S: A therapeutic approach to reactive ego disturbances in children in placement. Am J Orthopsychiatry 32:18–32, 1962

Frank DA, Klass PE, Earls F, et al: Infants and young children in orphanages: one view from pediatrics and child psychiatry. Pediatrics 97(4):569–578, 1996

Freud A, Burlingham DT: Infants Without Families. New York, International Universities Press, 1944

Gindis B: Navigating uncharted waters: school psychologists working with internationally adopted post-institutionalized children. Communique (National Association of School Psychologists) 27:6–9, 1998

Halfon N, Berkowitz G, Klee L: Mental health service utilization by children in foster care in California. Pediatrics 89:1238–1244, 1992

Halfon N, Mendonca A, Berkowitz G: Health status of children in foster care: the experience of the Center for the Vulnerable Child. Arch Pediatr Adolesc Med 149(4):386–392, 1995

Heneghan AM, Horwitz SM, Leventhal JM: Evaluating intensive family preservation programs: a methodological review. Pediatrics 97(4):535–542, 1996

Hochstadt NJ, Jaudes PK, Zimo DA, et al: The medical and psychosocial needs of children entering foster care. Child Abuse Negl 11(1):53–62, 1987

Hughes DA: Building the Bonds of Attachment. Northdale, NJ, Jason Aronson, 1998

Kagan RM, Reid WJ, Roberts SF, et al: Engaging families of court-mandated youths in an alternative to institutional placement. Child Welfare 66(4):365–376, 1987

Keck G, Kupecky R: Adopting the Hurt Child: Hope for Families With Special-Needs Kids. Colorado Springs, CO, Pinon Press, 1995

Kempe CH, Sliverman FN, Steele BF, et al: The battered child syndrome. JAMA 181:17–24, 1962

Lawder E, Poulin J, Andrews R: A study of 185 foster children 5 years after placement. Child Welfare 65(3):241–251, 1986

Lindsey D: Factors affecting the foster care placement decision: an analysis of national survey data. Am J Orthopsychiatry 61(2):272–281, 1991

Nickman, SL: Losses in adoption: the need for dialogue. Psychoanal Study Child 40:365–398, 1985

Nickman, SL: Adoption, in Comprehensive Textbook of Psychiatry, 10th Edition. Edited by Saddock BJ, Saddock VA. Baltimore, MD, Lippincott, Williams & Wilkins, 1999, pp 2368–2873

Pilowsky DJ: Psychopathology among children placed in family foster care. Psychiatr Serv 46(9):906–910, 1995

Reddy LA, Pfeiffer SI: Effectiveness of treatment foster care with children and adolescents. J Am Acad Child Adolesc Psychiatry 36:581–588, 1997

Rosenfeld AA, Wasserman S: Healing the Heart: A Therapeutic Approach to Disturbed Children in Group Care. Washington, DC, Child Welfare League of America, 1990

Rosenfeld AA, Pilowsky DJ, Fine P, et al: Foster care: an update. Journal of the American Academy of Child Psychiatry 36:448–457, 1977

Rosenfeld AA, Altman R, Kaufman I: Foster care, in Managing Care, Not Dollars: The Continuum of Mental Health Services. Edited by Schreter R, Sharfstein S, Schreter C. Washington, DC, American Psychiatric Press, 1997, pp 125–138

Rosenfeld AA, Wasserman S, Pilowsky DJ: Psychiatry and children in the child welfare system, in The Child Psychiatrist in the Community (Child and Adolescent Psychiatric Clinics of North America, Vol 7, No 3). Edited by Berkowitz SJ, Adnopoz JA. Philadelphia, PA, WB Saunders, 1998, pp 515–535

Ruff HA, Blank S, Barnett HL: Early intervention in the context of foster care. J Dev Behav Pediatr 11(5):265–268, 1990

Runyan DK, Gould CL: Foster care for child maltreatment: impact on delinquent behavior. Pediatrics 75(3):562–568, 1985

Simms MD: The foster care clinic. J Dev Behav Pediatr 10(3):121–128, 1989

Spitz RA: Hospitalism. Psychoanalytic Study of the Child 1:53, 1945

Steinhauer PD: The Least Detrimental Alternative. Toronto, ON, University of Toronto Press, 1991

Wald MS, Carlsmith JM, Leiderman PH: Protecting Abused and Neglected Children. Stanford, CA, Stanford University Press, 1988

Washington Social Legislation Bulletin 34:181, November 25, 1996

Wasserman S, Rosenfeld AA: Decision-making in child abuse and neglect. Bulletin of the American Academy of Psychiatry and the Law 13(3):259–271, 1985

Wyatt DT, Simms MD, Horwitz SM: Widespread growth retardation and variable growth recovery in foster children in the first year after initial placement. Arch Pediatr Adolesc Med 151(8):813–816, 1997

Zeanah CH, Larrieu JH: Intensive intervention for maltreated infants and toddlers in foster care. Child Adolesc Psychiatr Clin N Am 7(2):357–371, 1998

CHAPTER 11

Termination of Parental Rights

Diane H. Schetky, M.D.

Case Example 1

Mrs. Cutler is referred for assessment regarding her ability to care for and protect her 6-year-old daughter. Mrs. Cutler was born with congenital deafness and spent her early years in an abusive hearing family. She was then placed in an institution for the deaf that stressed lipreading. Her signing skills remained rudimentary, and she developed little by way of intelligible speech. At age 18, she moved into a halfway house where she met and married a man with a substance abuse problem. On learning that he was sexually abusing their daughter, she left him and promptly moved in with another man who had charges pending regarding sexual abuse of his daughters. A neglect petition was filed by the state, and her daughter was placed in foster care.

Case Example 2

Serena is a single mother of two toddlers living in public housing and receiving extensive support from her social worker around basic parenting issues. One day she calls 911 stating that her 3-year-old daughter, Jill, is covered with blood. The paramedics arrive and find Jill wrapped in a sheet that appears to have diluted blood on it; she is covered with blood from the waist down, but no source for the bleeding can be found. The child is taken to the hospital where it is noted that she is smiling and in no distress, but she will not say what happened. Her physical exam, including genital exam, is normal. About a month later, Serena takes Jill to the hospital complaining that there is blood in Jill's urine. An astute pediatrician decides to type the blood in her urine and finds that it is not the same type as the child's. A forensic consultation is sought.

Case Example 3

While high on cocaine, Gene Sylvester broke into the home of his estranged wife in the middle of the night. He entered her bedroom where she was asleep with their 3-year-old daughter, Lucy, and fatally shot his wife in the head. He fled, leaving Lucy with her mother's body and covered with blood and brain tissue. Lucy's grandmother assumes temporary custody of her and immediately gets her into counseling with a therapist skilled at working with traumatized children. At trial, Gene is sentenced to life in prison. The grandmother petitions the court to adopt Lucy, and the court appoints you as a guardian *ad litem* to represent the best interests of Lucy.

LEGAL ISSUES

Concurrent Permanency Planning

Chapter 10, "Foster Care and Adoption," reviewed the plight of children who are caught in the limbo of "permanent" foster care. In 1992, the W. K. Kellogg Foundation sought to hasten the exodus of children from foster care to permanent homes and set out the following goals:

- Family support to those at risk of losing custody of their children
- Coordinated assessment to determine the needs of the family
- One casework team in which a single caseworker or team works with the child and another with the biological parents through the permanency planning process
- One foster care placement until permanency is achieved
- One year to permanency

Out of these goals evolved the concept of concurrent permanency planning in which an alternative plan is put in place in the event the child cannot be reunited with his or her birth parents. This concept became codified in Public Law 96-272 (P.L. 96-272) under the Adoption and Safe Families Act of 1997 (Ford 1988). Under this law, states may petition for termination of parental rights if the child has been in foster care for 15 of the most recent 22 months. Exceptions are children living with relatives and when such a move would not be in the child's best interests.

Caseworkers practice "full disclosure" in which from the onset of entry into the system, birth parents are informed about the negative effects of separation on children, what their options are, and what is expected of them. Much of the success of concurrent planning lies with the expanded role of foster families, who are now called permanency planning families and who are expected to advocate for the birth parents and facilitate visits. They also participate in case reviews and are viewed as part of the treatment team. Caseworkers in these programs are given reduced case loads and are expected to provide support to the permanency planning families. Those states that have implemented concurrent planning programs have shown dramatic decreases in the amount of time children spend in foster care. Additional advantages to the plan are that it is child-focused and specific. In contrast, previous statutes regarding termination of parental rights were exceedingly vague and failed to define such terms as "reunification within a reasonable time."

There is currently a surge in the number of foster children being adopted in the United States. This surge is in part attributable to a 1996 law that established tax credits to families who adopt and bonus awards to states that increase their number of adoptions, in addition to concurrent planning. In addition, agencies are taking more aggressive steps to recruit adoptive families, including using the media and Internet to advertise the availability of children and sponsoring adoption fairs at which potential adoptive parents can preview children.

Discontinuing Reunification Efforts

The state is entitled to bring about a petition to terminate parental rights if it is determined that family reunification efforts are not succeeding and that termination of parental rights is in the child's best interests. Typical grounds for terminating parental rights include parents who are unwilling or unable to protect a child from jeopardy or to take responsibility for a child and failure to make a good-faith effort to rehabilitate and reunify with

a child. In addition, termination may occur if parents decide to relinquish parental rights or when parents cannot be located or have abandoned a child. Under P.L. 96-272, certain heinous crimes against children, such as murder, rape, or sexual abuse, may constitute grounds for automatically pursuing termination of parental rights.

The standard of proof for discontinuing reunification efforts requires only a preponderance of the evidence. In the 1982 case of *Santosky v. Kramer*, the U.S. Supreme Court decided that a higher standard of "clear and convincing evidence" is required to terminate parental rights. If the state discontinues efforts to reunify, it must give written notice of this decision to the parents, including the reasons for the decision.

Courts usually require demonstration that a parent's conduct or condition is such as to render him or her incapable of caring for the child and that such conduct or condition is not likely to change within the foreseeable future. The state must demonstrate that the plan for the reunification efforts is not consistent with the permanency plan for the child.

Due Process Rights

Parents

Parents are entitled to legal counsel in child protection proceedings and may request the court to appoint counsel for them. If indigent, the court must pay the costs for counsel. Parents are entitled to an evidentiary hearing or trial in which they may contest the allegations made against them.

Children

Recognizing that the child's interest is not always synonymous with the parent's or the state's, children in most states are entitled to representation by a guardian *ad litem* or an attorney during adjudication hearings and proceedings to terminate parental rights. The guardian *ad litem* (who may be an attorney, volunteer, or clinician) is entitled to records and may interview the child, parents, and foster parents. He or she may subpoena, examine, and cross-examine witnesses and is expected to act on behalf of the child's best interests. The guardian must make the child's wishes known and prepare a written report that includes the guardian's findings and recommendations.

Foster Parents

Foster parents must be provided with notice of hearings and be allowed the opportunity to be heard. They may testify but are not allowed to present evidence or witnesses, because they are not considered parties in the proceedings.

Special Situations

Rights of Unwed Fathers

The rights of unwed fathers were upheld in the case of *Stanley v. Illinois* (1972), which extended due process rights to the father of an illegitimate child in a custody proceeding. Many states now require parental notification and the birth father's consent if he can be identified and located, prior to terminating his parental rights. Recent case laws have taken into consideration the extent of the father's prebirth involvement and support as a weighting factor in determining his standing in adoption. Courts have also established that failure on the part of the unwed father to provide support can constitute abandonment.

Rights of Grandparents

Historically, courts have tended to recognize the rights of grandparents as derivatives of parental rights rather than inherent rights. Thus, termination of parental rights by extension would terminate the grandparents' rights. Grandparents, however, may petition the courts as third parties and request the right to visitation.

Indian Child Welfare Act of 1978

The Indian Child Welfare Act of 1978 gives authority to tribes to determine the best interests of Native American children. This act resulted, in part, from the United States' recognition of tribal sovereignty and the importance of Native American children's preserving their roots by remaining in their culture. Title I of the act recognizes that tribal courts have exclusive jurisdiction over custody proceedings, other than divorce, involving children residing on reservations. In the cases of children living off the reservation, it requires the state courts to transfer custody proceedings to the tribal courts. The act also requires that in termination of parental rights, that the burden of proof be beyond a reasonable doubt, which is higher than the clear and convincing standard used in the rest of the United States for termination of parental rights proceedings.

Experts who render opinions in these matters must be familiar with the culture of Native American children. In the case of *In re Adoption of H.M.O.* (1998), a decision awarding petition for adoption of a child was reversed on grounds that the expert witnesses who testified against the child's mother were not members of the child's tribe nor were they knowledgeable about tribal customs.

Alternatives to Termination of Parental Rights

Long-Term Foster Care

Long-term foster care may be an option for older children who resist adoption because of loyalty binds, who wish to maintain some contact with parents unable to care for them, or who want to remain with foster parents who are not in a position to adopt. There are also older children who drift from short-term to long-term foster care and who, because of their age, may have trouble finding an adoptive home. Some children may fear adoption and the possibility of yet another rejection and may not wish to be adopted.

Although long-term foster care may sound like a potential solution for a minority of children, it is not without problems. It is expensive; nationwide, foster care payments were roughly $3.1 billion between the years 1984 and 1996. Long-term foster care lacks stability. Foster parents often receive inadequate support both emotionally and financially, and placements may fall apart when children reach adolescence or when health or family problems arise within the foster parents' families. In addition, foster children may feel like they are second-class citizens and may live in fear of being rejected if their behavior is unacceptable.

Guardianship

Guardianship affords the rights and responsibilities of a parent except for the duty to support. It permits the child to maintain contact with the birth parent while relieving the parent of parental responsibilities. Such an arrangement might be preferred by a relative caring for a child who does not wish to alienate the child's parent by pursuing termination of parental rights and adoption. Guardianship is cost-effective for the state, since typically guardians receive no support for raising the child. Exceptions exist in a few states that have funds to support subsidized guardianship placements. Lack of financial support is often a deterrent to persons who wish to assume the responsibilities of guardianship.

Emancipation

Petitions for emancipation may be submitted to courts by teens or their parents. Emancipation requires the consent of the teen's parent or legal guardian and relieves them of any liabilities or responsibilities for the child. It is usually not considered unless there is evidence that the teen is competent, self-supporting, and able to live on his or her own or is married.

Open or Kinship Adoptions

Open or kinship adoption, as noted in Chapter 10, is becoming popular, particularly among Native Americans and African Americans who prefer to see children raised within their own communities and cultures. Such arrangements are often beneficial to children in that they promote continuity of care and their identity, avail them of community support, and allow them to maintain some contact with their birth parents. Unfortunately, some states are reluctant to make kinship placements with relatives because federal funds are not available to foster care programs for children in placements with relatives.

CLINICAL ISSUES

The Rationale for Terminating Parental Rights

Permanent placement is an alternative to indefinite foster care for children unable or unlikely to be returned home. The decision to terminate parental rights is based on the beliefs that 1) the child is entitled to have some adult function on a permanent basis in the role of nurturing parent, 2) the child is entitled to maintain such a relationship once it has been ratified by time, and 3) the child is entitled to a minimal level of freedom from abuse and exploitation within that relationship. When those rights are not being served by the relationship between child and parents and when they would be better served by severing that relationship and freeing the child for adoption, it is the child's right for that separation and reattachment to occur.

Assessing the Child's Needs

Special Needs

Does the child have special needs? A hyperactive child might require parents with exceptional patience and the ability to provide structure, whereas the child with a developmental delay might do best with parents who do not hold out high expectations for achievement from him. The child who is acting out sexually will probably do best with parents who can set limits but at the same time are not too prudish about sexual matters. Such a child might also do better in a home where there are no younger children.

Capacity for Object Relations

Many children who have experienced multiple placements develop attachment disorders that may jeopardize the success of subsequent placements, particularly adoptive ones. Others have learned to adapt a standoffish posture by way of protecting themselves from future losses. History of past and present attachments will often help differentiate what is a transient defensive posture from the inability to attach. If a child with attachment disorder is placed in an adoptive home, the adoptive parents are likely to become quite discouraged, feel unappreciated, and feel as if they have failed. However, new treatment is emerging for children with attachment disorders that holds promise (Hughes 1998).

Emotional or Intellectual Impairment

The extent of emotional or intellectual impairment is critical in determining what type of care, treatment, and remediation the child needs. Psychological testing can help document where the child is developmentally and subsequent gains made in placement. Some children who have experienced profound neglect show remarkable rebounds in their development when placed in nurturing and intellectually stimulating homes. It is imperative that adoption agencies level with prospective adoptive parents about the extent of a child's impairment and let them know what the prognosis might be. Severely disturbed children may need a period of time in therapeutic foster care before they can be considered for adoption. This also allows the clinician time in which to form a clearer picture of the child's diagnosis, for example, differentiating mental retardation from environmental deprivation, and adjustment disorders from more persistent conduct disorders.

Adoptability

Adoptability has increasingly become a function of who will have the child and finding the right fit. Previous barriers to adoption, such as Down syndrome or even being HIV positive, are diminishing as are prejudices against the physically handicapped or children of mixed races, and children with special needs now constitute almost 50% of adoptions. Among the most difficult children to place are older children with conduct disorders, acting-out behavior of a sexual nature, and attachment disorders. Adoptive parents need to be fully informed of the extent of the child's problems and provided with ample support. With high-risk children, one must always consider the risk of failed adoption and the devastating effect on these children of yet another rejection, although the rate of disrupted adoptions is only about 12% (Barth 1999).

Assessment of the Parent-Child Relationship

Chapter 9, "Parenting Assessment in Cases of Neglect and Abuse," covers parenting and child assessments and addresses some of the limitations of parent-child observations. These observations are only one part of the evaluation but can provide valuable information. Most children in foster care will have supervised visitation, and forensic examiners may gain new insights by observing these visits. Parents who have lost their children to custody of the state may be very defensive and angry and attempt to get their children to align with them. They may try to thwart a foster placement by turning the child against foster parents. Some parents flaunt their disrespect for authority by violating the parameters of supervised visits, for example, speaking inappropriately of legal proceedings, trying to convince the child of their innocence, berating the caseworker, or offering the child false promises of returning home.

Attachment problems may be evident as when the child is overly affectionate with a clinician or supervisor he has never met before or fails to react when his mother leaves the room. Children may have difficulty with transitions around a visit, and this does not necessarily indicate attachment problems or that a visit went poorly. Some children may be slow to warm up to parents they have not seen for a while or avoidant because they are angry that the parent has abandoned them. Children may be cranky and difficult because they are tired or physically ill. The child's reactions before and after visits must to be taken in context of his or her history, attachment issues, and what occurs during visitation. Children who have been previously traumatized by parents may react adversely to ongoing visits and show regressive behaviors. This may be exacerbated by parents who behave inappropriately during visits. If parents behave inappropriately while under observation, one must wonder how they react when alone with their child.

Visitation supervisors keep notes on visits, and these can be helpful sources of information to the forensic psychiatrist regarding recurring patterns of behavior and whether or not the parent is able to respond to guidance and limits.

Possible Contraindications to Terminating Parental Rights

For children staying with relatives who do not wish to adopt them, the benefit of preserving the relationship with relatives must be weighed against the need for permanency. Relatives may not wish to adopt for fear of alienating a parent. One needs to consider how intrusive the parent might be in the child's life and whether the contact is positive or negative. Age and health of the relative providing care must also be considered.

Children who remain strongly bonded to their birth parents, no matter how abusive they may be, often undermine foster care or adoptive placements. This is particularly so with older children who may identify with their parents' acting-out behaviors or who may have loyalty conflicts that interfere with forming attachments to adoptive parents. Other children may cling to fantasies, counter to reality, that their parents will improve and come to claim them.

The child who is acting out sexually or aggressively is not likely to be a good candidate for adoption and usually needs continued therapy and foster care before he is ready for adoption. Even if adoptive parents are willing to work with a child around these behaviors, there is risk that they may not appreciate what they are in for and have second thoughts once the child is placed with them.

The child who does not wish to be adopted is not likely to be a good candidate for adoption. Older children may be quite vocal about their wishes. They may resist adoption out of fear of the unknown or fear of another rejection, or they may not wish to leave their foster parents or sever ties with parents or siblings. Although courts are more likely to recognize visitation rights among siblings in foster care than in adoption, it may be possible in some cases for them to have continued visitation after adoption. How much weight to give to a child's wishes will depend on his or her maturity and the overt and covert reasons for the child's preference. With most adolescents one would give strong consideration to their wishes, and with school-age children, some consideration. It is important to explore the reasons behind their stated preferences. Preschoolers do not have sufficient maturity to make informed decisions about such matters, though it is always worthwhile to explore their feelings and fantasies about adoption.

Weighing the Child's Best Interests

Having assessed parent, child, the parent-child relationship, and the history, the forensic examiner must attempt to arrive at recommendations. Factors to consider include the child's need for permanency, continuity of relationships with siblings and extended family, capacity for attachment, and adoptability. One must consider the quality of the parent-child relationship and what impact severing of that relationship would have on the child.

Readiness for adoption is another factor, because courts may be reluctant to terminate parental rights if a child does not appear to be adoptable.

In terms of the parent, one needs to consider whether there is a relationship with the child that can be salvaged, whether the parent possesses requisite parenting skills and intelligence, and whether it is likely that the parent can be rehabilitated and, if so, in time to meet the needs of the developing child. Past history, willingness and ability to accept help, change, and maintain their gains are often good barometers of the future.

The question often arises about the potential trauma of removing children from foster parents to whom they have bonded. In some cases, foster parents may compete with relatives who wish to adopt a child. In the *Adoption of Hugo* (1998), foster parents, who had cared for 1-year-old Hugo since birth, wished to adopt him, but the court ruled that an aunt was better able to meet his special needs related to developmental delay. The case was appealed on grounds that the court ignored evidence that the child would be harmed if separated from foster parents and his sister, who also resided with them. The Supreme Court of Massachusetts upheld the decision of the trial court, stressing that the child's attachment to the caregiver is a factor to consider but not the determining factor in making a placement decision.

PITFALLS

Rescue Fantasies

Rescue fantasies are common among persons who work in child protection. It is easy to overidentify with a child and want to salvage him from an abusive or disadvantaged home environment. Clinicians may even fantasize about adopting particularly appealing children, and a few have even done so—in violation of their ethical codes. Such acting-out on the part of a clinician usually results from unresolved countertransference issues. More commonly, rescue fantasies take the form of wanting to see the child in a nurturing home and to shelter the child from the deficiencies of his or her home.

Bias

Bias may be apparent when value judgments polarize competing families. The clinician is privy to much information about the child's family of origin and, in contrast, knows very little about the foster family, which may tend to skew his or her thinking. Biases about lifestyles, fathers as primary parents, and adoptions by gays, lesbians, or single parents may also influence recommendations.

Fear of Doing Harm

Fear of doing harm to parents can be quite powerful. Clinicians are trained to be helpful and empathic, and it is difficult to arrive at the decision that nothing more can be done to bring about family reunification. It counters clinicians' notions of being healers and helpers and engenders anxiety about how such a recommendation will affect the parent. This is particularly difficult if parents suffer from conditions over which they have little control such as mental retardation or major mental disorders. There is a terrible finality in terminating parental rights, and, unlike making psychiatric diagnoses, forensic examiners do not have time in which to correct erroneous opinions. The danger is that our apprehension may lead to watering down of findings or stalling in order to buy time. The risk to the child is that of prolonging the search for permanency and leaving the child in limbo.

A tactful way to deal with recommendations to cease parental reunification efforts is to address the parent's limitations in the context of his or her own deprived childhood. It is possible to say, in some cases, that a mother truly loves her child and has tried to the best of her ability but that her parenting capacities have been limited by her own terribly abusive childhood or mental illness. Further, one might add that she needs to apply her limited emotional resources to her own healing and not be saddled with responsibilities for a child for whom she is not able to care.

Role Conflict

Role conflict may occur when the clinician is not clear where his or her advocacy lies and which hat he or she wears. Divided loyalties may also arise in child protective services cases when caseworkers attempt to advocate for a parent and then find themselves having to testify against him or her. Splitting the case between two or more workers may eliminate this problem. The guiding principle for forensic experts in dependency and neglect hearings is always the best interest of the child. Therapists who testify on behalf of parents often lack objectivity and the broad database of the forensic examiner and are not in a position to make recommendations about custody.

The Limits of Prediction

Prediction is usually most accurate if based on past behavior rather than speculation. Psychological profiles derived from the Minnesota Multiphasic Personality Inventory (MMPI) may be invoked in court to predict future parenting (see Chapter 6, "Psychological Testing in Child and Adolescent Forensic Evaluations"). This can be risky if the test was not valid, the parent does not conform to the profile in all ways, or data are taken out of context or are not integrated with other aspects of the evaluation.

CASE EXAMPLE EPILOGUES

Case Example 1

The psychiatrist could not help but feel sympathy for Mrs. Cutler, to whom life had dealt a bad hand. She also had to decide whether she held deaf parents up to the same standard of parenting as hearing parents. Mrs. Cutler's dependency issues were very real, and it was not clear to what extent they might be altered by psychotherapy. Her daughter was evaluated, and it was apparent that she had assumed a very parental role and was literally her mother's mouthpiece, as her mother relied heavily on her to negotiate with the outside world.

Mrs. Cutler was evaluated with the help of a translator. Her manner was angry and defensive, and she expressed her conviction that her boyfriend was not a sex offender and that he posed no threat to her daughter. Psychological testing showed borderline intelligence, low frustration tolerance, and emotional lability. The prognosis for change was felt to be guarded, but nonetheless, it was recommended that she pursue psychotherapy with the goal of gaining more independence. It was also recommended that she explore job training and develop more proficiency in signing. A year later, she continued in therapy, but she remained with her abusive boyfriend and little else had changed in her life. She and her ex-husband agreed to relinquish parental rights, and her daughter was placed in an adoptive home. In a subsequent case (*In re AP*), a Pennsylvania superior court established that whether or not a parent is disabled, the parent must meet "irreducible minimum parenting responsibilities" for a child to be returned home.

Case Example 2

Extensive review of both Serena's and her children's medical records showed misuse of medical services, particularly whenever her social worker was out of town. There were frequent trips to the emergency room with complaints that Jill was not breathing, but she always seemed fine when examined. Out-of-state records pointed to prior factitious illness in Serena. Serena, who is concrete in her thinking, denies knowledge of where the blood on her daughter came from, but her own history is replete with trauma involving blood. She discloses that she has great difficulty with reading, shopping, memory, and handling money. She also has had difficulty relating to the other single mothers in her housing complex, whom she believes talk about her. Her relationship with her own mother is highly conflicted, and her social worker is her sole support in life. She gets help around life skills and parenting while her children are in day care, but she does not think she needs these services.

Serena is massively overweight and moves about slowly. When observed with her daughters, she manages to get down on the floor with them but cannot keep up with their play. She treats them in a symbiotic fashion and has difficulty differentiating her own needs from theirs. Her knowledge of child rearing is rudimentary, and she has difficulty setting limits with her children. For example, Jill becomes frustrated because her mother is unable to help her complete a simple puzzle and turns to her and calls her "a baby." Psychological testing confirms borderline intelligence, poor organizational skills, and major issues around dependency. Jill is seen alone and shows no serious emotional or developmental problems. She states she can't remember how she came to be covered with blood.

The children are placed in foster care where they thrive. Jill ultimately reveals that her mother had smeared her with blood and laughs about the incident. The forensic psychiatrist makes diagnoses of Munchausen syndrome by proxy, mild mental retardation, and dependent personality disorder. The prognosis for Serena's ability to care for her children is felt to be poor, and it is recommended that the state not pursue parental reunification. In addition to evidence of parental neglect and limited cognitive skills, there is concern that her attempts to induce factitious illness in her daughters will escalate and result in physical as well as emotional harm to them if they are returned to her. Her attorney will not accept the diagnosis of Munchausen syndrome by proxy and insists on a second opinion from an expert on the disorder from "away" who "knows what he is talking about." The expert in Munchausen syndrome by proxy evaluates Serena and confirms the diagnosis and prognosis. Serena enters therapy at the urging of her attorney but shows little insight into her behavior or motivation for change. The court terminates her parental rights.

Case Example 3

You meet separately with all of the parties and find that Lucy, understandably, is terrified of her father and is closely bonded with her grandmother. Mr. Sylvester cannot understand the basis for his daughter's fears and comments, "I never laid on hand on her and she knows I never would." He wants to maintain parental rights so that he can have visitation with Lucy in prison like the other inmates in for murder who still get to see their kids. He insists he can still be a father to her from prison. This case clearly qualifies for automatic termination of parental rights under heinous crimes and you recommend adoption by the maternal grandmother and no further contact with the father. The court agrees, Lucy's name is changed upon being adopted, and with the help of extensive therapy and a devoted grandmother she does well.

ACTION GUIDELINES

Understand the Law

Laws regarding termination of parental rights and adoption vary from state to state and anyone who does this type of forensic work needs to be familiar with them. The states' assistant attorney general or the state's protective services office can direct you to appropriate statutes.

Careful Documentation

Successful terminations are built upon careful documentation of efforts to help parents and their failure to respond. This includes recording missed and canceled appointments and documenting recommendations that have been made to parents and whether or not they were acted upon. The forensic examiner needs to be able to give examples as to why a parent continues to be unable to care for or protect the child in question and why that parent's conduct or condition is harmful to the child. The judge who sees that no stone has been left unturned is more likely to terminate parental rights in that case than in a case where parents have not had the opportunity to avail themselves of services or visitations.

Time Is of the Essence

Children become less adoptable with age and their insecurities are likely to increase in foster care. If the forensic examiner is recommending additional services to a parent before discontinuing reunification efforts, he should be very specific and give a timeline on which goals are expected to be accomplished. He might also suggest that he re-evaluate the parent in 6 months.

Humility

Forensic examiners need to recognize the limits of their expertise and that they are but one cog in the wheel of justice. Factors other than their evaluations often have bearing on the outcome of a case.

Ethical Issues

Forensic examiners who do a lot of work for the state or particular agencies need to guard against becoming allied with their referral sources and strive towards objectivity and fairness in their evaluations.

We need to work toward the availability of support systems for families so that foster care and termination of parental rights do not become alternatives to intervention with multiproblem families. Programs need to be funded in such a way that they promote the integrity of the family rather than removal of children from troubled homes. We need to advocate for services to foster parents and give them more public recognition.

REFERENCES

Adoption of Hugo, 700 NE 2d 516 Mass (1998)

Barth R: Risks and rates of adoption disruptions, in Adoption Factbook III. Waite Park, MN, National Council for Adoption, 1999

Ford M: Three concurrent planning programs. St Paul, MN, North American Council on Adoptable Children, 1988

Hughes D: Building the Bonds of Attachment: Awakening Love in Deeply Troubled Children. Northvale, NJ, Jason Aronson, 1998

In re Adoption of HMO, 399977 WL, Mont (1998)

In re AP 728 A2d 375 PA Sup Ct (1999)

Santosky v Kramer, 455 US 745 (1982)

Stanley v Illinois, 405 US 645 (1972)

SUGGESTED READINGS

Bower J: Achieving permanence for every child: the effective use of adoption subsidies. St Paul, MN, North American Council on Adoptable Children, 1988

Derdeyn A, Rogoff A, Williams S: Alternatives to absolute termination of parental rights after long-term foster care. Vanderbilt Law Review 31(54):1165–1192, 1978

Katz L, Robinson C: Foster care drift: a risk assessment matrix. Child Welfare 70(3):347–358, 1991

Kessel S, Robbins S: The Indian Child Welfare Act: dilemmas and needs. Child Welfare 63:225–232, 1984

Langelier P, Nurcombe B: Residual parental rights: legal trends and controversies. Journal of the American Academy of Child Psychiatry 24 (6):793–796, 1985

Marshner C (ed): National Council for Adoption: Adoption Factbook III. Waite Park, MN, Park Press, 1999

Schetky D, Angell R, Morrison C, et al: Parents who fail: a study of 51 cases of termination of parental rights. Journal of the American Academy of Child Psychiatry 18:366–383, 1979

U.S. Department of Health and Human Services: Barriers to Freeing Children for Adoption. Washington, DC, Office of the Inspector General, 1991

Welty K: Achieving Permanence for Every Child: A Guide for Limiting the Use of Long-Term Foster Care as a Permanent Plan. St. Paul, MN, North American Council on Adoptable Children, 1997

CHAPTER 12

Transracial and Transcultural Adoption in the United States

Donna M. Norris, M.D.
Yvonne B. Ferguson, M.D., M.P.H.

Case Example 1

A Caucasian foster couple raised an African American child for the first 3 years of her life. When they sought to adopt the child, the African American paternal grandmother challenged the adoption and claimed the child should be placed with her.

Case Example 2

A 1-month-old biracial child, Timmy, was placed with Caucasian foster parents. Within the year, they applied to adopt Timmy, but the agency denied the petition after the child had been in the foster home for nearly 2 years. Although they did not have an African American home for Timmy, the agency "intended to find one."

Case Example 3

A long-married Caucasian couple was unable to conceive or to obtain a child from the United States. They sought an international adoption of a newborn. The parents were aware that there had been serious neglect and violence in the child's early history. When the child was 7 years old, the couple separated and initiated a battle for custody. There were inordinate demands by the adoptive mother for the child to reject the father. The child was quite emotionally distressed by these demands. The adoptive mother reacted angrily that the court would seriously consider the adoptive father as the custodian and was overheard to express the wish that the child be returned to the streets of her country rather than be placed in the custody of the father.

LEGAL ISSUES

Historically, private adoption agencies in the United States have either denied services to African Americans or devised different policies and practices based on race. Not until 1933 were there significant numbers of public child welfare agencies. Although most agencies in the North serviced African Americans, due to de facto segregation practices, African American children did not have access to the full spectrum of services, especially adoption and institutional services. Even after the Civil Rights movement, foster care, which was less labor-intensive for caseworkers than adoption or institutional care, continued to be the primary placement service offered to African American children (McRoy 1989).

Definitions

For the authors' purposes, *transracial adoption* (TRA) is the adoption of a child of a different race or ethnicity from the parents' race. This type of adoption is to be contrasted with *inracial adoption* (same-race adoption), which is still the norm and was the exclusive type of adoption in the United States before the 1950s. In practice, the overwhelming number of adoptive parents available for TRA in the United States are Caucasian, and the overwhelming number of children available for TRA are children of color. African American children are the most available children for this type of adoption in the United States (Binder 1998). This simplistic definition of TRA does not easily accommodate the various permutations of race on either side of the adoptive equation. For example, if a biracial child whose features are predominantly Caucasian is placed with an African American couple, is this a TRA? What do we call the placement of an African American child with a biracial couple? *Transcultural adoption* (TCA) is the adoption of a child of a culture different than the parents' culture. It is possible for an adoption to be both transracial and transcultural, as is the case in many international adoptions.

Historical Background

In the past 50 years, the sociopolitical and demographic complexion of the United States has been significantly transformed, and these changes have affected all aspects of American culture and lifestyle. Until recently, race has been a complicating factor, overtly and covertly, governing the child placement process for all children. The traditional practice has been inracial child placement. Whereas it has been difficult for non-Caucasian children to be placed with Caucasian parents on other than an emergency foster care basis, it has been even more difficult for the reverse to occur ("White woman awarded custody" 1999). With the new century, this country is faced with even greater challenges and changes in its population demographics (U.S. Bureau of the Census 1996).

Among married couples in the United States, 18.5% (5.3 million) are infertile. Despite new reproductive technologies (e.g., in vitro fertilization and intrauterine insemination), approximately 2% of American families (not all infertile) adopt approximately 50,000 nonrelated children annually (Kim 1996). Caucasian families in the United States desirous of adoption have sought domestic transracial and international transcultural adoptions, particularly involving Eastern European, Asian, and Latin American children. In a racially tense country such as the United States, whose history is replete with separation of the races, emotional rancor among professional groups has raged over the psychopolitical soundness of transracial adoption, but less so over transcultural adoption.

For a variety of reasons, the number of minority children in foster care has exploded, thereby creating a crisis in the delivery of appropriate care. Minority children experience more disrupted foster placements and remain in foster care longer than Caucasian children (Everett 1991). Proponents of transracial and transcultural adoption argue that it is discriminatory under the Fourteenth Amendment for minority children to be denied available adoptive homes, regardless of the parents' race, and that there is no evidence that Caucasian parents rearing African American children do them psychological harm (Bar-

tholet 1991; Clark and Clark 1958). Further, they note a consensus among experts that children in prolonged foster care and institutions do suffer emotional and behavioral problems. Opponents of this argument assert that transracial adoption is tantamount to "racial or cultural genocide." They maintain that nonminority parents cannot rear minority children to identify with their race, have racial pride, or eventually advocate for societal changes of racial injustices. Nor, they argue, can nonminority parents equip minority children with the requisite skills to combat the racism they will encounter on a daily basis. Skin color and other ethnic physical features can be the focus of verbal or nonverbal negative reactions by those of the majority and/or similar minority groups. Some argue that adoption agencies have not aggressively recruited minority adoptive parents. Other critics view the controversy of transracial adoptions as a power dynamic, with the majority population exercising control over a commodity, African American children (Kupenda et al., in press). There is little agreement among minority groups on the need for transracial and transcultural adoptions.

History of Transracial Adoption—A Social Experiment

Although a few isolated cases of transracial placements had occurred in the late 1940s, some states had prohibitive laws against such adoptions. Tensions were high among people of different races living together in this country, and it was not until the late 1960s that the U.S. Supreme Court struck down prohibitions against interracial marriages (*Loving v. Commonwealth of Virginia* 1967). At the time, black-white interracial marriages were still illegal in 17 states. Despite their illegality, black-white interracial unions occurred throughout the pre-1967 history of the United States, both in and out of wedlock (Rosenblatt et al. 1995).

By the 1950s, the pool of Caucasian babies began to shrink as a result of family planning. This trend grew stronger in the 1970s as a result of abortions and decreased shame associated with out-of-wedlock births. The remaining adoptable pool tended to be children who were older, had special needs, or were minorities whose mothers could not afford or did not desire abortions. This created a supply-and-demand crisis. North American adoption agencies began to make efforts to place African American and Native American children without restriction. Montreal's Open Door Society of 1962 and the Council on Adoptable Children, two parent groups, began experimentally recruiting families interested in transracial adoption (Kim 1980). The Child Welfare League of America and the Bureau of Indian Affairs continued a conceptual shift in placement practices with the emphasis ostensibly on the "child's best interest," placing 400 Native American children in Caucasian homes from 1958 to 1968. During the climate of social unrest and change in this country in the 1960s, the Bureau of Indian Affairs reversed its previous stand and the Child Welfare League of America revised and reversed its operating practices to emphasize a preference for inracial adoptions (Bartholet 1991).

The Indian Child Welfare Act of 1978 (P.L. 95-608) declared it in the best interests of Native American children to promote the stability and security of Indian tribes and families by the establishment of minimum federal standards for the removal of Indian children from their families and the placement of such children in foster or adoptive homes that will reflect the unique values of Native American culture: "It gives first priority for adoption to the child's extended family, second to its tribe, and third to other Indians." It went on to say that "an Indian tribe shall have jurisdiction exclusive as to any State over any child custody proceeding involving an Indian child who resides or is domiciled within the reservation of such tribe."

Against a backdrop of the burgeoning Civil Rights movement and black nationalism, African American children were placed in white adoptive homes in small numbers. Both good-faith intentions of breaking down segregation barriers and profit motives were operative in these early social experiments. A heated backlash erupted from vocal minorities, and in 1972 the National Association of Black Social Workers (NABSW) publicly denounced transracial adoption as "cultural genocide" (National Association of Black Social Workers 1972). There have always been informal adoptions (very common in African American extended families) and private adoptions of African American babies given up at birth. African Americans adopt at a higher rate than do Caucasian families (Wheeler 1993), but many of these adoptions are of the informal variety. Another source that began feeding the pool of children available for adoption was the foster care system.

The 1960s and 1970s saw the decimation of many minority families due to higher mortality rates, incarceration, substance abuse, unemployment secondary to racism, and inadequate preparation of minorities for the job market. The confluence of these forces increased single-parent families and homelessness, and in the 1990s, the HIV epidemic would contribute its share. The effect was the explosive expansion of the number of minority children in foster care (Everett 1991). Because of the income differentials between African American and Caucasians

and other race-based selection screens, often middle-class African American families desirous of adopting could not meet the eligibility criteria of some adoption agencies. To counter this, African American–run agencies specializing in African American adoptions sprang up and African American churches assisted in recruiting adoptive parents. From 1989 to 1990, only 382 inracial adoptions of predominantly African American children had occurred through such agencies, with a pool of 17,500 African American children in need of adoptive homes for that period (Bartholet 1994).

In the late 1970s, the National Association for the Advancement of Colored People and the National Urban League urged consideration of transracial adoptions. Later, in 1995, an advisory committee of the African American leadership group, Project 21, condemned adoption policies that would turn down stable, nurturing homes, of any race, interested in adopting African American children while adoption agencies spent protracted periods of time looking for same-race homes.

In 1980, Congress passed the Adoption Assistance and Child Welfare Act, which provides economic support to families who adopt special needs children. It requires that every child in foster care have a permanency plan within 18 months. The Multiethnic Placement Act of 1994 (MEPA) and Interethnic Adoption Provisions of 1994 prohibit discrimination in placement on the basis of race, color, or national origin of either the prospective parent or the child. The goal is to increase the number of adoptable children by facilitating the recruitment of potential parents.

History of Transcultural Adoption—Another Avenue

From the end of World War II until after the Korean Conflict, war orphans from Sweden, Japan, and Korea became available for adoption without the bureaucracy required by United States adoption agencies. These were the first transcultural-transracial adoptions. Operation Babylift occurred after the Vietnam War, bringing Vietnamese orphans to the United States. Asian sources of babies diminished following the summer Olympics in Korea in 1988, with media attention on the flow of children out of the country causing loss of face among Korean officials. United States citizens wishing to adopt then turned to Latin America and more recently to Eastern Europe (Wilkinson 1995). The changing attitude of other countries about adoption of their children, the Caucasian infant shortage in the United States, greater affluence of United States parents (adoption costs can be as much as $60,000), humanitarian desires to provide opportunities for children from impoverished or traumatic circumstances, and the initial underregulation of this adoptive pathway have paved the way for current trends (Simon 1994).

The United Nations 1993 Convention on the Protection of Children and Cooperation in Respect on Intercountry Adoption was signed at The Hague by many countries, including Burkina Faso, Cyprus, Colombia, Costa Rica, Ecuador, Lithuania, Mexico, Moldova, Paraguay, Peru, the Philippines, Poland, Romania, Sri Lanka, and Venezuela. The agreement brought safeguards for those children who are often illegally obtained by prohibiting the improper gain, abduction, sale, or trafficking in children (Jacot 1999).

CLINICAL ISSUES

Demographics of Transracial and Transcultural Adoptions

Among children initially placed in foster care, 50%–70% are returned to their parents. But in 1995, 600,000 children had spent all or part of the year in foster care, 40,600 had been in foster care for more than 5 years, and 50,000 children were declared legally free for adoption, that is, parental rights had been permanently terminated (Rosenfeld et al. 1997). African American children wait to be adopted significantly longer than do Caucasian children. Older children and sibling groups also have longer waits. Of all children waiting for adoption, 43% are African American, 40% are Caucasian, and 7% are Hispanic. Only 4% of these children were younger than 1 year old; 36% were 1–5 years old, 43% were 6–12 years old, and 17% were older than age 12. The median age at adoption was 7.4 years. Two out of three waiting children have special needs—medical, developmental, behavioral, or psychological—or are members of a minority. Many children whose parents' rights have been terminated are never adopted (Westat 1986).

In 1968, there were 733 TRAs. The number of African American children adopted annually by Caucasian parents increased to 2,574 in 1971. By 1975, as a result of outcries by the NABSW, the number of transracial adoptions had dropped to 831. By 1984, it is estimated there were 20,000 African American children in Caucasian homes, yet it is estimated that transracial adoptions make up only 1% of all adoptions (Stolley 1993). TRAs of foreign-born children have increased, rising from 5,663 in 1975 to 9,120 in 1988 (U.S. Bureau of Census 1996). African American–Caucasian biracial children are the most frequently placed group in transracial adoptions.

Adoptees from developing countries often arrive in the United States with marginal health status, further compromising the adjustment to their new homes. Between 1977 and 1997, the number of TCAs coming to the United States doubled; they came from Russia (3,816), China (3,597), South Korea (1,654), Guatemala (788), and Romania (621) (Jacot 1999). For 6 years (1980–1986), slightly more than half of the 50,441 children adopted into this country came from South Korea (Smith 1988). There may be factors within the sociocultural framework of that country which have contributed to this trend. There is little tolerance for illegitimacy or mixed heritage; therefore, adoption may present opportunities for education and vocational advancement, which might not be otherwise attainable. Korea has many requirements regarding adoptions of their children. The prospective parents must be a married couple between the ages of 25 and 45, have been married at least 3 years, not have more than four children in the household, and be free of any life-threatening diseases.

In China, where males are the preferred gender, the rules for adoptions out of country had been quite strict until 1991. The rules were relaxed after the orphanages were found to be overcrowded with infant girls, some of whom were being allowed to die ("Give Me Your Squalling Masses" 1996; Jacot 1999). Prior to 1991, there were probably no more than 100 Chinese babies coming into the United States each year for adoption. By 1995, U.S. parents found it much easier to adopt Chinese infant girls (Elegant 1998; "Give Me Your Squalling Masses" 1996).

Research

Most researchers have found that ethnoracial awareness begins in early childhood, between ages 3 and 5 years, but children do not understand the permanence of this classification. Between ages 6 and 9 years, development of racial and ethnic constancy occurs (Clark and Clark 1958). For the past several decades, the body of research on transracial and transcultural adoption can be broadly compartmentalized into studies of family integration, racial identity, self-esteem, school performance, and overall adjustment. These variables have been examined for both transracial and inracial adoptions. Researchers studying children placed at an early age have found no clear differences between the groups other than variance in their reference group orientation (Alstein and Simon 1992; Vroegh 1997). Transracial adoptees, many of whom are biracial, frequently referred to themselves as mixed or part Caucasian. In terms of family integration, the younger the child, the easier is the assimilation into the family.

The family's racial stance, which can be categorized as either racially dissonant or racially aware, can strongly influence the adoptee's ability to develop a healthy racial identity (Kallgren and Caudill 1993). In the racially dissonant family, the residence is generally in a predominantly Caucasian neighborhood, and the child usually attends a predominantly Caucasian school, with little opportunity to interact with or see positive role models of his or her race. In homes where adoptees' racial identities are denied, adoptees typically develop an unhealthy attitude toward their ethnic origins, which in turn contributes to poor self-image. Racially aware families, on the other hand, typically reside in racially and ethnically diverse neighborhoods and the child attends integrated schools and churches. These adoptees are actively involved with their birth cultures and tend to develop healthy racial identities and self-esteems.

Critics of early TRA research cited problems with flawed racial identity measures, selection of subjects who were Caucasian appearing, unsophisticated statistics, and problematic interviewers (Chimezie 1975; Vroegh 1997). These problems have been improved on in the past decade. The general findings are that at least three-quarters of the transracial adoptees are happy and feel a part of their families, about the same percentage as inracial adoptees. Some findings show that some transracial adoptees actually outperform their inracial counterparts on IQ tests. A 20-year study of 200 Caucasian parents and their predominantly African American adopted children in their early to mid-20s at the time of follow-up supports that the adoptees are happy with their racial identity and racial awareness and are comfortable with themselves (Simon 1993, 1994). About 20% of the TRA adoptees experienced problems during the preteen and teen years, for example, stealing or school-related problems, but this was no greater than for inracial adoptees (Barth and Berry 1988).

Several authors have described significant factors that affect the adjustment and successful adaptation of adopted children born in developing countries (Rutter and Garmezy 1983; Verhulst et al. 1990a, 1990b, 1992). In many cases, the limited diets and inadequate pre- and postnatal care available for pregnant mothers increase the risk that infants will be born in poor health. The marginal economic circumstances of these mothers also increase the likelihood that their children will be exposed to unhealthy living environments, including abuse and neglect. Additional stresses include adjustment to the loss of early caretakers and, depending on the age at placement, adaptation to a change in language.

A 17-year study investigated the long-term adjustment of 224 transcultural and inracial adoptees as adults, including Asians born in Korea and Vietnam, African Americans born in the United States but adopted by Caucasians, and Caucasians born in the United States and adopted by Caucasians (Brooks and Barth 1999). The original 1977 study design included transculturally/transracially adopted children from Korea, Vietnam, and Colombia, representing the largest numbers of transcultural adoptions in this country. The results indicated that most of the children, except the inracially adopted Caucasian males, demonstrated good adjustment as defined by educational performance, problem behavior, and the Global Assessment Scale. Caucasian and African American males experienced more adjustment difficulties, with lower academic performance; involvement with drugs, alcohol, and the police; and lower grade point averages, than did the females across all ethnic groups. This study supported the finding that transracial/transcultural adoption for these particular groups is not detrimental to the child's long-term adjustment.

PITFALLS

Political

Transracial and transcultural adoptions are thorny forensic matters for the child psychiatrist due to the political valence attached to intrafamilial mixing of the races in the United States. Although race and skin color are emotionally charged issues in other countries as well, they seem to assume greater importance in the United States because of its tragic history based on the dehumanizing treatment of the African American and Native American races by the Caucasian race before, during, and after slavery.

The forensic child expert must lay aside his or her political position on the subject of TRA or TCA and approach a requested evaluation from a position predicated on current evidence-based research. Each assessment is a unique situation, and the "interests of the child" must always supersede those of the parents, the extended family, or the race. An African American home is not, by definition, necessarily the best home for an African American child. Nor are all prospective Caucasian adoptive parents necessarily without bias or of such fortitude that they can provide a protective enough environment in which an African American child can thrive. Although TRAs and TCAs are not without problems, there is absolutely no crueler or more psychologically damaging practice than to deny children legally free for adoption a stable and loving home if one exists.

Legal

It is now illegal to delay the initiation of the process of obtaining the status "legally free for adoption" or to protract appropriate termination of parental rights of minorities because of unavailability of inracial adoptive parents. Some flexibility of adoption standards and subsidization of special needs adoptees may be reasonable and appropriate to increase the pool of inracial adoptive parents (e.g., considering older parents, single parents, or parents of lower income status). These should be viewed as maneuvers to level the playing field due to past discriminatory adoption criteria, not to lower the criteria bar beneath a minimum parental desirability standard. Parents who would otherwise be uninterested in adoption should never be coerced or "bought" for the sake of accomplishing inracial placement.

Clinical

In fairness to parents considering TRAs or TCAs, it is the duty of adoption agencies to make them aware of potential pitfalls. The risks of attachment disorder of childhood or adolescence, seen particularly in the new wave of Eastern European adoptees, are conditions that would challenge the most earnest of parents.

CASE EXAMPLE EPILOGUES

Case Example 1

In 1978, the U.S. Fifth Circuit held that race could have a determinative impact on child placement (*Drummond v. Fulton County* 1978). The trial court removed the child from her foster home and placed her with her grandmother. Although permitting the use of race in child placement, the appellate court ruled that race may not be the sole factor in child placement for adoption (Forde-Mazrui 1994). The court let the lower court's decision stand, although it found that the foster parents qualified in all other respects (Forde-Mazrui 1994). Today this ruling would be illegal under MEPA.

Case Example 2

Due to an adoptive mother's grassroots advocacy, Texas was the first state to ban race as a main criterion for adoption selection in 1993 (Wheeler 1993). The federal government followed suit with MEPA, which would have made this ruling, which went against the recommendations of professional organizations, such as the California Academy of Child and Adolescent Psychiatry, illegal.

Case Example 3

As seen often in divorce cases involving biological children, children who are adopted may also become the pawn of custody conflicts and may be particularly vulnerable due to their earlier losses. The judge would have ruled in the best interests of the child had he awarded custody to the father. Unfortunately, in this case, he did not.

ACTION GUIDELINES

General

The best interests of the child must always be the forensic goal in navigating the shoals of race and culture. There is no "formula family" prescribed by the state. There are single-parent, stepparent, same-sex, common law, biracial, bicultural, bireligious, blended, and extended forms to name a few. Research, albeit with its limitations, has generally shown positive outcomes for both transracial and transcultural adoptees when measures of family integration, scholastic achievement, self-esteem, racial and ethnic identity, and overall adjustment were used. The younger the child at the time of adoption, the easier the integration; the older the child at the time of adoption, the stronger the child's ethnoracial identity and the greater his curiosity about his race, country of origin, and birth parents.

Society, child welfare agencies, and the courts in the United States are at a confounding point in history. Equal protection and antidiscrimination laws, designed to protect the civil rights of racial and ethnic minorities and strictly applied to all other areas of daily life, have been selectively ignored in order to preserve inracial adoption as the normative child placement configuration. Ostensibly to allow adoption workers to find minority adoptive parents, excessive delays in placing minority children freed for adoption have taken place in the past at the expense of children's mental health and well-being. The forensic child expert has the awesome but instrumental task of evaluating the individual parties in a prospective transracial or transcultural adoption or custody dispute in an arena teeming with emotional and political acrimony and must do so without bias. Pediatricians, child psychiatrists, child psychologists, social workers, and teachers are important resources for these families. Some parents may have questions regarding the behavioral adjustment of their children or some other aspect of the adoption. It is important that prospective adoptive parents be encouraged to obtain resource materials to contribute to their own knowledge base and to help answer questions that their children may have about the adoption (Buettner 1997; Girard 1989; Haskins 1992; Hoobler and Hoobler 1994; Jordan-Wong 1992; Kraus 1992; MiNer 1998; Rogers 1994; Schwartz 1996; Sobol 1994). Supportive services to these families before a crisis arises are of significant preventive health benefit. Not until this country flushes out the powerful vestiges of racism that permeate the daily lives of its citizens and institutions, however, will the issues of color, race, and ethnicity in child placement be moot regardless of laws on the books.

The Role of the Forensic Child Expert

In the United States all adoptions must present for the court's approval. The standard of "best interests of the child" governs child placement in the probate and family court systems. This general standard is used for all children, whether contested custodial petitions between biological parents or the adoptions of children who are of racial and cultural groups other than those of the adoptive parents are involved. Contrary to the recommendations of child development experts, in many TRAs and TCAs, there may be little attention paid to maintenance of continuity of the child's relationship with caregivers or the developmental importance of expediency in decision making about adoptions (Goldstein and Goldstein 1996). Because the child's long-term psychological well-being should always be the primary concern, the court asks for the recommendations of mental health professionals and social service agencies for their best clinical judgments in these matters. The forensic child expert may be called on to answer questions concerning the effects of TRA and TCA, the return of the child to the birth parent (Kermani and Weiss 1995), or continuation of foster placement. The request may be made by the court, a parent(s), or the child's or parents' attorney to assist with adoptions. There could be a request for assistance in custody cases; for example, the adoptive parents of transracial or transcultural adoptees may divorce and contest custody or biological grandparents may contest custody. The evaluator should clarify what questions are being asked and determine if he or she is qualified to provide the answers. As with any forensic evaluation, the child should never be evaluated without consent of the custodial parent or authorization of the court, unless privilege and confidentiality are waived (American Academy of Child and Adolescent Psychiatry 1997).

History of Prospective Adoptive Parents

Foremost in the expert's history gathering is the consideration of the adoptive parents' motive for adopting

transracially or transculturally. Have they ever been foster parents, and if so, for how long and with how many children? If they are experienced foster parents, what has factored into their desire to adopt this child? Will they continue to be foster parents? If so, have they considered the ramifications for the prospective adoptee? Have any other foster children been of a race or culture other than that of the parents? Many adoptive parents will have had children; some will be childless. In the former case, are their children biological? Are they stepchildren in the home? Are they adults? If the prospective adoptive parents are childless, to what extent did the couple try to conceive? Is there any desperation in their quest for parenthood? Was an ethnic child their first choice or default option? What are the couple's ethnic origins, racial attitudes, educational backgrounds, and life experiences that may have prepared them for the vicissitudes encountered in parenting a child of a different race? Do any of the following apply for the adoptive parents: attendance at integrated schools, churches, or clubs; residence in multicultural neighborhoods; employment in multicultural workplaces; travels; volunteer work outside of their communities? Some Caucasians are naive about the random but predictable microtraumas that African Americans experience daily (Pierce 1989). Will they—can they—be sounding boards when their child reports these experiences at the end of a school day? Will they be overprotective, effectively stifling their child's ability to eventually cope with these stresses independently? Will they be prepared for the stares, the questions, the insensitive remarks, and the outright insults that will predictably be experienced? If the prospective adoptive parents are racially naive, to what extent are they willing to alter their lifestyle to accommodate a child of a different race? These are questions for all prospective parents of children from diverse cultures.

In many transracial/transcultural adoptions, there may be little information available regarding the mother's prenatal care, the complications of the child's birth, prematurity, low birth weight, abuse or neglect history, or other pertinent medical or family history. The parents may be unprepared to understand the significance of these residual medical and/or psychological factors on the child's health status. They may be completely shocked to find that their child has both physical and psychological problems stemming from the preadoption condition. Adoption specialists are finding that they are dealing with children returned to adoption agencies for replacement. This phenomenon, called *disruption*, seems more related to children who have been adopted from Eastern Europe (Seelye 1998).

History of Birth Parent(s)

Biological parents of transracial adoptees may either have relinquished their child for adoption or had their parental rights terminated. If the latter, it could have been for reasons having to do with child abuse or neglect driven by an underlying substance abuse problem or psychiatric illness. Like any other person(s) who has ever given up a child for adoption or not fought to block the child's adoption or fought and lost, the parent(s) may be plagued with guilt or resentment against the judicial or child welfare system. This may especially be true if child protective services has removed the child from their custody. In a case in which the birth parent is contesting the TRA of her child, foremost in the history gathering is determination of the reason the child was removed or given up. Would the parent be contesting the adoption if it were inracial? Did the parent exercise any permissible visitation rights and pay any designated portion of the child's support while in foster care? If countertransference issues impede the psychiatrist's ability to collect data in a nonjudgmental fashion, it would behoove him to seek appropriate consultation.

History of the Child

There is a double challenge in assessment of a transracial adoptee. Naturally there are adoption and abandonment issues, but there is also the sensitive issue of race. As with any child or adolescent evaluation, the first task is to establish rapport with the patient. This task can be painstaking if the forensic expert is viewed as an agent of others and vested with powerful authority to influence the adoptee's life arrangement. Establishing the ground rules is part of this process, especially rules having to do with the purpose of the consultation and confidentiality rules (when there is no confidentiality, it is important to disclose this fact to teens). It is important to ascertain why the adoptee does or does not want to be there. Demarcating the examiner's relationship with parents, school, and the court at the outset is important. Unlike the therapeutic setting in which there is the luxury of time to allow the adoptee's agenda to unfold in an evaluation, the forensic expert's agenda must be imposed.

The race issues do not need to be plunged into immediately, but they cannot be skirted or apologized for. Inquiring about the child's feelings about adoption in general can set the stage for approaching the subject of TRA. The examiner need not consider herself an expert in TRA; she need only be willing to be a student of the adoptee and his families. An open admission of ignorance goes a long way in establishing the doctor-patient relationship as long as the patient perceives sensitivity, honesty, and lack of arrogance and judgmentalness on the part of the examiner.

Attention must be paid to the quality of bonding that has developed between child and parent(s) as well as siblings and the potential psychological damage that could result from the disruption of such bond(s). In the case of newborn adoptions, which may be relevant to TRAs if a child was removed from a biological mother determined to be a substance abuser, the California Academy of Child and Adolescent Psychiatry (1994, p. 3) recommends that

> all newborn adoptions be finalized within the first four months of life, conforming with known developmental needs of the infant. Although adoption finalization at birth would be most preferential for the infant and adoptive parents, it is understood that biological parents need a reasonable amount of time to appropriately resolve their ambivalence about giving up their child, but this time period should not exceed this four month time period, to insure the psychological attachment of the parent and child, and to mitigate the possibility of developmental difficulties.

Although this position is congruent with conventional wisdom, there is no longitudinal research data on the outcome of children who have had early attachments disrupted with the intent to reattach to loving, nurturing adults (Griffith 1995). Psychological pain ensues when the bond is broken between child and psychological parents, but we just don't know how resilient children are in the above circumstances.

REFERENCES

Alstein HJ, Simon RJ: Adoption, Race, and Identity: From Infancy Through Adolescence. New York, Praeger, 1992

American Academy of Child and Adolescent Psychiatry: Practice parameters for child custody evaluation. J Am Acad Child Adolesc Psychiatry 36 (suppl):57S–68S, 1997

Barth P, Berry M: Adoption and Disruption: Rates, Risks, and Responses. New York, Aldine de Gruyter, 1988

Bartholet E: Where do black children belong? the politics of race matching in adoption. University of Pennsylvania Law Review 139(5):1163–1256, 1991

Bartholet E: Race matching in adoption: an American perspective, in The Best Interests of the Child: Culture, Identity, and Transracial Adoption. London, Free Association Books, 1994, pp 151–187

Binder RL: American Psychiatric Association resource document on controversies in child custody: gay and lesbian parenting, transracial adoptions, joint versus sole custody, and custody gender issue. J Am Acad Psychiatry Law 26(2):267–276, 1998

Brooks D, Barth RP: Adult transracial and inracial adoptees: effects of race, gender, adoptive family structure, and placement history on adjustment outcomes. Am J Orthopsychiatry 69(1):87–99, 1999

Buettner D: African Trek. Minneapolis, MN, Lerner Publications, 1997

California Academy of Child and Adolescent Psychiatry: Position paper on newborn infant adoptions. Sacramento, CA, California Academy of Child and Adolescent Psychiatry, 1994

Chimezie A: Transracial adoption of black children. Social Work 20:296–301, 1975

Clark KB, Clark MP: Racial identification and preference in Negro children, in Readings in Social Psychology. Edited by Macoby EE, Newcomb TM, Hartley EL. New York, Holt, Rinehart & Winston, 1958

Drummond v Fulton County Department of Family and Children's Services, 437 US 910 (1978)

Elegant S, Pao M: Bringing home baby: as any stroll through Manhattan's Upper East Side illustrates affluent Americans are bringing China's orphans to the United States in record numbers. Far Eastern Economic Review 161(32):54–55, 1998

Everett JE: Children in crisis, in Child Welfare: An Africentric Perspective. Edited by Everett JE, et al. New Brunswick, NJ, Rutgers University Press, 1991, pp 2–4

Forde-Mazrui K: Black identity and child placement: the best interests of black and biracial children. Michigan Law Review 92:925–967, 1994

Girard LW: We adopted you, Benjamin Koo. Niles, IL, Albert Whiteman & Company, 1989

Give me your squalling masses: coming to America. The Economist 338(7951):22(1), 1996

Goldstein J, Goldstein S: "Put yourself in the skin of the child," she said. Psychoanal Study Child 51:46–55, 1996

Griffith E: Forensic and policy implications of the transracial debate. Bulletin of the American Academy of Psychiatry and the Law 23(4):501–512, 1995

Haskins J: Count your way through China. Minneapolis, MN, Carolrhoda Books, 1992

Hoobler D, Hoobler T: The Chinese family album. New York, Oxford University Press, 1994

The Indian Child Welfare Act of 1978, Pub L 95–608

Interethnic Adoption Provisions of 1994, Pub L 104–188, §1808

Jacot M: Adoption: for love or money? UNESCO Courier, 1999, pp 37–39

Jordan-Wong J: A forever family. New York, HarperCollins, 1992

Kallgren CA, Caudill PJ: Psychol Rep 72:551–558, 1993

Kermani EJ, Weiss EA: Biological parents regaining their rights: a psycholegal analysis of a new era in custody disputes. Bulletin of the American Academy of Psychiatry and the Law 23(2):261–267, 1995

Kim SP: Behavioral symptoms in three transracially adopted Asian children: diagnosis dilemma. Child Welfare 59:213–224, 1980

Kim WJ: Transcultural/transracial adoption. AACAP News March–April 1996, p 33

Kraus J: Tall Boy's Journey. Minneapolis, MN, Carolrhoda Books, 1992

Kupenda AM, Thrash AL, Riley-Collins JA, et al: Law, life and literature: using literature to expose transracial adoption laws as adoption on a one-way street. 17 Buff Pub Int L J (in press)

Loving v Commonwealth of Virginia, 388 US 1, 6 n5 (1967)

McRoy R: An organizational dilemma: the case of transracial adoptions. J Appl Behav Sci 25(2):145–160, 1989

MiNer C: Rain forest girl. Childs, MD, Mitchell Lane Publisher, 1998

Multiethnic Placement Act of 1994: Pub L 103–382, 42 USC §471a

National Association of Black Social Workers: Position paper on transracial adoption, 1972

Pierce CM: Unity in diversity: thirty-three years of stress, in Black Students: Psychosocial Issues and Academic Achievements. Edited by Berry GL, Asamen JW. Newbury Park, CA, Sage, 1989, pp 296–312

Rogers F: Let's Talk About Adoption. New York, GD Putnam's Sons, 1994

Rosenblatt PC, Karis TA, Powell RD: Multiracial Couples: Black and White Voices. Thousand Oaks, CA, Sage Publications, 1995

Rosenfeld AA, Pilowsky DJ, Fine P, et al: Foster care: an update. J Am Acad Child Adolesc Psychiatry 36(4):448–457, 1997

Rutter M, Garmezy N: Developmental psychology, in Handbook of Child Psychology, Vol 4. Edited by Mussen PH. New York, Wiley, 1983, pp 775–911

Schwartz P: Carolyn's story. Minneapolis, MN, Lerner Publications, 1996

Seelye K: Specialists report rise in adoptions that fail. New York Times, March 4, 1998, p A12

Simon RJ: Transracial adoption: highlights of a twenty-year study. Reconstruction 2(2):130–131, 1993

Simon RJ: Transracial adoption: the American experience, in In the Best Interests of the Child: Culture, Identity, and Transracial Adoption. Edited by Gabor I, Aldridge J. London, Free Association Books, 1994, pp 136–150

Sobol H: We Don't Look Like Our Mom and Dad. New York, Coward-McCann, 1994

Smith L: Babies from abroad. American Demographics 10(3):38–42, 1988

Stolley KS: Statistics on adoption in the United States. Future Child 3:26–42, 1993

U.S. Bureau of the Census: Resident population of the United States: middle series projections, 2035–2050, by sex, race, and Hispanic origin with median age. Washington, DC, U.S. Government Printing Office, March 1996

Verhulst FC, Althaus M, Versluis-Den Bieman HJM: Problem behavior in international adoptees, I: an epidemiological study. J Am Acad Child Adolesc Psychiatry 29(1):94–102, 1990a

Verhulst FC, Althaus M, Versluis-Den Bieman HJM: Problem behavior in international adoptees, II: age at placement. J Am Acad Child Adolesc Psychiatry 29(1):104–111, 1990b

Verhulst FC, Althaus M, Versluis-Den Bieman HJM: Damaging backgrounds: later adjustment of international adoptees. J Am Acad Child Adolesc Psychiatry. 31(3):518–524, 1992

Vroegh K: Transracial adoptees: developmental status after 17 years. Am J Orthopsychiatry 67(4):568–575, 1997

Westat: Adoptive services for waiting minority and non-minority children. H4–11, H4–14. Rockville, MD, Westat, 1986, pp x–xi, 3.7–3.44

Wheeler DL: Black children, white parents: the difficult issue of transracial adoption. Chronicle of Higher Education 40:A8–A10, 1993

White woman awarded custody of black child in Florida adoption case. Jet 96(9):25, 1999

Wilkinson HS: Psycholegal process and issues in international adoption. American Journal of Family Therapy 23(2):173–183, 1995

PART III

Child Abuse

Allegations of abuse made by young children can have grave repercussions, resulting in loss of contact with a parent or even imprisonment of the alleged offender. Part III provides new and important information on memory in children that the forensic examiner needs to know in order to assess the credibility and reliability of statements made by children. Dr. Clark provides a framework for how memory develops in children in Chapter 13, and in Chapter 14, Drs. Bruck and Ceci review current research on the suggestibility of children. The latter discuss the implications of this emerging body of research on children's testimony in court. In Chapter 15, Dr. Quinn provides guidelines for assessing allegations of sexual abuse in children and discusses the importance of avoiding actions that might contaminate a child's statements.

No longer arcane, Munchausen syndrome by proxy is receiving increased attention in the media. In Chapter 16, Dr. Schreier, one of the foremost experts on this disorder, acquaints the reader with the dynamics of the bizarre condition that many clinicians and jurists have refused to accept in the past. He provides invaluable guidelines for how to conduct investigations once this condition is suspected. Sexual harassment of children and teens is also an old problem that is finally receiving attention; in Chapter 17, Drs. Benedek and Clark discuss the evolution of litigation for damages related to sexual harassment and how to conduct such a forensic evaluation. And in Chapter 18, Dr. Benedek and Ms. Brown conclude this part with an overview of child pornography, with emphasis on the pernicious effect of its availability over the Internet.

Although the issues continue to change, the basic forensic principles for assessing them do not. However, the forensic examiner needs to keep current on the literature in these new areas in order to recognize these conditions and to be able to provide effective scientifically based testimony and rebut the testimony of less informed experts.

CHAPTER 13

Developmental Aspects of Memory in Children

Beth K. Clark, Ph.D., A.B.P.P.

Case Example

A 5-year-old girl tells a friend that "my uncle tickles my vagina." After the friend tells their teacher, the police come to the 5-year-old's home to interview her. She runs away upon seeing them, yelling, "I can't remember anything." The child is then interviewed at a center specializing in the evaluation of sexually abused children. The evaluating clinician is experienced and asks open-ended questions. The parents are advised to avoid providing the child with information she does not already have. At the first interview, the child is asked to talk about her uncle. She indicates that he baby-sits for her and that they watch TV. She says that he holds her on his lap and tickles her on the vagina. At a second interview, she does not mention any tickling and reports that they play games while they watch *Sesame Street*. She says these games happened "one or two or eight" times around the time that Santa visits. She is able to talk about many things that have happened over the year in her kindergarten class, but she cannot remember the number of her classroom or her home address. She can describe her home environment but is not sure what kind of job her mother has. She thinks she may be a teacher (when in fact she is a businesswoman). During further interviews, the girl continues to report being tickled on the vagina and talks about a number of other activities she engaged in with her uncle, relating that these all happened at her home.

When the uncle is charged with child sexual abuse, his defense attorney moves to dismiss the case because the child has given inconsistent reports and has an unreliable and faulty memory. He cites in part evidence that the uncle did baby-sit for the child several times at his own home, not only at her house.

When a child makes a report that he or she has been abused, there are usually only two witnesses: the alleged perpetrator of the event and the child. As clinicians, we are often faced with the important and difficult task of assessing the reliability and quality of children's reports. It is essential for the examining clinician to have a working knowledge of how memory develops in children, as well as how memories are retained and recalled, and to understand which interview techniques elicit the most accurate reports. This chapter confines itself primarily to a discussion of the ability of children to remember and report autobiographical events—that is, events that occur in their own lives.

MEMORY DEVELOPMENT

We know that children, as a rule, do not remember things as well as adults do and that they forget more quickly. However, even infants have some ability to remember, and children's memory significantly improves over time. Many studies (e.g., Fivush and Shukat 1995; Zaragoza et al. 1995) have noted the variability of the development of memory between particular children, which underscores the need for careful individual assessment.

Infants and Toddlers (Ages 0–3)

Originally it was thought that very young children had poor memories, primarily because they did not have the verbal and/or neurological tools to encode an event.

However, with the advent of studies using nonverbal methods, there is now some evidence that children even younger than 1 year old can remember or at least recognize some things after a period of time passes. Children who learned a series of both novel and familiar tasks at this age could recall both types of tasks after 2–6 weeks and recalled a familiar task 1 year later (McDonough and Mandler 1994). Another group of 1- to 2-year-olds could recall a specific event 8 months later (Bauer et al. 1994). However, it is likely that these memories are implicit, that is, due to simple conditioning, as opposed to explicit memory, which involves an awareness that something has been remembered (Nelson 1994). Although there is some controversy in this area, there is a general consensus that infants and toddlers do not have the neurological maturity to be able to have an explicit memory of a particular event in their lives. As children move beyond this stage of development, they typically do not remember events occurring during it; this forgetting is the so-called infantile amnesia. This is likely due to a complex interaction of cognitive and linguistic development and socialization. The ability to form explicit memories is not available to infants, so the events are lost. In addition, the process of cognitive development is so rapid during this time that the changes are likely to affect the ability to retain earlier information. Memory is confounded by the lack of experience in remembering and by the social process of learning how to do so. Thus, adults or older children claiming to remember events occurring before the age of 3 should be approached with some skepticism. It does appear, however, that some preschoolers can report an event that happened to them during toddlerhood (Boyer et al. 1994). This is likely due to individual differences in cognitive and verbal ability during the preschool years, with those children who are more advanced more likely to be able to report.

Preschoolers (Ages 3–5 or 6)

By age 3, a qualitative change in the ability to remember appears in most children. As verbal abilities become more complex and children are exposed to contextual situations where they can learn to remember, there are advances in the three major requirements of memory. Children get better at encoding—specifically attending to a particular aspect of the environment long enough to take it into memory. They begin to be able to store events and experiences in short-term memory and, less effectively, in long-term memory. Finally, they become more able to retrieve memories by thinking about them or by responding to questions or prompts.

School-Age and Older Children

Although young children may understand at some level that there are mental processes involved in attempts to retrieve information and can be taught some of these processes, a major shift appears to take place beginning at age 6. At this point, children begin to use strategies in order to help them store and remember things. For example, at 7 or 8 they begin to more frequently use verbal rehearsal in order to retain information. These early strategies are somewhat limited and rigid; however, they become more sophisticated and flexible throughout childhood and into adolescence (Kail 1990).

Older children are better judges of how hard a memory task is and are much better predictors of how accurate their memories will be given the task (e.g., see Flavell et al. 1970). Acquiring knowledge about the world and accurately remembering it interact in interesting ways as children become older. The more knowledge they have, the more ability there is to form associations among points of knowledge, thus aiding storage, retention, and retrieval. As they are exposed to repeated and familiar events, children develop "scripts," or generic templates based on experience. Whereas this allows them more easily to recall familiar events, it also leads to difficulty in retaining some specific memories as they simply meld into a familiar script of the event (Kail 1990). Like adults, older children may not remember all actual details of events clearly over time, and they tend to elaborate or recall based not on their knowledge of the actual event but based on a script. Thus, some novel events may be remembered more easily because no script exists for them or because they fall so far outside the usual script. Also similar to adults, older children are quite accomplished at remembering the gist, or general meaning, of an event.

MEMORY RETENTION AND RECALL

Age

Because so many problematic allegations of sexual abuse are made by children of preschool age, an extensive amount of research has been done on how such children remember and report the events that occur in their lives. This section will focus on this population but will also refer to older children. A general rule is that retention and recall improve with age, with older children experiencing many of the same strengths and weaknesses as adults in their ability to accurately report an event. The reader is also referred to several other reviews of this subject (Ceci and Bruck 1995; Kuehnle 1996; Poole and Lamb 1998). Also, see Chapter 14, "Reliability and Suggestibility of Children's Statements," for a more complete review of how suggestibility affects memory.

We know that preschool children generally remember less than older children and adults. A review of the literature highlights a difficulty that many clinicians experience when interviewing preschoolers: for every positive discovery about a child's capacity to remember and report, there is a negative attached. For example, because of their greater dependency on context in remembering, preschool children recall more completely when asked more specific questions, but as recall increases, it becomes less accurate and includes erroneous detail.

Suggestibility

One of the greatest problems with children's memory is that it can be influenced by suggestions at any point in the encoding, storage, and retrieval processes (see Chapter 14). However, as mentioned above, memory can also be enhanced by cues. Thus, the first report given by a child about an event, especially if it is one that is not inappropriately influenced by the adult who is taking the report, may be the most accurate, though not the most complete. Cueing the child may produce more recall; however, it may also result in more mistakes in recollection and/or report. Thus the clinician is faced with a constant dilemma regarding how to effectively interview these children: Should one ask only open-ended questions, and when, if ever, should one sacrifice accuracy for completeness?

As in the Case Example, young children can be quite accurate within and across interviews, but they tend to be less consistent than older children. It is important to note that this lack of consistency is often a function of the questions children are asked by adults, as opposed to any problems with their memory. Confusing questions bring confused answers. This is particularly observable when reviewing direct and cross-examination of young children by attorneys who are unschooled in how to ask questions that young children can understand. Children's testimony is at times called into question not because they cannot give an age-appropriate account of what happened to them, but because they are unable to answer poorly worded and ill-conceived questions. Unfortunately, mental health clinicians and others who must interview children in forensic contexts are not immune to this problem.

Salience

Preschoolers, by virtue of having a rather idiosyncratically self-centered view of the world, may report what was salient to them, as opposed to what the interviewer wants to elicit. For example, in response to the request, "Tell me about your trip to Florida," the child might respond, "We went to Disneyworld." On a different day, the child might answer, "I rode on Dumbo and ate ice cream." In the Case Example, the child reports both sitting on her uncle's lap and playing games with him while watching TV. Both responses can be accurate, but they are not consistent.

Multiple Reports

Children who make allegations that they have been sexually abused are often interviewed a number of times—by law enforcement officers, protective services workers, therapists, and evaluators. Multiple interviewing should raise a concern that a child's memories of events may be affected by the numerous times the child has been asked to recount what occurred. It is clear that if children are asked to report under free recall conditions, their reports can be very stable across repeated interviews. In a free recall session, the child is asked very open-ended questions about the event, such as: "Tell me everything you remember about what happens when your uncle babysits for you." The data on free recall are robust enough that some authors suggest that if a child gives highly inconsistent narratives in free recall sessions, one might question their motivation, their capacity to accurately report, or whether they had been subject to external influence (Poole and White 1995). However, being able to retrieve and verbally report memories with minimal prompts (as opposed to simply recognizing an external depiction or description of an event) are very sophisticated tasks, which is why young children give less information than older children in free recall situations.

Both children and adults tend to remember more information over time if they are questioned repeatedly in a free recall context. In this context, frequent retelling of the event does not appear to do much harm, and carefully performed repeated interviews may actually help children retain their memories over a period of time. This makes sense when we think, for example, of how repeating information learned for a test over a number of days or weeks helps a student to retain it. However, the chance of inaccurate reports rises with the addition of at least two factors. First, interviews containing leading questions, or questions that give children information that they may not have or that suggest the answer, or interviews that are misleading increase the chances of incorrect reports emerging. Second, the longer the passage of time between the occurrence of the event and the interview, the less accurate the report. Thus, a child who is interviewed many months after an alleged event and is then given faulty information or is unduly influenced during several interviews cannot be expected to give a very reliable report.

Young children who have experienced repeated events can confuse them and when reporting, combine details of one event into the report of another. Again, the report may be accurate in terms of what happened to the child, but the child may not be able to give such details as how many times something occurred, what time of day it happened, where it transpired, and which events occurred at which times, because there may have been numerous events at different times and locations.

Source Memory

Young children also have difficulty in what is often called *source memory*, that is, they tend to confuse where a memory came from. Therefore, it may make little difference to them whether they actually remember something happening, whether someone told them about it, or whether they imagined it. Ceci and colleagues (1994) demonstrated this problem in a study in which preschool children were asked to think about events that had actually occurred to them in the past and about others that had not occurred. The children were then interviewed weekly, by an adult who showed them a card with the event pictured and asked them to tell whether the particular event had ever happened to them. The children were asked open-ended questions about details remembered about each possible event. At the end of 10 weeks, each child was asked if the events had occurred. Fifty-eight percent of the preschoolers indicated that at least one event that had not happened had actually happened to them; 25% endorsed the majority of the events that had not happened as having happened to them. Many children told detailed stories and, perhaps most disturbingly, were highly resistant to debriefing, even after they were told by such trusted figures as parents that the event did not happen. Ceci and colleagues concluded that these results indicated that the children actually came to believe the false events were true memories. This is of particular concern because in this study the interview techniques used were quite open-ended and not leading. However, a recent study by Pezdek and Roe (1997) presents some different findings. In this study, attempts

were made to plant, erase, or change memories of being touched in groups of 4- and 10-year-olds. Attempts to plant or erase memories were unsuccessful for most children in both groups. Consistent with other research, it proved easier to change an actually experienced memory of being touched. The authors hypothesized that this may have been due to the greater discrepancy between the child's actual experience and what they were being told in the plant-and-erase conditions than in the alteration condition. In any event, it is clear that preschoolers are susceptible to mistakes in recall based on source memory problems.

Stress

There is controversy over whether and how stress affects memory. Whereas some studies have shown no or little effect of stressful events on children's memory, others have concluded that stress reduces the ability to remember accurately, while still others have found that stress actually enhances memory. At this point, it cannot be definitively stated how memory and stress are related.

As children get older and develop memory skills similar to adults, reporting of events tends to be affected primarily by social and intrapsychic factors and less by developmental limitations. Factors that influence memory recall in most of us, such as motivational issues, social influence, passage of time, attention, and psychological defense mechanisms, come to the fore.

SUMMARY

Understanding the development of memory and the research on memory retention and recall are crucial for effective interviewing not only with children who have made allegations of sexual abuse but also with all children evaluated in the forensic context. It is clear that preschool and early school-age children present the greatest challenge for the clinician. As children mature in verbal and cognitive skills, and as they benefit from more experiences in the social world, their abilities to encode, remember, and report events improve. Actual memory becomes less of an issue, and social and intrapsychic factors involved in recall become more important. Careful, informed, and conservative interview techniques are the best way to provide the most forensically useful information about children of any age.

CASE EXAMPLE EPILOGUE

Case Example

At a preliminary examination, the prosecutor is able to establish from witnesses that the uncle has both held the child on his lap while watching television and has also played games with her. She brings in evidence that indicates that the child's memory is at a level appropriate to her age and development and that the things she cannot remember are not typically things that children at her level do remember. The prosecutor notes that the child has not been unduly influenced by other parties and that her reports were as a result of free recall sessions with a skilled clinician. The child testifies that she was frightened by the police and was too scared to talk to them, but that she liked the lady at the clinic. The prosecutor argues that the issue of faulty and inconsistent memory is not grounds to dismiss the case. The judge agrees and binds the case over for trial.

ACTION GUIDELINES

The research on memory retention and recall indicates the need for caution in clinical settings. Although it may be tempting to conclude that obtaining reliable reports, especially from preschool children, is a futile exercise, it is more compelling to realize that the research places the onus clearly on the clinician to use appropriate interview techniques in order to allow the child to provide the best report possible. This is not the child's problem; it is the interviewer's challenge. A working and up-to-date knowledge of the current research findings in this area is essential if one is to interview children who make allegations of sexual abuse. What follows are some clinical considerations that flow from the research.

Assess the Child's Developmental Level Carefully

It is extremely important to understand at what stage the child is in his general development, not only his memory development. This can and should be part of a general assessment of his developmental level. Data on language development and the extent of abstract cognitive abilities are especially important. Psychological testing may be helpful in determining developmental level (see Chapter 6, "Psychological Testing in Child and Adolescent Forensic Evaluations"). In one case, a child had supposedly made a very detailed allegation of abuse to her mother. However, testing indicated that the child was extremely concrete and had verbal abilities well below expected for her age, and it was determined that she would have been unable to have made the allegations in the manner in which they were reported by the mother.

One method of assessing memory is to ask the child to tell about important events that have occurred in the recent and distant past. For example, the child may be asked to tell everything she remembers about her last birthday, or about events like Christmas or Hanukkah, the first day of the school year, or summer vacation. Then the accuracy of the recall can be checked independently by asking parents what occurred. Short-term and incidental memory can be assessed by asking the child about events that have occurred earlier in the clinical interview. For instance, the clinician might take the child to another office and ask her what toys she had used in the playroom. Information about the level of sophistication with which the child can encode, retain, and report events can be determined by observing how much breadth and detail the child can report after this relatively short period of time. In addition, the clinician can see how the child responds to open-ended and more specific questions in a context removed from interviewing the child about the actual events in question in the forensic setting.

Because of the above-mentioned source memory problems, children should be asked how they remember an event. It is important to assess whether they were told about it by someone else, saw a picture or movie of it, saw it happen to someone else, or actually had it happen to them.

Tests have been developed that assess several aspects of memory in school-age and sometimes younger children. These tests may be a helpful adjunct to a full evaluation of memory development. Tests of some utility include the Test of Memory and Learning (Reynolds and Bigler 1994) and the Children's Memory Scale (Cohen 1997).

Review All Available Data

Placing the child's report in context is of vital importance. The clinician needs to know as much as possible about what the child said first and subsequently, to whom it was said, and what the interviewer or parent said. Thus the clinician should review all available data such as police reports and protective services records and, if possible, review the records or speak to any persons to whom the child has reported.

Consider Interview Questions Carefully

Allowing a child to freely recall events clearly produces the most accurate reports. However, because very young children give more information when cued, the clinician must deal with the issue of whether to ask specific questions or provide the child with prompts. This is a serious dilemma: Does one take the risk of getting an inaccurate report that may be harmful to a person being accused, or does one risk missing important information about actual abuse, placing the child at further risk?

At the very least, interview questions should proceed from the open-ended to the more specific. More specific questions can be crafted using information that the child has already provided, as opposed to using questions that give the child information the interviewer may be unsure whether they have had prior to the evaluation. The decision to use leading questions must ultimately be left to the interviewer and should be based on the particular circumstances of the evaluation and its outcome. However, using leading questions should clearly be a careful clinical decision, as opposed to a result of poor interviewing techniques. If such questions are used, the questions and their answers should be documented, preferably verbatim. Any reports or testimony about information received following leading questions should be accompanied by statements making clear that this information may be less accurate than information obtained under free recall conditions.

Methods for Improving Recall and Reporting of Events

Some evidence has emerged that prior practice and training in how to recall and report events improve both accuracy and breadth of recall. In particular, the work of Karen Saywitz and her colleagues (Saywitz and Snyder 1996) has shown promise. They have developed a technique they call "narrative elaboration." School-age children were shown five ways to remember an event, each represented by a picture on a card: People, Setting, Actions, Conversation/Affective State, and Consequence. The children viewed an event or had something occur to them and were taught to use the above strategy for organizing their narrative report of the event. They were then interviewed, first under a free recall condition: "When you tell me what happened to you, tell as much as you can about what really happened, even the little things, without guessing or making anything up." After they had given as much information as they could, each card was presented with the prompt, "Does this help remind you of anything more?"

Saywitz and colleagues found that children interviewed in this way remembered about one-third more information than control subjects, with girls performing better than boys. The most information obtained was on the physical appearance of the persons in the event. The most errors (nearly 75%) occurred on the Consequences card. This card was an attempt to help the child remember what type of things ensued after the event. It was concluded that the concept may have been too abstract for the age of the children in the study. Saywitz and colleagues have subsequently refined the cards, and have adapted the technique for use with preschool children, although with somewhat mixed results. Still, the concept of training children to be more effective reporters is a promising one, especially when employing procedures where careful, open-ended interview questions are used.

REFERENCES

Bauer PJ, Hertsgaard A, Dow GA: After 8 months have passed: long-term recall of events by 1-to 2-year-old children. Memory 4:353–382, 1994

Boyer M, Barron L, Farrar MJ: Three-year-olds remember a novel event from 20 months: evidence for long-term memory in children? Memory 4:417–445, 1994

Ceci SJ, Bruck M: Jeopardy in the Courtroom: A Scientific Analysis of Children's Testimony. Washington, DC, American Psychological Association, 1995

Ceci SJ, Crotteau-Huffman M, Smith E, et al: Repeatedly thinking about non-events. Consciousness and Cognition 3:388–407, 1994

Cohen M: Children's Memory Scale Manual. Odessa, FL, Psychological Assessment Resources, 1997

Fivush R, Shukat JR: Content, consistency, and coherence as they relate to early autobiographical recall, in Memory and Testimony in the Child Witness. Edited by Zaragoza MS, Graham JR, Hall GCN, et al. Thousand Oaks, CA, Sage, 1995, pp 5–23

Flavell JH, Friedrichs AG, Hoyt JD: Developmental changes in memorization processes. Child Development 37:283–299, 1970

Kail R: The Development of Memory in Children. New York, WH Freeman, 1990

Kuehnle K: Assessing Allegations of Child Sexual Abuse. Sarasota, FL, Professional Resource Press, 1996

McDonough L, Mandler JM: Very long-term recall in infants: infantile amnesia reconsidered. Memory 4:339–352, 1994

Nelson K: Long-term retention of memory for preverbal experience: evidence and implications. Memory 4:467–475, 1994

Pezdek K, Roe C: The suggestibility of children's memory for being touched: planting, erasing, and changing memories. Law and Human Behavior 21:95–106, 1997

Poole D, Lamb E: Investigative Interviews of Children. Washington, DC, American Psychological Association, 1998

Poole DA, White LT: Tell me again and again: stability and change in the repeated testimonies of children and adults, in Memory and Testimony in the Child Witness. Edited by Zaragoza MS, Graham JR, Hall GCN, et al. Thousand Oaks, CA, Sage, 1995, pp 24–43

Reynolds CR, Bigler ED: Test of Memory and Learning. Austin, TX, PRO-ED, 1994

Saywitz KJ, Snyder L: Narrative elaboration: test of a new procedure for interviewing children. Journal of Consulting and Clinical Psychology 6:1347–1357, 1996

Zaragoza MS, Graham JR, Hall GCN, et al: Memory and Testimony in the Child Witness. Thousand Oaks, CA, Sage, 1995

CHAPTER 14

Reliability and Suggestibility of Children's Statements

From Science to Practice

Maggie Bruck, Ph.D.

Stephen J. Ceci, Ph.D.

In the past decade, there has been an explosion of developmental research on the accuracy of children's autobiographical memory and on their suggestibility (e.g., Ceci and Bruck 1993, 1995; Fivush 1995; Nelson 1993). This research was primarily motivated by forensic matters concerning the ability of young children to provide accurate eyewitness testimony, particularly in cases of sexual abuse.

Although in most cases children's reports of sexual abuse are probably reliable, there were a number of criminal trials in the 1980s and 1990s that raised fundamental concerns about the impact of suggestive questioning on the reliability of young children's reports of sexual abuse (see Ceci and Bruck 1995 and Nathan and Snedeker 1995 for case descriptions). In these cases, young children accused parents, teachers, or other caretakers of sexual abuse. Their reports involved claims of ritualistic abuse, pornography, multiple victims and perpetrators, involving presumably painful insertions of utensils and tools. Because of the absence of medical evidence and adult eyewitnesses in these cases, the major issue before the jury was whether or not to believe the sometimes fantastic and uncorroborated claims of the children. Prosecutors argued that children do not lie about sexual abuse, and therefore must be believed. The defense tried to argue that the children's reports were the product of repeated suggestive interviews by parents, law enforcement officials, social workers, and therapists. However, because there was no direct scientific evidence to support the defense's arguments, and in light of the belief common at that time that children do not lie about sexual abuse, many of these cases resulted in convictions.

Our studies and those of other researchers have begun to fill this empirical vacuum by examining the sociological and psychological factors that might influence children's testimonies in such cases. The major findings of this research present a profile of both the strengths and weaknesses of children's recall that are primarily moderated by the factor of age. Because of the forensic issues regarding the testimony of young children, most of the research has focused on children 7 years and younger.

In this chapter, we will not review in any detail the empirical work on children's suggestibility, as this has been done previously in numerous publications (Ceci and Bruck 1993, 1995; Poole and Lamb 1998). Rather, we will highlight the major findings and then discuss some forensic applications in terms of cases that we have consulted on. Before addressing these major issues, we first define the major concepts of autobiographical memory and suggestibility.

Autobiographical memory refers to the recall of personally experienced events. Recalling the details of last week's vacation or recalling the details of a friend's murder more than 40 years ago are both instances of autobiographical recall. In the absence of external influences, recall can be quite accurate and detailed. However, memory is not like a tape recorder. Certain types of errors, such as omissions, distortions, and confabulations, commonly occur due to natural memory processes. Each of these types of errors increases with the passage of time from the target event.

Recall errors can also occur because of external factors; of specific interest in this chapter are errors that occur as a result of a variety of suggestive interviewing techniques. Suggestibility refers to the tendency to accept and then report information provided implicitly or explicitly by others through suggestive techniques. For example, if a child who has never had a bike accident is told by an interviewer that an accident did happen and that he should think hard to remember the accident, sometimes this will result in the child's subsequently making the false claim that he was hurt while riding a bike. In other words, the child incorporates the inaccurate suggestion of the interviewer into his own autobiographical report.

SUMMARY OF MAJOR SCIENTIFIC FINDINGS

Autobiographical Memory

Four salient aspects of young children's recall of experienced events are summarized. First, with the emergence of productive narrative language skills around age 2 years, children can remember salient, personally experienced events over long periods of time (Fivush 1993; Peterson and Rideout 1998). Second, although forgetting occurs at all ages, younger children show steeper forgetting curves than older children (Brainerd and Reyna 1995; Brainerd et al. 1990). Third, when asked open-ended questions—such as "What did you do at school today?"—preschool children often provide little information, although what they do provide is accurate. In this sense their free recall is characterized as accurate but incomplete (Fivush 1993; Goodman et al. 1987). Fourth, in order to elicit reports from young (preschool) children about their past, interviewers often use an array of focused retrieval strategies, such as the use of specific questions (e.g., "Did you have recess at school today?"). However, the use of such strategies increases the number of errors in children's reports (e.g., see Peterson and Bell 1996). These four findings indicate that in the absence of any previous prompting or suggesting by adults, children's spontaneous non-prompted statements are likely to be accurate, especially for recently experienced events.

Suggestibility

Children's reports that emerge as a result of suggestive interviewing can often be inaccurate. They can come to report events that never happened. In our work, we have described the "architecture" and process of suggestive interviewing techniques (Ceci and Bruck 1995). In this characterization, the concept of interviewer bias is the defining feature of many suggestive interviews. Interviewer bias is a term used to characterize those interviewers who hold a priori beliefs about the occurrence of certain events and, consequently, mold the interview to elicit statements from the interviewee that are consistent with these prior beliefs. One of the hallmarks of interviewer bias is the single-minded attempt to gather or accept only confirmatory evidence and to avoid all avenues of disclosure that may produce negative or inconsistent evidence. Thus, while gathering evidence to support his or her hypothesis, an interviewer may fail to gather any evidence that could potentially disconfirm that hypothesis. The biased interviewer does not ask questions that might provide alternate explanations for the allegations (e.g., a biased interviewer would not ask, "Did your mommy and daddy tell you that this happened or did you see it happen with your eyes?"). Nor does the biased interviewer ask about events that are inconsistent with the hypothesis or that might prompt the child to answer in a certain way that would call the child's accuracy and previous allegations into question (e.g., a biased interviewer would not ask, "Who else besides your teacher touched your private parts? Did your mommy touch them too?"). And the biased interviewer does not challenge the authenticity of the child's report when it is consistent with the hypothesis (e.g., the biased interviewer would not say, "It's important to tell me only what you saw, not what someone may have told you." or "Did that really happen?" or "It's OK to say you don't remember or you don't know."). Biased interviewers also ignore inconsistent or bizarre evidence or else interpret it within the framework of their initial hypothesis (e.g., a biased interviewer who was told by a child that the defendant took him to the moon in a spaceship might try to twist this into a more feasible account of going on a space ride at an amusement park with the defendant). It is important to note that within this context, a biased interviewer may be a police officer, a therapist, and even a parent. It takes no special skills to be a biased interviewer.

Interviewer bias influences the entire architecture of interviews, and it is revealed through a number of different component features that are potentially suggestive. For example, in order to obtain confirmation of their beliefs, biased interviewers may not ask children open-ended questions such as "What happened?" but quickly resort to a barrage of very specific questions, many of which are repeated and leading. When interviewers do not obtain information that is consistent with their suspicions, they may repeatedly interview children about the same set of suspected events until they do obtain such information, sometimes reinforcing responses consistent with their beliefs and ignoring information that is inconsistent with their beliefs. "Stereotype induction" is another strategy used by biased interviewers. Here the interviewer gives the child information about some characteristic of the suspected perpetrator. For example, children may be told that a person who is suspected of some crime "is bad" "or does bad things." Interview bias is also reflected in the use of some techniques that are specific to interviews between professionals and children. One of these involves the use of anatomically detailed dolls and line drawings in investigations of sexual abuse. When interviewers suspect abuse, before the children have made any allegations, they sometimes ask children to show on the dolls how they have been sexually abused.

The current research in the field of children's suggestibility examines the degree to which these and other interviewing techniques, when used in isolation or in combination, result in tainted and unreliable reports from young children. The following is a summary of the major findings:

1. There are reliable age effects in children's suggestibility, with preschoolers being more vulnerable than older children to a host of factors that contribute to unreliable reports. Despite these significant age differences, it is nonetheless important to point out that there is still concern about the reliability of older children's testimony when they are subjected to suggestive interviews. There is ample evidence that children older than age 6 years are influenced by suggestive questioning about a wide range of events (e.g., Goodman et al. 1989; Poole and Lindsay 2001; Warren and Lane 1995) and that even adults' recollections are impaired by suggestive interviewing techniques (e.g., Hyman et al. 1995; Loftus and Pickrell 1995). Thus, age differences in suggestibility are a matter of degree.

2. When children incorporate false suggestions into their reports, they often lose the source of the information and make source monitoring errors; that is, they cannot correctly distinguish between suggested and experienced events (Johnson et al. 1993) and, conse-

quently, inaccurately report that they actually witnessed the suggested information. These types of errors reflect false beliefs. Although source monitoring errors occur at all ages, they are most prominent in children younger than age 6 years (e.g., Ackil and Zaragoza 1995; Parker 1995; Poole and Lindsay 1995, in press).

Suggestibility effects can also result from social factors such as the child's compliance or acquiescence to the perceived wishes of the interviewer. The child reports what he or she thinks the interviewer wants to hear rather than what actually happened. Finally, suggestibility may initially reflect compliance, but with time and additional interviews, the false reports may become false beliefs. That is, what begins as a recognized attempt to please an interviewer by making an inaccurate claim can become tomorrow's false memory, wherein the child actually comes to believe the inaccurate claim.

3. Errors that children make as a result of suggestive techniques involve not only peripheral details but also central events that involve their own bodies. At times children's false reports can be tinged with sexual connotations. In research studies, young children have made false claims about "silly events" that involved body contact (e.g., "Did the nurse lick your knee?" "Did she blow in your ear?"), and these false claims persisted in repeated interviewing over a 3-month period (Ornstein et al. 1992). Young children falsely reported that a man put something "yucky" in their mouth (Poole and Lindsay 1995, 2001). Preschoolers falsely alleged that their pediatrician had inserted a finger or a stick into their genitals (Bruck et al. 1995a) or that some man touched their friends, kissed their friends on the lips, and removed some of the children's clothes (Lepore and Sesco 1994). A significant number of preschool children falsely reported that someone touched their private parts, kissed them, and hugged them (Bruck et al. 2000b; Goodman et al. 1990; Goodman et al. 1991; Rawls 1996). In addition, when suggestively interviewed, children will make false allegations about nonsexual events that could have serious legal consequences were they to occur. For example, preschool children claimed to have seen a thief at their day care (Bruck et al. 1997).

4. A range of interviewing techniques can negatively influence the accuracy of children's reports. These include verbal dimensions of the interview (e.g., the way questions are asked, the number of times questions are repeated, and the use of reinforcement/ punishment), but they also include nonverbal tech-

niques such as the use of dolls, line drawings, and props. Young children who are interviewed with these media tend to make more errors (of commission) than do children who are interviewed without these media (e.g., Bruck et al. 1995a, 2000b; Gordon et al. 1993; Salmon et al. 1995; Steward and Steward 1996).

5. The "mix" of suggestive interviewing techniques in conjunction with the degree of interviewer bias can account for variations in suggestibility estimates across and within studies. If a biased interviewer uses more than one suggestive technique, there is a greater chance for a tainted interview than if he or she uses just one technique. For example, the effects of stereotype induction paired with the repeated use of misinformation had greater detrimental effects on the accuracy of young children's reports than using only repeated misinformation or stereotype induction (Leichtman and Ceci 1995). In another study (Bruck et al. 1997), we constructed highly suggestive interviews that combined a variety of suggestive techniques (visualization, repeated questioning, repeated misinformation) to elicit children's reports of true events (helping a visitor in the school; getting punished) and false events (helping a woman find her monkey; seeing a thief taking food from the day care). After two suggestive interviews, most children had assented to all events, a pattern that continued to the end of the experiment. Thus, it appears that combining multiple suggestive techniques results in higher levels of inaccurate reports than commonly observed when only a single suggestive technique is used.

6. Real-world interviewers unfortunately appear to use many of the techniques that laboratory researchers have demonstrated to be deleterious to children's accuracy, such as strongly suggestive questions, invocation of peer pressure, and introducing information not previously provided by the child. For example, Lamb and his colleagues (1996) have examined interviews with alleged sexual abuse victims by investigators in Israel and in the United States. A small minority of the interviewers' utterances invited open-ended responses from the child. A much larger proportion of their utterances were leading or suggestive (e.g., Lamb et al. 1996; Sternberg et al. 1999).

7. Suggestive interviewing affects the perceived credibility of children's statements. Subjective ratings of children's reports after suggestive interviewing reveal that these children appear highly credible to trained professionals in the fields of child development, mental health, and forensics (e.g., Leichtman and Ceci 1995, Ceci et al. 1994a, 1994b); these professionals cannot reliably discriminate between children whose reports are accurate from those whose reports are inaccurate as the result of suggestive interviewing techniques. Another line of study suggests that even well-trained professionals cannot reliably differentiate between true and false reports of sexual abuse (Realmuto et al. 1990), even when they are provided with extensive background information about the case (Horner et al. 1993a, 1993b)

The major reason for this lack of accurate discrimination between true and false reports is perhaps due to the fact that suggestive techniques breathe authenticity into the resulting false reports. Children's false reports are not simple reflections or monosyllabic responses to leading questions. Under some conditions, their reports become spontaneous and elaborate, going beyond the suggestions provided by their interviewers. For example, in the study by Bruck et al. (1997), children's false reports contained the prior suggestion that they had seen a thief take food from their day care, but the reports also contained nonsuggested details such as chasing, hitting, and shooting the thief (also see Bruck et al. 1995b).

In sum, the existing scientific literature suggests that when children's false statements emerge from suggestive interviews, there is no "Pinocchio" test that can be used even by the most qualified professionals to definitively ascertain whether or not the event occurred.

8. Even though suggestibility effects may be robust, the effects are not universal. Thus, even in studies with pronounced suggestibility effects, there are always some children who are highly resistant to suggestion, and there are also some adults who are highly suggestible. Further, although suggestibility effects tend to be most dramatic after prolonged and repeated interviewing, some children incorporate suggestions quickly, even after one short interview (Garven et al. 1997; Thompson et al. 1997). Despite the variation in suggestibility, social scientists have not identified a particular cognitive, personality, or temperament style that can predict on an individual level which child will or will not fall sway to suggestive interview techniques. To date the strongest determinant is age.

9. Finally, although we have concentrated on the conditions that can compromise reliable reporting, it is also important to acknowledge that a large number of studies show that children are capable of providing accurate, detailed, and useful information about actual events, some of which are traumatic (e.g., see

Fivush 1993 and Goodman et al. 1992 for a review). What characterizes these studies is the neutral tone of the interviewer, the limited use of misleading questions (for the most part, if suggestions are used, they are limited to a single occasion), and the absence of any motive for the child to make a false report. When such conditions are present, it is a common (although not universal) finding that children are much more immune to suggestive influences, particularly about sexual details. When such conditions are present in actual forensic or therapeutic interviews, one can have greater confidence in the reliability of children's allegations. It is these conditions that we must strive for when eliciting information from young children.

The Accuracy of Interviewers' Reports of Their Interviews With Children

In light of the above findings, it is crucial to have an accurate record of the context in which a child's statements were made. For example, although an interviewer might later state that the child reported that she was touched by a man, the evaluation of the reliability of this statement differs depending on the context it was elicited in; for example, see the following:

Context A

> Adult: What happened at school today?
> Child: The man with a moustache touched me.

Context B

> Adult: What happened at school today?
> Child: Nothing.
> Adult: Tell me.
> Child: Nothing happened.
> Adult: Did you see the man?
> Child: No.
> Adult: Did you see the man with the moustache?
> Child: Yes.
> Adult: Did he touch you?
> Child: What?
> Adult: He touched you didn't he?
> Child: Yeah, the man with a moustache touched me.

Because of the importance of the context in which a child's reports are made, it is crucial to electronically record interviews, particularly the first interview. Hearsay evidence and diaries or logs do not substitute for objective electronic recordings for several reasons. First, when asked to recall conversations, most adults may recall the gist (the major ideas, the content), but they cannot recall the exact words used or the sequences of interactions between speakers. This linguistic informa-

tion rapidly fades from memory, minutes after the interactions have occurred (see Rayner and Pollatsek 1989 for a review). Bruck et al. (1999) videotaped interviews of mothers interviewing their 4-year-old children about a play activity that had taken place in the laboratory. Three days later, mothers were asked to recall the conversation. The mothers could not remember much of the actual content of the interview, omitting many details that had been discussed, but much of what they did recall was accurate. Most importantly, the mothers were particularly inaccurate about several aspects of their conversation: they could not remember who said what (e.g., they could not remember if they had suggested that an activity had occurred or if the child had spontaneously mentioned the activity). They could not remember the types of questions they had asked their children. For example, although some mothers in this study remembered that they learned that a strange man came into the room when the child was playing, they could not remember if the child spontaneously gave them this information or if they obtained it through a sequence of repeated leading questions that the child assented to with monosyllabic utterances. These findings have been replicated in a study in which mental health trainees interviewed young children about a special school activity (Bruck 1999). Warren and Woodall (1999) obtained similar results with experienced investigators who provided summaries immediately after the interview with a child. In this study, when asked what types of questions they had used to elicit information from the children, most of the interviewers answered that they had asked primarily open-ended questions, while few stated that they had asked specific questions, and only one reported asking any leading questions. Their estimates were highly inaccurate, as more than 80% of the questions asked by these interviewers were specific or leading.

Diaries and hearsay testimony do not substitute for electronic recordings because of the selectivity with which information gets remembered or ignored. It would be impossible to accurately remember or to write down an ongoing conversation, and thus, some information does get excluded. However, the omissions may reveal the bias of the recorder. In addition, events may have been omitted because they were judged to be unimportant at the time, but they in fact might be crucial for the understanding of the child's disclosures.

Finally, interviewer bias can contaminate the accuracy of recall or written logs. Sometimes interviewers will report with confidence that children made statements; however, a review of the actual interviews reveals that the reported statements were not made; rather, the interviewers' reports were merely consistent with their own biases or beliefs of what actually happened (Bruck 1999; Langer and Abelson 1974). These data provide empirical justification for the argument that every attempt should be made to electronically record interviews with young children.

APPLICATION OF THE SCIENCE TO THE COURTROOM

Over the past decade, we have been involved in a number of legal cases that raise issues about the reliability of children's allegations. Our participation in these cases has taken a number of forms. For a few, we provided expert testimony in criminal or civil trials. For others, we have written amicus briefs[1] or affidavits to courts. We have also provided advice or acted as consultants to attorneys about whether there is an issue of suggestibility of children in the case at hand. Although most of our work has been for the defense, as described below, we have also been experts or consultants for the prosecution. Before we provide some examples, it must be understood that in applying scientific principles to cases involving young child witnesses, we are not drawing conclusions about the truthfulness of the child's statement. Rather, we attempt to examine the conditions under which children make reports and then refer to the scientific literature to examine if there is a risk that such conditions sometimes eventuate in false reports. The following are a number of issues that we have encountered in our forensic work.

The Nature and Time Course of Children's Disclosures

When evaluating a child's allegations of sexual abuse, it is of primary importance to understand the evolution of the child's report. The following pattern has raised the most concerns regarding allegations of abuse. The child is initially silent—he does not make any unsolicited or spontaneous statements about abusive acts. Rather, the allegations emerge once an adult suspects that something has occurred and starts to question the child. At first, the child denies the event happened, but with repeated questioning, interviewing, or therapy, the child may eventually come to make a disclosure. Sometimes after the disclosure is made, the child may recant, only to later restate the original allegation after further questioning.

This was the pattern that occurred in numerous day care cases (e.g., *Massachusetts v. Amirault LeFave* 1998; *People v. Raymond Buckey et al.; State v. Michaels; State v. Robert Fulton Kelley Jr.*) and in other cases where children made accusations against parents (e.g., *People v. Scott Kniffen et al.*). For example, the *Amirault* case resulted in the conviction and imprisonment of a day care owner and her two adult children for multiple types of sexual abuse, involving pornography, ritualistic abuse, and penetration. There were no adult witnesses to the abuse. The only evidence was the claims of dozens of young preschool children. None of the child witnesses in *Amirault* spontaneously reported abuse to their parents. Even when their parents first directly asked them about abusive acts at the day care, all the children denied that anything had happened. Some children disclosed abusive acts within the first month of questioning by parents, police officers, social workers, and therapists; other children did not disclose until many more months of questioning. Some children recanted earlier allegations in subsequent interviews or sometimes within the same interview.

There are two different interpretations of the evolution of the allegations of sexual abuse made by the child witnesses in cases such as *Amirault*. The first interpretation is that the progression from silence to denial to disclosure to recantation to restatement is common, and perhaps even diagnostic, of sexual abuse. Some professionals claim that sexually abused children deny and recant because they are afraid (due to threats), ashamed, or even believe themselves to be culpable (see Bradley and Wood 1996 for a review). These descriptions characterize the beliefs of the interviewers in many cases. For example, in *Amirault*:

> One mother testified that the police said "just because they say no doesn't mean no; that they are afraid and sometimes it takes time for them to say what happened."

> One therapist/evaluator wrote that although Carol "had not yet revealed touching or penetration, they cannot be ruled out at this time. A gradual, piece by piece disclosure is common in children of this age."

However, there is little scientific evidence to support the view that most children may not readily or consistently disclose sexual abuse when directly asked about it and that many will also recant their earlier allegations. In

---

[1] The term *amicus brief* is a shortened form of *amicus curiae*, which is Latin for "friend of the court." This term describes a person or organization that is not a party to a lawsuit as plaintiff or defendant but that has a strong interest in the case and wants to present an opinion or relevant material.

the study by Bradley and Wood (1996), it was found that among 234 validated cases of child sexual abuse, 5% of the children denied the abuse when questioned by child protective services workers and only 3% recanted their earlier reports of abuse. Jones and McGraw (1987) found a recantation rate of 8% among 309 validated sexual abuse cases seen at a child protective services agency. One factor that appears to predict nondisclosure of sexual abuse is the supportiveness of the caretaker: children whose parents do not doubt their children's claims and who have no motivation to protect the alleged abuser are most likely to have children who will readily disclose when first asked about sexual abuse (Lawson and Chaffin 1992).

The discrepancy between the patterns of disclosure of the children in some cases, such as *Amirault*, and those reported in the scientific literature (e.g., the children in legal cases show high rates of denial and high rates of recantation) raise the following hypotheses. First, low recantation rates (and denial rates) reported in the scientific literature might be the result of sample bias; all of the children studied in these field studies had already come to the attention of interviewers, so perhaps their disclosures were already solidified. Maybe there are high numbers of abused children who never come to the attention of interviewers precisely because they have been denying it. If true, then the low rates of denial observed among the children in these studies could be an underestimate of the denial rate in the population of abused children. To whatever extent this possibility is true, we have no way of knowing. On the other hand, there is the hypothesis that allegations can emerge as a result of suggestive interview techniques. This hypothesis requires an analysis of the record to document how the children were questioned. We have found in a number of our cases that the children were subjected to a variety of suggestive practices that included repeated interviews, repeated leading questions, selective reinforcement, peer pressure, and demonstrations with anatomically detailed dolls and line drawings, among others. This pattern provides evidence for the hypothesis that the children's allegations were a product of suggestive questioning. Based on the scientific literature, there is a high risk that the use of these techniques can result in false reports.

Contrast these day care cases to one that involved a 5-year-old boy who was traveling by airplane between the West and East Coasts and because of foul weather had to make an unscheduled layover in one of the major airline hubs. The parents were promised that the child would be properly supervised in a hotel for the night and then would be put on a plane first thing in the morning. The young child was housed with an adolescent boy. On the bus the next morning, the young child announced to the

passengers that he had been abused by the adolescent (who was also on the bus). Later, he told a woman sitting next to him on the plane the same story. Then on landing, he ran into his mother's arms with the same story. In this case, the child made three identical allegations without any prompting, without any suggestive interviewing, and without any prior motivation to do so. Under such circumstances, the reliability of these statements must be considered very seriously, even if there is later interviewing that may be suggestive in nature. That is, the child's initial disclosure statements were spontaneous and consistent. Even though there was the threat of the adolescent perpetrator on the bus, the child still told his story. Although experts for the defense tried to argue that the child's statements were tainted by later suggestive interviews (several weeks after the initial disclosures), reviews of the videotapes revealed that the child spontaneously repeated his story and that the interviewing techniques, although not the best, were not that suggestive. This case also exemplifies another important principle—the child's first disclosure and the circumstances surrounding it are the first and often most important focus of examination.

In much of our casework, interviewers and mental health professionals defend their suggestive interviewing practices by stating that abused children must be urged in a variety of ways to disclose or else they will remain silent and at risk for further harm. Sometimes, interviewers assure themselves of the safety of actively pursuing children until they assent to abuse, by stating that children cannot be influenced to "lie" about sexual abuse (Faller 1984; Sgroi 1982). Although it is the case that a variety of suggestive techniques elicit true disclosures about events that children initially find unpleasant to discuss, these very same methods also can result in false disclosures, even of a criminal nature (Bruck et al. 1997).

To summarize, if a child's indicting statements are made in the absence of any previous suggestive interviewing and in the absence of any motivation on the part of the child or adults to make incriminating statements, then the risk that the statement is inaccurate is quite low. If, however, the child initially denies any wrongdoing when first asked about a criminal action, but later (after one or more suggestive interviews) comes to make allegations, there is a risk that the statements are not accurate but the result of the suggestive interviews.

The Accuracy of Interviewers' Notes, Parents' Diaries, and Hearsay Testimony

As shown in the previous section, knowledge of the exact wording of each question asked of children during investigative interviews—as well as the number of times questions are repeated and the tone of questioning—is necessary to determine whether strategies recognized as capable of affecting the reliability and accuracy of children's reports were applied (consciously or unconsciously) by interviewers. Without electronic recordings of interviews, this information cannot be preserved. Because suggestive interviews can have lasting effects on the accuracy of children's memory and reports, the failure to record all interviews makes it impossible to support any claims that children's reports are accurate or reliable and free of suggestive influences.

In light of these data, it is important to determine how the child's statements were recorded. In most cases we have worked on, most of the statements are not electronically preserved, unfortunately. Sometimes, there are notes of interviews or diaries in the file. Other times, hearsay testimony is presented at trial. When there is no electronic preservation of interviews, the scientific literature warns us to be very cautious in interpreting the child's statements. The following examples indicate why this approach is justified. The following is a brief excerpt from a police detective's written report of an interview with a 9-year-old child.

> On other occasions, Britt said that a man would put his privates in his butt, and that at the same time, a woman would make him put his mouth on her privates, and yet on another occasion, they would hang him and his brother from the ceiling, on a hook, while being tied up.

It appears from this report that the child made spontaneous and detailed statements about the abuse without any prodding or suggestion. However, we were able to compare the written report with the audiotaped transcript of the actual interview:

> Adult: When you were on the floor tied up, did they ever try to stick a penis up your butt?
> Child: Yes.
> Adult: Okay, when you were tied up, Britt, on the floor, and a man was sticking his penis into your butt, was a lady doing something to you at the same time?
> Child: No.
> Adult: Would that ever happen?
> Child: Yes.
> Adult: What would the lady be doing?
> Child: I can't remember.
> Adult: Would she be doing anything with your mouth?
> Child: (pause) Yes…
> Adult: Would she make you do something with your mouth on her privates?
> Child: Yes…

> Adult: At any time when you were any of these places where the strangers were, did they ever hang you up to the ceiling?
> Child: Yes.
> Adult: What would they use to hang you up from? (Long pause) Remember?
> Child: A hook.

Although the police report is accurate in terms of the gist, it is inaccurate in terms of how the events were reported and who in fact initially provided information about the events. It is possible that the official report was influenced by the bias of the investigator as evidenced by his omissions that the child was prodded and not forthcoming. It should also be noted that such errors are also made by unbiased interviewers who cannot recall whether children's statements were spontaneous or the result of suggestive interviewing techniques (Bruck et al. 1999; Warren and Woodall 1999).

In the next example, the interviewer was an expert witness for the prosecution. The following example is taken from her report of a pretrial evaluation of a preschool child and shows how adults can also make source monitoring errors (they forget who said what). The expert wrote in her report: "He informed me [the defendant] drank the pee-pee. That's how she got crazy."

The following was the actual interaction, taken from recorded transcriptions:

> Dr. L: Did she drink the pee-pee?
> Child: Please, that sounds just crazy. I don't remember about that. Really don't.

As can be seen, the above expert witness reversed the child's and her own statements, testifying that the child told her what, in reality, she had suggested to the child.

In some cases in which there were no electronic records, we were still able to detect elements of inaccuracy, incompleteness, and inconsistency of the police's, mental health professionals', and parents' reports. The following examples are taken from the *Amirault* case. According to the police report of October 4, 1984, Sue made the following statement:

- After saying that AC touched her vagina, Sue later denied the statement.
- After saying that Tooky told her to take her pants down, Sue said he was only fooling.
- Some bad guys at school.
- Sue was asked what school she liked the best. She answered Fells Acres. When asked why, she replied, "We did Play-Doh."

The social services report of the same interview contained the following information:

- Sue told her mother that her vagina was touched by AC.
- Sue told her father that Tooky asked her to take her pants down.
- "As Sue was not volunteering, Officer Healy asked her directly about bad guys at school."

There is no reference in this report to Sue's statement that she liked Fells Acres Daycare because they did Play-Doh.

It is for these reasons that it is crucial to electronically preserve all interviews with child witnesses, particularly the first one.

Although it is true that many of the errors that occur in our case examples are common and made by unbiased interviewers, in the case examples, it is our hypothesis that the errors do reflect the biases of the interviewers and the note-takers. They have come to believe that the child was abused, and their recollections of the children's statements or their recording of the children's statements are deeply colored by these beliefs. Thus, interviewer bias is detrimental in terms of the potential not only for tainting the statements of children but also for tainting the statements and memories of the interviewers themselves.

SUMMARY

We have concluded on the basis of both our laboratory work and our forensic work that unless investigators and other adults are very careful in the interviewing procedures that are used with children suspected of having been abused, one can never make an accurate determination of whether or not abuse occurred. There are a number of interviewing procedures that have the potential to make nonabused children look like abused children. Using these procedures, children may not only come to falsely report acts of sexual abuse but also to believe that they experienced the events they reported. These children's memories may be permanently tainted by the sexualized suggestions of their interviewers. These children can appear highly credible to subsequent interviewers, to family, and to jurors. There are no valid scientific tests to determine which of the children's reports were accurate, once the children have been subjected to suggestive interview methods. Thus when children undergo extremely suggestive interviews, a determination of reliability and accuracy of any of the allegations of abuse is impossible.

REFERENCES

Ackil JK, Zaragoza MS: Developmental differences in eyewitness suggestibility and memory for source. J Exp Child Psychol 60:57–83, 1995

Bradley A, Wood J: How do children tell? the disclosure process in child sexual abuse. Child Abuse Negl 20:881–891, 1996

Brainerd C, Reyna VF: Learning rate, learning opportunities, and the development of forgetting. Dev Psychol 3:251–262, 1995

Brainerd C, Reyna VF, Howe ML, et al: The development of forgetting and reminiscence. Monogr Soc Res Child Dev 55:1–93, 1990

Bruck M: Interviewer bias creates tainted reports. Paper presented at Society for Research on Child Development, Albuquerque, NM, April 1999

Bruck M, Ceci SJ, Francoeur E, et al: Anatomically detailed dolls do not facilitate preschoolers' reports of a pediatric examination involving genital touch. J Exp Psychol Appl 1:95–109, 1995a

Bruck M, Ceci SJ, Francoeur E, et al: "I hardly cried when I got my shot!": influencing children's reports about a visit to their pediatrician. Child Dev 66:193–208, 1995b

Bruck M, Ceci SJ, Hembrooke H: Children's reports of pleasant and unpleasant events, in Recollections of Trauma: Scientific Research and Clinical Practice. Edited by Read D, Lindsay S. New York, Plenum, 1997, pp 199–219

Bruck M, Ceci S, Francoeur E: The accuracy of mothers' memories of conversations with their preschool children. J Exp Psychol Appl 5:1–18, 1999

Bruck M, Ceci SJ, Francoeur E: Anatomically detailed dolls do not facilitate preschoolers' reports of touching. J Exp Psychol Appl 6:74–83, 2000

Bruck M, Melnyk L, Ceci SJ: Draw it again Sam: the effects of repeated drawing on the accuracy of children's reports and source monitoring attributions. J Exper Child Psychol 77:169–196, 2000

Ceci SJ, Bruck M: The suggestibility of the child witness: a historical review and synthesis. Psychol Bull 1(13):403–439, 1993

Ceci SJ, Bruck M: Jeopardy in the Courtroom: A Scientific Analysis of Children's Testimony. Washington, DC, American Psychological Association, 1995

Ceci SJ, Crotteau-Huffman M, Smith E, et al: Repeatedly thinking about non-events. Conscious Cogn 3:388–407, 1994a

Ceci SJ, Loftus EW, Leichtman M, et al: The role of source misattributions in the creation of false beliefs among preschoolers. Int J Clin Exp Hypn 62:304–320, 1994b

Faller KC: Is the child victim of sexual abuse telling the truth? Child Abuse Negl 8:473–481, 1984

Fivush R: Developmental perspectives on autobiographical recall, in Child Victims and Child Witnesses: Understanding and Improving Testimony. Edited by Goodman GS, Bottoms B. New York, Guilford, 1993, pp 1–24

Fivush R: Language, narrative and autobiography. Conscious Cogn 4:100–103, 1995

Garven S, Wood JM, Shaw JS, et al: More than suggestion: consequences of the interviewing techniques from the McMartin preschool case. J Appl Psychol 83:347–359, 1997

Goodman GS, Aman C, Hirschman J: Child sexual and physical abuse: children's testimony, in Children's Eyewitness Memory. Edited by Ceci S, Toglia M, Ross D. New York, Springer-Verlag, 1987, pp 1–23

Goodman GS, Wilson ME, Hazan C, et al: Children's testimony nearly four years after an event. Paper presented at the annual meeting of the Eastern Psychological Association, Boston, MA, April 1989

Goodman GS, Rudy L, Bottoms B, et al: Children's concerns and memory: issues of ecological validity in the study of children's eyewitness testimony, in Knowing and Remembering in Young Children. Edited by Fivush R, Hudson J. New York, Cambridge University Press, 1990, pp 249–284

Goodman GS, Bottoms BL, Schwartz-Kenney B, et al: Children's testimony about a stressful event: improving children's reports. Journal of Narrative and Life History 1:69–99, 1991

Goodman GS, Batterman-Faunce JM, Kenney R: Optimizing children's testimony: research and social policy issues concerning allegations of child sexual abuse, in Child Abuse, Child Development, and Social Policy. Edited by Cicchetti D, Toth S. Norwood, NJ, Ablex, 1992, pp 65–87

Gordon B, Ornstein PA, Nida R, et al: Does the use of dolls facilitate children's memory of visits to the doctor? Applied Cognitive Psychology 7:459–474, 1993

Horner TM, Guyer MJ, Kalter NM: The biases of child sexual abuse experts: believing is seeing. Bulletin of the American Academy of Psychiatry and Law 21:281–292, 1993a

Horner TM, Guyer MJ, Kalter NM: Clinical expertise and the assessment of child sexual abuse. J Am Acad Child Adolesc Psychiatry 32:925–931, 1993b

Hyman I, Husband T, Billings F: False memories of childhood experiences. Applied Cognitive Psychology 9:181–197, 1995

Johnson MK, Hashtroudi S, Lindsay DS: Source monitoring. Psychol Bull 144:3–28, 1993

Jones D, McGraw JM: Reliable and fictitious accounts of sexual abuse in children. Journal of Interpersonal Violence 2:27–45, 1987

Lamb ME, Hershkowitz I, Sternberg KJ, et al: Effects of investigative utterance types on Israeli children's responses. International Journal of Behavioral Development 19:627–637, 1996

Langer E, Abelson R: A patient by any other name... clinician group difference in labeling bias. J Consult Clin Psychol 42:4–9, 1974

Lawson L, Chaffin M: False negatives in sexual abuse disclosure interviews: incidence and influence of caretaker's belief in abuse in cases of accidental abuse discovery by diagnosis of STD. Journal of Interpersonal Violence 7:532–542, 1992

Leichtman MD, Ceci SJ: The effects of stereotypes and suggestions on preschoolers' reports. Dev Psychol 31:568–578, 1995

Lepore SJ, Sesco B: Distorting children's reports and interpretations of events through suggestion. J Appl Psychol 79:108–120, 1994

Loftus EF, Pickrell J: The formation of false memories. Psychiatric Annals 25:720–725, 1995

Massachusetts v Amirault LeFave, 424 Mass 618 (1998)

Nathan D, Snedeker M: Satan's Silence—Ritual Abuse and the Making of a Modern American Witch Hunt. New York, Basic Books, 1995

Nelson K: Events, narratives, memory: what develops? in Memory and Affect in Development: The Minnesota Symposia on Child Psychology. Edited by Nelson C. Hillsdale, NJ, Lawrence Erlbaum, 1993, pp 1–24

Ornstein P, Gordon BN, Larus D: Children's memory for a personally experienced event: implications for testimony. Applied Cognitive Psychology 6:49–60, 1992

Parker J: Age differences in source monitoring of performed and imagined actions on immediate and delayed tests. J Exp Child Psychol 60:84–101, 1995

People v Scott Kniffen et al, Kern County (California) Sup Ct No 24208

People v Raymond Buckey et al, Los Angeles Sup Ct No A7509000

Peterson C, Bell M: Children's memory for traumatic injury. Child Dev 67:3045–3070, 1996

Peterson C, Rideout R: Memory for medical emergencies experienced by 1- and 2-year-olds. Dev Psychol 34:1059–1072, 1998

Poole DA, Lamb ME: Investigative Interviews of Children: A Guide for Helping Professionals. Washington, DC, American Psychological Association, 1998

Poole DA, Lindsay DS: Interviewing preschoolers: effects of nonsuggestive techniques, parental coaching and leading questions on reports of nonexperienced events. J Exp Child Psychol 60:129–154, 1995

Poole DA, Lindsay DS: Children's eyewitness reports after exposure to misinformation from parents. J Exp Psychol Appl 7:27–50, 2001

Rawls J: How question form and body-parts diagrams can affect the content of young children's disclosures. Paper presented at the NATO Advanced Study Institute, Recollections of Trauma: Scientific Research and Clinical Practice, Port de Bourgenay, France, June 1996

Rayner K, Pollatsek A: The Psychology of Reading. Englewood Cliffs, NJ, Prentice-Hall, 1989

Realmuto G, Jensen J, Wescoe S: Specificity and sensitivity of sexually anatomically correct dolls in substantiating abuse: a pilot study. J Am Acad Child Adolesc Psychiatry 29:743–746, 1990

Salmon K, Bidrose S, Pipe M: Providing props to facilitate children's events reports: a comparison of toys and real items. J Exp Psychol 60:174–194, 1995

Sgroi S: Handbook of Clinical Intervention in Child Sexual Abuse. Lexington, MA, Lexington Books, 1982

State v Michaels, 136 NJ 299, 642 A2d 1372 (1994)

State v Michaels, 136 NJ 299, 642 A2d 1372 (1994)

State v Robert Fulton Kelley Jr, Superior Criminal Court, Pitt County, North Carolina, #91-CRS-4250–4363 (1991–1992). no 933 SC65

Sternberg K, Lamb M, Esplin P, et al: Using a scripted protocol in investigative interviews: a pilot study. Applied Developmental Science 3:70–76, 1999

Steward MS, Steward DS: Interviewing young children about body touch and handling. Monogr Soc Res Child Dev 6(1):1–214, 1996

Thompson WC, Clarke-Stewart KA, Lepore S: What did the janitor do? suggestive interviewing and the accuracy of children's accounts. Law and Human Behavior 21:405–426, 1997

Warren A, Lane P: The effects of timing and type of questioning on eyewitness accuracy and suggestibility, in Memory and Testimony in the Child Witness. Edited by Zaragoza M. Thousand Oaks, CA, Sage, 1995, pp 44–60

Warren A, Woodall C: The reliability of hearsay testimony: how well do interviewers recall their interviews with children? Psychology, Public Policy, and Law 5:355–371, 1999

CHAPTER 15

Interviewing Children for Suspected Sexual Abuse

Kathleen M. Quinn, M.D.

Case Example 1

A 5-year-old girl and her 3-year-old sister had attended a local day care center when they had first moved to town. After 6 months the mother removed them due to concerns that the head teacher used physical punishment described by the older girl as hitting her on the face. Shortly thereafter, the mother was called by another mother, who stated that there were also concerns that sexual abuse had occurred at the center. The 5-year-old and 3-year-old were interviewed together by the local department of human services and police. The first two interviews were unstructured and included the protective services worker sitting on the floor with the children whispering questions and answers. Puppet play was used in an attempt to understand the girls' vocabulary concerning body parts.

Case Example 2

A couple who have been divorced for several years were engaged in a visitation battle in domestic relations court over their children, ages 9 and 7. The mother had restricted the father's visitation in the past because of her ex-husband's history of physical abuse toward herself and the children and his alcoholism. Now sober and in Alcoholics Anonymous, the father insisted on visitation. The court awarded a limited visitation plan, beginning with a half a day a week and a gradual increase to alternating full weekends. Three months into the resumption of the visitation the mother and the 9-year-old girl alleged the child had been approached sexually by her father. The 7-year-old boy made no allegation. A report was made by the mother to the local department of human services. A motion to terminate visitation was filed by the mother's attorney in domestic relations court.

Case Example 3

A 3-year-old boy alleged his teenage stepbrother had touched his bottom. The child was not yet toilet trained, and the intake worker taking the complaint found that the stepbrother assisted the 3-year-old in the bathroom. The mother, who reported the allegation, stated that the 3-year-old had immature language skills.

CRITICAL ISSUES

What Is Child Sexual Abuse?

Child sexual abuse (CSA) describes a wide range of acts. Legal and research definitions require two elements: 1) sexual acts involving a child, and 2) an "abusive condition," such as coercion, significant age differences, or a caretaking relationship between the participants. Such conditions indicate an unequal power relationship, and imply lack of consent (Finkelhor 1994).

Sexual acts involving a child refer to acts done for sexual stimulation. Such acts are usually classified as contact sexual abuse or noncontact sexual abuse. *Contact sexual abuse* involves touching of the sexual areas of either the child's body or the perpetrator's body. *Noncontact sexual abuse* may include exhibitionism, voyeurism, or the child's involvement in the production of pornography. Contact with the child's genitals for caretaking purposes (e.g., washing or application of ointments) is excluded in the definition of CSA.

Controversy continues in the assessment of whether some acts constitute sexual abuse. For example, when is sexual activity between peers abuse? How old must an adolescent be to consent to intercourse? When is over-stimulation and overexposure to adult sexual acts abuse? A community standard, including the consideration of the age difference between the participants, their relationship, and legal definitions, will aid in defining what is abuse (Finkelhor 1979).

How Frequently Does Child Sexual Abuse Occur?

Sexual abuse occurs in secret. Therefore, existing statistics must be viewed as estimates of the incidences of CSA. There are three official sources of data compiled on the incidence of CSA brought to professional attention: 1) The National Incidence Study of Child Abuse and Neglect, 2) state child protective agencies, and 3) law enforcement agencies.

As of 1994, over 3 million children were reported to child protective services in the United States with allegations of abuse and neglect, of which 11% were allegations of CSA. One million of these reports were substantiated, of which 15% were for CSA (Wiese and Daro 1995). Compared with other forms of child maltreatment, CSA allegations have a higher rate of substantiation (McCurdy and Daro 1994). On the bases of this data, 150,000 substantiated cases of CSA, or 2.4 cases per 1,000, are brought to the attention of child protective services agencies annually (Finkelhor 1994).

Surveys of adult survivors of CSA provide the most complete estimate of child sexual abuse. Disclosure rates remain low due to secrecy and shame (Russell 1986). If the rates of sexual abuse against minors is as great as that reported by adults in retrospective surveys, approximately 500,000 new cases of child sexual abuse occur each year (Finkelhor 1994).

LEGAL ISSUES

Laws

Legal definitions of CSA are found in child sex offense, incest, and child protection statutes (Bulkley 1985). Sexual activity with children by adults is a crime in every state. Both the age of the child and of the perpetrator as well as their relationship often determines the nature of the offense and resulting penalties. Consenting intercourse may be specifically prohibited if the adult is a parent or legal guardian or someone acting in a position of authority over a child, such as a foster parent, teacher, or household member.

Numerous inconsistencies exist in the laws across states. The age at which children can legally consent to sexual activity ranges from 11 to 17 years. Penalties for perpetrators range from minimum sentences of several months to life imprisonment or death. In addition, the definition of prohibited acts varies widely.

Civil statutes, mandatory reporting laws, and juvenile or family court jurisdiction acts exist for the protection of abused and neglected children. Statutory definitions in every state can be interpreted to include sexual abuse. Legal action may be brought against both the actively abusive parent as well as a complicitous spouse.

All 50 states have mandatory reporting acts that require certain professionals working or caring for children to report suspected abuse or neglect to public child protective agencies and/or the police. Mandatory reporting statutes vary as to the specific level of risk that will trigger the required report—an injury (harm standard) or risk of injury (endangerment standard). Each statute will indicate whether the allegation must be directly from the child or whether it can come from a third party, and it will specify a time limit within which a professional must make a report in order to discharge the duty. All state reporting acts are available at the Web site of the National Clearinghouse on Child Abuse and Neglect Information: www.calib.com/nccanch. The purpose of reporting laws has been to establish a comprehensive public policy mechanism for child protection designed to encourage reports of abuse to protect children and to designate one agency to handle abuse and to offer services to children and families. In most states a mental health professional or other named professional can be charged with a violation of criminal law for failure to report known or suspected cases of child abuse. Failure to report may also make the professional liable for civil damages in a malpractice case. All state statutes provide the mandated reporter with immunity from suits for negligence or defamation if a suspected case of abuse is reported in good faith.

Although reports of abuse have increased dramatically in recent years due to both increased public awareness and the reporting acts, child abuse, including sexual abuse, is still significantly underreported. Despite protections and possible sanctions, many professionals fail to report suspected abuse. In a review of 12 studies, an average of 40% of psychologists failed to report at least one case of suspected abuse (Brosing and Kalichman 1992). Mandated reporters must follow the child protection laws in their states to avoid both criminal and civil liability. Professionals encountering cases raising issues concerning abuse should consult with knowledgeable colleagues and/or legal counsel to determine their responsibility for reporting. They may also consult with the legal department of the designated human services agency to determine if a hypothetical set of facts meets criteria for reporting. Mandated reporting of abuse is a well-recognized exception to confidentiality. In addition to professionals caring for children, almost half the states require "any person" to report suspected abuse or neglect. In addition, in the wake of concerns about false allegations of CSA, some states have passed statutes making it illegal to knowingly make a false accusation of CSA.

Legal Interventions

The development of research concerning the impact of testifying on children and the evolution of case law has affected current legal interventions. Beginning in the 1980s, researchers began to study the effect on children of testifying. Testimony by children in juvenile court in which procedures are more informal is generally well tolerated and often gives the child an antidote to the sense of powerlessness produced by abuse (Runyan 1993). Certain factors make testimony in either juvenile or criminal court more stressful, including 1) lack of maternal support, 2) multiple testimony appearances, and 3) harsh questioning (Goodman et al. 1992; Lipovsky 1994).·

Evolution of case law has clarified that the Sixth Amendment (confrontation clause) does not guarantee the defendant the absolute right to face-to-face confrontation. Two recent U.S. Supreme Court cases, *Coy v. Iowa* (1988) and *Maryland v. Craig* (1990) have clarified that exceptions to confrontation can be recognized but must be based on an adequate demonstration of the necessity of finding that the child witness is physically or psychologically unavailable. Several states have statutes authorizing courts to declare witnesses psychologically unavailable. Clinicians may become involved in assessing a child who is refusing to testify or appears traumatized by the prospect of testifying before a defendant. The legal standard of declaring a child unavailable for testimony is high and does not include mere discomfort or reluctance.

Alternative testimonial approaches available include videotape depositions and closed-circuit television at the time of trial as well as, in some states, explicit state laws authorizing the judge to protect child witnesses from developmentally inappropriate questions.

It is settled that the confrontation clause permits admission of reliable history (*Idaho v. Wright* 1990). Three major hearsay exceptions commonly used in abuse trials are 1) "excited utterances," or *res gestae*, 2) statements made to a physician during diagnoses and treatment, and 3) residual hearsay—an exception permitting such evidence when it can be shown to be reliable. For example, in *White v. Illinois* (1992) the Supreme Court stated "[t]here can be no doubt" of the medical diagnosis or treatment exception being firmly rooted as an exception to the exclusion of hearsay evidence.

CLINICAL ISSUES

Validation of Complaint

When faced with a case with an allegation of sexual abuse, the clinician is presented with a number of problems in attempting to assess the complaint. First, few of the cases have any physical corroboration. Even when the offender has confessed to sexual acts, including penetration, the physical exam may be normal (Kerns and Ritter 1992; Muram 1989). In a recent review of 21 studies of children who were allegedly sexually abused, normal findings were reported in 26%–73% of girls and 17%–82% of boys. Findings that were diagnostic of sexual abuse (genital trauma, sexually transmitted diseases, or sperm) were found in only 3%–16% of the child victims (Bays and Chadwick 1993). Several reasons exist for the lack of physical findings in sexually abused children, including 1) delay in seeking the medical exam, 2) rapid healing, 3) sexual acts, such as fondling, deep kissing, oral sodomy, and cunnilingus, that do not leave physical findings, and 4) elasticity of hymenal and anal tissue.

A second problem in the validation of sexual abuse complaints is that of false negatives and retractions. The clinician must assess the clinical credibility of both denials and retractions. Has the child sensed the negative impact of her statements on her own life and that of her family? Is a later disclosure related to lowered resistance, better or worse interviewing, or the parroting of an adult's earlier allegation? The clinician should anticipate these questions and develop, when possible, data to answer these concerns. Recantations and later disclosures are common. Sorenson and Snow (1991) found that in a sample of 116 high-certainty cases, 72% of children initially denied sexual abuse, but over the course of several interviews, all but 4% disclosed. A total of 22% of the children in this sample recanted during the disclosure process. Similarly, Lawson and Chaffin (1992) examined disclosures of 22 children found positive for sexually transmitted disease. Only 43% of these children disclosed, and only 17% did so when their parents were unsupportive. However, a more recent study by Bradley and Wood (1996) challenges the assumption that gradual disclosure of sexual abuse is the norm. Studying 234 cases of validated sexual abuse, they found that denial of abuse occurred in only 6% of cases and recantation in 4%. Most of the children disclosed sexual abuse in the first interview.

Third, in attempting to validate an allegation of sexual abuse, the clinician may be confronted with the problem of interviewing children of special populations who have unique needs. These special populations may include those with sensory losses (e.g., deafness), mental disabilities (e.g., retardation), and/or communication challenges (e.g., language disabilities); children whose first language is not English; or preschoolers. These children often require interviewing techniques that the average clinician does not possess.

Fourth, the alleged victim may not appreciate the abusive nature of the alleged events. Approximately 40% of victims of substantiated maltreatment are age 5 years and younger. These children may not appreciate that they are indeed victims of abuse.

Fifth, behavioral problems cited as the bases for sexual abuse allegations may overlap with other sources of a child's problem. Children express distress with a wide range of signs and symptoms. In addition, families with multiple problems may expose the child to multiple stressors. The clinician must be cautious in using behavioral indicators as support for sexual abuse allegations. However, sexual behavior continues to be one of the most valid indicators of sexual abuse in children (Kendall-Tackett et al. 1993). Ongoing research involving the Child Sexual Behavior Inventory (Friedrich et al. 1992) indicates that sexually abused children exhibit a wider range and greater frequency of sexual behaviors than either nonabused, nonclinical controls or psychiatric nonabused patients. However, both developmental norms and clinical diagnoses must be considered. For example, 43.5% of 2- to 6-year-old boys in the normative group touched their mother's breasts, whereas 48.8% of 2- to 6-year-old abused boys were reported as displaying the same behavior (Friedrich 1993). In a related study, parents with children with attention-deficit/hyperactivity disorder (ADHD) frequently reported their children as having problems with boundaries and increased levels of masturbation. However, as a group, children with ADHD exhibited less sexual interest and less sexual aggression than children who had been sexually abused (Friedrich 1994). Clinicians must remember that sexual behavior in children is influenced by a number of variables, such as the child's developmental level, mental health history, exposure to sexuality, and life stresses.

Finally, the alleged perpetrator is often well known to the child. Younger victims are more likely abused by members of their intimate social network. Although these demographics may lessen eyewitness issues, validation is made more complicated by the child's (and family's) divided loyalties. Sexual abuse by strangers is no more than 10%–30%, as reported in adult retrospective surveys.

All of these factors make investigating an allegation of abuse a complex problem, and one that deserves the highest degree of care to objectivity and up-to-date research in order to provide the clinical and judicial systems the best set of data.

The Evolution of Interviewing Practices

The professional history of CSA has been characterized by its "discovery" and subsequent polarization and denial in professionals and the public. Freud discovered the origins of neuroses in the seduction theory and then replaced his recognition of CSA by the Oedipus complex. Similarly, the 1970s and 1980s were times of rediscovery of childhood sexual abuse and developing methods to investigate it, as well as a backlash against investigators and complainants.

Due to its secrecy, as well as frequent lack of physical evidence, sexual abuse allegations require that the alleged victim be interviewed. Modern interviewing recommendations in the early 1980s were primarily based on the pioneering work of Sgroi and colleagues (1982). By the mid-1980s, Jones and McQuiston (1985, 1986) proposed an interview protocol, as well as directing interviewers to assess the child's emotional and behavioral functioning, the family dynamics, and collateral sources.

Conte and colleagues (1991) undertook a systematic national study of child interview practices. The survey indicated that the most commonly used medium in the interviews was the anatomical doll. The survey authors expressed concerns that some of the interviewers' beliefs about credibility indicators were not empirically based nor consistently held between interviewers.

By the late 1980s and 1990s, guidelines for practice were developed by the multidisciplinary organization American Professional Society on the Abuse of Children (APSAC) (1990, 1995) and the American Academy of Child and Adolescent Psychiatry (1990, 1997). The goal of guidelines for investigating, interviewing, and the use of anatomical dolls has been to standardize practices and inform clinical practices with research findings. Guidelines are not intended to establish a legal standard or rigid standard of practice. Guidelines endorse support for flexibility based on professional judgment in individual cases.

A parallel phenomenon in the 1990s to guidelines for investigatory interviewing was a backlash against investigatory methods, those who do the investigations, and those who bring the allegations. The dangers of the backlash included the complete denial or minimization of the existence of sexual abuse. The backlash against child protection is often enunciated in highly critical, often strident materials describing the child protective system as out of control and on "witch hunts" to find abuse at any cost. The positive aspects of the backlash included the increased scientific bases of investigatory techniques, greater appreciation of the impact of development on both the allegations and adequate investigatory techniques, and increased adherence to basic forensic principles in the investigation of CSA, including objectivity and documentation.

Role of the Investigator

The primary goal of investigatory interviewing is to document the chronology, psychosocial context, and consistency of an allegation. The data gathered should be as uncontaminated as possible for use by the mental health and judicial systems. *Contamination* occurs when the source of the child's memory of the alleged event becomes distorted or falsified by factors inside or outside the interview. Contamination cannot be eliminated, as memory is reconstructive, not reproductive, but can be minimized by maintaining objectivity, role definition, and appropriate interview techniques.

Objectivity or independence is a key aspect of investigatory interviewing. The interviewer must strive to not ally himself or herself with any particular individual involved in the investigation of the allegation, thereby maintaining external independence. Similarly, the investigator must maintain internal independence by being open, honest, and unbiased in gathering data and hearing the child's account of his or her experience (White et al. 1988). Interviewers should utilize the same principles as scientific investigators by ruling in or out alternate hypotheses (Ceci and Bruck 1995; and see also Chapter 14, "Reliability and Suggestibility of Children's Statements") as well as acknowledging the limitations of their data.

Interviewers must be careful to avoid role confusions. The interviewer must remember that he or she is a forensic examiner, not a therapist or child advocate for any particular case. Techniques of investigation must not be mixed with those of therapy during the assessment of child sexual abuse. In some states, it is a violation of the mental health professional's code of ethics to do both within one case. There needs to be a sharp demarcation between evaluation and therapy. For example, the interviewer must be careful not to provide an emotional interpretation of the events revealed by the child. Comments such as "I'm sorry this awful thing happened to you" may make the child feel better and may make the interviewer feel he or she is building a stronger relationship with the child; however, in reality, such comments are potentially contaminating in that they are mixing investigation with therapy by providing a value judgment concerning the report of the child's experiences.

A second role confusion often exhibited by interviewers is mixing investigation with inappropriate advocacy. Statements to the referent, such as "I'm sure she'll tell me what happened," demonstrate a lack of independence on the part of the interviewer. Promising to the child that "nothing like this will ever happen again" is an empty promise in that the interviewer has no way of providing total protection to the child once he or she leaves the office. In addition, telling a child after a disclosure that "things will be better now" is likewise a potentially empty promise, because the child who experiences the court proceedings may find that things do not get better for a long time. In fact, things may actually get worse for the child.

A third role confusion to avoid is being the judge or jury. Interviewers must remember that the judge or jury makes the ultimate decision regarding the legal issues. It is not the interviewer's role to decide that Uncle Joe is guilty. The interviewer can have opinions and can provide data from the interview to support these opinions, but it is not the interviewer's responsibility to indicate guilt or innocence in a court of law.

In summary, clinicians receiving a referral of a case involving an allegation of CSA must define their role for themselves and all participants. In addition, clinicians must clearly understand who has hired them and who will see the data they gather. This is the issue of *agency*. In forensic evaluations, the evaluator may be hired by a parent or parent's attorney to assess the allegation or may be the agent of an institution (protective services or the court). The agent initiating the evaluation will see the data, may request a report, or may require testimony. The evaluator of a CSA allegation must provide the data in the form requested and structure the evaluation to provide objective, comprehensive data.

Interviewing Children— A Developmental Perspective

Clinicians must bring a developmental perspective to interviewing a child about allegations of abuse. There are well-documented age-related differences in memory, suggestibility, reasoning, knowledge, range of experience, and emotional maturity (see Chapters 13, "Developmental Aspects of Memory in Children," and 14, "Reliability and Suggestibility of Children's Statements"). The evaluator should plan to screen each child developmentally early in the investigatory interview and should tailor the interview to the child's level of functioning and interpret responses from a developmental perspective. Failure to bring a developmental perspective to the investigatory interview may promote omissions, inconsistencies, or distortions in the child's statements. Such errors in interviewing are more the function of the incompetence of the interviewer than the incompetence of the child (Saywitz and Camparo 1998).

Several writers have proposed questioning strategies (Boat and Everson 1988; Bull 1995; Faller 1993; Sternberg et al. 1997; Yuille et al. 1993). All agree that the interviewer should start with an open-ended inquiry and progress to more focused questions when open-ended ones are inadequate to make a determination about the allegations. Interviews that initially model the use of open-ended questions appear to aid disclosure. In the work of Sternberg et al. (1997), two-thirds of the children who were exposed to open-ended questions throughout the interview process described core details of the alleged incident.

Both appellate court decisions (*Massachusetts v. Amirault LeFave* 1998; *State v. Michaels* 1993) as well as professional literature have described what *not* to do. Techniques to be avoided or minimized include: 1) leading questions ("George touched your pee pee, didn't he?"); 2) repetitive questioning and/or interviewing; 3) questions promoting pretending, speculation, or use of fantasy ("Let's make believe…"); and 4) manipulation of the emotional tone to direct the interview.

Professionals regard the child interview as an essential part of determining the likelihood of sexual abuse. The child is always seen alone. Whereas there are some who suggest that children may be interviewed with a supportive adult present (Boat and Everson 1988; Sgroi et al. 1982), others are adamantly opposed (White et al. 1988) because of the problem with parental contamination. Even with the most understanding and supportive parent, there are factors that may contaminate the child's disclosure. The child may feel the need to satisfy the perceived expectations of the parents or not hurt their feelings by revealing the experience. Children may also feel they will get into trouble if sensitive information is revealed in front of the parent, because the parent has always lectured them on not letting anyone touch their private parts. When the reasons for interviewing the child alone are explained to parents, the overwhelming majority become supportive of such independent interviews.

When custody and visitation are at issue in addition to a sexual abuse complaint, the child should be seen for additional appointments in order to observe the child's interaction with each parent. The clinician performing this set of interviews should be the one doing the custody or visitation assessment. The purpose of this set of interviews is not to further determine the credibility of the allegation but rather to observe the quality of the overall relationship between the child and each parent. These data are often helpful in recommending the nature and frequency of any contact between the child and the alleged perpetrator. Much resistance should be anticipated in attempting to set up such appointments, and on occasion, the clinician may determine such an appointment is contraindicated due to the child's level of distress and/or resistance.

Parental Interviews

Psychosocial Issues

There are a number of psychosocial issues that must be clarified either in the intake or during the parental interviews. Especially in cases involving divorce, visitation, or custody, a chronology of escalating allegations should be documented to ascertain if previous attempts by the complainant have not been successful in changing the visitation and custody arrangements. The possible utility of the allegation as perceived by the complainant and child should be assessed, especially as it relates to custody and visitation changes. The complainant's potential for deceptive motives should be addressed, including the possibility of that person's having a major mental illness, which may lead him or her to distort reality. The clinician should also be aware of any person involved in the case who repeatedly sexualizes relationships.

The child's baseline sexual behavior and sexual knowledge as well as the presence of overstimulation should be assessed. A listing of those individuals who come in contact with the child should be made. A good history of the child's symptoms should be made, including the date of initial appearance, any increases or decreases in symptom severity, and the coexistence of other stresses that have occurred. The clinician should also investigate the child's fears or alienation, which might be fueling the allegation.

Family History

A thorough family history is necessary. This history should include a review of each parent's family of origin; the parents' dating, marriage, divorce, and remarriage history; a review of each child's history in the family and the presence of significant others; history of abuse or neglect of any member (adult or child); and an evaluation of significant mental and physical health problems of all family members. Efforts to obtain a description of the family's daily living patterns, their traditions concerning privacy and nudity, their approach to sexuality and sex education, and the child's exposure to sexually explicit materials and activities need to be made.

Child's History

Information should be gathered regarding the child's own history, including prenatal, birth, developmental, medical, caregiving, school, significant separations, and present living circumstances. Significant behavioral or emotional problems should be investigated also.

Child Interviews

Number of Interviews

The child is to be interviewed two to three times. If only one interview is conducted, there is a problem of trying to judge consistency of the complaint as well as allowing the child time to feel comfortable enough to reveal sensitive secrets. Having more than three interviews increases the chance that the child will feel coerced into elaborating the story or may increase the degree of contamination of the child's story by the interviewer.

Environment and Materials

The interview environment needs to be quiet and private, away from telephones and beepers. The room should have toys appropriate for the child's age and developmental level. There should not be an overabundance of toys, which may distract the child, causing the interviewer to have a more difficult time in getting the child to pay attention to the abuse interview.

Materials that are felt to be *inappropriate* for use in a clinical evaluation of sexual abuse include materials that have been designed to promote sexual education and/or abuse prevention, such as puppets, media materials (e.g., newspapers, TV footage), or lineups of suspected perpetrators.

Free Play

There are two major parts of a CSA interview: free play and the structured interview. The free play portion is designed to achieve several goals: 1) to allow the child and interviewer to become comfortable in the room and with each other; 2) to establish a positive rapport between the two; and 3) to allow the interviewer to informally assess the child's developmental levels.

The developmental abilities to be assessed include the child's suggestibility, ability to deceive, cognitive style and level, and language and speech abilities. It should be remembered that children's memory, as is adults' memory, is basically divided into two types: free recall and recognition. When a child is able to reveal information through free recall by open-ended, nonleading questions, there is more likelihood that the information is coming from the child's own memory unless there is proof of prior contamination factors.

In assessing a child's ability to deceive or distort, the clinician must assess if the child appears to be pursuing a goal by lying (e.g., change of custody or visitation), if the child echoes the adult's report, and if the child's presentation is consistent with a mental disorder that could compromise a child's capacity to perceive reality.

The level of sexual knowledge must be part of a sexual abuse assessment. Efforts must be made to match that expected for that child with what is known about his or her cultural and class background and in light of ongoing research.

Anatomical Dolls

The anatomical dolls are widely used as aids in investigatory interviews involving allegations of CSA. Concerns have been raised about whether or not the anatomical dolls might suggest sexual material, overstimulate nonabused children, or be used by poorly trained, overzealous interviewers. Research regarding how suggestive the anatomical dolls are is conflicted (Everson and Boat 1994; Bruck et al. 2000). Research from the 1980s and 1990s indicates:

1. Explicit sexual positioning of dolls (e.g., penile penetration of orifices) is uncommon in nonreferred, presumably nonabused children. However, it may occur due to prior sexual exposure or in some demographic groups. Four- and 5-year-old boys from lower socioeconomic status (SES) families are somewhat more likely to enact explicit sexual acts with dolls compared with younger children, girls, or children from higher SES families (Boat and Everson 1994). A child's explanation of what he or she is demonstrating may clarify the diagnosis of maltreatment versus overstimulation and overexposure.

2. The mouthing or sucking of a doll's penis is very rare before about age 4 and infrequent after age 4 in nonreferred, presumably nonabused children (Everson and Boat 1990).

3. If a child's positioning of the dolls indicates a detailed knowledge of sexual acts, the probability of sexual abuse is increased.

4. Manual exploration of a doll's genitals, including digital penetration of a doll's vagina or anal opening, is rather common behavior in young, presumably non-abused children (Boat and Everson 1994). Diagnostic concern is raised if such a demonstration is associated with negative emotional expression (fear, anxiety, anger), behavioral regression, obsessive repetition (Terr 1981), or verbal disclosure of maltreatment.

Everson and Boat (1994) have detailed the appropriate use of the dolls as including the following:

1. The anatomical model in which the dolls are used to document the child's vocabulary for body parts, utilizing questions such as "What do you call this part?" "What is it for?" "Is it for anything else?" "Has anything happened to your _____?" "Has it ever been hurt?"
2. A demonstration aid in which the dolls are used as a prop to show what occurred; caution should be exercised in using the dolls as a demonstration aid in children under approximately 3.5 years who may not be developmentally capable of using the dolls to represent themselves (DeLoache 1995).
3. A memory stimulus—the dolls may serve as a prop and concrete cue to recall specific acts of a sexual nature.
4. A screening tool—the child may be given the opportunity to examine and handle the dolls while the evaluator observes the child's play, emotional reactions, and remarks.
5. An icebreaker—the role of the dolls may be as a stimulus to start a conversation about body parts and sexual issues.

The dolls are not a "test" for abuse. Evaluators who use them should possess training or knowledge and experience to conduct forensic interviews of children suspected of having been sexually abused. The evaluator should know the child's history concerning exposure to, and use of, the dolls. The number of dolls presented depends on their specific use in the interview. A formal interview protocol is not required (American Professional Society on the Abuse of Children 1995). Detailed documentation of the interview process should be preserved.

Documentation

Documentation methods should be complete and detailed. Written notes done at the time of the interview or audiotapes can preserve both the questions and replies. Preservation of a verbatim record of all portions of the interview is preferred to demonstrate the methods of interviewing and the child's behavior and verbal statements. The videotape recording of the interview, if available, offers several advantages, including reduction of the number of interviews, preservation of evidence of abuse, and incentives to use proper interview techniques; a videotape may also encourage confession, and the videotape may be used by experts to review methods of investigation (Myers 1997). Opponents of videotaping have argued that videotaping may be dissected by the defense to show inconsistencies or incompleteness of children's statements or interviewer error. In general, expert testimony concerning the natural history and developmental issues related to disclosure and the adequacy of an investigation are often sufficient to rehabilitate the evidence.

CREDIBILITY

The investigating clinician should document and discuss factors that argue for or against the validity of the allegation. The strongest validation criteria are based on documenting explicit sexual experiences with a progression of sexual acts over time described by the child. The interviewer should look for sexual experiences beyond the child's expected knowledge or experience, a description told from the child's viewpoint and vocabulary, and an emotional response consistent with the nature of the abuse. The assessment of a sexual abuse complaint should also include possible motivations for the issuance of a false sexual abuse complaint by either the child or the adult (Quinn 1988).

The two most common reasons to view an allegation of CSA as not credible are a recantation by the child and the existence of improbable elements in a child's disclosure. As described earlier, recantations are common even in high-certainty cases and should be assessed for their own credibility. Recent interest in high-profile cases with bizarre and improbable elements has prompted a small literature on this little-studied aspect of CSA allegations. Everson (1997) has written that the existence of improbable or fantastic elements in a child's account should not prompt an automatic dismissal of the child's account. He details possible sources of the implausible accounts: the event, the assessment process, and influences outside the assessment process. He describes 24 specific mechanisms to explain implausible elements in a child's account of abuse. Severe abuse produces more implausible and fantastic allegations (Dalenberg 1996). Fantasy elements should not automatically lead evaluators to suspect the entire allegation.

CASE EXAMPLE EPILOGUES

Case Example 1

Several months after the first set of interviews, the investigators became concerned that their techniques would be criticized. They redid the interviews, this time separating the children and using an interview protocol that contained a series of questions surveying the child's knowledge of body parts and screening for abuse. The children were much less forthcoming at the time of the second set of interviews, denying all sexual abuse. Due to the inconsistencies between the interviews and the poor techniques used initially, the prosecutor decided not to include these children in the pending lawsuit against the day care. Repetitive nightmares and sexualized play suggested that the children had been abused in some way.

Case Example 2

The social worker for the department of human services initially worked up the case by interviewing the girl in her mother's home and made no attempt to interview the father. However, a psychiatrist associated with the domestic relations court consulted with the worker and recommended an interview of the child at a neutral site (the social worker's office) and contact with the father. A series of two interviews with the girl revealed a consistent history of fondling and nudity within the father's home. The disclosure was noted to be in age-appropriate language with unique details such as who said what to whom. The social worker, after her initial skepticism that this might be a false allegation, concluded that the abuse was substantiated. The case was scheduled to be heard in domestic relations court to determine what, if any, contact between the father and daughter would be permitted.

Case Example 3

The intake worker, on hearing this history, decided that additional expertise would be required on this case. She called the local hospital-affiliated sex abuse team and asked to speak to the coordinator. The two professionals decided that a senior member of the sexual abuse team with experience in early childhood development and special needs children would interview the child while the social service personnel watched behind a one-way mirror. The two interviews, which were conducted over the next several days, appeared to indicate that the 3-year-old was describing hygienic touching as opposed to abuse. The family readily decided to change their handling of the 3-year-old's toileting. No other overstimulating or inappropriate experiences were detailed during the evaluation. The 3-year-old was also referred for a speech and language assessment.

ACTION GUIDELINES

A. General principles

1. Document the chronology, context, and consistency of the complaint.
2. Maintain objectivity.
   a. External independence: not allying oneself with any particular individual involved in the investigation.
   b. Internal independence: not allowing oneself to be biased relative to the allegations.
3. Gather uncontaminated data for the court system.

B. Interviewer requirements

1. Be skilled in managing parental behaviors, emotions, and reactions.
2. Be comfortable interacting with children.
3. Have knowledge of basic child development principles.
4. Be skillful in managing a wide range of children's behaviors.
5. Remain current with regard to child witness and child sexual abuse literature.
6. Establish interview format.

C. Avoiding role confusion

1. Maintain evaluation stance rather than engaging in therapeutic procedures.
2. Avoid emotional interpretation of events to child.
3. Remember who is trier of fact (judge/jury).
4. Maintain independence by avoiding inappropriate advocacy.

D. Triaging intake

1. Determine whether evaluation by clinician is mandatory or voluntary. If possible, get court-appointed status.
2. Determine ability to perform requested evaluations; learn the legal issues at stake.
3. Assess amount of time available for necessary procedures and availability for any court procedures.
4. Inform participants of financial considerations.
5. Assess divorce, custody, and visitation arrangements.
6. Obtain pertinent court information.
7. Assess quality of any previous evaluations, including who did it, what kind of training the person has, techniques utilized, availability of written report, who received feedback, and contaminative influences.

8. Determine levels of documentation to be utilized (e.g., audiotaping, videotaping, written report, etc.).

E. Interviews

1. Arrange for parental interviews, separate and balanced, if parents are seen separately.
2. Obtain psychosocial, family, and childhood histories from each parent.
3. Make appointments for the child's interview, informing parent of need to see child alone.
4. Prepare interview room with minimum number of toys and desired evaluation materials.
5. Establish free play period for child, with goals of a) making child comfortable and relaxed with interviewer, b) rapport building, c) informal developmental assessment of memory, suggestibility, capacity to lie, cognitive style, and level of sexual knowledge.
6. Guide child through interview from open-ended to focused questions.

F. Ancillary services

1. Arrange for psychological testing, if indicated.
2. Refer for medical exam if not already done.

G. Assessment of contamination

1. Review interviews for interviewer's behaviors that may have affected child's responses.
2. Judge technical, system, and/or parental factors that may have influenced child (videotaping, intensive questioning, etc.).

H. Report writing

1. Write a *complete* report, including
   a. referral information
   b. time, place, and participants of each contact
   c. background information
   d. behavioral observations
   e. type of procedures utilized in evaluation
   f. information gathered from interview
   g. testing report if done
   h. impressions
   i. diagnosis
   j. recommendations
2. Include degree of factors that may have affected child's responses in past as well as present evaluations.

REFERENCES

American Academy of Child and Adolescent Psychiatry: Guidelines for the Evaluation of Child and Adolescent Sexual Abuse, Revised Edition. Washington, DC, American Academy of Child and Adolescent Psychiatry, 1990

American Academy of Child and Adolescent Psychiatry: Practice parameters for the forensic evaluation of children and adolescents who may have been physically or sexually abused. J Am Acad Child Adolesc Psychiatry 36(10), supplement, October 1997

American Professional Society on the Abuse of Children: Guidelines for Psychosocial Evaluation of Suspected Sexual Abuse in Young Children. Chicago, IL, American Professional Society on the Abuse of Children, 1990 (Available from APSAC, 407 South Dearborn Avenue, Suite 1300, Chicago, IL 60605)

American Professional Society on the Abuse of Children: Guidelines for the Psychosocial Evaluation of Suspected Sexual Abuse in Young Children. Chicago, IL, American Professional Society on the Abuse of Children, 1995 (Available from APSAC, 407 South Dearborn Avenue, Suite 1300, Chicago, IL 60605)

Bays J, Chadwick D: Medical diagnoses of the sexually abused child. Child Abuse Negl 17:91–110, 1993

Boat B, Everson M: Interviewing young children with anatomical dolls. Child Welfare 57:337–352, 1988

Boat BW, Everson MD: Anatomical doll exploration among nonreferred children. Child Abuse Negl 18:139–153, 1994

Bradley A, Wood K: How do children tell? the disclosure process in child sexual abuse. Child Abuse Negl 20(9):881–891, 1996

Brosing CL, Kalichman SC: Clinician's reporting of suspected child abuse. Clin Psychol Rev 12:155–168, 1992

Bruck M, Ceci S, Francoer R: Children's use of anatomically detailed dolls to report genital touching in a medical examination. J Exp Psychol Appl 6:74–83, 2000

Bulkley J: Child Sexual Abuse and the Law, 5th Edition. Washington, DC, American Bar Association, 1985

Bull R: Innovative techniques for questioning children, especially those who are young and those who are learning disabled, in Memory and Testimony in the Child Witness. Edited by Zaragoza MS, Graham JR, Hall GCN, et al. Thousand Oaks, CA, Sage, 1995, pp 179–194

Ceci SJ, Bruck M: Jeopardy in the Courtroom. Washington, DC, American Psychological Association, 1995

Conte J, Sorenson E, Fogarty L, et al: Evaluating children's reports of sexual abuse: results from a survey of professionals. Am J Orthopsychiatry 61:428–437, 1991

Coy v Iowa, 487 US 1012 (1988)

Dalenberg CJ: Fantastic Elements in Child Disclosure of Abuse. 9 APSAC Advisor 9(2):1, 5–10, 1996

DeLoache J: The use of dolls in interviewing young children, in Memory and Testimony in the Child Witness. Edited by Zaragoza MS, Graham JR, Hall GCN, et al. Thousand Oaks, CA, Sage, 1995, pp 160–178

Everson MD: Understanding bizarre, improbable and fantastic elements in children's accounts of abuse. Child Maltreatment 2:134–149, 1997

Everson MD, Boat BW: Sexualized doll play among young children. J Am Acad Child Adolesc Psychiatry 29:736–742, 1990

Everson MD, Boat BW: Putting the anatomical doll controversy in perspective. Child Abuse Negl 18:113–129, 1994

Faller KC: Child Sexual Abuse: Intervention and Treatment Issues. Washington, DC, U.S. Department of Health and Human Services, 1993

Finkelhor D: Sexually victimized children. New York, Free Press, 1979

Finkelhor D: Current information on the scope and nature of child sexual abuse. Future Child 4(2):31–53, 1994

Friedrich WN: Sexual behavior in sexually abused children. Violence Update 3 (5), 1, 7–11, 1993

Friedrich WN: Psychological assessment of sexually abused children: the case for abuse-specific measures. Paper presented at the American Psychological Association Annual Conference, Los Angeles, CA, August 12, 1994

Friedrich WN, Grambach P, Damon L, et al: Child Sexual Behavior Inventory: normative and clinical comparisons. Psychol Assess 4:303–311, 1992

Goodman GS, Taub EP, Jones DPH, et al: Testifying in criminal court. Monogr Soc Res Child Dev 57:1–159, 1992

Idaho v Wright, 497 US 805, 110 S Ct 3139 (1990)

Jones D, McQuiston M: Interviewing the sexually abused child. Denver, CO, C.II. Kempe National Center for the Prevention and Treatment of Child Abuse and Neglect, 1985

Jones D, McQuiston M: Interviewing the Sexually Abused Child, 2nd Edition. Denver, CO, CH Kempe National Center for the Prevention and Treatment of Child Abuse and Neglect, 1986

Kendall-Tackett KA, Williams LM, Finkelhor D: The impact of sexual abuse on children: a review and synthesis of recent empirical studies. Psychol Bull 113:164–180, 1993

Kerns DL, Ritter ML: Medical findings in child sexual abuse cases with perpetrator confessions. Presented at the annual meeting of the Ambulatory Pediatric Association, Baltimore, MD, May 7, 1992. Published in American Journal of Diseases of Children 146:494, 1992

Lawson L, Chaffin M: False negatives in sexual abuse disclosure interviews. Journal of Interpersonal Violence 7:532–542, 1992

Lipovsky JA: The impact of court on children. Journal of Interpersonal Violence 9(2):238–257, 1994

Maryland v Craig, 497 US 836 (1990)

Massachusetts v Amirault LeFave, 430 Mass 169, 714 NE2d 805 (1988)

McCurdy K, Daro D: Current trends in child abuse reporting and fatalities: the results of the 1993 annual fifty-state survey. Working paper no. 808. Chicago, IL, National Committee for Prevention of Child Abuse, April, 1994

Muram O: Child sexual abuse: relationship between sexual acts and genital findings. Child Abuse Negl 13:211–216, 1989

Myers JEB: The Backlash. Thousand Oaks, CA, Sage, 1994

Myers JEB: Evidence in Child Abuse and Neglect Cases, 3rd Edition. New York, Wiley Law Publishers, 1997

Quinn KM: The credibility of children's allegations of sexual abuse. Behav Sci Law 23:181–200, 1988

Runyan DK: The emotional impact of societal interventions into child abuse, in Child Victims, Child Witnesses. Edited by Goodman GS, Bottoms BL. New York, Guilford, 1993

Russell D: The Secret Trauma: Incest in the Lives of Girls and Women. New York, Basic Books, 1986

Saywitz K, Camparo L: Interviewing child witnesses: a developmental perspective. Child Abuse Negl 22(8):825–848, 1998

Sgroi S, Porter F, Blick L: Validation of sexual abuse, in Handbook for Clinical Intervention in Child Sexual Abuse. Edited by Sgroi S. Lexington, MA, Lexington Books, 1982, pp 39–80

Sorenson T, Snow B: How children tell: the process of disclosure in child sexual abuse. Child Welfare 70:3–15, 1991

State v Michaels, 625 A2d 489 (NJ S Ct App Div 1993), Aff.'d, 642 A2d 1372 (1994)

Sternberg KJ, Lamb ME, Hershkowitz I, et al: Effects of introductory style on children's abilities to describe experiences of sexual abuse. Child Abuse Negl 21(11):1133–1146, 1997

Terr L: Forbidden games: post-traumatic child's play. Journal of the American Academy of Child Psychiatry 20:740–759, 1981

White S, Quinn KM: Investigatory independence in child sexual abuse evaluations. Bulletin of the American Academy of Psychiatry and the Law 16:269–273, 1988

White S, Santilli G, Quinn KM: Child evaluator's roles in child sexual abuse assessments, in Sexual Abuse Allegations in Custody and Visitation Cases. Edited by Nicholson EB, Bulkley J. Washington, DC, American Bar Association National Legal Resource Center for Child Advocacy and Protection, 1988

White v Illinois, 502 US 346, 112 S Ct 736 (1992)

Wiese D, Daro D: Current Trends in Child Abuse Reporting and Fatalities: The Results of the 1993 Annual Fifty-State Survey. Chicago, IL, National Committee for Prevention of Child Abuse, 1995

Yuille JC, Hunter R, Joffe R, et al: Interviewing children in sexual abuse cases, in Child Victims, Child Witnesses. Edited by Goodman GS, Bottoms BL. New York, Guilford, 1993

CHAPTER 16

Forensic Issues in Munchausen by Proxy

Herbert A. Schreier, M.D.

Case Example[1]

A 7-year-old boy, Ian, is brought in by his mother, Mrs. Ferris, to an emergency room at a major medical center with a history of vomiting and diarrhea of 7 days' duration. He does not appear dehydrated or ill, as would be expected by the reported frequency of episodes and lack of oral intake. Mrs. Ferris gives a long history of feeding difficulties and missed school because of illnesses and multiple workups at other medical centers. Ian is admitted, and on the ward his condition deteriorates and he has severe episodes of vomiting. Intravenous fluids are started, and on the eighth day he has the first of two unexplained cardiac arrests; the second one occurs 6 days later. During the resuscitation, the mother at first appears calm; then a nurse overhears her "gleefully" describing the action to a friend over a phone close to the nurse's station. Though Mrs. Ferris never leaves the hospital, it is later recalled that she appeared more interested in talking with the nurses and other parents than in her child.

In the second month of Ian's hospitalization, his gastrostomy drainage bag begins filling up with more fluid than he is being given. Over a 7-day period it actually reaches a high of 3,600 milliliters (ml) of fluid when he has only taken in 1,200 ml.

Despite being very familiar with Munchausen by proxy (MBP), and the peculiarities of the presentation in this case, Ian's physician confers with colleagues in two other institutions trying to figure out what might be causing the findings. One gastroenterologist who had experience with more than 15 cases of MBP suggests yet another procedure requiring surgery; the other correctly suggests MBP, and the child improves

immediately after being separated from his mother. The mother mounted a campaign among other parents on the unit, trying to convince them that she was being persecuted by the hospital and physicians, who blamed her when they could not figure out what was wrong with her son.

Six years later I was consulted by a genetic counselor at our hospital who was trying to assist with a diagnosis of a 7-month-old infant who weighed 7 pounds, the same as his birth weight (failure to thrive). Multiple procedures including biopsies were performed but turned up nothing. She wondered if, because the mother had a history of "pseudo-seizures," she could be an MBP case. I attended a case conference on this child and immediately recognized his half-brother's name—Ian. The mother had remarried and now had two children with a different last name. When, as I suggested, the child was hospitalized and separated from the mother, he gained 2 pounds over a weekend.

The history of events since Ian's hospitalization is as follows: After a court hearing on Ian, the mother was ordered into therapy with a psychologist affiliated with a university clinic. She admitted to having MBP but not to harming her child (!) and was said to be "improved" after 6 months of therapy. The judge, against the wishes of child protective services and the district attorney and without asking for either an outside evaluation or a report from the consultant who was familiar with the disorder, returned Ian, who as a result of his cardiac arrests was now wheelchair bound. The medical records indicate that this child only came to the emergency room on one subsequent occasion, where it was found that he had a too-high

---

[1] For purposes of further disguising the material, there have been minor changes to the details of this case. It has been updated since appearing in *Hurting for Love* (Schreier and Libow 1993).

161

level of an anticonvulsant. Mrs. Ferris, as noted, was seen for pseudo-seizures, which appeared to have resolved when she became pregnant. This next child exhibited moderately severe failure to thrive but improved once his mother became pregnant with her third child. The third child was then nearly starved to death over a 7-month period.

CLINICAL ISSUES

Overview

Factitious disorder by proxy, popularly known as Munchausen by proxy (MBP), in which a parent or caretaker repeatedly falsifies symptoms or actually induces illness in an infant or child, frequently while in a hospital, is one of the most perplexing disorders in all of psychiatry. First described in England by Roy Meadow in 1977, there have been hundreds of reports in the scientific literature and much popular attention to it in the media. The disorder is overwhelmingly found in women, who appear to all the world as wonderful and caring mothers. Yet at the very same time, they may be repeatedly causing grave harm to their children. Because there are several other conditions in which a parent may fabricate symptoms or directly harm a child, it is important to explore the motivation for this behavior. Motivation is also important in evaluating prognosis for treatment of the mother and crucial in planning for the current and future disposition of the child. For example, many case studies and series indicate that this disorder involves persistent (Rosenberg 1995) or compulsive (Schreier 1992) harm-causing behavior that is knowingly and wantonly carried out. Horrific consequences including death, at times to only one but not infrequently serially or simultaneously to several children, are the norm.

Typically, as a result of the mother's elaborate production of symptoms or illness, the child is hospitalized and then harmed through invasive procedures related to attempts by physicians to understand and treat a confusing clinical picture. The aim of the perverse behavior on the parts of these mothers involves a need to be close to and in a relationship with the medical staff, and/or be the center of attention. This relationship is one of needy dependency that involves manipulation and also appears to contain elements of sadistic cruelty, not only toward the child but also toward the people whose life's work is to cure and protect children.

Case analyses repeatedly find difficulties in suspecting the mother's agency that go well beyond our inability to think that anyone, especially a mother, could repeatedly (and with premeditation) suffocate, starve, or poison a child. Detection is difficult even when these otherwise seemingly competent women leave glaring clues to their actions. Their skills may resemble those seen in impostors, and they may very effectively mimic caring and knowledgeable mothers. They may also exhibit psychopathic behavior and the kind of object relations found in female forms of perversion (Schreier and Libow 1993).

The interpersonal aspects of this disorder suggest that individuals who are seen as powerful are targeted and they may be especially susceptible to the manipulations of these women. These include people in the legal and health care professions who see themselves as altruistic and have a need to be seen as intelligent, caring, and able to function independently when solving complex problems. Despite training that aims at developing an ability to adopt a neutral and inquisitive stance toward patients, psychiatrists and other professionals are often not proficient at detecting lying, especially the manipulation of the truth these women may demonstrate.

Prevalence and Morbidity

Because MBP is often described as rare, some discussion of epidemiology is needed. Extrapolation from a carefully designed study done in England (McClure et al. 1996) suggests that at least 600 new cases of MBP presenting with just two conditions—acute life-threatening events (i.e., apnea) or nonaccidental poisoning—would be expected to occur each year in the United States. Further, although the histories reported in the literature clearly represent more serious cases, they indicate a death rate as high as 9%–10%, similar to the rate found by an informal survey of pediatric gastroenterologists and neurologists done at our institution. In suffocation cases, it is frequently found that one, two, or more siblings have died of sudden infant death syndrome (SIDS) or unexpectedly of mysterious causes. There are cases involving the deaths of nine children by one woman, and recently a woman was tried and convicted (25 years after the fact) of suffocating all five of her biological children. Some number of deaths from suffocation in the past erroneously attributed to SIDS may have fostered the idea of familial risk of SIDS (Firstman and Talen 1997).

Definitions

Guidelines have been proposed by the American Professional Society on the Abuse of Children (APSAC) to address some of the problems with the DSM-IV (and its Text Revision, DSM-IV-TR [American Psychiatric Association 2000]) diagnosis of factitious disorder by proxy (Ayoub et al. 1998). They stress that MBP consists of *two* components. The first is the identification of the victimization of the child. The second is the identification of the psychological motivations and the characteristics of the perpetrating parent or caretaker. In addition, the committee noted that the family often plays a role in MBP, either through passive support or directly participating in the deception that is at the core of the child's victimization. The committee recognized that a child victimized by abuse, regardless of the motivations, needs immediate protection and that one needs to consider whether falsification plays a role. They coined the term *pediatric condition* (illness, impairment, or symptom) *falsification* (PCF), defined as child maltreatment in which an adult falsifies physical and/or psychological signs and/or symptoms in a victim causing that person to be regarded as ill or impaired by others.

Falsification includes but is not limited to the following forms of deception: directly causing a condition, over- or underreporting signs and symptoms, creating a false appearance of signs and symptoms, and/or coaching the victim or others to misrepresent the victim as ill.

> Only the imagination and sophistication of the perpetrator limit the number and extent of the presenting symptoms. The presence of a valid illness does not preclude concurrent exaggeration or falsification. PCF through psychological or developmental symptoms has been described but appears to be less common. (Ayoub et al. 1998, p. 8)

Persons who intentionally falsify history, signs, or symptoms in a child to meet their own self-serving psychological needs have been diagnosed with factitious disorder by proxy and should be coded as such (300.19, DSM-IV-TR, p. 517).

Differential Diagnosis

Conditions that are not MBP include those in which parents who are overwhelmed or overly anxious, in order to get assistance with caring for their child, may blatantly falsify symptoms on one or two occasions. Other examples include children who are truant and present with illnesses resulting in missed school time, in which the primary motivation is the parent's wish to keep the child dependent and at home. These situations do not involve ongoing deception and manipulation of doctors, and serious illness fabrication is absent. In child neglect and failure to thrive (both commonly found as part of MBP), if the issue is the parent's inability to cope with the child and the parent's failure to feed or care for the child adequately, this also is not MBP. Yet another category of parents who may result in confusion in diagnosing MBP are

parents of chronically ill children who appear "difficult" because of psychological issues of their own, not because of manipulation of authorities or impostoring or because they disagree with the medical staff and may appear to interfere with treatment. Parental "difficulty" may also represent an expression of frustration or appropriate advocacy for their children. These are *not* examples of MBP, though at times it may be difficult to sort out the issues. If a child is being harmed, then action must be taken to protect that child, as has always been expected of people caring for children.

It should be noted that there is *no* particular psychological profile or checklist of symptoms that definitively confirms or excludes the diagnosis of MBP; rather, there are common patterns that should raise suspicion but should be examined on a case-by-case basis. Personality problems are found quite often, but perpetrators may appear relatively healthy on the usual psychological tests and in interviews, especially to the uninformed examiner. Psychotic delusions of illness in one's child may be mistaken for MBP, but if they are the source of the illness falsification, then the correct diagnosis should be delusional disorder (by proxy), somatic type. Up to three-quarters of mothers exhibited somatizing problems when younger, and about one-third will have had factitious disorders. Regarding motivation, it should be noted that contrary to the DSM-IV-TR definitions, external incentives such as monetary gain or seeking revenge on an abandoning spouse *may* be present along with the dynamics described above and do not preclude the diagnosis.

So-called doctor-shopping *may* be a sign of MBP when the motivation is not to actually get help for the child but to subject the child to the abuse of repeated investigations and needless procedures by doctors, to gain attention, to maintain the relationships with these powerful figures, or to evade suspicions aroused by their behavior with former doctors or hospitals. However, doctor-shopping need not always be present. Physicians and other health care providers may have long-term relationships with the children being victimized and indeed may be supportive of the mother, even after the falsification and the mother's hand in it are uncovered.

It is important to note that the specific immediate physical consequence of the abuse is not necessarily representative of the seriousness of the MBP condition or of the potential for future harm to the child. Perpetrators have been known to switch from seemingly mild abuse to life-threatening forms, and the characteristics of those more likely to do the latter are poorly understood. Furthermore, there is a fairly high recidivism rate of abuse in MBP (and this obviously relates only to the cases felt to be "mild" enough to consider returning the child). Mothers have been known to continue their harm-inducing behavior even during supervised visits while the child is in protective custody.

Management

The inability to consider the possibility that a mother is involved in MBP is the most difficult obstacle in the management of this disorder, so case evaluators must first overcome this obstacle. Another obstacle is the involvement of well-meaning "expert" evaluators who are not familiar with MBP and "experts for hire" who will devise their own novel explanations to serve a client (see Chadwick and Krouse 1997).

The usual issue is often an error of logic, such as using the statements of, or records provided by, someone accused of pathological lying as the only source of information about a case. Those inexperienced with the disorder may expect that psychological test data with minimal findings make an MBP process unlikely. This is not the case. Inexperienced therapists who treat or evaluate cases of MBP are just as likely as any other professional to be manipulated by the mother. Case evaluators need to have access to *all* case material and *all* treating persons, not just those offered by a hiring attorney.

Protective service workers and guardians *ad litem* need to be aware of or have access to persons knowledgeable about MBP in order to question evaluations that suggest the mother's wellness, improvement with treatment, or lack of dangerousness. One evaluator described a mother as having a "mild case of MBP." This was based on a misreading of the potential lethality of the methods of abuse and also reflected a lack of understanding regarding the possibility of a mother going from relatively mild abuse to very severe methods without warning. The issue is not what was done to the child, but aspects of the mother's psychopathology. In the same case, a treating psychologist relied on the mother's own word over a year's time that the child continued to have illnesses outside of her care and declared that she therefore doubted the diagnosis of MBP. Independent, outside verification of the facts concerning a child's condition is *essential* in deciding upon the future potential harm to a child. A forensic examiner who fails to insist on this displays his or her lack of experience with this disorder.

It is unwise to attempt to diagnose an MBP case without proper coordination of the various agencies involved. The workers ideally should meet face-to-face. This meeting should include 1) as many physicians involved in the child's care as possible; 2) someone who has gathered information from as many prior treating parties as possible; 3) if the abuse takes place in the hospital, a representative from administration or the hospital's legal department; and 4) a nursing supervisor, a child protective services worker, a social services worker, and a representative from law enforcement and/or the district attorney's office. A detailed plan should be worked out for either further investigations or confronting the parent. It is not unusual for doctors with doubts about a particular case to hear details of importance to their diagnosis for the first time at such meetings. It is essential that all agencies involved in these cases document their findings and opinions in the utmost of detail.

If covert surveillance is indicated, it should be decided who will be in charge (hospital personnel, unless it is a public hospital, or the police). If this is called for, steps should be taken to guard the parents' privacy as best as possible, and nurses who might be "recruited" by the mother should be encouraged to excuse themselves during the time the surveillance is taking place. They should be warned of the need to act totally professionally in the interest of the child.

Several hospitals have instituted an MBP team that can review a case and make recommendations. A consultation liaison psychiatrist, psychologist, or other professional familiar with the disorder in all its presentations, along with a county child protective worker, should be a part of this team and brought in on a case as early as possible.

Treatment

Not a great deal has been published about the treatability of people diagnosed with MBP. Anecdotal reports gleaned by the author over the years suggest that this is a very difficult condition to treat. The most common experience, as reported in the case presented here, is that the therapist becomes susceptible to the same ministrations as the physician. This often leads to the mother returning to court to start the processes of custody all over again. It is the contention of APSAC that no one should undertake treatment of a person diagnosed with MBP unless they are fully aware of the potential dynamic issues, feel competent to deal with personality disorders, and/or have ongoing supervision by someone with more experience treating such people. It is very valuable for a team of professionals involved in a treatment program to meet and to have a consultant from outside available to help resolve questions.

LEGAL ISSUES

Reluctance to Accept Diagnosis

Though MBP was described over 22 years ago, there is little uniformity in how it is treated in different jurisdictions in the United States and even within a particular jurisdiction in a state. Many factors are involved in a district attorney's decision about whether to press forward with any criminal procedure, and in the case of MBP the problems are usually greater. First and foremost is the disbelief of the prosecutors, or the difficulty they would anticipate in getting a judge and jury to see that a woman who looks so "good" could do such dastardly things to a helpless child. For example, in the case of Yvonne Eldridge, who was honored at the White House for her work with foster care children, a hearing officer handed down a decision to revoke her foster care license, finding that she had murdered and/or caused intentional harm to several children entrusted in her care. The county district attorney *refused* to charge her. Publicity and private urgings led to a state prosecution on a few of the possible charges. After long preparations for the trial and many delays, a jury convicted her after just 5 hours of deliberation. However, the sitting judge incorrectly allowed her to be released on bail after she served only one day of her sentence and allowed her to remain free while she mounted an appeal for a new trial. Months later he found in her favor and granted her a new trial based on poor representation, though he did not interview the defense attorney to find out if some of his actions were deliberate strategies.

Further, trials of MBP cases tend to be very expensive, involving as they do multiple experts. Experts who are knowledgeable about the disorder are difficult to find, whereas there appears to be a surfeit of "experts" who will testify that a completely strange presentation of an illness is a real possibility. This has been particularly true in repeated apnea cases, where the very idea of the genetics of multiple SIDS cases in families may have come from the inability of researchers to see the possibility that a mother would suffocate several of her children (Firstman and Talen 1997).

Standards of Proof and Admissibility of Evidence

A higher standard of proof (beyond a reasonable doubt) in criminal trials may also play a role in district attorneys' reluctance to take these cases. However, as the disorder becomes better known, there is a lessening reluctance for criminal prosecutors to be involved. A number of researchers have recommended that the threat of criminal prosecution be used as a "club" to gain an admission from the perpetrator and that this would make the protection of the child in juvenile court easier. However, because of the satisfaction people with MBP obtain from being litigious, this has not turned out to be particularly useful. Recently it has been my experience that there is now a greater willingness to try these cases in criminal court.

MBP in the Courtroom

As the standards for the admissibility of scientific evidence are currently in a state of flux, judges have varied enormously in their decisions on whether or not to allow testimony that a mother has been diagnosed with MBP into evidence. Some jurisdictions seek to balance relevance against the prejudicial nature that testimony about MBP may incur. Though prior codes of federal evidence (the so-called *Kelly-Frye* standard) have been applied to MBP as far back as 1981, in a murder trial (*People v. Phillips*), and upheld at the appellate court, MBP has been treated in a variety of ways since, including not being admissible unless the mother raised the issue of her good character. Parenthetically, *Phillips* upheld the ability of a psychiatrist to diagnose the mother with MBP based on his reading of the literature and the records and without interviewing the mother.

Daubert has replaced *Kelly-Frye* concerning the hard sciences, and the recent *Kumho* case (*Kumho Tire Co., Ltd. v. Carmichael* 1999), discussed in Chapter 33, "Psychic Trauma and Civil Litigation," may apply more stringent standards of scientific evidence which go beyond the expert's mere clinical experience. Traditionally an expert opinion on whether a witness is lying is inadmissible because it exceeds the ability and specialized knowledge of an expert and juries can decide for themselves. However, in *United States v. Shay* (1995), the First Circuit Court reversed a lower court's decision to exclude expert testimony on Munchausen disorder (not by proxy) because lying is characteristic of the condition.

As in most cases of MBP that come to trial, there is usually only circumstantial evidence, and the mother's appearance can be more persuasive of her innocence despite the weight of numerous abuses, especially those "accomplished" by doctors. The jury should be able to hear that this very picture is not at all uncommon and has been repeatedly documented through confessions. Without this understanding, even the most horrendous reported abuse of a child (e.g., 40 unnecessary operations and 200 hospitalizations) may lead a jury to doubt the mother's agency when she appears loving and caring.

Preparation for Court

Once the most difficult problem in MBP—that of suspecting it to begin with—is overcome, the issue of gathering data sufficient to first protect the child and then adjudicate the case poses major and in some ways unique issues for medical and legal personnel. The best one can do in a chapter of this length meant for a disparate audience is to highlight the particular issues that distinguish the pursuit of typical MBP cases from those of the more common forms of child abuse.

These cases most often involve indirect evidence, and the medical and social service people involved as well as the prosecutors must be ready to present a believable *res ipsa loquitor* argument (i.e., given the weight of the evidence, the only possible conclusion is that the mother is causing the symptoms). Peculiar illnesses or unexpected deaths in siblings or others in a mother's care, lack of symptoms in the index child when the mother is absent, or the appearance of symptoms only in the mother's presence require careful documentation. Legal personnel will often be called upon to ask the courts for enforced separation from the sickly child, in order to note changes in his or her condition away from the suspected perpetrator, as few mothers will volunteer to this so-called "separation test." The test must be for a sufficient length of time to be valid. All tests must be done with the utmost of care in fairness to the mother and the child. The possibility of false positives, such as food causing a reading in a stool sample that might be mistaken for a laxative, or the child having a rare disease (see Chapter 3 in Schreier and Libow 1993), must be carefully considered.

As professional opinions and hearsay are often admissible evidence, these must be gathered with great care, either through direct contact with physicians or hospitals or a very careful review of their records. It is often best to speak with other caretakers, as MBP mothers very frequently misquote what has been told to them or they may utilize a letter written by a doctor that may be somewhat exaggerated because it was requested to prod a social agency. Furthermore, these other caretakers may have been misinformed by a false family history given by the mother or may have recorded symptoms in the child that were reported as if they were actually witnessed. Although tedious, a careful review of prior charts can ultimately be the most important aspect in a case.

The U.S. Supreme Court, in a pre-MBP case in 1972, upheld evidence of prior criminal behavior, which is usually excluded from criminal prosecution. The court said that in "the crime of infanticide…evidence of repeated incidence is especially relevant because it may be the only evidence to prove the crime" (DiMaio and Bernstein 1974, p. 753). The introduction of other incidents of abuse appears to be rarely contested in the cases I have participated in or reviewed.

Covert Surveillance

Probably the most controversial aspect of MBP is the possible need to use covert video surveillance (CVS) in order to save the life of a child. The balance between the mother's right to privacy and the imminent threat to the child is of the utmost importance. Interestingly, the legal issues appear less controversial than the public ones; and in both England and the United States there appears to be a lessened expectancy of privacy when one is in a hospital. Several institutions are including the possibility of being videotaped in their consent to admission. Private institutions appear to present less of a difficulty than either public institutions or cases in which the physician is working for the state. The most conservative approach is to obtain a search warrant and allow the police to do the surveillance. This was done in a Seattle case, but only after the child became seriously ill from a bacteria found in saliva and passed through her gastric tube on two occasions and no explanation could be found for her extreme failure to thrive. The mother was discovered on camera to be diluting her child's formula.

The Federal Bureau of Investigation has suggested not having sound on the camera, so as not to pick up on the mother's private conversations, and focusing the camera only on the child. The latter is problematic, as in several cases the recorded abuse took place outside the bed area of the infant.

Though a detailed discussion is beyond the scope of this presentation, three aspects are worth noting. First, videotaped surveillance has been used in successfully prosecuting a murder in a California case. Second, as with the unit run by David Southall in England, when the guidelines are carefully prescribed, the effectiveness of CVS in saving lives is considered quite high. In a published report, CVS was successful in documenting abuse in 33 of 39 cases (Southall et al. 1997). Based on conviction or confessions, the suspicion rate was even more accurate, 37 of 39. For those still not convinced of the usefulness of CVS in saving lives, it should be noted that 28 of the 39 patients who were surveilled had a total of 41 siblings. "Twelve had died suddenly and unexpectedly. Death was attributed to SIDS in 11 of these children. After surveillance, four parents admitted deliberate suffocation in eight of their children!" (Southall et al. 1997, p. 738).

It should also be noted that in one series CVS was useful in making a *bona fide* medical diagnosis in cases that aroused suspicion of MBP (Hall et al. 2000). It is apparent that these investigatory roles are not ones that most medical personnel will take to easily. The problem is compounded by the ability of MBP mothers to find staff members in a hospital who believe that they are being wrongly accused or persecuted. Educational programs in hospitals and involving judges and others likely to be involved in such cases are essential. At least one hospital has set up a committee to monitor investigations when suspected MBP is reported to them. Few hospitals have been willing to tackle the thorny issue raised by CVS. In the United States there are no standards for monitoring the videos (e.g., hospitals have been known to not look at tapes until the day following the monitoring, which can be extremely risky).

Liability Issues

There are, of course, mandated reporting demands on professionals to protect children, and the possibility of a suit by the nonabusing parent of a child victim against a hospital and staff for not vigorously protecting a child certainly exists. The danger of false diagnosis has received attention elsewhere, and the number of such cases may increase. MBP accusations have now appeared with increasing frequency in divorce proceedings involving custody. Given the contentious bent of people with this disorder, there is the likelihood that forensic experts could come under fire and be sued for damages as well. Physicians have been sued for malpractice for misdiagnosing MBP, as well as for violating a mother's constitutionally protected right to have access to her family. In a recent federal court case, reporting doctors and an expert hired by the prosecution were sued for violating the mother's civil rights to due process through their court testimony. However, Judge Wexler of the U.S. District Court for the Eastern District of New York stated "it is without question that these doctors are entitled to absolute witness immunity with respect to their testimony in court regarding Ellen Storck's MBP. That such testimony is alleged to have been without basis and contradictory to acceptable medical practice is irrelevant" (*Storck v. Suffolk County et al.*).

PITFALLS

- Failure to suspect MBP and lack of familiarity with the disorder.
- Not being aware of the ability of the perpetrators to con staff and other professionals.

- Allowing the mother unsupervised visits. If the visits are supervised, not cautioning the visit supervisors about what to expect. Not having the supervisors keep careful written observations.
- Failure to review *all* medical records and interview all other available caretakers.
- Failure to anticipate and prepare with great care for the possibility of going to court either as witness or defendant.
- Minimizing parental pathology and being overly optimistic about prognosis.

CASE EXAMPLE EPILOGUE

At the trials of the mother who was accused of starving her infants, one nearly to death, the father testified that he believed his wife. There was a community outpouring of support for the family, particularly from their church. The mother's lawyer argued unsuccessfully for the return of the children to the mother after her original therapist testified that she did not have MBP and did not harm her children. At her criminal trial, in which the issue of MBP was permitted to be raised in a hypothetical question as to what might motivate a woman to engage in this kind of abuse, MBP was not offered as a diagnosis for the mother. She was sentenced to 90 days in a state psychiatric forensic unit for evaluation and then ordered into therapy with a local expert in MBP who felt she made progress. The mother became pregnant by another man and the baby was immediately placed into custody pending the outcome of an evaluation of her relationship during visitations over a 6-month period. She will continue to be on probation and see her therapist.

The case presentation hallmarks many features of MBP cases: the intense power of the process, even in the hospital; cognitive slippage in the mother's thinking, as she increases the child's fabricated stomach drainage to impossible amounts; the likelihood of professionals, such as inexperienced therapists and court personnel, to be fooled by MBP perpetrators; the passive and sometimes active support of spouses, despite possible grave risk to their own children by the stance they take.

ACTION GUIDELINES

A. Team management is essential and should include joint meetings with all of the treating staff.
B. Develop a plan involving people knowledgeable about MBP in the investigation of the case.
C. Compile a list of possible factitious illnesses and consider means of symptom induction.

D. Preserve samples of toxicology studies, using a high degree of security.

E. Careful review of all medical records and contact with all prior providers of treatment is essential. Records of siblings and mother may be extremely valuable.

F. Ask involved staff to document their observations of mother's behavior.

G. Only involve evaluators who are truly familiar with all or most aspects of MBP.

H. Consider the use of covert surveillance. It is best to have a protocol for exactly how this will be implemented in advance of needing it.

I. Be ready to document, for the courts if necessary, the importance of separation of the child from the mother for diagnostic purposes.

J. Monitors need to be trained to be exceedingly cautious and document all behavior of the mother. Typically the mother will want to spend more time talking to them than visiting with her child.

REFERENCES

American Psychiatric Association: Diagnostic and Statistical Manual of Mental Disorders, 4th Edition, Text Revision. Washington, DC, American Psychiatric Association, 2000

Ayoub D, Alexander R, Beck D, et al: Definitional Issues in Munchausen by proxy. APSAC Advisor 11(1):7–11, 1998

Chadwick DL, Krouse HF: Irresponsible testimony by medical experts in cases involving the physical abuse and neglect of children. Child Maltreat 2(4):331–341, 1997

DiMaio VJM, Bernstein CG: A case of infanticide. J Forensic Sci 19:745–754, 1974

Firstman R, Talen J: The Death of Innocents: A True Story of Murder, Medicine, and High-Stakes Science. New York, Bantam Books, 1997

Hall DE, Eubanks L, Meyyazhagan S, et al: Evaluation of covert video surveillance in the diagnosis of Munchausen syndrome by proxy: lessons from 41 cases. Pediatrics 105(6):1305–1312, 2000

Kumho Tire Co., Ltd. v Carmichael, 119 S Ct 1167 (1999)

McClure RJ, Davis PM, Meadow SR, et al: Epidemiology of Munchausen syndrome by proxy, non-accidental poisoning, and non-accidental suffocation. Arch Dis Child 75:57–61, 1996

Meadow R: Munchausen syndromy by proxy: the hinterland of child abuse. Lancet [2]:343–345, 1977

People v Phillips, 175 Cal Rptr 703 (Ct App 1981)

Rosenberg D: From lying to homicide: the spectrum of Munchausen by proxy, in Munchausen Syndrome by Proxy: Issues in Diagnosis and Treatment. Edited by Levin AV, Sheridan MS. New York, Lexington Books, 1995

Schreier HA: The perversion of mothering: Munchausen syndrome by proxy. Bull Menninger Clin 56:421–437, 1992

Schreier HA: Factitious presentation of psychiatric disorder by proxy. Child Psychology and Psychiatry Review 2(3):108–115, 1997

Schreier HA, Libow JA: Hurting for Love: Munchausen by Proxy Syndrome. New York, Guilford, 1993

Southall DP, Plunkett MC, Banks MW, et al: Covert video recording of life-threatening child abuse: lessons for child protection. Pediatrics 100(5):735–760, 1997

Storck v Suffolk County et al, 97 Civ 2880

United States v Shay, 57 F3d 126 (1st Cir 1995)

Yorker B: Legal issues in factitious disorder by proxy, in The Spectrum of Factitious Disorders. Edited by Feldman M, Eisendrath S. Washington, DC, American Psychiatric Press, 1996

CASES[2]

People v Phillips, 175 Cal Rptr 703 (Ct App 1981). *MBP allowed in a murder case, and appeals court upholds the mother being diagnosed with MBP without her being interviewed by the expert witness.*

Commonwealth v Robinson, 565 NE2d 1229 (1991). *Circumstantial evidence leads to conviction, though MBP not admitted.*

Tanya Thaxton Reid v State of Texas, 964 SW2d 723 (1998). *Expert testimony regarding MBP admitted for motive. Also admitted was case of another child who had similar symptoms to the deceased until removed from mother's care. Murder conviction upheld on appeal.*

Jessica A., 515 NYS2d 370 (1987). *Conviction through res ipsa loquitor reasoning.*

SUGGESTED READINGS

Artingstall K: Tactical Aspects of Munchausen Syndrome by Proxy and Munchausen Syndrome Investigation. Boca Raton, FL, CRC Press, 1998

Kinscherff R, Ayoub C: Legal issues in Munchausen by proxy, in The Treatment of Child Abuse: Common Ground for Mental Health, Medical, and Legal Practitioners. Edited by Reece R. Baltimore, MD, Johns Hopkins University Press, 2000

---

[2] For a more complete annotated bibliography of cases, see Kinscherff and Ayoub.

Meadow R: False allegations of abuse and Munchausen by proxy. Arch Dis Child 68:444–447, 1993

Parnell TF, Day DO (eds): Munchausen by Proxy Syndrome: Misunderstood Child Abuse. Thousand Oaks, CA, Sage, 1998

Plum HJ: Legal considerations, in Munchausen Syndrome by Proxy: Issues in Diagnosis and Treatment. Edited by Levin AV, Sheridan MS. New York, Lexington Books, 1995

Yorker B: Legal issues in factitious disorder by proxy, in The Spectrum of Factitious Disorders. Edited by Feldman M, Eisendrath S. Washington, DC, American Psychiatric Press, 1996

CHAPTER 17

Clinical and Forensic Aspects of Sexual Harassment in School-Age Children

Elissa P. Benedek, M.D.

Beth K. Clark, Ph.D., A.B.P.P.

Case Example 1

Amy, an eighth-grader in a public middle school, is sent to a forensic psychiatrist for evaluation after reporting to her parents that she was teased by male peers calling her "slut, prostitute, whore, and weenie." She reports to the psychiatrist that she believes her older brother is jealous of her academic performance and has started a schoolyard rumor that she eats "hot dogs/penises." She says that at first she was only teased by her brother's circle of friends, but now at all school athletic events a large group of students yell, "Weenie." They make obscene hand gestures and "roll their tongues in their mouths" when she passes by. Her mother complains to the psychiatrist that the school administration has done nothing to stop this, and the school administrator advised her, "Boys and girls just do that kind of thing." The administration has taken no action and states it has no future plans to address the issue.

Case Example 2

Sally, a 17-year-old girl, is in treatment for severe depression. She recently lost 15 pounds and her school grades have declined precipitously. Sally's treating psychiatrist is baffled by her unresponsiveness to supportive psychotherapy and antidepressants. Fortunately, Sally has developed a good rapport with her psychiatrist, and during a therapy session, she confesses that her math teacher, under the guise of after-school tutoring, has involved her in a sexual relationship. Sally reports that she enjoys the relationship but feels ashamed and guilty. The treating psychiatrist recognizes that the sexual relationship plays a part in Sally's current depression. The psychiatrist

calls a forensic colleague for consultation about ethical and treatment responsibilities to Sally's parents and to Sally.

The behaviors that may constitute sexual harassment have a history as long as that of the workplace. However, legal definitions of sexual harassment in the workplace have developed only over the course of the last few decades. The definition of sexual harassment in the school is still unclear. The parameters of the definition of sexual harassment may be static or they may change, depending on Supreme Court decisions. Indeed, the number of recent court decisions reflects the rather fluid status of sexual harassment as it applies to children.

The number of requests made to child and adolescent psychiatrists for forensic assessment of children, adolescents, and their parents who allege sexual harassment in the classroom has increased dramatically since the Supreme Court decision in *Davis v. Monroe County Board of Education* (1998).

LEGAL ISSUES

Definitions of Sexual Harassment

Current definitions of sexual harassment are stated in Title VII of the Civil Rights Act of 1964 and in Title IX of the Educational Amendment of 1972. Title VII states it is "illegal to discriminate against employees on the basis of race, color, religion, sex, or national origin." The inclusion of sex-based discrimination in Title VII may have been accidental, because it was the result of an amendment by a legislator hoping to make the act so unacceptable that it would be defeated (Shrier 1996). Title IX prohibits discrimination in educational programs that are recipients of federal monies. In 1972, the Equal Employment Opportunity Act was passed establishing the role of the Equal Employment Opportunity Commission (EEOC) in enforcing antidiscrimination measures in the workplace. A number of legal decisions have also shaped contemporary thinking. This area of the law is also an area that is likely to continue to evolve. The issue of sexual harassment in schools arose as one facet of the many evolving new decisions in this area.

Courts recognize two categories of sexual harassment in the workplace: 1) Quid pro quo harassment is harassment that links sexual favors to a condition of employment (e.g., a supervisor tells an employee that he or she must agree to a sexual relationship in order to receive a promotion or raise or to remain employed) and 2) harassment that creates a hostile work environment (i.e., a workplace that is permeated with discriminatory intimidation, ridicule, and insult that is sufficiently severe or pervasive to alter the conditions of the victim's employment and create an abusive working environment) (*Harris v. Forklift Systems, Inc.* 1993). Comparable categories of sexual harassment in schools are based on adult sexual harassment, that is, quid pro quo and hostile environment. These serve as the models for Supreme Court decisions with regard to sexual harassment in the schools.

School Sexual Harassment

Legal Issues

Sexual harassment in schools is a contemporary legal frontier in which schools have been compared to employment settings for children. A recent Supreme Court decision reflects the view of schools as the workplace locus of employment of children, adolescents, and young adults, and prior decisions with regard to employment harassment set precedents for school decisions.

In May 1999, the Supreme Court held, in a 5 to 4 decision, that schools may be held liable for sexual harassment of students. This decision followed an earlier decision regarding schools' strict liability for teacher-student harassment. That case centered on a 1990 case, *Gebser v. Lago Vista Independent School District* (1998). In a 5 to 4 decision, the court set what it considered a high hurdle for students to meet in suing school districts for harassment by teachers. In that case, a teacher was sexually involved with a student and the school was held liable for the

teacher's behavior. The court ruled that "a teacher's sexual overtures toward a student are always inappropriate."

In *Davis v. Monroe County Board of Education* (1999), the Supreme Court held, in a 5 to 4 decision, that schools may be held liable for peer sexual harassment, or sexual harassment of students by students. Their reasoning followed the earlier decision regarding schools' liability for teacher-student harassment. Briefly, the facts of the case centered around LaShonda Davis, a fifth-grader who claimed that a classmate began taunting her, asking her for sex in crude terms, and touching her breasts and genital area. On one occasion, the classmate also put a doorstop in his pants and behaved in a sexually suggestive manner. This harassment continued for months. Despite repeated complaints by LaShonda's mother to the school administration, the school did not intervene and even declined to reassign seats so that LaShonda and the harassing boy would not sit next to each other. LaShonda's grades dropped, and she wrote a suicide note. The family pressed criminal charges, and the boy pleaded guilty to sexual battery in juvenile court. The family subsequently sued the school. The lower federal court held that Title IX did not apply to student-on-student sexual harassment. The case was appealed to the Supreme Court.

Controversies

In *Davis*, the majority opinion was authored by Justice Sandra Day O'Connor. The opinion held that schools must know of the harassment and respond with "deliberate indifference" to behavior "so severe, pervasive, and objectively offensive that it denies the victims equal access to education" guaranteed by Title IX. Ordinary acts of "teasing and name calling among school children" are not a cause for action. Justice Kennedy authored a vehement 34-page dissent. He took issue with the majority's premise that "sex discrimination" or "sex harassment" was the proper way to describe what he called at various points "immature, childish behavior" and "inappropriate behavior by children who are just learning to interact with their peers." Kennedy stated that the court had taken the analogy between school and workplace too far. "The norms of the adult workplace that have defined hostile environment sexual harassment are not easily translated to peer relationships in schools," he wrote, "where teenage romantic relationships and dating are a part of everyday life." He added: "A teenager's romantic overtures to a classmate (even when persistent and unwelcome) are an inescapable part of adolescence."

Public reaction to the ruling was, of course, mixed. Supporters of Justice Kennedy raised a concern that schools would react precipitously to avoid liability in response to trivial transgressions. They cited the case of a North Carolina school district's decision to suspend a 6-year-old boy for kissing a 6-year-old girl on the cheek. On the other hand, the National School Board Association supported the Supreme Court's decision, noting that it set a high liability standard and that many schools already had sexual harassment and discrimination policies in place.

Equal Employment Opportunity Commission Definition of Harassment

Sexual Harassment

The EEOC, along with other groups, has defined sexual harassment. That definition is perhaps the most widely known definition of sexual harassment and defines sexual harassment in the workplace (see "Definitions of Sexual Harassment" section earlier in this chapter). The EEOC definition is similar to that in Title VII and Title IX.

Hostile Environment Harassment

The Office of Civil Rights expanded and adapted the EEOC definition to apply it to the school environment in a March 13, 1997, release of a report titled, "Guidance in the Federal Register." Its definition was written expressly for schools and defines a hostile environment in schools as follows: "Hostile environment harassment, which includes unwelcome sexual advances, requests for sexual favors, and other verbal, non-verbal, or physical conduct of a sexual nature by an employee, by another student, or by a third party is behavior that is sufficiently severe, persistent, or pervasive to limit a student's ability to participate in or benefit from an education program or activity or to create a hostile or abusive educational environment" (Department of Education 1997, p. 12038).

It is important to note that definitions of peer sexual harassment do overlap somewhat with criminal definitions of sexual assault—such as some of the behaviors defined as sexual harassment (touching, grabbing, pinching in a sexual way, pulling clothing off or down, forcing a kiss, or forcing other unwelcome behavior, e.g., rape)—and may blur the boundaries between harassment and criminal behavior and allow for prosecution in a criminal case and recovery of damages in a civil case.

CLINICAL ISSUES

Forensic clinicians will most often encounter sexual harassment of school-age children when attorneys representing parties in civil suits approach these mental health professionals. The clinician will typically be asked to assess the presence and extent of mental and emotional damage sustained by the child plaintiff, and sometimes by his or her family, as a result of alleged sexual harassment. Concerns may be raised about problems characteristic of adolescent psychopathology, such as depressive or anxious behavior, social or emotional withdrawal, suicidal gestures or attempts, drug and alcohol abuse, eating disorders, risky sexual behavior, and other acting-out behavior. The clinician's task is to determine whether any of these conditions exist and to what extent they may be related to the sexual harassment alleged in the lawsuit. Clinicians may also be asked to speak to developmental issues regarding the nature and impact of harassment.

Brief Review of the Literature

The subject of unwanted sexually oriented behavior and teasing occurring in school-age populations was brought to the fore in recent years by a survey conducted by the American Association of University Women (AAUW) and published in the popular press (American Association of University Women 1993). The results of the survey indicated that 81% of the respondents—students in grades 8 to 11—reported having been subjected to what the study defined as sexual harassment. Slightly more girls (85%) than boys (76%) reported being harassed, and the behavior occurred most often during the middle school or junior high years. Twenty-five percent of girls and 10% of boys said that they had been harassed by a teacher or school employee. Interestingly, many students said that they had also harassed others. Attention was further directed to this issue by papers published by the Wellesley Center for Research on Women (e.g., Stein et al. 1993), which has also published guides for schools regarding policy making and prevention issues (e.g., Stein and Tropp 1994). These studies obtained similar results to the AAUW survey, finding that, of 342 urban high school students, 87% of girls and 79% of boys also reported harassing others. They found that girls are more often subject to more overt forms of harassment and that boys more often use sexually harassing behaviors. Girls perceived being sexually harassed as more threatening than did boys. The authors indicate that the incidence of peer harassment is so pervasive that it appears to be the norm.

When defining sexual harassment, the studies have included a broad range of behaviors, such as sexual comments and looks; showing sexually oriented pictures or notes; "mooning" someone; touching or brushing up against someone in a sexual manner; pulling down, snapping, or grabbing clothing; and forcing unwanted kisses or other behavior.

However, there is little literature on the actual clinical assessment of a child who complains of having been sexually harassed or on any particular characteristics these children might show. When an adult, such as a teacher, is the harasser, there may be a fine line between what is defined as harassment and behavior that would fall into the category of sexual abuse or assault. The literature on sexual abuse of children by adult authority figures would thus certainly be relevant in such a case. Similarly, familiarity with some of the literature regarding the effects of sexual harassment on adults may be helpful (e.g., O'Donohue 1997). However, it should be noted that this literature generally indicates that there are a broad range of responses to sexual harassment on the part of adults and that there is no "typical" pattern.

Studies of college students who have been harassed can be reviewed (e.g., Paludi 1990). In one study (Houston and Hwang 1996), 80 female college students were asked about their experiences of sexual harassment in high school. They found that women who reported having an overprotective mother, who had had unwanted sexual contact during childhood, and who reported few positive behaviors between their parents reported experiencing a greater number of sexual harassment incidents than women who had not experienced any of these problems. Other than this, we know little about such questions as what type of harassment causes the most severe problems, what type of adolescents are most likely to be significantly affected by harassment, and whether harassment causes any particular symptoms more often than others.

Clinical Considerations

The Developmental and Social Context

As noted above, cases of teacher-student harassment are often indistinguishable from cases in which an adult sexually assaults a minor in some manner. Clinical assessment of these cases can be conducted as outlined in Chapter 4, "Introduction to Forensic Evaluations." In some cases, allegations regarding harassment by a teacher or school employee may be more verbal in nature. They may consist of grossly inappropriate or unwanted sexually oriented comments, in or outside of the classroom, or of pervasive "put-downs" or displays of favoritism toward one gender. The courts have yet to fully define where such behavior crosses into harassment, but the clinician

should be aware that he or she may need to understand the issue of how a school setting can be made a hostile environment by responsible adults.

The Supreme Court decision and dissent in *Davis v. Monroe County* highlights a number of issues to consider in the clinical evaluation of cases in which allegations of peer harassment are made. As the studies show, sexually oriented teasing, touching, and taunting are extremely common in adolescent groups. Other kinds of teasing and bullying are also prevalent. There are "in groups" and "out groups" and rumors circulate regularly.[1] Some of this may be defined as inappropriate and potentially harmful behavior and requires intervention by school personnel and parents as it comes to their attention. However, especially in younger adolescent groups, such as middle school populations, these behaviors are closely intertwined with development and must be considered in this context. Early adolescence, of course, is a time when sexual development proceeds at a fast pace. Young teens are extremely aware of their own and others' sexual maturation, yet they often do not have the emotional maturity to avoid inappropriate language and behavior. At this age, they are also exquisitely self-conscious and may be quite vulnerable to comments aimed at their sexuality or body. The clinician must attempt to understand the behavior of the alleged harasser and his or her target in light of a working knowledge of adolescent development and an understanding of the context in which the harassment occurs. The issue of whether a particular behavior reaches the level of sexual harassment is, of course, a question of fact in a legal case. What does set it apart, according to the courts, is that it is behavior that is objectively offensive to a child, is based on his or her gender, and is severe and pervasive enough to interfere with the child's ability to participate in school activities. The clinician who fails to seriously consider an allegation of peer sexual harassment with the excuse that "boys will be boys" or that it is merely immature behavior will likely be unable to perform an objective evaluation. Likewise, the clinician who fails to understand the complexity of such behaviors in adolescent development and who assumes all behavior is harassment will have a similar problem.

Diagnostic Issues

In assessing a child for damages associated with peer sexual harassment, the clinician must be aware of what "normal" adolescent behavior is. Crying in one's room or having emotional outbursts is fairly common in a middle school child, even if that child has not behaved in this

---

[1] In the authors' experience, the "hot dog" rumor mentioned in the clinical example is apparently a kind of adolescent "urban myth," which seems to circulate somewhat frequently among young teens.

way before. However, symptoms such as escalating problems with appetite and sleep and destructive temper tantrums that significantly impair the child's ability to carry on his or her daily activities are another matter. The clinician must evaluate each case while giving consideration to the cognitive, temperamental, emotional, and sexual maturation of the parties involved, as well as the context in which it occurs, the pervasiveness of the behavior, and the response of the social environment.

The diagnosis of posttraumatic stress disorder (PTSD) has become a common consideration when evaluating children who complain of mental and emotional damage resulting from traumatic events. The threshold for a PTSD diagnosis is that the trauma must be quite severe, involving actual or threatened death or serious injury or a threat to the physical integrity of the child. In addition, the response to the threat must be extreme, involving intense fear, helplessness, or horror. Given these threshold criteria, and given the research findings regarding the pervasiveness of sexually harassing behaviors in everyday adolescent life, it would likely be rare that a diagnosis of PTSD would be appropriate in a peer sexual harassment case. However, a broad range of other diagnostic possibilities, including other anxiety disorders, adjustment reactions, depression, eating disorders, substance abuse, conduct disorders, or no diagnosis, should be considered.

Forensic clinicians frequently must deal with controversial social issues in their practice. Peer sexual harassment is such an issue, and it is an evolving area with only a few judicial guidelines and even less research. A cautious, objective, and thorough approach is likely to serve well.

Components of Assessment

The assessment of a child who alleges that he or she has been sexually harassed should be conducted in a manner similar to any other child forensic evaluation (see also Chapter 4, "Introduction to Forensic Evaluations"). A thorough review of all case documents should be made, including case pleadings, depositions, and school and medical records. Documents reflecting both sides of the case should be reviewed in the interest of acquiring as objective a view as possible. It is often essential to interview the child's parents in order to obtain accurate information about the child's developmental history and temperament. Because many adolescents are hesitant to be forthcoming about themselves to interviewers, speaking with the parents can add information that the child may withhold or underplay. Careful attention should be paid to the cultural and ethnic background of the child

and his or her family, especially in terms of how these factors affect the perception and reaction to sexual harassment.

Both parents and child should be asked for a full developmental history, including a sexual history. The quality of the marriage and the manner in which the parents relate to each other should be assessed, as should any parental history of sexual abuse or harassment. Data on parenting styles and sibling relationships should be obtained. For instance, in Case Example 1, the child's brother and his friends were responsible for initiating the harassment. A history of peer relationships is important to take. This should include when, whether, and how the child has been teased and how the child has responded, whether the child has had difficulties with bullying or teasing others, and under what circumstances this occurred. The child's basic temperament should be assessed, including such areas as reaction to change, emotional responsiveness, activity level, and sociability. The developmental history should include an exploration of the child's move from latency into adolescence, where the child is in developmental maturity, and how the child and the parents have handled this transition. An understanding of the child's concept of his or her own body image, as well as any discomfort, is helpful. Any history of previous traumas, harassment, or abuse should be thoroughly assessed. Information about how the child typically deals with social and emotional problems can be quite helpful when determining whether the child's response to the alleged harassment is consistent with or different from his or her "normal" adolescent coping mechanism.

A report by the child about what happened should be taken in as much detail as possible so that a full understanding of the event or events and their context is obtained. Interview data from both parents and child on how the alleged harassment has affected the child is essential. This should include questions about psychiatric symptoms, day-to-day behavior changes, and any changes in such things as school attendance and participation in school and social activities. Data should be gathered on how parents, peers, and school personnel have responded to the situation. For example, an over- or underreaction by parents may affect the child's ability to cope with the situation.

Psychological testing may be used as an added source of data regarding issues of personality and psychopathology (see Chapter 6, "Psychological Testing in Child and Adolescent Forensic Evaluations"). Finally, a thorough mental status and symptom history should be obtained from both child and parents. The symptom history should include questions about all characteristic adolescent pathological behaviors, such as problems with appetite, mood, sleep, or drugs or alcohol. A thorough assessment will provide the clinician with a full picture of the child and his or her environment, both before and after the incidence of harassment, thus allowing for informed expert opinion on the presence and extent of any damages sustained and on the presence of exacerbating or mitigating factors to the damages.

PITFALLS

Countertransference Issues

In evaluating a child for sexual harassment, it is critical to remain objective. The conduct of the teacher or peer harasser as described may appear to be clearly egregious. However, as in most forensic cases, there are two sides to every issue. It is critical to maintain objectivity and for the evaluator not to become too empathic with the child or too angry at the alleged harasser.

Crystal Ball Gazing

The court will decide the ultimate issue. The forensic evaluator can shed light on the emotional condition of the child or adolescent who alleges harassment, not on the ultimate issue of whether the harassment did or did not occur or whether the report of the child or adolescent is credible. Other chapters have made it clear that the forensic psychiatrist is neither a crystal ball gazer nor a truth detector.

Dual Agency

As in other forensic situations, the forensic clinician must decide which role to assume—that of a therapist or that of an evaluator. There are expressed and implicit ethical prohibitions against wearing both hats.

Reputation

In order to preserve a reputation as an objective evaluator, the clinician must attempt to diversify a forensic practice and evaluate plaintiffs and defendants in harassment cases. This is not always possible, but the clinician should make it clear to all consulting attorneys that the evaluation will be objective.

CASE EXAMPLE EPILOGUES

Case Example 1

The conduct that Amy alleges appears to meet the Office of Civil Rights definition of sexual harassment, because it includes verbal and nonverbal harassment by peers. In examining Amy's school record, it was clear there was a drop in her grades between the eighth and tenth grades and that there was a connection between the drop in her grades and the behavior she alleged. There were no other confounding variables. The forensic psychiatrist could not opine on the credibility of Amy's complaints nor could she opine on Amy's emotional condition and the relation between Amy's anxiety and depression and the behavior of her classmates. However, she could note Amy's clear depressive disorder and recommend a course of treatment.

Case Example 2

A forensic psychiatrist met with Sally's treating clinician regarding Sally's sexual relationship. In the opinion of the forensic psychiatrist, Sally's sexual relationship came under the heading of dangerous behavior, because the sexual relations were not consensual given the disparity of ages and the fact that Sally was a minor. Because of the sexual relationship, Sally was exposed to a number of risks including sexually transmitted disease, AIDS, and unwanted and unanticipated pregnancy. The forensic psychiatrist encouraged the treating psychiatrist to urge Sally to share the relationship with her parents in a joint session. Such a session would serve both to bring the relationship into the open and to allow Sally and her parents to work on a solution in a supportive therapeutic atmosphere. However, if this was not possible in a brief period of time, the consultant psychiatrist recommended that Sally be told that confidentiality would be violated and Sally's parents would be informed of this dangerous liaison.

ACTION GUIDELINES

A. Take a complete sexual history from parents and child.
B. Review documents from school (e.g., grades, counselor reports).
C. Review all prior mental health reports.
D. Limit reports to diagnosis and treatment plan and psychiatric and psychological issues. Do not comment on veracity of allegations of harassment.
E. Obtain psychological tests if appropriate.
F. Seek consultation if unclear.

REFERENCES

American Association of University Women: How Schools Shortchange Girls. Washington, DC, American Association of University Women Educational Foundation and National Education Association, 1992

American Association of University Women: Hostile Hallways: The AAUW Survey on Sexual Harassment in America's Schools. New York, Louis Harris & Associates, 1993

Civil Rights Act of 1964 (Title VII), 42 USC §2000e–2(a) (1964)

Davis v Monroe County Board of Education, 526 US 629 (1999)

Department of Education, Office of Civil Rights: Guidance in the Federal Register, 1997

Equal Employment Opportunity Commission: Guidelines on Sexual Harassment. 29 CFR §1604.11(B) (1980a)

Equal Employment Opportunity Commission: Title VII Guidelines on Sexual Harassment, 45 Fed Reg. (219: Rules and Regulations), 74676-74-677 (1980b)

Equal Employment Opportunity Commission: Equal Employment Opportunity Commission Guidelines, 29 CFR §1604.11(A)(a) (1987)

Gebser v Lago Vista Independent School District, 524 US 27–4 (1998)

Harris v Forklift Systems, Inc., 114 S Ct 367 (1993)

Houston S, Hwang N: Correlates of objective and subjective experiences of sexual harassment in high school. Sex Roles 34:189–204, 1996

O'Donohue W: Sexual Harassment: Theory, Research and Treatment. Boston, MA, Allyn & Bacon, 1997

Paludi MA (ed): Ivory Power: Sexual Harassment on Campus. Albany, NY, SUNY Press, 1990

Shrier DK (ed): Sexual Harassment in the Workplace and Academia. Washington, DC, American Psychiatric Press, 1996

Stein N, Tropp L: Flirting or Hurting? A Teacher's Guide on Student-to-Student Sexual Harassment in Schools. Wellesley, MA, Center for Research on Women, 1994

Stein N, Marshall N, Tropp L: Secrets in Public: Sexual Harassment in Our Schools. Wellesley, MA, Center for Research on Women, 1993

Title VII, §703(a)(2), 42 USC at 2000

CHAPTER 18

Children and Pornography

Old Problems, New Technology

Elissa P. Benedek, M.D.
Catherine F. Brown, Ed.M.

Case Example 1

A 14-year-old boy, Allen, was brought in for a clinical forensic evaluation after it was alleged that he had brutally strangled, raped, and murdered his 12-year-old neighbor. At first he denied participation in the murder and rape and accused a neighborhood gang of raping his neighbor and then strangling her to prevent her from talking. When the scenario he described proved impossible (there was no forensic evidence of rape to support his claims of gang rape and murder), Allen retracted his story. He admitted to the murder and rape but reported that the idea for the rape emerged from a television program he had viewed several months before. A forensic clinician was asked, in a civil suit, to evaluate Allen and, specifically, to provide information for the defense on the effects of television viewing on children, adolescents, and Allen in particular.

Case Example 2

Barbara, a 13-year-old computer genius, had purposefully downloaded materials of a sexually explicit nature from the Internet. During treatment by a child psychiatrist whom her parents had arranged for her to see after they discovered her Web-surfing preoccupation, she admitted a history of downloading erotic material. Barbara asked the psychiatrist whether she would tell Barbara's parents about the extent of this behavior. The child psychiatrist requested a consultation with Dr. Zak, a forensic child psychiatrist, because of her concerns about violating Barbara's confidentiality by talking to her parents.

Case Example 3

An 8-year-old boy had been kidnapped and sexually abused by an older male friend of his mother's. After a cross-country flight, Carl was identified from a picture on a milk carton and was returned home. In a clinical examination, Carl told the examiner that Mr. Smith (the man who had abducted him) had first employed him to do minor household tasks but later on showed him sexually explicit videotapes. The boy explained that Mr. Smith had supplemented the videotapes with a personal, persuasive narrative: He told Carl that his strength and muscular development would be enhanced by participating in the same sort of sexual behavior that Carl had viewed on the tapes. He photographed Carl engaging in sexual acts. Carl was reluctant to discuss this behavior with his mother, a single parent, and accepted the word of his newfound friend. The forensic examiner was asked on the stand whether the videotapes and photographs had contributed in any way to the boy's involvement in mature sexual activity.

Electronic technologies that permit one- and two-way communication at lightning-fast speeds via the broadcast media and computers linked by networks are among the most pivotal innovations of the twentieth century. Such technologies have opened vast new windows into our universe. Through live and recorded programs, television has given us front-row seats for man's first steps on the moon, shown us the delicate beauty of Earth when viewed from afar, and educated us about peoples and environments most of us will never see firsthand. It also has exposed millions of Americans to cultural events and icons, from Shakespeare to Sinatra, that are inaccessible for many people because of cost, location, or time. The Internet unites computer users throughout the world, facilitating communication, information exchange, entertainment, and commercial transactions in a manner that is hastening the rate at which our planet is effectively shrinking. If such technologies did not exist, our lives would be far less rich and much more tedious.

These extraordinary inventions, however, have an ugly underbelly. Although they do indeed facilitate entertainment, education, communication, and commerce, they also can harm the youngest members of our society. One way they do so is by exposing them to obscene and pornographic material. Often, that exposure occurs even though children have not sought it out. On the Internet, for example, the frequency of unwanted exposure is surprisingly high, according to a report in the *Journal of the American Medical Association.* A telephone survey of 1,501 randomly selected youths ages 10–17 found that 19% of those who said they were regular Internet users had received unwanted sexual solicitations. Twenty-five percent of the youths who received these communications said that the contact had seriously distressed them (Mitchell et al. 2001). Undeniably, there is no turning the clock back on the pervasiveness of television and the Internet in American society, although, perhaps, as clinicians, educators, and parents, we wish at times that we could.

The task for us as forensic clinicians is to lend our expertise to the continuing debate about the effects of these new technologies as we deal with children and adolescents who have been victimized by being willing or unwilling participants in the production of pornographic programs or have been harmed by exposure to such materials on television or the Internet. Forensic child psychiatrists can serve in many roles in this new arena, such as conducting evaluations of children victimized by participating in or viewing pornography or advising legislators and courts as experts with regard to the damages caused by participating in or viewing pornography.

DEFINITIONS AND LEGAL ISSUES

The question of definition always lies at the heart of public discussion, academic inquiry, legal decisions, and policy making about pornography, erotica, and obscenity. Pronouncements by government officials, educators, and parents about what is pornographic, what is obscene, and

what is erotic are often highly subjective. For example, in an admission that has become a cliché, Supreme Court Justice Potter Stewart had to concede in one opinion that he could not define pornography, but he knew it when he saw it (*Jacobellis v. Ohio* 1964). To state that the definition of pornography is subjective, however, does not mean that it is completely idiosyncratic. The term *pornography* derives from the Greek *porne*, meaning whore, and *graphein*, meaning to write. Thus, pornography literally means the writings of harlots or depictions of acts of prostitutes (Webster's Collegiate Dictionary 1994). *Erotica* is derived from the name of the Greek god Eros and refers to sexual love. It is often used to refer to literary or artistic works that have a sexual quality or theme. The term *obscenity* is derived from the Latin *ob*, meaning to, and *caenum*, meaning filth (Webster's Collegiate Dictionary 1994). Indeed, obscenity has traditionally been associated with filth, offensiveness, disgust, shame, and the idea of insulting or breaching an accepted moral standard (*Roth v. United States* 1957).

According to the Federal Communications Commission's (FCC) definition of *indecency*, broadcast programs are indecent if they contain "language or material that depicts or describes in terms patently offensive, as measured by contemporary standards for the broadcast medium, sexual or excretory activities, or organs" (Federal Communications Commission 1993). Indecency has been further defined by the FCC and the courts through a series of cases relating to the broadcast media. The broadcast media have always been thought to present two special problems to distinguish them from print media and therefore have been subject to broader regulations than print media.

The first of these problems relates to children. The Supreme Court reasoned in *Federal Communications Commission v. Pacifica Foundation* (1978) that "broadcasting is uniquely accessible to children, even those too young to read." Written material may be incomprehensible to a kindergartner or a first grader, for example, but a broadcast containing sexually explicit language can capture a child's interest and can enlarge a child's vocabulary in an instant. Second, because broadcasting has comparatively few programming choices due to the finite width of the electromagnetic spectrum and number of cable channels, most audiences comprise both children and adults. To elaborate, in 1978 Justice Powell, concerning *Pacifica*, wrote, "Sellers of printed and recorded matter and exhibitors of motion pictures and live performances may be required to shut their doors to children. But such a requirement has no effect on adults' access."

While the age and number of children watching television in any time period can only be estimated and is not known with absolute certainty, Congress and the FCC have made the assumption that fewer unsupervised children are in the audience during nighttime hours and thus have "channeled" the airing of indecent material to those hours.

This rule does not pertain to programs broadcast over cable television. Currently, adult programming can be seen and heard in many homes that do not subscribe to cable channels that carry such programming because the signal is not scrambled or is incompletely scrambled. The Telecommunications Act of 1996 had addressed this problem of "signal bleed," but in May 2000 the Supreme Court struck down the provision in the law requiring cable providers that air sexually explicit material to scramble their signal fully or restrict such programming to certain "safe harbor" hours when children were unlikely to be in the viewing audience (10 A.M. to 6 P.M.). Stating that this provision was a violation of free speech under the First Amendment, the Court noted that the law included a less-restrictive option, which requires cable operators to provide blocking devices to subscribers who ask for them. That the ruling was controversial among the justices, however, is evident by the fact that the vote was 5 to 4 (*United States et al. v. Playboy Entertainment Group, Inc.* 2000).

In *Sable Communications of California, Inc. v. Federal Communications Commission* (1989), the court addressed the "exposure of children to sexually explicit telephone services." A case arose when, after a decade of experimenting with various regulatory measures designed to restrict access by children to so-called dial-a-porn services, Congress passed a law prohibiting the transmission of obscene and indecent expression for commercial purposes (Child Protection and Obscenity Enforcement Act of 1988). The Supreme Court responded with a steaming rebuke unanimously invalidating the law as it is applied to indecent communications: "Sexual expression which is indecent but not obscene is protected by the First Amendment..." (*Sable Communications of California, Inc. v. Federal Communications Commission* 1989). The court found that for the government to regulate indecent expression, it must do so only in furtherance of a "compelling" state interest and "by narrowing down regulations designed to serve those interests without unnecessarily interfering with First Amendment freedoms." Strict scrutiny is the highest form of scrutiny applied by the court to any regulation of expression. That the expression was sexually explicit and involved commercial activity, that is, the telephone lines, was irrelevant.

To summarize, each of the definitions above represents a different perspective that could be applied to the same visual or auditory depiction. For example, a picture or message may be pornographic to some viewers but may not necessarily be obscene (disgusting, insulting). Similarly, what is obscene to some will be erotic (literary or artistic) to others. Imagine a magazine layout featuring a photo of a nude woman with accompanying text stating that the woman has had enjoyable sexual relations with many partners and that posing for male viewers of this magazine thrills her. Such a photo may be considered pornographic by the definition above because, for some viewers, the layout and description may suggest that the woman is a whore. Others might view the photo of the woman as intended solely for the pleasure of male viewers and find the description erotic as she has portrayed one aspect of sexual love. The definition of obscenity is based on community standards of morality; most likely the layout would not be considered obscene or indecent in most communities in the United States (*Miller v. California* 1973). Whether pornography, obscenity, or indecency is harmful or harmless and to whom is difficult to state with certainty. It depends on definition, viewer, context, and current law.

When an audience is not limited to consenting adults, courts have traditionally interpreted the First Amendment to permit greater regulation or even prohibition of any sexually explicit expression. This is particularly true when young children are involved. For example, the Supreme Court has found repeatedly that states may not only criminalize the depiction of children in sexually explicit films and photographs, but also may prohibit the distribution and possession of those films and photographs in an attempt to eliminate any market for child pornography (*New York v. Ferber* 1982). In most media, it is possible to restrict access by children to sexually explicit expression without foreclosing access by adults. However, it is difficult but not impossible to do so on the Internet. On the Internet, sexually explicit material can be distributed throughout the world to an audience that includes both adults and children. It is difficult for the server or information provider who is genuinely concerned about distribution to children to distinguish who is receiving a "hit" from the Internet. Many responsible providers, however, require that users enter personal information, such as a credit card number, to effectively block out children from their sites. Nonetheless, it is clear that certain individuals have kidnapped or "hit-mapped" Web pages for the explicit purpose of enticing children to view pornography. Thus, the Internet might pose even more risk to children than broadcast television. In broadcast television, channeling, or limitation of sexually explicit material to periods outside of safe harbor hours, is one method of preventing children from viewing pornographic material. There are no safe harbor hours on the Internet; it is open for business to anyone around the clock. In addition, television programs are now rated by age and content categories, and parents can use this information to monitor and control the viewing habits of their children. They can do this automatically if they have purchased a television set equipped with what is known as a V-chip and programmed it to block broadcasts with ratings acknowledging sexual content (S), suggestive dialogue (D), or violence (V). Effective July 1, 1999, the Federal Communications Commission, carrying out a mandate from Congress, required manufacturers to include a V-chip in half their newly manufactured televisions with screens that measure 13 inches or larger diagonally. Unfortunately, it seems that the V-chips have few users, even among those parents whose new sets are equipped with a V-chip (Greenman 1999), suggesting there is no substitute for parental involvement in children's media habits. The reasons that the V-chip has not yet caught on are unclear. It may be that many parents are still unaware of its existence or that it is difficult to program. Some parents may feel they do not need it or believe that such screening accomplishes little in a society drenched with sexually explicit messages and images in virtually every medium.

As they acquire the skills to use the Internet, young children easily learn how to access sexually explicit material. Even an innocent search can unearth pornographic sites. Contemporary productions consist of images, action, and music that make these sites inviting to young eyes and ears. By clicking on a hyperlink, a child or adolescent can proceed from one site to another with ease.

Software is available to control access by minors to certain information on the Internet. Information providers such as Web site hosts can segregate audience members by requiring that potential users of a site provide some evidence of their age, that is, a credit card number or a driver's license number. Some adult Internet sites also contain bold warning screens acknowledging the fact that the material to be accessed is "adult" and require a password that is supplied to users only upon proof—not just affirmation—of age. Some Internet service providers, such as Erols, have taken some steps in limiting access to pornographic sites, using their commonsense professional judgment rather than legal compulsion. Parents can also purchase and install software on their home computers that is designed to block access to pornographic and other sites judged harmful to children.

Screening devices, however, do not provide complete protection. The fact that they are imperfect, however, is acceptable by current legal standards. Complete protection has never been a requirement in indecency regulations in the broadcast and print media because it could result in restricting adults to exposure to "only what is fit for children." Instead, the courts have required that measures to control indecency be reasonably effective in enhancing parental control over children's viewing.

PUBLIC HEALTH AND CLINICAL ISSUES

In 1986 Surgeon General C. Everett Koop convened a surgeon general's workshop on pornography and public health. The workshop that generated this report was not the first government-sponsored effort to examine the question of the social and public health effects of pornography. In the late 1960s, the Commission on Obscenity and Pornography was formed, and after funding much research and holding many hearings, it released its report in 1970. The commission's findings were summarized in the report's introduction: "[E]mpirical research designed to clarify the question has found no evidence to date that exposure to explicit sexual materials plays a significant role in the causation of delinquent or criminal behavior among youth or adults. The Commission cannot conclude that exposure to erotic materials is a factor in the causation of sex crime or sex delinquency" (Report of the Commission on Obscenity and Pornography 1970).

This report was criticized, both by commission members (Cline 1970) and others, for flaws in the design of some commissioned research, misinterpretations of some of the research, and limitations of the scope of much of the research. Despite criticisms, however, the general conclusion of the commission, that pornography had no marked social effects, continued to be the generally accepted and cited wisdom in this area.

In response to a growing concern over child pornography, both houses of Congress held hearings on the issue in 1977. During these hearings, witnesses estimated that between 300,000 and 600,000 children were involved in the production of pornography at that time and that more than 260 child pornographic publications were being produced. Subsequent to these hearings, the federal government and nearly all state governments enacted laws against the production, distribution, and possession of child pornography.

In 1979 the British government formed the Committee on Obscenity and Film Censorship. The conclusions of this committee were similar to those of the 1970 United States Commission on Obscenity and Pornography. Unlike its American counterpart, however, the committee produced a report that was criticized for its failure to include what were considered relevant research studies (Court 1980).

Next, the Canadian government convened the Special Committee on Pornography and Prostitution, which delivered its report in 1985. This committee found that whereas individual research projects identified some of the harmful effects of exposure to pornography on children and adolescents, the research was contradictory and inconclusive and could not be relied on as a guide for policy formation ("Pornography and Prostitution in Canada," 1985).

The United States Attorney General's Commission on Pornography was formed in 1985 in response to a number of concerns: 1) continuing criticism of the findings of previous commissions; 2) recent technological advances and changes in social standards that allowed both youth and adults easier access to pornography; 3) recent research indicating that the content of both hard-core and traditional soft-core pornography had changed in the 1970s and 1980s to include considerably more sexually violent material; and 4) preliminary research suggesting that these new forms of pornography had differing effects on viewers' attitudes and behaviors than the pornography studied earlier. These developments called for a reassessment of the possible impact of the changes in the content of pornography, the technology used to produce and view it, and potential users of pornography. Moreover, a new research approach had emerged, emphasizing that the underlying message communicated by the pornography might have at least as much effect as the explicitness of the sexual content—that is, that the message might add to viewing and treating women and children in a humiliating, degrading fashion.

Surgeon General Koop was asked to testify before the Attorney General's commission with regard to 1) what was known about pornography to a reasonable degree of certainty and the effects of pornography on the mental and physical health of children, adolescents, and young adults in the United States; 2) what additional effects are justifiably suspected and how these effects could be verified or refuted; and 3) what actions could and should be taken by those in the medical, mental health, and public health fields to combat the effects of pornography.

The participants in the Surgeon General's 1986 workshop were asked to reach consensus on the effects of pornography as a public health concern. They agreed that the following statements were supported by "directly relevant social science data" and demonstrated theory (Report of the Surgeon General's Workshop on Pornography and Public Health 1986):

- Children and adolescents who participate in the production of pornography experience adverse, enduring effects.
- Prolonged use of pornography increases beliefs that less common sexual practices are more common.
- Acceptance of coercive sexuality appears to be related to sexual aggression.
- In laboratory studies measuring short-term effects, exposure to violent pornography increased punitive behavior toward women.

Research Issues

Designing and executing research to isolate the specific effects that exposure to pornography may have on children and adolescents is a formidable task because of the methodological and ethical barriers inherent in doing such investigations. Exposure to pornography is only one of many independent factors potentially affecting a child, and attempting to isolate its unique effects may contribute to a clinician's oversimplifying a complex situation. It is important to note that the effect on a child of any particular influence, such as exposure to indecency, obscenity, or pornography, is the result of many interacting factors, including age, maturity, and parental influence. Exposure to pornography does not occur in a vacuum. Moreover, conducting investigations regarding exposure to pornography while protecting the child or adolescent subjects from potential harm creates a number of vexing ethical dilemmas.

Even if one were willing to study the multiple variables to produce specific emotional and behavioral effects on a child or adolescent, there are ethical constraints that inevitably limit the kind of research design that can be used, because the exact short- and long-term effects on children of exposure to pornography are unknown and because exposing youth to pornography for experimental purposes could conceivably produce short- and long-term emotional problems. Exposure in the laboratory violates basic ethical and moral issues. The researcher, therefore, is caught in a catch-22 situation. It is impossible to know exactly what effects different types of materials (videotapes, computer-generated materials) might have on children. It is also impossible to conduct the investigations as long as adverse effects are hypothesized. If it could be demonstrated that problematic short-term effects could be controlled by debriefing, one could not be assured that there would be no long-term effects. Because of these serious ethical constraints, interested researchers are reluctant to test many propositions related to the effects of pornography on children.

One source of information about the effects of pornography on children and adolescents is clinical studies on children who come to the attention of mental health professionals or the juvenile justice system. These reports are valuable, highlight relevant issues, and provide direction for more controlled investigations. However, clinical studies are limited in that they cannot isolate the specific effects of the variable being considered, such as exposure to indecency, obscenity, or pornography from other potentially influential variables. With clinical data alone, it is impossible to isolate the etiology of a particular problem. In addition, the patients who are available for clinical studies generally are children who already have identified problems. Those authors who contribute to clinical reports are often biased with regard to what influences and factors in a child's life they use to illustrate the points they wish to make. Clinical accounts are not proof, but they are, nonetheless, valuable reminders of how devastating certain influences can be on susceptible children.

Laboratory studies might provide another source of valuable information about the effects of exposure to pornography. The attraction of this approach is that it is "scientific" in the sense that a hypothesis can be directly tested and findings amassed to support global theories. However, the drawback of such an approach is that it is not "ecological"; it is artificial. Phenomena evident in the laboratory may not be evident in the real world. Laboratory aggression against women in multiple studies, for example, has been shown to be linked to exposure to sexually violent materials, thus suggesting a theory of a synergistic effect between the viewing of violence and sex and aggression (Malamuth 1989). Laboratory work in this area has been conducted using college students as subjects, but no laboratory studies are available involving children and adolescents. In addition, it is difficult to judge whether the strength of an effect that will produce statistically significant group differences in a controlled laboratory study reflects a difference of significant magnitude in the real world. A difference of 2.5 on a 7-point attitude rating scale completed by a large number of college students, for instance, may produce a highly significant statistical effect in a controlled study. Whether this difference really translates into an attitudinal difference of notable proportions in the real world is another question.

A third type of social scientific evidence that is commonly considered when attempting to assess the effects of pornography is that of examining relationships or changes in social indicators. This strategy involves examining the correlation between two indicators under different conditions, for example, the possible incidence of sexual abuse and the distribution of sexually oriented videotapes in a particular state. As in laboratory studies, it is difficult in correlational studies to control all the variables that may be related to any observed correlation or shift, and correlation does not mean causation.

A literature search conducted on *Medline* and *PsycInfo* in 1997 uncovered few studies of direct relevance to the effects of child exposure to pornography. This was not surprising given the ethical constraints discussed above. Although the literature is scarce, it is one of the tools that help us arrive at certain conclusions about child exposure to pornography.

Clinical Issues

Child pornography is defined as any visual reproduction of the sexual abuse of children. It is difficult to obtain figures regarding the pervasiveness of child pornography. In the late 1980s, child pornography allegedly constituted 7% of the pornography market (Franklin et al. 1989).

Sexual exploitation of children as subjects in the pornography industry has been linked to a variety of adverse short- and long-term emotional, behavioral, and somatic consequences in children, as well as similar consequences in adults who were exploited as children (Finkelhor and Brown 1986). These authors have theorized that adverse effects can be caused by several factors, including traumatic sexualization, betrayal, powerlessness, and stigmatization. Traumatic sexualization is a result of a child's being involved in and rewarded for developmentally inappropriate sexual behavior. Betrayal results from the manipulation of a child by a trusted adult. Powerlessness results from a sense of vulnerability felt because of the repeated invasion of a child's body and an inability to stop the abuse. Finally, stigmatization can occur as a result of the child's blaming himself or herself for the abuse. Other serious effects can include eating disorders, depression, mistrust, hostility, conduct disorders, and a large variety of behavioral consequences.

Evidence about the role and effect of pornography in sexually exploited children necessarily comes exclusively from clinical studies. Burgess (1984) completed extensive interviews with 62 children referred by law enforcement agencies when the children's participation in sex and pornography rings was discovered. Burgess et al. noted several possible limitations to the generalizing of the results of their interviews to all children involved in such activities. Most notably, their sample might not have been representative of the total population, because only those children referred by law enforcement agencies were interviewed. Burgess et al. also identified a list of symptoms exhibited by children involved with pornography, including being uncommunicative, withdrawn, inattentive, and fearful. It is impossible to isolate the effects of participation in the production of pornography from those caused by other forms of sexual exploitation that are often experienced by those same children. However, clinical experience indicates almost unequivocally that the effects of such involvement are adverse and harmful. For example, children and adolescents involved in pornography also may be involved in prostitution and other sexual activity with adults (Burgess and Clark 1984). Many come from homes where they have experienced prior neglect and abuse. Thus, as we have discussed earlier, the specific effects of involvement with the production of pornography cannot be isolated cleanly. Involvement with pornography production is only one of the many influences operating in the lives of these children.

Children up to age 9 years frequently confuse expressed parental sexual activity with violence because they do not understand what sex is, and sexual behavior looks violent to them because of the intense, repetitive, and unfamiliar movements. Children hearing sexual cries, grunts, or moans often associate them with reactions to pain rather than sounds stimulated by pleasure. In a therapeutic play room, children have been heard to comment, "My daddy hurt my mommy last night," and it was clear that the child was referring to parental sexual activity and not physical or sexual abuse, as evidenced by the child's verbalization and play behavior. Children viewing explicit sexual activity on television may perceive it as violence. This may be as traumatizing as seeing actual violence. Sleep disturbances, nightmares, and regressive behavior may result.

The literature supports the hypothesis that the prolonged use and viewing of pornography increases beliefs that less-common sexual practices are more common. Zillman and Bryant (1988) have researched this area extensively. In a series of studies of college students, those who viewed pornography over a 6-week period believed that certain forms of sexual behavior (fellatio, cunnilingus, and anal intercourse) were more common in the general population than those who were not exposed to pornography during the same period.

Pornography may be the primary means by which many children and adolescents learn about the sexual behavior of couples. It is possible to see how pornographic materials can affect children's perceptions about how common certain behaviors are. The pornography that portrays sexual aggression as pleasurable for the victim increases the acceptance of the use of coercion in sexual relations. Malamuth (1989) has completed a series of studies that show that exposure to pornographic rape scenes in which the assault resulted in a female vic-

tim's sexual arousal altered males' assessments of a later rape depiction. His studies compared, among other variables, the effects of materials in which the victim was aroused by an attack, the victim resisted and abhorred the attack, or two people were involved in a mutually consensual sexual act. Those subjects viewing a scene in which the victim was aroused by the attack saw the victim of a later rape depiction as having suffered less than those who viewed a victim who abhorred the attack or a person involved in mutually consensual act did.

The forensic assessment of the child or adolescent exposed to pornography is similar to forensic assessment discussed in Chapter 17, "Clinical and Forensic Aspects of Sexual Harassment in School-Age Children." During any clinical evaluation, a child or adolescent should be routinely queried about television viewing habits, including the viewing of videotape programs and the use and misuse of the Internet. Also, the child or adolescent should be asked whether friends or family members participate in the production of pornographic material, access and/or download Internet pornographic material, or watch pornographic videos or adult programs on cable television. If the child or adolescent volunteers or responds in the affirmative to any of these queries or volunteers relevant information, the area should be explored extensively. The child or adolescent should be queried about the nature of the participation, that is, what he or she did, saw, and felt while participating and afterward. In addition, the child or adolescent should be asked about his or her extent of participation. The nature of parental involvement and knowledge also should be elicited. For example, Jane, a 16-year-old girl, was photographed in the nude and insisted that her parents knew nothing of her participation in this activity, despite the fact that her father had driven her to the studio, sat outside the studio door while the pictures were being taken, and had lunch with Jane and the photographer, who discussed the shoot in depth. Jane herself claimed to be shocked when her seminude pictures appeared in a teenage magazine under the caption, "Teen Date Rape." Jane maintained that stance of denial throughout the clinical evaluation and seemed unable to link her current depression and eating problems to her participation as a model in pornographic pictures beginning at age 6 with her parents' knowledge and support.

Child and adolescent statements should be verified with historical information. Such information can be obtained from pediatricians, schoolteachers, and parents. Mindy, a 13-year-old girl who used the Web proficiently and regularly to purchase character dolls with money she earned from doing household chores, volunteered, in a clinical evaluation for attention-deficit/hyperactivity disorder, that her favorite Web pages had recently been corrupted with ads for pornographic dolls. Her father confirmed this report and added that she had solicited his help in finding alternative sites to use for her purchases of character dolls. In contrast, Sam, a 14-year-old boy, downloaded pornographic material from his computer and sold it to his classmates for profit at his junior high school. His parents were unaware of his thriving business until the evaluator brought it to their attention. Sam offered this information in response to explicit questions about his use of the Internet during the course of his evaluation.

PITFALLS

Lack of Information

Clinicians must be careful in evaluating children and adolescents for exposure to pornography (which may include viewing pornography or participation in its production) and reaching conclusions in legal situations where there is a paucity of research data to support their conclusions. The current limitations of testimony based only on clinical observation must be acknowledged, but support from the literature, though not as conclusive as we might wish, may also be acknowledged.

Countertransference

Clinicians must be wary of the host of feelings evoked during the evaluation of children and adolescents who have been exposed to pornography and present as seriously emotionally and mentally disturbed. The etiology of their disturbance is multifactorial, and these young patients are not helped by the clinician's responding to feelings of horror, disgust, or anger, wish to rescue, or attribution of all symptomatology to exposure to pornography.

CASE EXAMPLE EPILOGUES

Case Example 1

The forensic evaluator was able to shed light on the effects of television viewing on children and adolescents with regard to the relationship between television and obscenity. The literature supported the effects of television in this area. With regard to television's serving as a model for the rape and subsequent murder of Allen's neighbor, the evaluator informed Allen's attorney that Allen had a long prior history of lying to escape the consequences of his behavior and that although he claimed to have viewed a television program, he could provide no details with regard to the name of the program, the date of the program, or the plot and story line with the exception of the fact that he had viewed a boy rape and murder a neighbor. The clinician informed the attorney that there was reason to doubt Allen's version of the events in question.

Case Example 2

Dr. Zak was respectful of her obligation to maintain Barbara's confidentiality. However, she was also concerned about the effects that extensive viewing of erotica might have on Barbara and her relationship with her peers and her family. She discussed with Barbara the importance of sharing this material with her parents in a joint session. Barbara agreed to do this, so there was no need to violate Barbara's confidentiality.

Case Example 3

Carl had clearly been influenced to participate in sexual behavior by Mr. Smith. Mr. Smith had carefully groomed him by showing him videotapes and rewarding Carl for his participation in sexual activity. Mr. Smith's manner of enticing Carl was congruent with the available literature on sexual abuse and the initiation of children and adolescents into premature sexual activity by victimizers. The forensic examiner was quite comfortable citing the literature in this area in her testimony.

ACTION GUIDELINES

A. Encourage professional organizations dealing with children and adolescents to adopt policy statements urging parental supervision of children and adolescents as they interact with new technologies such as the Internet.

B. Encourage professional mental health workers to publish clinical experiences with children and adolescents who have had negative experiences related to their exposure to pornography on network television, cable television, videotape programs, or the Internet.

C. Encourage professional mental health workers to document and publish their clinical and research work that relates to children and adolescents who have been victimized by being subjects in pornographic publications.

REFERENCES

Burgess AW: Response patterns of children and adolescents exploited through sex rings and pornography. Am J Psychiatry 141:656–662, 1984

Burgess AW, Clark ML: Child Pornography and Sex Rings. Lexington, MA, Lexington Books, 1984

Child Protection and Obscenity Enforcement Act of 1988, Pub L No 100-690, sec 7524, 102 Stat 4502

Cline VB: 1970 Minority Report of the U.S. Commission on Obscenity and Pornography. New York, Bantam Books, 1970

Court JH: Pornography and the Harm Condition. Adelaide, Australia, Flinders University, 1980

Federal Communications Commission: Enforcement of Prohibition Against Broadcast Indecency, 18 USC 1464, §FCC Rcd 704, n 10 (1993) [http://www.fcc.gov/mmb/enf/indecl.html]

Federal Communications Commission: New Indecency Enforcement Standards to Be Applied to All Broadcast and Amateur Radio Licensees, FCC No 87153, 62 Rad Reg 2d (P&F) 1218 (1987)

Federal Communications Commission v Pacifica Foundation, 438 US 726 (1978)

Finkelhor D, Brown A: Initial and long-term effects: a conceptual framework, in Source Book on Child Sexual Abuse. Edited by Finkelhor D. Beverly Hills, CA, Sage, 1986, pp 180–198

Franklin M, Osanka F, Lee J: Sourcebook on Pornography. Lexington, MA, Lexington Books, 1989

Greenman C: The V-chip arrives with a thud. New York Times, November 4, 1999, p D-1

Jacobellis v Ohio, 378 US 184 (1964) (Stuart J, concurring)

Malamuth NM: Sexually violent media, thought patterns, and antisocial behavior, in Public Communication and Behavior, Vol 2. New York, Academic Press, 1989, pp 159–204

Malamuth NM: Pornography's impact on male adolescents. Adolescent Medicine: State of the Art Reviews 4:563–576, 1993

Mitchell JK, Finkelhor D, Wolak J: Risk factors for and impact of online sexual solicitation of youth. JAMA 285:3011–3014, 2001

Miller v California, 413 US 15 (1973)

New York v Ferber, 458 US 747 (1982)

Pornography and Prostitution in Canada: Report of the Special Select Committee on Pornography and Prostitution. Ottawa, ON, Canada, Supply and Services, 1985

Report of the Surgeon General's Workshop on Pornography and Public Health. Washington, DC, U.S. Public Health Service, U.S. Department of Health and Human Services, 1986, pp 13–29

Report of the U.S. Commission on Obscenity and Pornography. Washington, DC, U.S. Government Printing Office, 1970, p 27

Roth v United States, 354 US 476 (1957)

Sable Communications of Calif, Inc, v FCC, 492 US 115 (1989)

Telecommunications Act of 1996, Pub L 104-104, sec 505, 110 Stat 136, 47

United States et al. v Playboy Entertainment Group, Inc., No 98-1682 (2000)

Webster's Collegiate Dictionary, 10th Edition. Springfield, MA, Merriam-Webster, 1994

Zillman D, Bryant J: Effects of prolonged consumption of pornography on family values. Journal of Family Issues 4:518–544, 1988

SUGGESTED READINGS

Attorney General's Commission on Pornography: Final Report. Washington, DC, U.S. Department of Justice, 1986

Cate FH: Cybersex: regulating sexually explicit expression on the Internet. Journal of Behavioral Sciences and the Law 14:145–166, 1996

Committee on Commerce, Science, and Transportation: Commercial Distribution of Material Harmful to Minors on World Wide Web: Report of the Committee on Commerce, Science, and Transportation on S1482, June 25, 1998, Washington DC, U.S. Government Printing Office, 1998

Corne S, Briere J, Esses LM: Women's attitudes and fantasies about rape as a function of early exposure to pornography. Journal of Interpersonal Violence 7:454–461, 1992

Franklin M, Osanka F, Lee J: Sourcebook on Pornography. Lexington, MA, Lexington Books, 1989

Liebert RM, Sprafkin J, Davidson E: The Early Window: Effects of Television on Children and Youth. Needham Heights, MA, Allyn & Bacon, 1988

Malamuth NM: Pornography's impact on male adolescents. Adolescent Medicine: State of the Art Reviews 4:563–576, 1993

Page RM, Hammermeister J, Scanlan A, et al: Psychosocial and health-related characteristics of adolescent television viewers. Child Study Journal 26:319–331, 1996

Strasburger VC: Adolescent sexuality and the media. Pediatr Clin North Am 36:747–773, 1989

Yates A: Childhood sexuality, in Child and Adolescent Psychiatry: A Comprehensive Textbook, 2nd Edition. Edited by Lewis M. Baltimore, MD, Williams & Wilkins, 1996, pp 221–235

PART IV

Youth Violence

The current surge in youth violence in the United States is akin to the canaries in the mine telling us that there is something very unhealthy about our environment. Although violence among youth had been escalating for some time, it took several tragic school shootings to get people to think about it as a public health problem that might have identifiable causes and be amenable to prevention and intervention. We know that the causes of violence are multifaceted, and just as there are many causes, there are many ways in which we as citizens and clinicians can intervene.

We are also becoming increasingly aware of how violence can be transmitted from one generation to the next.

In Chapter 19, Dr. Perry discusses the effect of violence on the child's developing brain, which may set the stage for subsequent conduct disorders, dissociative disorders, and posttraumatic stress disorder. Witnessing violence often results in altered states of arousal in children. Dr. Dickstein surveys the toll that domestic violence takes on children and reminds us of the importance of thinking and asking about domestic violence in Chapter 20. A large body of research has emerged on the impact of media and community violence on children, and this is reviewed by Dr. Al-Mateen in Chapter 21.

Nearly 80,000 American youths have died from gun violence since 1979, which is more than the number of American troops killed in the Vietnam War. Dr. Ash reminds us in Chapter 22 of how readily children have access to weapons and that many routinely carry them "for protection." As is well known, the risks of handgun ownership far outweigh their value for self-defense. Dr. Ash provides suggestions for how to take a weapons history and promote a rational assessment of the risks of carrying weapons. In Chapter 23, Dr. Schetky summarizes the literature on risk factors for youth violence, discusses common pitfalls in assessing the risk of violence in youths, and offers guidelines for these evaluations. Dr. Cornell concludes this part in Chapter 24 with a discussion of which prevention and intervention programs appear to offer the most hope for decreasing youth violence.

CHAPTER 19

Neurodevelopmental Impact of Violence in Childhood

Bruce D. Perry, M.D., Ph.D.

We humans are the most complex and puzzling of living creatures. We can create, nurture, protect, educate, and enrich. Yet we also degrade, humiliate, enslave, hate, destroy, and kill. A man can tenderly hold his newborn and moments later beat the baby's mother. Violence permeates our history. In all societies and in every culture, past and present, violence has played a role in shaping our sociocultural evolution. Although no society has been able to break free from violence, there is tremendous variation in the type and degree of violence across cultures and time. In some cultures, random street violence has been suppressed with oppressive institutional violence; in others, interfamilial violence is rare but intrafamilial violence—violence to spouses and children—is rampant.

Today, despite remarkable advances in technology, social justice, and education, violence continues to be a permeating and pervasive element of American society. We are bathed in violent images. Violence fascinates *and* repulses us. Whether journalist, producer, politician, or scholar, we consider, comment on, and analyze violence. We have academic conferences, congressional hearings, special documentaries; we issue opinions, create task forces, start programs, blame guns, blame Hollywood, blame parents. Yet no simple solutions emerge. We continue to be shocked, enraged, and confused by the horrors of violence in our homes, schools, and streets.

How can we truly begin to understand the heterogeneity and complexity of the violence that surrounds us—random violence and institutionalized violence, the violence in behaviors, the violence in ideas, the violence in words? Can we ever understand the detached adolescent killing his classmates in school, mothers killing their infants, husbands killing wives, children, and themselves? Can we understand random bombing of civilians in the name of God? Can we understand systematic or institutionalized rape, torture, slavery, and genocide?

Violence and its associated factors are complex and multidimensional. This chapter considers only one of many perspectives from which to examine violence: the effects of violence and fear on the development of the child. More specifically, violence-related neurodevelopmental changes and functional consequences of these alterations in the brain will be reviewed. This view is presented with the hope that some of the devastating costs of violence to the individual child, family, community, and society can be illustrated from a neurodevelopmental perspective.

NEURODEVELOPMENT AND ADAPTATION TO A VIOLENT WORLD

Millions of children are victims of, or witnesses to, violence in the home, community, or school (see Perry 1997; Chapter 20, "Domestic Abuse as a Risk Factor for Children and Youth," and Chapter 21, "Effects of Witnessing Violence on Children and Adolescents," this volume). While the majority of homes, communities, and schools are safe, far too many children experience violence in one or more of these settings. For some children, a safe community and school may help buffer the impact of violence in the home. The highest-risk children, however, are safe nowhere; their home is chaotic and episodically abusive, their community is fragmented and plagued by gang violence, and the schools are barely capable of providing structure and safety from intimidation and threat, let alone education. These children must learn and grow despite a pervasive sense of threat. These children must adapt to this atmosphere of fear. Persisting fear and the neurophysiological adaptations to this fear can alter the development of the child's brain, resulting in changes in physiological, emotional, behavioral, cognitive, and social functioning. The core principles of neurodevelopment provide important clues about the mechanisms underlying the observed functional changes in children exposed to violence.

Cortical Modulation and Use-Dependent Development of the Brain

As the brain grows and organizes from the "inside out" and the "bottom up," the higher, more complex areas begin to control and modulate the more reactive, primitive functioning of the lower parts of the brain (see Figure 19–1). The person becomes less reactive, less impulsive, and more thoughtful. The brain's impulse-mediating capacity is related to the ratio between the excitatory activity of the lower and more primitive portions of the brain (brainstem and diencephalon; see Figure 19–1) and the modulating activity of the higher (subcortical and cortical) areas. Any factors that increase the activity or reactivity of the brainstem (e.g., chronic traumatic stress) or decrease the moderating capacity of the limbic or cortical areas (e.g., neglect, brain injury, mental retardation, Alzheimer's disease, alcohol intoxication) will increase an individual's aggression, impulsivity, and capacity to be violent (see Figure 19–1).

A key neurodevelopmental factor determining this moderating capacity is the brain's amazing capacity to organize in a "use-dependent" fashion. This means that the more any neural system is activated, the more it will change. The more a child practices piano, the more she will "build in" the motor-vestibular neural systems mediating this behavior, and, of course, the better she will become at playing piano. When an infant or toddler is spoken to, the neural systems responsible for speech and language will be activated. Frequent and repetitive talking or singing will help the child's brain develop the capacity for language; the infant or toddler living in a setting where no one speaks or sings to them will develop language slower and may even have profound communication delays. During development, repetitive and patterned sensory experiences result in corresponding neural system organization and, thereby, functioning (Courchesne et al. 1994). The brain develops functions and

capacities that reflect the patterned repetitive experiences of childhood. This is true for a host of functions associated with violent behaviors.

The capacity to moderate frustration, impulsivity, aggression, and violent behavior is age-related. With a set of sufficient motor, sensory, emotional, cognitive, and social experiences during infancy and childhood, the mature brain develops—in a use-dependent fashion—a mature, humane capacity to tolerate frustration, contain impulsivity and channel aggressive urges. A frustrated 3-year-old (with a relatively unorganized cortex) will have a difficult time modulating the reactive, brainstem-mediated state of arousal and will scream, kick, bite, throw, and hit. However, the older child when frustrated may feel like kicking, biting, and spitting, but has built in the capacity to modulate and inhibit those urges. All theoretical frameworks in developmental psychology describe this sequential development of ego functions and superego, which simply are cortically mediated, inhibitory capabilities that modulate the more primitive, less mature, reactive impulses of the human brain. Loss of cortical function through any variety of pathological processes (e.g., stroke, dementia) results in regression—a loss of cortical modulation of arousal, impulsivity, motor hyperactivity, and aggression, which are all mediated by lower portions of the central nervous system (brainstem, midbrain). Conversely, any deprivation of optimal developmental experiences that leads to underdevelopment of cortical, subcortical, and limbic areas will necessarily result in persistence of primitive, immature behavioral reactivity and predispose to violent behavior.

A growing body of evidence suggests that exposure to violence or trauma alters the developing brain by altering normal neurodevelopmental processes. Trauma influences the pattern, intensity, and nature of sensory, perceptual, and affective experience of events during childhood (see Perry 1994, 1997, 1999; Perry et al. 1995b). Threat activates the brain's stress response neurobiology. This activation, in turn, can affect the development of the brain by altering neurogenesis, migration, synaptogenesis, and neurochemical differentiation (Lauder 1988; McAllister et al. 1999). Indeed, the developing brain is exquisitely sensitive to stress. For example, rats exposed to perinatal handling stress show major alterations in their stress response later in life (Plotsky and Meany 1993; Vaid et al. 1997; Vallee et al. 1997). These animal models suggest that early exposure to consistent, moderate stress can result in resilience, whereas exposure to unpredictable or chronic stress results in functional deficits and vulnerability to future stressors.

The human brain develops and, once developed, changes in a use-dependent fashion (for review see Perry

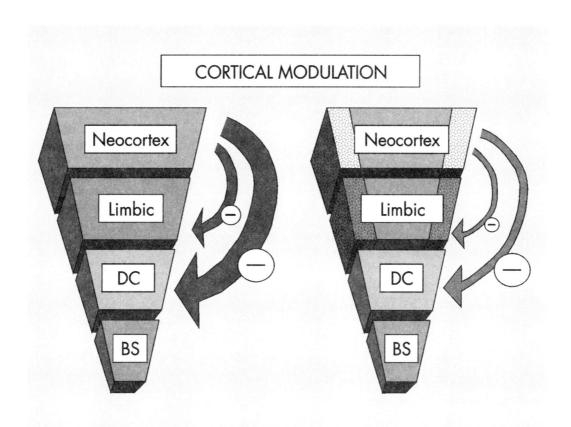

FIGURE 19–1. Cortical modulation.

The brain develops in a sequential and hierarchical fashion. As the more complex limbic, subcortical, and cortical areas organize, they begin to modulate, moderate, and control the more primitive and reactive lower portions of the brain so that by adulthood *(left image)* there are powerful inhibiting systems capable of regulating impulsivity. During childhood and with any event that can inhibit cortical functioning (e.g., brain injury, Alzheimer's disease, alcohol intoxication), the capacity of these cortical modulating systems is compromised *(right image)*. Furthermore, any developmental experiences that alter the development of cortical, subcortical, or limbic systems (e.g., emotional or cognitive neglect, mental retardation) will decrease the cortical modulation capacity and increase the likelihood of impulsive aggressive behaviors. Abbreviations: DC = diencephalon; BS = brainstem.

Source. Adapted from Perry 1997.

1999, 2001; Perry and Pollard 1998; Perry et al. 1995b). Neural systems that are activated in a repetitive fashion can change in permanent ways, altering synaptic number and microarchitecture, dendritic density, and the expression of a host of important structural and functional cellular constituents, such as enzymes or neurotransmitter receptors (Brown 1994; Courchesne et al. 1994; McAllister et al. 1999). The more any neural system is activated, the more it will modify and build in the functional capacities associated with that activation. The more someone practices the piano, the more the motor-vestibular neural systems involved in that behavior become ingrained. The more someone is exposed to a second language, the more the neurobiological networks allowing that language to be perceived and spoken will modify. And the more threat-related neural systems are activated during development, the more they will become built in.

In summary, then, exposure to violence activates a set of threat responses in the child's developing brain; in turn, excess activation of the neural systems involved in the threat responses can alter the developing brain; finally, these alterations may manifest as functional changes in emotional, behavioral, and cognitive functioning. The roots of violence-related problems, therefore, can be found in the adaptive responses to threat present during the violent experiences. The specific changes in neurodevelopment and function will depend on the child's response to the threat, the specific nature of the violent experience(s), and a host of factors associated with the child, his or her family, and the community (see Perry 2001; Perry and Azad 1999).

The Child's Response to Threat

When the child perceives threat (e.g., anticipating an assault on self or loved one), his or her brain will orchestrate a total-body mobilization to adapt to the challenge. The child's emotional, behavioral, cognitive, social, and physiological functioning will change. These responses to threat are heterogeneous and graded. The degree and nature of a specific response will vary from individual to individual in any single event and across events for any given individual. In animals and in humans, two primary but interactive response patterns, hyperarousal and dissociative, have been described (Perry 1999; Perry et al. 1995b). Most individuals use various combinations of these two distinct response patterns during any given traumatic event. The predominant response patterns and combinations of these primary styles appear to shift from dissociative (common in babies and young children) to hyperarousal during development.

THE HYPERAROUSAL CONTINUUM: "FIGHT OR FLIGHT" RESPONSES

Neural Systems Regulating the Neurobiological Response to Threat

Reticular Activating System

The initial phase of the hyperarousal continuum is an alarm reaction that begins activation of the central and peripheral nervous system. A network of ascending arousal-related neural systems in the brain, consisting of locus coeruleus noradrenergic neurons, dorsal raphe serotonin neurons, cholinergic neurons from the lateral dorsal tegmentum, mesolimbic and mesocortical dopaminergic neurons, and others, forms the reticular activating system (RAS). Much of the original research on arousal, fear, and response to stress and threat was carried out using various lesion models of the RAS (Moore and Bloom 1979). The RAS is an important, multisystem network involved in arousal, anxiety, and modulation of limbic and cortical processing (Munk et al. 1996). These key brainstem and midbrain monoamine systems, working together, provide the flexible and diverse functions necessary to modulate the variety of functions related to anxiety regulation.

Locus Coeruleus

A key component of the RAS network is the locus coeruleus (LC) (Aston-Jones et al. 1996; Murberg et al. 1990). This bilateral nucleus of norepinephrine-containing neurons originates in the pons and sends diverse axonal projections to virtually all major brain regions, enabling its function as a general regulator of noradrenergic tone and activity (see Aston-Jones et al. 1996). The LC plays a major role in determining the "valence" or value of incoming sensory information, increasing in activity if the information is novel or potentially threatening (Abercrombie and Jacobs 1987a, 1987b). The ventral tegmental nucleus (VTN) also plays a part in regulating the sympathetic nuclei in the pons and medulla (Moore and Bloom 1979). Acute stress results in an increase in LC and VTN activity and release of norepinephrine, which influences the rest of the brain and body. These brainstem catecholamine systems (LC and VTN), which coordinate with all key areas of the brain, play a critical role in regulating arousal, vigilance, affect, behavioral irritability, locomotion, attention, the response to stress, sleep, and the startle response.

Activity of the LC mirrors the degree of arousal (i.e., sleep, calm-alert, alarm-vigilant, fear, and terror) related to stress or distress in the environment (internal and external). Fear increases LC and VTN activity, increasing the release of norepinephrine in all of the LC and VTN terminal fields throughout the brain. The LC tunes out noncritical information and mediates hypervigilance. This nucleus orchestrates the complex interactive process that includes activation of autonomic nervous system tone, the immune system, and the hypothalamic-pituitary-adrenal (HPA) axis, with resulting release of adrenocorticotropin and cortisol. Sympathetic nervous system activation can be regulated by the LC, which results in changes in heart rate, blood pressure, respiratory rate, glucose mobilization, and muscle tone. All of these actions prepare the body for defense—to fight against or run away from the potential threat.

Hippocampus

Another key system linked with the RAS that plays a central role in the fear response is the hippocampus, located at the interface of the cortex and the lower diencephalic areas. It plays a major role in memory and learning. In addition, it plays a key role in various activities of the autonomic nervous and neuroendocrine systems. Stress hormones and stress-related neurotransmitter systems (i.e., those from the locus coeruleus and other key brainstem nuclei) target the hippocampus. In animal models, various hormones (e.g., cortisol) appear to alter hippocampus synapse formation and dendritic structure, thereby causing actual changes in gross structure and hippocampal volume as defined using various brain imaging techniques (see McEwen 1999 for review). Repeated stress appears to inhibit the development of neurons in the dentate gyrus (part of the hippocampus) and atrophy of dendrites in the CA3 region of the hippocampus (Sapolsky and Plotsky 1990; Sapolsky et al. 1990). These neurobiological changes are likely related to some of the observed functional problems with memory and learning that accompany stress-related neuropsychiatric syndromes, including posttraumatic stress disorder (PTSD) (see Perry and Azad 1999).

Amygdala and Emotional Memory

In the recent past, the amygdala has emerged as the key brain region in the processing, interpreting, and integration of emotional functioning (Davis 1992a, 1992b). In the same fashion that the LC plays the central role in orchestrating arousal, the amygdala plays the central role in the central nervous system (CNS) in processing afferent and efferent connections related to emotional functioning (Phillips and LeDoux 1992; Sapolsky et al. 1990). The amygdala receives input directly from sensory thalamus, hippocampus (via multiple projections), entorhinal cortex, sensory association areas of cortex, polymodal sensory association areas of cortex, and from various midbrain and brainstem arousal systems via the RAS (Selden et al. 1991). The amygdala processes and determines the emotional value of simple sensory input, complex multisensory perceptions, and complex cognitive abstractions, even responding specifically to complex, socially relevant stimuli. In turn, the amygdala orchestrates the response to this emotional information by sending projections to brain areas involved in motor (behavioral), autonomic nervous system, and neuroendocrine areas of the CNS (Davis 1992a, 1992b; LeDoux et al. 1989, 1990). In a series of landmark studies, LeDoux and colleagues have demonstrated the key role of the amygdala in emotional memory (LeDoux et al. 1989, 1990). In the response to threat, therefore, the amygdala and its related neural systems will have alterations in activity relative to the nonthreat state.

Hypothalamic-Pituitary-Adrenal Axis

As with central neurobiological systems, stress, threat, and fear influence HPA regulation. Abnormalities of the HPA axis have been noted in adults with PTSD (Murberg et al. 1990). Chronic activation of the HPA system in response to stress has negative consequences. The homeostatic state associated with chronic HPA activation wears the body out (Sapolsky and Plotsky 1990; Sapolsky et al. 1990). Hippocampal damage, impaired glucose utilization, and vulnerability to metabolic insults may all result from chronic stress (see McEwen 1999 for review).

THE DISSOCIATIVE CONTINUUM

Infants and young children are not capable of effectively fighting or fleeing. In the initial stages of distress an infant will manifest a precursor form of a hyperarousal response. In these early alarm stages, the infant will use its limited behavioral repertoire to attract the attention of a caregiver. These behaviors include changes in facial expression, body movements, and, most important, vocalization (i.e., crying). This is a successful adaptive strategy if the caretaker comes to feed, warm, soothe, fight for, or flee with, the infant.

Unfortunately, for many infants and children these strategies are not effective. In the absence of an appropriate caregiver reaction to the initial alarm outcry, the child will abandon the early alarm response. The converse of use-dependent development occurs—disuse-related extinction of a behavior. This defeat response is well characterized in animal models of stress reactivity and "learned helplessness" (Miczek et al. 1990). This defeat reaction is a common element of the presenting emotional and behavioral phenomenology of many neglected and abused children (Carlson et al. 1989; Chisholm et al. 1995; George and Main 1979; Spitz 1945). Indeed, adults, professional or not, often puzzle over the emotional nonreactivity, passivity, compliance, and hypalgesia of many abused children.

In the face of persisting threat, the infant or young child will activate other neurophysiological and functional responses. This involves activation of dissociative adaptations. Dissociation is a broad descriptive term that includes a variety of mental mechanisms involved in disengaging from the external world and attending to stimuli in the internal world. This can involve distraction, avoidance, numbing, daydreaming, fugue, fantasy, derealization, depersonalization, and, in the extreme, fainting or catatonia. In our experiences with young children and infants, the predominant adaptive responses during the trauma are dissociative.

Children exposed to chronic violence may report a variety of dissociative experiences. Children describe going to a "different place," assuming the personae of superheroes or animals, a sense of "watching a movie that I was in" or "just floating"—classic depersonalization and derealization responses. Observers will report these children as numb, robotic, nonreactive, "daydreaming," "acting like they were not there," or "staring off in a glazed look." Younger children are more likely to use dissociative adaptations. Immobilization, inescapability, or pain will increase the dissociative components of the stress response patterns at any age.

Neurobiology of Dissociation

In animals, the defeat response is mediated by different neurobiological mechanisms than the fight-or-flight response. What little is known about the neurobiology and phenomenology of dissociative-like conditions appears to most approximate the defeat reaction described in animals (Blanchard et al. 1993; Henry et al. 1993; Miczek et al. 1990). As with the hyperarousal response, there is brainstem-mediated CNS activation that results in increases in circulating epinephrine and associated stress steroids. A major difference in the CNS, however, is that vagal tone increases dramatically, decreasing blood pressure and heart rate (occasionally resulting in fainting) despite increases in circulating epinephrine.

Dopaminergic systems, primarily mesolimbic and mesocortical, play an important role in defeat reaction models in animals. These dopaminergic systems are intimately involved in the "reward" systems, affect modulation (e.g., cocaine-induced euphoria) and, in some cases, are co-localized with endogenous opioids that mediate pain or other sensory processing. The opioid systems are clearly involved in altering both perception of painful stimuli and sense of time, place, and reality. Opioids appear to be major mediators of the defeat reaction's dissociative behaviors (e.g., Abercrombie and Jacobs 1988). Indeed, most opiate agonists can induce dissociative responses in humans.

The capacity to dissociate in the midst of terror appears to be a differentially available adaptive response—some people dissociate early in the arousal continuum, some only in a state of complete terror (see Table 19–1). The determinants of individual differences in the specific stress response to threat have yet to be well characterized. In its most common form, however, the child and adult response to trauma is an admixture of these two primary adaptive patterns, arousal and dissociation.

STATES BECOME TRAITS: THE CLINICAL PRESENTATION OF CHILDREN EXPOSED TO VIOLENCE

A current working hypothesis regarding the effects of traumatic events on the neurobiology of the developing child posits that the specific symptoms a child develops will be related to the intensity and duration of the adaptive style (or combination of adaptive responses) present during the threat. If the neurobiology of the specific response (hyperarousal or dissociation) is activated long enough, there will be molecular, structural, and functional changes in those systems (Perry 1994, 1997, 2001; Perry and Pollard 1998; Perry et al. 1995b). Any factors

that prolong the original threat response will increase the likelihood of long-term symptoms, whereas any factors that decrease the threat response will decrease the risk for long-term problems.

If a child dissociates in response to a severe trauma and stays in that dissociative state for a sufficient period of time, he or she will alter the homeostasis of the systems mediating the dissociative response (i.e., opioid, dopaminergic, HPA axis). A sensitized neurobiology of dissociation will result, and the child may develop prominent dissociative-related symptoms (e.g., withdrawal, somatic complaints, dissociation, anxiety, helplessness, dependence) and related disorders (e.g., dissociative disorders, somatoform disorders, anxiety disorders, major depression).

If the child exposed to violence uses a response that is predominantly hyperarousal in origin, the altered homeostasis will be in a different set of neurochemical systems (i.e., adrenergic, noradrenergic, HPA axis). This child will be vulnerable to developing persistent hyperarousal-related symptoms and related disorders (e.g., PTSD, attention-deficit/hyperactivity disorder, conduct disorder). These children are characterized by persistent physiological hyperarousal and hyperactivity (Perry et al. 1995a, 1995b). They are observed to have increased muscle tone, a low-grade increase in temperature (frequently), an increased startle response, profound sleep disturbances, affect regulation problems, and generalized (or specific) anxiety (Kaufman 1991; Ornitz and Pynoos 1989; Perry 1994). In addition, our studies indicate that a significant portion of these children have abnormalities in cardiovascular regulation (Perry 1994; Perry et al. 1995a; see Figure 19–2).

The specific symptoms a child develops following exposure to violence, then, can vary depending upon the nature, frequency, pattern, and intensity of the violence, the adaptive style of the child, and the presence of attenuating factors such as a stable, safe, and supportive home. Within this heterogeneity, however, certain trends emerge. Observations from clinical work suggest that there are marked gender differences in the response to violence (Perry et al. 1995a, 1995b). Females are more likely to dissociate, and males are more likely to display a classic fight-or-flight response. As a result, more males will develop the aggressive, impulsive, reactive, and hyperactive symptom presentation (more externalizing), whereas females will be more anxious, dissociative, and dysphoric (more internalizing).

Children raised with persisting violence are much more likely to be violent (e.g., Halperin et al. 1995; Hickey 1991; Koop et al. 1992; Lewis et al. 1989; Loeber et al. 1993). This can be explained, in part, by the persis-

TABLE 19–1.   Continuum of adaptive responses to threat

Internal state	Arousal continuum	Dissociative continuum	Regulating brain region	Cognitive style	Sense of time
Calm	Rest	Rest	Neocortex Cortex	Abstract	Extended future
Arousal	Vigilance	Avoidance	Cortex Limbic	Concrete	Hours to days
Alarm	Resistance (crying)	Compliance (robotic)	Limbic Midbrain	Emotional	Minutes to hours
Fear	Defiance (tantrums)	Dissociation (fetal rocking)	Midbrain Brainstem	Reactive	Seconds to minutes
Terror	Aggression	Fainting	Brainstem Autonomic	Reflexive	None

Note.   Different children have different styles of adaptation to threat. Some children use a primary hyperarousal response, others a primary dissociative response. Most use some combination of these two adaptive styles. In the fearful child, a defiant stance is often seen. This is typically interpreted as a willful and controlling child. Rather than understanding the behavior as related to fear, adults often respond to the oppositional behavior by becoming angry and more demanding. The child, overreading the nonverbal cues of the frustrated and angry adult, feels more threatened and moves from alarm to fear to terror. These children may end up in a primitive "mini-psychotic" regression or in a very combative state. The behavior of the child reflects his or her attempts to adapt and respond to a perceived (or misperceived) threat.

  When threatened, a child is likely to act in an immature fashion. Regression, a retreat to a less mature style of functioning and behavior, is commonly observed in all of us when we are physically ill, sleep deprived, hungry, fatigued, or threatened. During the regressive response to the real or perceived threat, less-complex brain areas mediate our behaviors. If a child has been raised in an environment of persistent threat, the child will have an altered baseline such that the internal state of calm is rarely obtained (or only artificially obtained via alcohol or drug use). In addition, the traumatized child will have a sensitized alarm response, overreading nonthreatening verbal and nonverbal cues as threatening. This increased reactivity will result in dramatic changes in behavior in the face of seemingly minor provocative cues. All too often, this overreading of threat will lead to a fight-or-flight reaction—and increase the probability of impulsive aggression. This hyperreactivity to threat can, as the child becomes older, contribute to the transgenerational cycle of violence.

tence of this fight-or-flight state—and by the profound cognitive distortions that can accompany a persisting state of fear. A young man with these characteristics may misinterpret a behavior as threatening and will, being more reactive, respond in a more impulsive and violent fashion. He is, literally, using the original (childhood) adaptive fight-or-flight response in a new context, but now, later in life, in a maladaptive fashion.

ALTERED NEUROBIOLOGY IN CHILDREN EXPOSED TO VIOLENCE

Few studies have examined the neurobiological effect of trauma and violence in children. Several studies have utilized brain-regulated peripheral measures, including psychophysiology (e.g., startle, heart-rate regulation), or peripheral measures related to catecholamine or neuroendocrine functioning. In all of these studies, the findings have suggested a dysregulated, sensitized stress response neurobiology in children and adolescents following exposure to trauma or violence (for review see Perry and Azad 1999; Perry and Pollard 1998). These findings are consistent with the hypothesis that the orig

inal adaptive neurophysiological states associated with the response to threat become, over time and in a use-dependent fashion, traits (Perry et al. 1995b).

  In one of the first studies to examine brain-related physiological responses in traumatized children, Ornitz and Pynoos (1989) demonstrated an increased startle response, a finding suggesting sensitized brainstem and midbrain catecholamines (Davis 1992a, 1992b). Similarly altered brainstem catecholamine and neuroendocrine functioning was suggested by a pilot study of sexually abused girls. Following abuse, these girls exhibited greater total catecholamine synthesis, as measured by the sum of the urinary concentration of epinephrine, norepinephrine, and dopamine, when compared with matched control subjects (DeBellis et al. 1994a, 1994b). In our laboratory, altered platelet alpha$_2$-adrenergic receptor number and cardiovascular functioning were demonstrated in children exposed to traumatic violence, suggesting chronic and abnormal activation of the sympathetic nervous system (Perry 1994; Perry et al. 1995b). In our clinic populations, evidence of brain-mediated alterations of cardiovascular functioning has been demonstrated in various ways (Figures 19–2 and 19–3). In both the acute and chronic posttraumatic period, resting heart rate is different from that of comparison popula

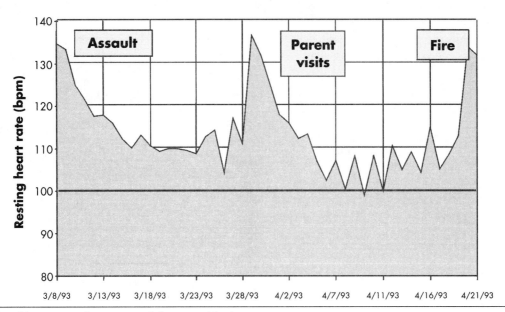

FIGURE 19–2. Hyperarousal symptoms following a life-threatening event.

In the 3 days following the ATF assault on the Branch Davidian compound in Waco, Texas, 21 children were released. All of these children were in harm's way during the assault. A clinical team led by ChildTrauma Clinic personnel lived and worked with these children for the 6 weeks following their release. These children had various PTSD-related symptoms. Reenactment behaviors and cue-specific increases in anxiety were observed in the presence of stimuli associated with the assault, including white vans and a helicopter. The physiological hyperarousal was illustrated by the profound increases in resting heart rate observed in all of the children throughout the 6 weeks of the standoff. Five days after the original raid, the group's average resting heart rate was 134 (the group average should have been approximately 80). In the middle of the period of standoff, many of these children visited with a parent released from the compound. These visits resulted in dramatic changes in the children's behavior (e.g., return of bed-wetting, hiding under beds, aggressive behavior) and in their resting heart rates, indicating that these visits were, in some regard, distressing to the children. During these visits, the children were reminded by their parents that they were "in the hands of the Babylonians," inducing fear and confusion. When these visits stopped, the children improved. When the children were told about the fire, their distress increased dramatically. It should be noted that the normal resting heart rate for a group of comparison children is approximately 90 beats per minute—the Davidian children for the entire period of the standoff and beyond never had resting heart rates below 100.
Source. From Perry et al., in preparation—a.

tions. In other studies, clonidine, an alpha$_2$-adrenergic receptor partial agonist, has been demonstrated to be an effective pharmacotherapeutic agent (Perry 1994), further suggesting altered LC functioning in children exposed to violence.

Little research on the neurobiology of dissociation in children exists. In our preliminary studies, traumatized children with dissociative symptoms demonstrated lower heart rates than comparably traumatized children with hyperarousal symptoms. Using continuous heart rate monitoring during clinical interviews, male, preadolescent children exposed to violence exhibited a mild tachycardia during nonintrusive interviews and a marked tachycardia during interviews about specific exposure to trauma ($n = 83$; resting heart rate = 104; interview heart rate = 122). In comparison, females exposed to traumatic events tended to have normal or mild tachycardia that decreased during interviews about the traumatic event ($n = 24$; resting heart rate = 98; interview heart rate = 82). This gender difference was associated with differences in emotional and behavioral symptoms, with

males exhibiting more externalizing and females more internalizing symptoms (Perry et al. 1995a; see Figure 19–3). In a recent case series with 10 children with severe dissociative symptoms (e.g., fainting, catatonia, bradycardia), naltrexone, an opioid antagonist, improved dissociative symptoms (Perry et al., in preparation—a). The hypothesized therapeutic site of action is the opioid receptors regulating LC activity (Abercrombie and Jacobs 1988).

These indirect studies all support the hypothesis that use-dependent alterations in the key neural systems of the brain are related to the stress response following exposure to violence in childhood. More recently, using newer methods that allow more direct examination of the brain supports the notion that prolonged threat alters the developing brain. Preliminary studies by Teicher and colleagues (1997) have demonstrated altered EEG findings in a sample of abused children that suggest hippocampal, limbic, and cortical abnormalities (see also Ito et al. 1993). DeBellis (1999a; 1999b), in a series of landmark studies, demonstrated altered cortical develop-

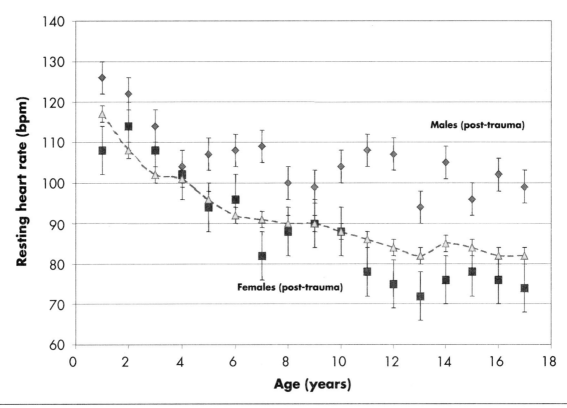

FIGURE 19–3. Resting heart rate in traumatized children.

Over a 5-year period, each child referred to the ChildTrauma Clinic, which specializes in working with traumatized or maltreated children, had a resting heart rate taken at first presentation. These resting rates were plotted by age and gender (total $n = 526$; traumatized males are the *gray diamonds* ±SEM, $n = 320$; traumatized females are the *black squares* ±SEM, $n = 206$). The *gray triangles* are values from normal pediatric population norms in which there are no observed gender differences. In young children, there do not appear to be any gender differences; by age 5, however, gender differences emerge, with males having higher resting heart rates (consistent with persistent hyperarousal) and females having somewhat lower resting heart rates (consistent with persistent dissociative adaptations). These resting rates are pretreatment.
Source. From Perry et al., in preparation—a.

ment in children with PTSD. In 44 subjects with PTSD, the intracranial and cerebral volumes were smaller than those of matched control subjects (DeBellis 1999a). These differences were related to the severity and time of onset of symptoms.

Clearly more research is indicated; however, all studies to date suggest that exposure to violence in childhood alters brain development and that the abnormalities are more prominent if the traumatic exposure begins early in life and is severe and chronic.

CLINICAL IMPLICATIONS

There are profound clinical implications of persistent fear states in children. These children will have impaired capacities to benefit from social, emotional, and cognitive experiences. This is explained by three key principles of brain functioning: 1) the brain changes in response to experience in a use-dependent fashion; 2) the brain inter-

nalizes and stores information from any experience in a state-dependent fashion, and 3) the brain retrieves stored information in a state-dependent fashion.

Use-Dependent Learning: State-Dependent Storage and Recall

As described above, the brain changes in a use-dependent fashion. All parts of the brain can modify their functioning in response to specific patterns of activation. These use-dependent changes in the brain result in changes in cognition (this, of course, is the basis for cognitive learning), emotional functioning (social learning), motor-vestibular functioning (e.g., the ability to write, type, ride a bike), and state-regulation capacity (e.g., resting heart rate). No part of the brain can change without being activated—you can't teach someone French while she is are asleep or teach a child to ride a bike by talking with him.

One of the most important elements of understanding children exposed to violence is that all humans process, store, retrieve, and respond to the world in a state-dependent fashion (see Table 19–1). When a child is in a persistent state of low-level fear that results from exposure to violence, the primary areas of the brain that are processing information are different from those in a child from a safe environment. The calm child may sit in the same classroom as a child in an alarm state, both hearing the same lecture by the teacher. Even if they have identical IQs, the child that is calm can focus on the words of the teacher and, using neocortex, engage in abstract cognition. The child in an alarm state will be less efficient at processing and storing the verbal information the teacher is providing. This child's cognition will be dominated by subcortical and limbic areas, focusing on nonverbal information—the teacher's facial expressions, her hand gestures, or at what times she seems distracted. And, because the brain internalizes (i.e., learns) in a use-dependent fashion, this child will have more selective development of nonverbal cognitive capacities. The children raised in the vortex of violence have learned that nonverbal information is more important than verbal information.

This means that hypervigilant children from chronic violence settings frequently develop remarkable nonverbal skills in proportion to their verbal skills ("street smarts"). Indeed, often they overread (misinterpret) nonverbal cues (e.g., eye contact means threat, a friendly touch is interpreted as an antecedent to seduction and rape); interpretations that are accurate in the world they came from but now, hopefully, out of context. During development, these children spent so much time in a low-level state of fear (mediated by brainstem and midbrain areas) that they were focusing consistently on nonverbal cues. In our clinic population, children raised in chronically traumatic environments demonstrate a prominent Verbal > Performance split on IQ testing ($n = 108$; WISC Verbal = 8.2; WISC Performance = 10.4 Perry et al., in preparation—b). In a separate study of 400 children removed from their parents by child protective services, IQ testing demonstrated that only 2% of the children had a significant Verbal > Performance split (V score 12 or more points greater than P score), whereas 39% demonstrated a significant Performance > Verbal split (P score 12 or more points greater than V score) (Perry et al., in preparation—b).

This is consistent with the observations of teachers that many of the maltreated or traumatized children they work with are often judged to be bright but can't learn easily. Often these children are labeled as learning disabled. These difficulties with cognitive organization contribute to a more primitive, less mature style of problem solving—with aggression often being employed as a tool.

This principle is critically important in understanding why a traumatized child—in a persistent state of arousal—can sit in a classroom and not learn. This child has different parts of the brain controlling his functioning compared with a child who is calm. The capacity to internalize new verbal cognitive information depends on having portions of the frontal and related cortical areas being activated. This, in turn, requires a state of attentive calm—a state the traumatized child rarely achieves.

Children in a state of fear retrieve information from the world differently than children who feel calm (see Table 19–1). As a child moves along the continuum of arousal (see Table 19–1), the part of the brain that is orchestrating functioning shifts. An excellent illustration of this is in how the sense of time is altered in alarm states. In such children, the sense of future is foreshortened, and the critical time period for the individual shrinks. The threatened child is not thinking (nor should she think) about months from now. This has profound implications for understanding the cognition of the traumatized child. Immediate reward is most reinforcing. Delayed gratification is impossible. Consequences of behavior become almost inconceivable to the threatened child. Reflection on behavior—including violent behavior—is impossible for the child in an alarm state. Cut adrift from the internal regulating capabilities of the cortex, the brainstem acts reflexively, impulsively, and aggressively to any perceived threat. Eye contact for too long becomes a life-threatening signal. Wearing the wrong colors or a particular hand gesture—cues that to the calm adult reading about another "senseless" murder in the paper are insignificant—are, to the hypervigilant, armed adolescent born and raised in the vortex of violence, enough to trigger a "kill or be killed" response.

THE FUTURE: IMPEDIMENTS TO PROBLEM SOLVING AND PREVENTION

There are many important and effective treatment approaches to the child traumatized by violence. Yet even with optimal clinical techniques, treatment of maltreated children would overwhelm the entire mental health and child welfare communities in this country. Today the number of children who would benefit from intervention far outstrips the meager resources our society has dedicated to children exposed to violence. Even as we develop more effective and accessible intervention models, we must focus on prevention.

A society functions as a reflection of its child-rearing practices. If children are ignored, poorly educated, and not protected from violence, they will grow into adults who create a reactive, noncreative, and violent society. In a brilliant analysis of this very process, Hellie (1996) describes a dark age in Russia (1600–1700) characterized by excessive brutality, violence, and pervasive fear that for generations inhibited creativity, abstraction, literacy, and the other elements of humanity. All societies reap what they have sown.

Today in the United States, despite the well-documented adverse effects of domestic, community, school, and media violence, we continue to seek short-term and simplistic answers. In order to minimize the many destructive pathways that come from violence in childhood, we need to dedicate resources of time, energy, and money to these complex problems. And we need to help provide the resource-predictable, safe, and resource-rich environments our problem solvers require. Too often the academic, public, and not-for-profit systems asked to address these problems are resource-depleted yet have a mandate to "do something." Unfortunately, the solutions that arise from this reactive approach to complex problems are very limited and, typically, short-sighted (see Table 19–2).

Our problem solvers must understand the indelible relationship between early life experiences and cognitive, social, emotional, and physical health. Providing enriching cognitive, emotional, social, and physical experiences in childhood could transform our culture. But before our society can choose to provide these experiences, it must be educated about what we now know about child development. Education of the public must be coupled with continuing research into the effect of positive and negative experiences on the development of children. All of this must be paired with the implementation and testing of programs that can enrich the lives of children and families and programs to provide early identification of, and proactive intervention for, at-risk children and families.

TABLE 19–2.   Continuum of adaptive responses to threat in a living group (family, organization, community, or society)

Social-environmental pressures	Prevailing cognitive style	Prevailing affective tone	Systemic solutions	Focus of solution	Rules, regulations, and laws	Child-rearing practices
Resource-surplus Predictable Stable/safe	Abstract, creative	Calm	Innovative	Future	Abstract, conceptual	Nurturing, flexible, enriching
Resource-limited Unpredictable Novel	Concrete, superstitious	Anxiety	Simplistic	Immediate future	Superstitious, intrusive	Ambivalent, obsessive, controlling
Resource-poor Inconsistent Threatening	Reactive, regressive	Terror	Reactionary	Present	Restrictive, punitive	Apathetic, oppressive, harsh

Note. In the same fashion as an individual, living groups experience threat and challenges to their survival. Similar to an individual, the cognition of a group moves down a gradient under threat. When there are no external threats and resources are plentiful and predictable *(Row 1)*, the group has the luxury of thinking in abstract ways to solve any of its current problems (e.g., Bell Labs from 1940 to 1965). The focus of the solution can be the future, and the least powerful members of the living group (e.g., children and women) can be treated with the most flexible, nurturing, and enriching approaches. When resources become limited and there are economic, environmental, or social threats *(Row 2)*, the group, organization, or society becomes less capable of complex, abstract problem solving. The solutions tend to reflect the immediate future (e.g., the next funding cycle, the next election cycle), and all aspects of functioning in the group become more regressed. The least powerful are ignored or controlled to minimize any excessive drain on the most powerful. In a group, organization, or society under direct threat *(Row 3)*, the focus of all problem solving becomes the moment. The solutions tend to be reactive and regressive. The least powerful are ignored, and, if they get in the way, they are harshly dealt with. The more out of control the external situation is, the more controlling, reactive, and oppressive the internally focused actions of this group will become. In each of these situations, the prevailing child-rearing styles will create children who will reinforce that group or society's structure: in a safe and abstract-thinking group the children will be more likely to receive and benefit from enrichment and education, thereby optimizing their potential for creativity, abstraction, and productivity. In contrast, children raised in groups or societies under threat will be more likely to be raised with harsh or distant caregiving. The result will be impulsive, concrete, and reactive adults who are perfectly positioned to fit in and contribute to a reactive, oppressive, and aggressive group or society.

The problems related to violence are complex, and they have complex effects on our society. Yet there are solutions to these problems. The choice to find solutions is up to us. If we choose, we have some control of our future. If we, as a society, continue to ignore the laws of biology, and the inevitable neurodevelopmental consequences of chronic exposure to violence in childhood, our potential as a humane society will remain unrealized. The future will hold sociocultural devolution—the inevitable consequence of the competition for limited resources and the implementation of reactive, one-dimensional, and short-term solutions. This need not be. Parents, caregivers, professionals, public officials, and policy makers do have the capacity to make decisions that will increase or decrease violence in our children's lives. Hopefully, an appreciation of the devastating effects of violence on the developing child will help all of us make the good decisions and difficult choices that will create a safer, more predictable, and enriching world for children.

REFERENCES

Abercrombie ED, Jacobs BL: Single-unit response of noradrenergic neurons in the locus coeruleus of freely moving cats, I: acutely presented stressful and non-stressful stimuli. J Neurosci 7:2837–2843, 1987a

Abercrombie ED, Jacobs BL: Single-unit response of noradrenergic neurons in the locus coeruleus of freely moving cats, II: adaptation to chronically presented stressful stimuli. J Neurosci 7:2844–2848, 1987b

Abercrombie ED, Jacobs BL: Systemic naloxone administration potentiates locus coeruleus noradrenergic neuronal activity under stressful but not non-stressful conditions. Brain Res 441:362–366, 1988

Aston-Jones G, Valentino RJ, Van Bockstaele EJ, et al: Locus coeruleus, stress and post traumatic stress disorder: neurobiological and clinical parallels, in Catecholamine Function in Post Traumatic Stress Disorder: Emerging Concepts. Edited by Murberg M. Washington, DC, American Psychiatric Press, 1996, pp 17–62

Blanchard DC, Sakai RR, McEwen B, et al: Subordination stress: behavioral, brain and neuroendocrine correlates. Behav Brain Res 58:113–121, 1993

Brown JW: Morphogenesis and mental process. Dev Psychopathol 6:551–563, 1994

Carlson V, Cicchetti D, Barnett D, et al: Disorganized/disoriented attachment relationships in maltreated infants. Dev Psychol 25:525–531, 1989

Chisholm K, Carter MC, Ames EW, et al: Attachment security and indiscriminately friendly behavior in children adopted from Romanian orphanages. Dev Psychopathol 7:283–294, 1995

Courchesne E, Chisum H, Townsend J: Neural activity-dependent brain changes in development: implications for psychopathology. Dev Psychopathol 6(4):697–722, 1994

Davis M: The role of the amygdala in conditioned fear, in The Amygdala: Neurobiological Aspects of Emotion, Memory, and Mental Dysfunction. Edited by Aggleton JP. New York, Wiley-Liss, 1992a, pp 255–306

Davis M: The role of the amygdala in fear-potentiated startle: implications for animal models of anxiety. Trends Pharmacol Sci 13:35–41, 1992b

DeBellis MD, Chrousos GP, Dorn LD, et al: Hypothalamic-pituitary-adrenal axis dysregulation in sexually abused girls. J Clin Endocrinol Metab 78:249–255, 1994a

DeBellis MD, Lefter L, Trickett PK, et al: Urinary catecholamine excretion in sexually abused girls. J Am Acad Child Adolesc Psychiatry 33:320–327, 1994b

DeBellis MD, Baum AS, Birmaher B, et al: Developmental traumatology, part I: biological stress symptoms. Biol Psychiatry 45:1259–1270, 1999a

DeBellis MD, Keshavan MS, Clark DB, et al: Developmental traumatology, part II: brain development. Biol Psychiatry 45:1271–1284, 1999b

George C, Main M: Social interactions of young abused children: approach, avoidance and aggression. Child Dev 50:306–318, 1979

Halperin JM, Newcorn JH, Matier K: Impulsivity and the initiation of fights in children with disruptive behavioral disorders. J Child Psychol Psychiatry 36(7):1199–1211, 1995

Hellie R: Interpreting violence in late Muscovy from the perspective of modern neuroscience. Paper presented at the 28th National Convention of the American Association for the Advancement of Science, Boston, MA, November 1996

Henry JP, Liu YY, Nadra WE, et al: Psychosocial stress can induce chronic hypertension in normotensive strains of rats. Hypertension 21:714–723, 1993

Hickey E: Serial Murderers and Their Victims. Belmont, CA, Wadsworth Publishing, 1991

Ito Y, Teicher MH, Glod CA, et al: Increased prevalence of electrophysiological abnormalities in children with psychological, physical, and sexual abuse. Journal of Neuropsychiatry 5:401–408, 1993

Kaufman J: Depressive disorders in maltreated children. J Am Acad Child Adolesc Psychiatry 30(2):257–265, 1991

Koop CE, Lundberg G: Violence in America: a public health emergency. JAMA 22:3075–3076, 1992

Lauder JM: Neurotransmitters as morphogens. Prog Brain Res 73:365–388, 1988

LeDoux JE, Romanski L, Xagoraris A: Indelibility of subcortical emotional memories. J Cogn Neurosci 1:238–243, 1989

LeDoux JE, Cicchetti P, Xagoraris A, et al: The lateral amygdaloid nucleus: sensory interface of the amygdala in fear conditioning. J Neurosci 10:1062–1069, 1990

Lewis DO, Mailouh C, Webb V: Child abuse, delinquency, and violent criminality, in Child Maltreatment: Theory and Research on the Causes and Consequences of Child Abuse and Neglect. Edited by Cicchetti D, Carlson V. Cambridge, England, Cambridge University Press, 1989, pp 707–721

Loeber R, Wung P, Keenan K, et al: Developmental pathways in disruptive child behavior. Development and Psychopathology 5:103–133, 1993

McAllister AK, Katz LC, Lo DC: Neurotrophins and synaptic plasticity. Annu Rev Neurosci 22:295–318, 1999

McEwen BS: Stress and hippocampal plasticity. Annu Rev Neurosci 22:105–122, 1999

Miczek KA, Thompson ML, Tornatzky W: Subordinate animals: behavioral and physiological adaptations and opioid tolerance, in Stress: Neurobiology and Neuroendocrinology. Edited by Brown MR, Koob GF, Rivier C. New York, Marcel Dekker, 1990, pp 323–357

Moore RY, Bloom FE: Central catecholamine neuron systems: anatomy and physiology of the norepinephrine and epinephrine systems. Annu Rev Neurosci 2:113–153, 1979

Munk MHJ, Roelfsema PR, Konig P, et al: Role of reticular activation in the modulation of intracortical synchronization. Science 272:271–273, 1996

Murberg MM, McFall ME, Veith RC: Catecholamines, stress and post-traumatic stress disorder, in Biological Assessment and Treatment of Posttraumatic Stress Disorder. Edited by Giller EL. Washington, DC, American Psychiatric Press, 1990, pp 27–65

Ornitz EM, Pynoos RS: Startle modulation in children with post-traumatic stress disorder. Am J Psychiatry 147:866–870, 1989

Perry BD: Neurobiological sequelae of childhood trauma: post-traumatic stress disorders in children, in Catecholamines in Posttraumatic Stress Disorder: Emerging Concepts. Edited by Murberg M. Washington, DC, American Psychiatric Press, 1994, pp 253–276

Perry BD: Incubated in terror: neurodevelopmental factors in the "cycle of violence," in Children, Youth and Violence: The Search for Solutions. Edited by Osofsky J. New York, Guilford, 1997, pp 124–148

Perry BD: Memories of fear: how the brain stores and retrieves physiologic states, feelings, behaviors and thoughts from traumatic events, in Splintered Reflections: Images of the Body in Trauma. Edited by Goodwin JM, Attias R. New York, Basic Books, 1999, pp 26–47

Perry BD: The neuroarcheology of childhood maltreatment: the neurodevelopmental costs of adverse childhood events, in The Cost of Child Maltreatment: Who Pays? We All Do. Edited by Franey K, Geffner R, Falconer R. San Diego, CA, Family Violence and Sexual Assault Institute Press, 2001, pp 15–39

Perry BD, Azad I: Post-traumatic stress disorders in children and adolescents. Curr Opin Pediatr 11:121–132, 1999

Perry BD, Pollard R: Homeostasis, stress, trauma, and adaptation: a neurodevelopmental view of childhood trauma. Child Adolesc Psychiatr Clin N Am 7:33–51, 1998

Perry BD, Pollard RA, Baker WL, et al: Continuous heart-rate monitoring in maltreated children [abstract]. New Research: Annual Meeting of the American Academy of Child and Adolescent Psychiatry, New Orleans, LA, November 1995a

Perry BD, Pollard R, Blakely T, et al: Childhood trauma, the neurobiology of adaptation and "use-dependent" development of the brain: how "states" become "traits." Infant Mental Health Journal 16(4):271–291, 1995b

Perry BD, Schick S, Dobson C: Syncope, bradycardia, cataplexy and paralysis: evidence of a sensitized opioid-mediated dissociative response following childhood trauma (in preparation—a)

Perry BD, Dobson C, Mann D, Schick S: Altered cognitive development in children exposed to chronic threat (in preparation—b)

Phillips RG, LeDoux JE: Differential contribution of amygdala and hippocampus to cued and contextual fear conditioning. Behav Neurosci 106:274–285, 1992

Plotsky PM, Meaney MJ: Early postnatal experience alters hypothalamic corticotrophin-releasing factor (CRF) mRNA, median eminence CRF content and stress-induced release in adult rats. Mol Brain Res 18:195–200, 1993

Sapolsky RM, Plotsky PM: Hypercortisolism and its possible neural bases. Biol Psychiatry 27:937–952, 1990

Sapolsky RM, Uno H, Rebert CS, et al: Hippocampal damage associated with prolonged glucocorticoid exposure in primates. J Neurosci 10:2897–2902, 1990

Selden NRW, Everitt BJ, Jarrard LE: Complementary roles for the amygdala and hippocampus in aversive conditioning to explicit and contextual cues. Neuroscience 42:335–350, 1991

Spitz R: Hospitalism: an inquiry into the genesis of psychiatric conditions in early childhood. Psychoanal Study Child 1:53–74, 1945

Teicher M, Ito Y, Glod CA, et al: Preliminary evidence for abnormal cortical development in physically and sexually abused children using EEG coherence and MRI. Ann NY Acad Sci 821:160–175, 1997

Vaid RR, Yee BK, Shalev U, et al: Neonatal nonhandling and in utero prenatal stress reduce the density of NADPH-diaphorase-reactive neurons in the fascia dentata and Ammon's Horn of rats. J Neurosci 17:5599–5609, 1997

Vallee M, Mayo W, Dellu F, et al: Prenatal stress induces high anxiety and postnatal handling induces low anxiety in adult offspring: correlation with stress-inducing corticosterone secretion. J Neurosci 17:2626–2636, 1997

Domestic Abuse as a Risk Factor for Children and Youth

Leah J. Dickstein, M.D.

Case Example 1

Five-year-old Sasha is referred to Dr. Clinton by his kindergarten teacher because he is not talking in school. He was adopted a year earlier from Russia, and the teacher at first attributed his silence to language problems. However, his mother, Mrs. Williams, reports that he speaks English well at home. His mother reluctantly agrees to a psychiatric consultation. Dr. Clinton meets with Sasha on a warm summer day and finds it odd that he is wearing a long-sleeved shirt. Sasha will not talk to Dr. Clinton but immerses himself in playing with the dollhouse where he depicts parents fighting and hitting each other. He carries on a monologue, but when approached directly about his home life, he shuts down. Curious about the long-sleeved shirt, Dr. Clinton asks him to roll up his sleeve. Sasha complies and Dr. Clinton finds recent cigarette burns on his forearm.

Case Example 2

Brandon is taxing his third-grade teacher with his impulsive and inappropriate behavior, which appears to be escalating. He is displaying highly sexualized behavior and is calling his female classmates "bitch" and other derogatory names. A referral is made to child protective services to rule out sexual abuse. They, in turn, request a consultation by a child psychologist, Dr. Thurlow.

Case Example 3

An attorney contacts Dr. Cushing regarding the attorney's 16-year-old client, Darlene, who is facing possible criminal charges in the death of her 1-month-old son, Joey, and who may be tried as an adult. He requests an evaluation regarding the matter of waiver and wonders about exculpatory factors in the case. Darlene has been in an abusive relationship with her 20-year-old boyfriend, Ray, who allegedly threw Joey into his crib because he was crying and interrupting his viewing of a Monday night football game on TV. Joey suffered a subdural hematoma from the blow and was found dead the next morning. The attorney wonders whether their abusive relationship was a factor in Darlene's failure to seek help.

LEGAL ISSUES

Reporting Where Minors Are Involved

In 1994, Tomkins reported that an estimated 3 million children witnessed their mothers being abused. In addition, children from homes in which there is domestic violence are themselves likely to become victims of violence. According to Jones (1996), Kuhlman, Lehto, and Mazura all emphasized that "whether liability for failure to report is based on a civil and/or criminal statute, most

Call 312–464–5066: Jean, for free copies of the American Medical Association treatment protocols on domestic violence, child abuse, and the mental health effects of family violence (American Medical News, September 23/30, 1996, pp. 20–21).

The author wishes to make a special acknowledgment to Jim Jones, Law Professor at the University of Louisville, for his expertise, reference and resource materials, and wonderful caring attitude.

hold the nonreporting physician actually must have recognized the patient intentionally was abused and still not have reported the battering before being held responsible for not doing so" (Jones 1996, p. 195).

Mandatory child abuse reporting laws went into effect in 1974, and early on statutes *singled out* the physician as a mandated reporter because it was felt that physicians had the necessary training and expertise to identify child abuse and that they often saw child abuse cases but chose not to report them. McAfee (1995) reported that more than 85% of Americans felt they could tell a physician if they were a victim of family abuse—a much higher percentage than those reporting they could tell the police (Jones 1996). The members of four professions are now mandated to report suspicions of child abuse or neglect: medicine, social service and other mental health, school, and law enforcement. The exact wording of child abuse reporting statutes varies from state to state. The professional who fails to report the abuse or violence may be held liable for injuries to the victim suffered after the time when the professional should have acted. However, they are considered liable only for injuries that occurred *after* the report should have been made.

Landeros v. Flood (1976) is the leading pro-liability decision reflecting negligence liability when failure to report child abuse occurs. In this case, the mother of an 11-month-old girl, Gita Landeros, took her to a California hospital for treatment. The child had been severely battered, but Flood, the examining physician, did not report her condition to the authorities. A physician at another hospital later saw the child, correctly diagnosed the continued abuse, and reported it. Flood was held liable for the subsequent abuse.

The *Tarasoff* ruling, where applicable, also applies to potential child abuse victims concerning the professional's duty to warn of possible threats by an abuser toward a child; thus both a failure to report and a *Tarasoff* claim could be charged against the professional. Physicians and other health professionals must understand and accept that they "owe a duty to the abuse victims they care for" (Jones 1999, p. 57). Davidson (1996) noted that "courts often treat abuse victims the same, regardless of whether they are children or spouses."

Child abuse is, like all domestic violence, not a private issue and can only be stopped by being taken seriously via mandatory reporting and punishment for violating reporting laws. Victims of abuse are often reluctant to report their victimization because of fear of retaliation by the perpetrator, self-blame, or loyalty to the perpetrator. The health professional must follow the law to protect those victims, and disclosure for reasons of safety must take precedence over patient confidentiality.

Resistance to Reporting

In a recent study of 400 family medicine, general internal medicine, and obstetrics/gynecology physicians (Rodriguez et al. 1999), about 79% reported they routinely screen injured patients for domestic abuse, 10% screened new patients, 9% screened patients at routine checkups, and 11% screened at the first prenatal visit. Obstetricians/gynecologists (17%) and other physicians practicing in public clinics (37%) were most likely to report this screening; internists and health maintenance organization (HMO) physicians were least likely to screen. Professionals who fail to report may do so because of concerns about patient confidentiality, anxiety about not knowing what to do about abuse, failure to ask about or recognize abuse, or fear of liability or repercussions. Possibly, they may not want to be bothered with the paperwork and possible court appearances. Many physicians fear that asking patients will result in a torrent of emotion or cause more problems.

Inform Family of Reporting

Clinicians should inform the family when they plan to report abuse or suspected abuse and explain that they are mandated reporters.

Battery as a Defense

Battery may be invoked as a defense by women who kill their batterers, or, as is discussed in Case Example 3, by women who are unable to intervene when a child is being abused.

Legislative Reforms

Major efforts to enable and encourage battered women to avoid using violence against their batterers include the Violence Crime Control and Law Enforcement Act of 1994, the largest crime bill in United States history; the American Medical Association's (AMA's) Physicians' Campaign Against Family Violence, begun in 1991; and Save-A-Shelter (1999)—sponsored by the AMA and the AMA Alliance—a national relief effort urging medical societies and alliances to "adopt" abuse shelters, transition homes, rape crisis centers, and other safe havens to help abuse victims. All these efforts are directed at the medical recognition, treatment, elimination, and education of the public about domestic violence.

Overview of Domestic Violence

Brief History

Given that its manifestations are similar to those of many other disorders, domestic violence is the "great mimic" of the late twentieth century, as tuberculosis was in the early 1900s (Dickstein 1988). The Association of American Medical Colleges' publication, *Academic Medicine*, in January 1997, included a supplement, Educating the Nations' Physicians About Family Violence and Abuse (Alpert et al. 1997). At the December 1996 AMA House of Delegates Meeting, Resolution 303 was amended to read "Education of Medical Students and Residents About Domestic Violence Screening" (American Psychiatric Association 1997).

Definition

Domestic violence most often takes the form of spousal abuse but often overlaps with child abuse. In 95% of cases, women are the victims in physical, emotional, psychological, sexual, and economic forms of abuse. There is no typical woman victim; 2 to 4 million women are victims annually. Abuse often begins in utero, because pregnant women are the most common victims (Uva 1997). All forms of abuse are used to perpetuate fear, intimidation, inappropriate control, and power by the perpetrator, who almost always is a man. No age group is immune, including the elderly, the most recently identified at-risk group.

Domestic abuse occurs among all racial, ethnic, socioeconomic, and religious groups. Perpetrators may be highly respected in their professional roles while abusing spouses and children and "acting out" behind closed doors. A recent book by Dr. Abraham Twerski, rabbi-psychiatrist, concerns domestic violence in the Jewish community. Sexual orientation—whether heterosexual, homosexual, or bisexual—does not affect the occurrence of violence; violence is prevalent in all sexually intimate relationships, whether formal marital bonds exist or partners simply live together (or live apart yet have a significant relationship).

Among women who do not work outside the home, vulnerability to violence can be greater and the ability to leave can be less, although, with courage, they often take the children and escape to family or friends or to the more than 1,500 women's shelters nationwide. (However, animal shelters still outnumber women's shelters!)

Prevalence

- The Federal Bureau of Investigation estimates that, in the United States, a woman is battered every 15 seconds and approximately 2 million people annually are battered by their spouses.
- Of the 18,692 homicides in the United States in 1984, 8.4% (i.e., 1,570 victims) involved one spouse killing the other (Boxer et al. 1997). Children are often witnesses to these homicides.
- Of all murdered women, 30% are killed by their known male partners.
- If a woman leaves an abusive situation, she runs a 75% higher risk that her former partner will murder her.
- Two of three victims return to the violent home from temporary shelters, and those who don't become part of the growing homeless population.
- Almost half of all injuries suffered by women seen in emergency rooms are due to battering, yet only 4% of those injuries are recognized as being caused by battering and the woman offered appropriate treatment.
- Seeking an end to battering is a cause of half the suicide attempts by African American women, and of one out of four suicide attempts by all women (Gaines and Kraska 1997).
- A handgun in the home is 43 times more likely to be used to kill a family member than to be used in self-defense. In addition, more than 1.7 million people annually are confronted by a spouse with a gun or a knife (Kellermann and Reay 1986).

Clearly, these statistics highlight the fact that some form of domestic violence occurs in at least half of the homes in the United States annually. Clinicians must be well informed of their state's laws, reporting procedures, and referral agency resources to offer patients.

Dynamics

Domestic abuse is a behavior learned throughout the life cycle—in childhood, adolescence, and adulthood—by victims, observers, and perpetrators. Ninety-five percent of abuse against girls and 80% of abuse against boys is perpetrated by men. Victimizers, and at times victims, lack effective verbal and nonverbal communication skills. Equally pertinent, these people have been stereotypically socialized as to sex role, that is, *mis*-socialized about "appropriate" roles for women and men, and these myths too often lead to potential and actual abuse. Common myths that perpetuate abuse include the beliefs that women are raised to be helpless in regard to caring for themselves while simultaneously being expected to be inordinately pleasing and helpful to others, at whatever cost to themselves. These women victims are taught early to suppress anger and assertiveness and instead to cry, overeat, and use alcohol and illicit and prescribed tranquilizers to numb their emotional pain. Abusing men are *mis*-socialized to be all-powerful, that is, to abuse power and to control at any price, and to perceive women as helpless and powerless. They deny their normal and vulnerable dependency feelings in order to maintain the appearance of being in control at all times and at any price. They may turn to alcohol or substance abuse to deal with their feelings, and, in turn, intoxication may lead to increased behavioral disinhibition and more violence.

Finkelhor (1988) identified three aspects of male sex-role socialization that increase the likelihood of abuse of women:

1. Men have difficulty acquiring nonsexual, intimate, interpersonal relationships, whereas women learn this behavior early, as they are more likely to care for small children.
2. Men are socialized to choose younger, smaller, less powerful individuals as sex partners, whereas women seek older, more powerful partners.
3. Men are socialized to feel that weakness and subordination are erotic stimuli.

Effects on Children and Adolescents

Physical Risk

In 1987, New York book editor Hedda Nussbaum revealed herself to be a domestic violence victim when police found her live-in partner, another professional, attorney Joel Steinberg, had abused her for years and beaten to death their 6-year-old adopted daughter, Lisa. The Nussbaum case is an infamous and tragic example of the effects of domestic violence on children. Despite the fact that they were both professionals, Steinberg severely abused his wife to the point that she was isolated from all contacts. Furthermore, she was physically beaten so severely, over time, that she was psychologically unable to protect herself and/or their adopted child. This couple did not fit the stereotype of being poor and uneducated, but they did fit the stereotype of the abuser isolating the victim to the point she could neither function nor defend herself or her child; furthermore, no one in their environs either noted her changed behavior or acted responsibly to report what they observed.

The documented physical abusers of adolescents are most often fathers; the abuse usually begins in adoles-

cence, related to interpersonal conflicts about adolescent developmental tasks and to parental midlife crises. In addition, adolescent male children who attempt to intervene in spousal abuse are at risk for being abused. Abusers of prepubertal children are usually single-parent, low-income mothers from ethnic minority groups.

Emotional Harm

One study found that children who witnessed family violence demonstrated similar behavioral and social maladjustment as child abuse victims (Jaffe et al. 1986).

Children exposed to high levels of family and marital conflict are also at increased risk for becoming violent in the future (Farrington 1989; McCord 1979). Studies of psychiatric disturbance in abused children and adolescents who have been referred for treatment have found the following: impulsivity (Martin and Beezley 1977), hyperactivity or depression (Martin and Beezley 1977), conduct disorders, learning disabilities (Salzinger et al. 1984), substance abuse (Kaplan 1996), and a high incidence of nightmares and night terrors (Cuddy and Belicki 1992). There are increases in suicide attempts (Kaplan 1996) and increases in self-mutilation and running away. Additionally, delinquent and violent adolescents frequently have histories of physical abuse (Truscott 1993).

Interventions

Recognition

Recognition of abuse within a family must begin with the clinician's awareness of how common it is and how stereotypical thinking about victims and perpetrators can prevent a timely diagnosis of abuse. The clinician should interview the child or adolescent patient separately from the parent(s) and/or caretaker(s) in order to take an in-depth history and conduct a thorough physical examination. Generally, the observed injuries are more severe than could reasonably be attributed to the claimed cause, from diagnosed subdural hematomas to burns and soft-tissue bruises resembling the article used to inflict the injury. The story of how the injuries occurred may be inconsistent with findings and may change over time. Physical, medical, and emotional neglect must be evaluated according to developmental and situational expectations (e.g., no immunizations or winter clothing, failure to thrive). The possibility that sexual abuse is also occurring may need to be explored.

Asking the Right Questions

All clinicians evaluating children and adolescents for all forms of abuse must be specifically trained to conduct examinations. The child needs to be given permission to talk about possible abuse, and the clinician needs to avoid leading questions (see Chapter 15, "Interviewing Children for Suspected Sexual Abuse").

Therapy for the Child Witness or Victim

The forensic clinician needs to be aware of effective treatments, as he or she is often asked to make recommendations to the court in this regard. Treatment of the child or adolescent begins with crisis intervention when the clinician first becomes aware of the abuse and becomes involved professionally. A basic principle of treatment includes helping the child realize that the person(s) who abused him or her are at fault and the child is not, even though the child or adolescent may be compliant regarding the abuse. The clinician must repeatedly make it explicitly clear that adults should protect, not abuse, children and adolescents. Another basic treatment focus is helping the child understand that though the abuser or the child victim may be taken out of the home, once again, it is not the child's fault.

Treatment modalities are of major importance to the potential healing of the victim and include: general medical care when necessary; individual supportive psychotherapy, peer group therapy, psychoeducation, and cognitive behavioral therapy as indicated—in stages of readiness and need; and pharmacotherapy when indicated. To begin family and/or group therapy too early and without individual treatment of the adult in-home perpetrator can be dangerous. Issues in treatment of the child victim include managing anger, learning trust, understanding the uses and abuses of power, and improving self-esteem.

Responses to violence vary by age, type of abuse, and chronicity of abuse, and treatment needs to be tailored to the child's unique experience.

> Preschool child witnesses are more affected and show more reactive behaviors such as generalized fears, regression, clinging and irritability. Schoolage children evidence sleep, somatic and school problems. Adolescents may run away, become delinquent, marry early or become pregnant. (Pelcovitz and Kaplan 1994, p. 750)

Witnessing chronic parental violence can result in posttraumatic stress disorder, type 2, as described by Terr (1991), with denial, dissociation, attention-deficit/hyperactivity disorder, conduct disorders, and depression (Braun 1986). Children may react differently depending on whether they witnessed physical or verbal abuse or actually experienced it. Reactions also vary by sex: among children who witness abuse, females are more likely to show withdrawal, passivity, and depression, whereas boys externalize the abuse with aggression. Boys are more likely to be targets of both parents' aggression because mothers see their sons as similar to their fathers and because boys are more likely to defend their mothers, thus invoking their fathers' rage.

Perpetrators

Treatment programs for perpetrators must be on a long-term basis, always designed to first protect the child or adolescent from any further abuse. Individual, group, family (in some but not all cases), and marital therapy; pharmacotherapy and substance abuse treatment; violence control; and parenting and child development education are often necessary for the parent-perpetrators and passive parent victim-observers of child abuse. Treatment for parents is often challenging because of the parents' own early abuse experiences and consequent abusive life experiences. A pioneering Boston, Massachusetts, program, EMERGE, for adult male perpetrators remanded by the courts to learn about gender roles and issues and effective and appropriate verbal and nonverbal communication, has proven very effective. Only after perpetrators have made substantial progress and gained insight into their personal lives and coping skills, or lack thereof, should family therapy be considered (Dickstein 1999).

Spousal Victims

Therapy for spousal victims must be easily available and safety parameters need to be established. Spousal victims, long used to suffering in silence, must be constantly encouraged to recognize that in order to care appropriately and safely for their children, they must first develop healthier self-esteem by caring for themselves.

Reporting

As already described, reporting in a timely manner is mandatory for all clinicians. Domestic violence assistance guidelines must be developed by all county and state police departments, in coordination with local government offices for women, and made available in the form of handout materials at multiple sites where women, men, adolescents, and children can easily and readily gain access to them.

Information on domestic abuse should be made available to victims, including the following sources of help: county and city police; 24-hour crisis hot lines as well as adult, child, and spousal abuse hot lines; legal assistance, such as the Legal Aid Society; and counseling and support groups. Information on how to obtain an emergency protective order and emergency housing, including shelters, should also be supplied.

SUMMARY

Domestic abuse as a risk factor for children and youths is a major health concern, and possibly an underrecognized public health epidemic. Improved clinician training, together with education of teachers, parents, children, and everyone in the community, must become a priority. To do less is tantamount to sanctioning the senseless, harmful, and often tragic subsequent development of traumatized children and youths who, without recognition of the abuse and effective treatment, will become psychiatrically impaired adults—adults who will often be unable to care effectively and appropriately for themselves, those with whom they attempt to relate, or their future progeny.

In light of our current general medical and psychiatric research data, diagnostic acumen, and effective treatment modalities, all clinicians must assume appropriate responsibilities to treat patients correctly.

PITFALLS

Denial

Treating professionals may fail to consider or ask about the possibility of domestic violence in patients' lives because of denial.

Stereotypes

Dangerous stereotypes (e.g., domestic violence only occurs among the poor or uneducated, and usually only among minority group members) can result in failure to ask about abuse. Clinicians may fail to consider that men may also be victims of domestic abuse.

Countertransference

Clinicians who have not come to terms with abuse, or the possibility of abuse, in their own lives may fail to ask about it. They may overidentify with certain patients and fail to consider the possibility of the occurrence of abuse among the educated and economically privileged (e.g., among physicians and health professionals), in which abuse may more likely be well hidden and denied.

Attributing Symptoms and Findings to Other Causes

Clinicians may fall prey to accepting glossed-over explanations of the discovered trauma or abuse and fail to interview and examine the patient about suspicious injuries without the accompanying adult present.

Minimizing Extent of Abuse

The clinician may minimize the extent of abuse and its emotional impact on the victim or on the children who witness it.

CASE EXAMPLE EPILOGUES

Case Example 1

Dr. Clinton meets again with Sasha's mother, who keeps sunglasses on throughout the interview. He confronts her with his findings. She tearfully breaks down and reveals a long and sordid history of domestic abuse; she says that Sasha's father burned him as a warning not to disclose the abuse in school. As she removes her sunglasses to dry her tears, Dr. Clinton notices that she has a black eye. She states she was fearful of seeking help or disclosing the abuse because her husband had threatened her that he would take Sasha, their only child, from her and that she would never see him again.

Dr. Clinton tells her he must report the abuse and plans are made to get her and Sasha to a safe house. He agrees to continue to work with Sasha.

Case Example 2

Brandon demonstrates his uninhibited behavior in Dr. Thurlow's office, and she wonders if he might have attention-deficit/hyperactivity disorder. However, she also considers a study on normative sexual behavior (Friedrich et al. 1991) that found that exposure to family violence can have a dysregulating effect on children, resulting in increased aggressive and sexual behavior (see Chapter 19, "Neurodevelopmental Impact of Violence in Childhood"). Brandon denies any history of sexual abuse. When asked where he learned his sexual vocabulary, he says from his dad, who uses the same terms to refer to his mother. He goes on to detail the fights and mutual name-calling that are almost daily occurrences in his home. He is also exposed to a lot of violence and sexuality on TV, which is poorly monitored in his home. Dr. Thurlow details her concerns in her report to child protective services and recommends treatment for all of the family members.

Case Example 3

Darlene is seen and relates how she left her abusive home at age 14 and quit school to move in with Ray, whom she could talk to, and who seemed to treat her well. Things changed when she became pregnant. Ray lost his job, began drinking more, and became very possessive of her. He criticized her housekeeping and cooking and had little sympathy for her morning sickness. He once threw a plate of eggs at her because they were not cooked to his satisfaction. He began berating her verbally and cut her off from her friends. After their baby was born, she felt very alone and depressed. She stayed in the relationship in hopes she could please Ray and because she didn't feel she could raise their baby alone.

She described Ray's hurling their baby into the crib, hearing Joey's head strike the crib frame, and how the baby then stopped crying. She wanted to go check on him, but Ray wouldn't let her; he yelled at her to "Leave Joey alone and let him sleep." She said she pleaded with him, but he became more angry and threatening and she felt afraid. She breaks down in tears and now tries to blame herself for not calling 911.

Dr. Cushing laments the fact that more neonatal services were not provided to this high-risk family. He notes in his letter to the referring attorney that Darlene's history of abuse, her immaturity, passivity, and dependency, and Ray's domination all made it difficult for her to call for help. He notes that years of emotional abuse undermined her sense of self and ability to assert herself, and that she never had the opportunity for treatment in the past. Finally, he underscores the fact that she has never been violent.

ACTION GUIDELINES

Consider Domestic Abuse

Early diagnosis of domestic violence can be made if patients, in this instance, children and adolescents, are questioned carefully and empathically during the first and follow-up evaluation and treatment appointments. If the children and adolescents' presenting symptoms persist, clinicians must, in a supportive manner, ask again about domestic violence experiences.

Explore Impact

Clinicians need to encourage the child's trust and explore the effect of family violence on the child. A child requires ongoing support regarding his or her disclosures and the aftermath on the family's functioning.

Be Familiar With Reporting Laws

Clinicians and their staff must be familiar with reporting laws in their state and have prearranged reporting procedures that are easily accessible. Furthermore, they must be prepared to testify in court and carefully document disclosures and physicians' findings.

REFERENCES

Alpert EJ, Cohen S, Sege RD: Family violence: an overview. Acad Med 72 (1 suppl):S3–S6, 1997

American Psychiatric Association: APA delegate summary of American Medical Association House of Delegates meeting, American Psychiatric Association, Washington, DC, February 25, 1997

Boxer B, Wyden R, Morella C: The Domestic Violence Identification and Referral Act 5.101, HR 884, in J Haynes Douglas NOW Legal Defense and Educational Fund Meeting Announcement and Issue Update, March 12, 1997, p 3

Braun B: Treatment of Multiple Personality Disorder. Washington, DC, American Psychiatric Press, 1986

Cuddy M, Belicki K: Nightmare frequency and related sleep disturbance as indicators of a history. Dreaming: Journal of the Association for the Study of Dreams 2:15–22, 1992

Davidson H: Family Violence: A Clinical and Legal Guide. Washington, DC, American Psychiatric Press, 1996

Dickstein L: Spouse Abuse and Other Domestic Violence, in The Violent Patient. Psychiatr Clin North Am 11:611–627, 1988

Dickstein L: Domestic violence, in Medical Management of the Violent Patient. Edited by Tardiff K. New York, Marcel Dekker, 1999, pp 359–380

Farrington DP: Early predictors of adolescent aggression and adult violence. Violence Vict 4:79–100, 1989

Finkelhor D: Many myths said to surround child sex abuse. Psychiatric News, January 1988, pp 28–29

Friedrich WN, Grambsch P, Broughton D, et al: Normative sexual behavior in children. Pediatrics 88:456–464, 1991

Gaines L, Kraska P: Drugs, Crime and Justice: Contemporary Perspectives. Prospect Heights, IL, Waveland Press, 1997

Jaffe P, Wolfe D, Wilson S, et al: Similarities in behavioral and social maladjustments among child victims and witnesses to family violence. Am J Orthopsychiatry 56:142–146, 1986

Jones J: Battered spouses' damage action against non-reporting physicians. DePaul Law Review 45:191–262, 1996

Jones J: Kentucky tort liability for failure to report family violence. Northern Kentucky Law Review 26(1):43, 1999

Kaplan S (ed): Child abuse (special issue). Child Adolesc Psychiatr Clin North Am 3(4), 1994

Kaplan S: Family Violence: A Clinical and Legal Guide. Washington, DC, American Psychiatric Press, 1996

Kellermann AL, Reay DT: Protection or peril? an analysis of firearm-related deaths in the home. N Engl J Med 314: 1557–1560, 1986

Landeros v Flood, 17 Cal.3d 399, 413–414 (1976)

Martin HP, Beezley P: Behavioral observations of abused children. Dev Med Child Neurol 19:373–387, 1977

McAfee O: Physicians and Domestic Violence. JAMA 273:1790–1791, 1995

McCord J: Some child-rearing antecedents of criminal behavior in adult men. J Pers Soc Psychol 37:1477–1486, 1979

Pelcovitz D, Kaplan SJ: Child witnesses of violence between parents: psychosocial correlates and implications for treatment. Child Adolesc Psychiatr Clin North Am 3:745–758, 1994

Rodriguez MA, Bauer HM, McLoughlin E, et al: Screening and intervention for intimate partner abuse: practices and attitudes of primary care physicians. JAMA 282:468–474, 1999

Salzinger S, Kaplan S, Pelcovitz D, et al: Parent and teacher assessment of children's behavior in child maltreating families. Journal of the American Academy of Child Psychiatry 23:458–464, 1984

Terr L: Childhood traumas: an outline and overview. Am J Psychiatry 148:10–20, 1991

Truscott D: Adolescent offenders: comparison for sexual, violent and property offences. Psychol Rep 73:657–658, 1993

Uva J: Family violence: how residents can break the cycle (letter). JAMA 277:288, 1997

SUGGESTED READINGS

Finkelhor D, Gelles R, Hotaling G, et al (eds): The Dark Side of Families: Current Family Violence Research. Newbury Park, CA, Sage, 1983

Fritsch TA, Frederich KW: Mandatory reporting of domestic violence and coordination with child protective services. Domestic Violence Report 3(4), April/May 1998

Gerteis M: Through the Patient's Eyes: Understanding and Promoting Patient-Centered Care. San Francisco, CA, Jossey-Bass, 1993

Horowitz K, Weine S, Jekel J: PTSD symptoms in urban adolescent girls: compounded community trauma. J Am Acad Child Adolesc Psychiatry 34:1353–1361, 1995

Jaffe P, Wolfe D, Wilson S: Children of Battered Women, Newbury Park, CA, Sage, 1990

Kinard EM: Emotional Development in Physically Abused Children: A Study of Self-Concept and Aggression. Palo Alto, CA, R & E Research Associates, 1982

Koop C, Lundberg G: Violence in America: a public health emergency. JAMA 267:3075–3076, 1992

McKay M: The link between domestic violence and child abuse: assessment and treatment considerations. Child Welfare 73:29–39, 1994

Shaffer T: Legal interviewing and counseling in a nutshell. Eagen, MN, West Group, 1997

Twerski A: The Shame Borne in Silence: Spouse Abuse in the Jewish Community. New York, Mikov Publications, 1996

CHAPTER 21

Effects of Witnessing Violence on Children and Adolescents

Cheryl S. Al-Mateen, M.D.

TYPES OF VIOLENCE

Violence has been declared a public health problem by the Centers for Disease Control. A juvenile's history of exposure to violence affects our assessment of his potential to perpetrate violence. It may also affect clinical treatment when the youth is encountered in the juvenile justice system. In addition to violence in the home, which is discussed in Chapter 20, "Domestic Abuse as a Risk Factor for Children and Youth," children often witness violence in the media and the community. For the purposes of this chapter, community violence includes both war and terrorism in the community at large, as well as neighborhood violence.

Children and adolescents can be exposed to violence in multiple settings. The remotest form in which violence can be witnessed is through the media, such as in the movies, on television, and in music. However, video and computer game violence is not remote, as the player is actively involved. Violence moves closer, with potential threat to the individual, in situations of community and domestic violence. Finally, a child may become a direct victim or perpetrator of violence.

LEGAL ISSUES

Exposure to media violence has been cited as contributory in various crimes. Strasburger (1995) describes one case in which a 7-year-old found his parents' .357 Magnum and ammunition, loaded it, and accidentally killed his 3-year-old sister. He reports two different instances in which children set fires, imitating Beavis and Butthead. Michael Carneal, a 14-year-old who had only fired a handgun once before, fired eight shots—hitting a different teenager each time, killing three and wounding five. He learned to shoot by playing video games (Grossman and DeGaetano 1999).

The role of the forensic mental health professional includes both the assessment of exposure of the juvenile to violence as well as recognizing the effects of this exposure. This chapter focuses on the assessment of the exposure to violence, the psychosocial effects of witnessing its different forms, and the ways these experiences may contribute to the later perpetration of violence.

EXPOSURE TO VIOLENCE

Community Violence

War and Terrorism

The child and adolescent psychiatrist may evaluate and treat children and adolescents who have emigrated from such diverse war zones as Cambodia, the Middle East, the Balkans, or central Africa. Children raised in war have experienced an extreme most others cannot imagine. Their lifestyle is focused on basic survival and their attempts to obtain food, water, shelter, electricity, and basic health (Gabarino et al. 1992). Malnutrition may have placed the child at risk for disease as well as disruption of the growth and development of neurological and other systems.

Children raised in terrorism may experience, witness, or hear of rape, torture, and murder on an impromptu or organized basis by individuals or the military. They may have been targeted for genocide. Children may have been recruited or know others who committed violent and cruel acts in defense of their families, neighborhoods, or culture.

Children living in these environments have witnessed air raids, missile attacks, interrogations, arrests, and the imprisonment of (or other separation from) parents. Youngsters experience psychological distress when a parent is imprisoned for political purposes, even when full details are hidden from the child. It is particularly important with refugee families to obtain a specific history of exposure to organized violence, optimally through the use of direct interview or play techniques (Almqvist and Brandell-Forsberg 1995).

Studies of children in Vietnam, the Middle East, and Bosnia have found that children exposed to war show increased aggression (Almqvist and Brandell-Forsberg 1995). Preschoolers are more likely to develop symptoms than older children (Gabarino et al. 1992; Weine et al. 1995). As there are less mature neurological resources, the child is less capable of understanding the overwhelming events around him. This is consistent with known neurophysiological changes in the brain as a result of exposure to violence between the ages of 6 months and 6 years (Kostelny and Gabarino 1994; see Chapter 19, "Neurodevelopmental Impact of Violence in Childhood").

Parents are the most important factor in protecting the child's cognitive and emotional development from this overwhelming stressor (Gabarino et al. 1992). Children who live in communities where there is war or terrorism experience chronic, repetitive stressors but often do not reveal the full extent of these experiences to their parents. Parents may also underestimate their children's reactions to such experiences (Almqvist and Brandell-Forsberg 1995).

The child who is raised with a foundation of religious or nationalist ideology as a support and as the basis for the family's struggle can find this ideology helpful for coping. It can also be protective against the need for the use of violence as a means of revenge (Gabarino et al. 1992; Kostelny and Gabarino 1994). Removal of the refugee family to a safe and supportive environment can result in a decrease in psychiatric symptoms with good functioning over time (Sack et al. 1993).

Immediate Community—Neighborhood Violence

Chronic community violence has been defined as "frequent and continual exposure to the use of guns, knives, drugs, and random violence" (Osofsky 1995). It is generated from an interaction of poverty, racism, marginality, hopelessness, the drug economy, gangs, rage, and the availability of weaponry (Bell 1997; Gabarino et al. 1992). The effects of community violence are not only from seeing the violent acts but also from protective limitations placed on a child's activities. These include restricting outside play or having to sleep, do homework, or watch television on the floor to avoid stray bullets from drive-by shootings (Gabarino et al. 1992). Many violent events that take place in neighborhoods and schools are witnessed by children, who are often emotionally close to the victims (Jenkins and Bell 1997). The effects of violence in a child's immediate community are quite similar to the effects of war and terrorism described earlier (Gabarino et al. 1992).

Children who are most likely to be able to cope effectively with dangerous environments are those whose parents are not overwhelmed by stressors as well (Fick et al. 1997). This, however, is difficult, as parents in neighborhoods with high levels of violence are more likely to be living in poverty, to have low-birth-weight babies, to be unmarried, and to have begun child-rearing as teenagers. These multiple stressors increase the likelihood that the parent may develop depression, becoming emotionally inaccessible or neglectful. Even parents who do not experience a significant psychiatric reaction to such stressors may be severely taxed emotionally and, as a result, affect the child's coping mechanisms. A parent who is traumatized may fail to recognize or acknowledge the level of trauma the child is experiencing. In studies of both war and community violence, it becomes apparent that parents are not aware of every traumatic experience a child has (Richters and Martinez 1993a).

Many children raised in violent communities may not have the predictable lifestyle and socialization through community institutions available to those in less violent settings (Hill 1995). As a result, their sense of safety is eroded, and they can have an increased sense of fatalism and of having no future. These young people often believe that they will die before they reach age 20. Feeling no other option than a need to immediately leave their mark on the world, these children and adolescents may engage in risk-taking, immortalizing behaviors as a result. There is also likely to be an increase in the use of violence to solve interpersonal conflicts (Hill 1994). Children who experience their first trauma before age 11 are more likely to develop psychiatric symptoms than those who experience their first trauma as teenagers (Davidson and Smith 1990). Exposure to endemic violence impairs the development of a sense of trust, and chronic exposure may lead to more severe problems. Exposure to high levels of community violence is related to conduct and emotional problems and increases the likelihood of the child becoming a perpetrator of violence in the future (Cooley-Quille et al. 1995; Gabarino et al. 1992).

Media Violence

Children and adolescents at the dawn of the new millennium have a wide range of venues available to vicariously experience violence. Violence can be found on broadcast, cable, and pay-per-view television, in movies in theaters and to rent, in music, in computer and video games, and over the Internet. With the development of computer graphics and special effects, the violence seen by children today is far more realistic than that in the 1960s and 1970s (Heath et al. 1989).

The maligning of violence in the media is of a different nature than is maligning community violence. Interpersonally, there are no positive aspects of war, or neighborhood or domestic violence. No agency champions the need for drive-by shootings. The media, however, has the capacity to teach, entertain, and foster positive development. When used to teach positive social themes, its beneficial potential is unlimited. Public service announcements and dramatic renditions of social issues provide a forum for discussion and enlightenment. As technology skills develop through the use of computers, self-confidence grows and problem-solving and motor skills improve. Music and the other arts serve as an outlet of expression for the composers' and listeners' emotions. The media are useful (American Medical Association 1996). Because of these positive characteristics, the media's negative aspects are not as easily recognized. This is seen most readily in parents of today's young and school-age children—this group has always had television, and, as a result, its members may have difficulty recognizing some of its insidious effects.

The American Academy of Pediatrics identifies violence in the media to be the "most easily remediable…factor" that contributes to violence (American Academy of Pediatrics 1995). The first governmental hearings on television violence were held in 1952 (Grossman and DeGaetano 1999). The media in the United States are more violent than that in the rest of the world (American Academy of Pediatrics 1995; Strasburger 1995). It has been noted that only Japan approaches the United States in the amount of violence depicted in entertainment. Japan, however, is not as violent a country as the United States. What is clear is that the nature of Japanese media violence is different. "Bad guys" commit most of the violence and "good guys" suffer from the violence; as a result, violence is seen as villainous and wrong, with painful consequences. The audience identifies more with the hero, who is not violent (Iwao et al. 1981).

Television and Movies

Television violence can be defined as "any overt depiction of the use of physical force—or the credible threat of such force—intended to physically harm an animate being or group of beings…also includes certain depictions of physically harmful consequences against an animate being or group that occur as a result of unseen violent means" (Mediascope, Inc. 1996b). Merely the presence of television in a community can increase the level of verbal and physical aggression seen in both adults and children (Williams 1986). In the 3 years (1994–1997) of the National Television Violence Study, which reviewed thousands of hours of television, 60% of all television programs (including broadcast, basic, and premium cable, excluding public broadcasting) consistently showed violence (Federman 1997, 1998; Wilson et al. 1996).

Currently, it is estimated that a child will have witnessed 8,000 murders via the media by the end of elementary school (Cloud 1999). Physiological arousal is seen in children watching violent television (Gröer and Howell 1990), with effects as noted in Chapter 19. Effects on the child's growing brain may be seen in children watching unlimited amounts of television, regardless of content (Healy 1998). These include lowered attention span and academic performance.

The television parental guidelines rating system was implemented in January 1997. Shows were rated with regard to their intended audience. Shows intended for children can be rated TVY (for all children) or TVY7 (for children over 7 years old). General audience shows are rated TVG (general), TVPG (parental guidance), TV14 (children over 14 years old), or TVMA (mature audiences). Children's programming shows consistently higher levels of violence throughout the day than dramas, comedy, movies, music videos, or reality-based shows. Significant levels of violence are seen in shows rated TVY and TVY7 (Federman 1998). Advertisers have even begun to use violence in marketing. One print example is using a black male model with abdominal scars consistent with knife and bullet wounds to advertise jeans (Hickey 1998).

The literature on television violence has wavered at times between whether the potential cathartic effect of watching violent television outweighs potential negative effects (Dill and Dill 1998; Vos Post 1995). In their review, Grossman and DeGaetano (1999) list immediate and long-term reactions to television violence. They describe "intense fear, crying, clinging behaviors, and stomachaches" (p. 36) as the former, with "nightmares and difficulty sleeping, concern about being hurt or killed, and aversion to common animals" (p. 36) as the latter.

There are three reported major effects of television violence (Molitor and Hirsch 1994). The first is a direct effect. Children and adults who watch a lot of violence on television may become more aggressive and develop favorable attitudes towards the use of aggression as a means of problem solving. Children who are more aggressive are more likely to be affected by violence on television. Some studies have found significant modeling effects of reports of violence in the media, including highly publicized suicides (Phillips and Carstensen 1986). Children imitate what they see on television, including the violent heroes (American Medical Association 1996). Television viewing is positively correlated with aggression in both boys and girls from age 8 through later in life (Eron and Huesmann 1984; Heath et al. 1989).

The second and third effects are indirect. It is thought that repeated exposure to violent scenes on television can desensitize those that watch the violence, resulting in an increased appetite for violence (American Medical Association 1996). Finally, in "The Mean World Syndrome" (Gerbner and Signorielli 1990), children and adults who watch a great deal of violence on television see the world as a meaner and more dangerous place. Children have a more emotional response to shows with realistic violence such as news reports and realism shows (American Medical Association 1996).

Children under age 8 have difficulty distinguishing between fantasy and reality on television—they believe all commercials and may not recognize that a character is a different person from the actor playing him (American Academy of Pediatrics 1995). They are more likely to imitate an unrealistic or fantasy character than one who is realistic (Perry and Bussey 1977). This causes even more concern about the cartoon violence in TVY-rated shows. Preschoolers who watch violent television have less imaginative play and spend more time imitating the aggressive acts they see on television. This diminishes the creative and developmental benefits of play. This effect is enhanced if the child is re-creating scenes from a television show with toys based on the show's characters (National Association for the Education of Young Children 1990).

Children in special education programs who are identified as emotionally disturbed have a higher baseline rate of aggressive behavior; they are also more likely to watch television shows with aggression than regular students or those classified as learning disabled do. These children are less able to distinguish the fantasy aspects of television from reality and are more likely to identify with and imitate the violent characters. These factors are additive, with the end result being that these children appear to be more vulnerable to the negative effects of television violence (Gadow and Sprafkin 1993).

Mediating comments by adults and education about the unreal nature of television violence can help children assess their viewing more critically (Molitor and Hirsch 1994; Voojis and van der Voort 1993). Children whose parents are actively involved in their television viewing are less interested in shows designated as violent (Federman 1997). Some teens deliberately watch only the violent scenes of movies on videocassette (Pennell and Browne 1999). In her discussion of television violence, Tepperman (1997) reported Centerwall's finding that up to one-third of a group of felons indicated they had deliberately imitated criminal behaviors they had seen on television.

Television violence does not affect all children equally nor does it incite violence in all individuals. Violence has been found most likely to facilitate imitative violence if the criteria in Table 21–1 are met (American Medical Association 1996; Federman 1998). The more realistic the violence is, the more likely it is to beget viewer violence. The use of violence is reinforced most strongly if it can be seen as justified, that is, perpetrated by the protagonist in fighting "the bad guy." The viewer who feels that the violent situation on television is reminiscent of his or her life is more likely to become violent. Of note is the conflict in the literature regarding humor. Some reviewers indicate that corrective humor is helpful. Others indicate that humor associated with violence helps increase the desensitization (Strasburger 1995). In addition, if the violence is associated with a sexual conquest, or if the viewer was already angry when watching the violence, the chance of imitative violence is increased (Comstock and Strasburger 1990; Strasburger 1995).

The literature concludes that exposure to violence in the media is correlated with serious aggressive behavior (Heath et al. 1989). This direct contribution is seen only in some individuals and may be of small magnitude. However, if the small magnitude is the difference

TABLE 21–1.   Sensational violence—media factors that foster violent behavior

Graphic or realistic violence
Use of gun or knife
Lack of consequences/reward for violence
Violence seen as justified
Identification with the perpetrator
No critical commentary
Violence related to sexual conquest

Source.   Adapted from American Medical Association 1996; Federman 1998.

between nonviolence and violence, then it cannot be considered negligible (Rosenthal 1986).

Music and Music Videos

"Older people are used to listening to rhythm and blues or rock and roll where the words were everything. Rap is about the beat. I just let my body go and dance." These are the words of a teenager attempting to explain the differences between today's forms of music and those which today's adults listened to in their youth; they are confirmed by the scientific literature. Teens listen to between 20 and 40 hours of music per week (Strasburger 1995). Music has long been one form of conscious or unconscious rebellion to adult society. The provocative nature of many types of music has long served as part of music's purpose in development (Strasburger 1995). Rap and heavy metal exist on a continuum with their more extreme forms, gangsta rap and industrial rock. Often, the beat of these forms of music is more prominent than the lyrics. Many adults have become concerned about these lyrics because of their themes of violence, suicide, or homicide; the worry is that adolescents who listen to these forms of music are being instructed to engage in forms of violence against themselves and/or others. Many youths focus, instead, on the rhythm (the beat), as the lyrics may be almost unintelligible on first listen. The emotional flavor of the music also serves as a release, which many teens will use to verbalize their mood.

The lyrics are more prevalent in alternative music, where, as in rhythm and blues or rock and roll, they often focus on romantic feelings. The types of music that fall under the broad category of "metal" are differentiated by the type of beat and the instruments used. Heavy-metal musicians may use more guitar, whereas industrial artists may use more metallic, banging sounds, with a more difficult to discern beat. Punk is a form of metal that often uses an "angrier" beat. The various forms of rap describe life experiences, reactions to these experiences, and relationship issues through poetry accompanied by a beat.

They range from the more positive descriptions of "hip-hop" to the often profoundly violent and negative characterizations that may be found in gangsta rap. Adolescents from different cultural backgrounds may listen to different forms of music. Parents often become concerned when their child listens to music that is perceived as coming from another cultural background.

For the clinician, it is most useful to inquire regarding what kinds of music the young person listens to. Many will listen to a variety. One should not assume, because the adolescent listens to a form of rap or metal, that the juvenile is automatically at risk for perpetrating violence. It is most informative to learn what aspect of the music the teen enjoys. The evaluator should delve most deeply into the music history of those who are preoccupied with the more extreme forms with the goal of understanding whether the chosen form of music is an expression of marginalism, depression, or some other area of concern (Strasburger 1995).

Music has even more affective impact when accompanied by visual images. Music videos are available in several genres including rock, rap, rhythm and blues, and country. Concern about videos relates to the connection of sex and violence (Strasburger 1995) and the portrayal of violence. Rock and rap videos are most likely to depict episodes of violence (DuRant et al. 1997). Similarly, the carrying of weapons, often by children, is most often seen in rock and rap videos. Country videos are least likely to portray weapon carrying.

The images of women in videos frequently involve sex and violence, which can contribute to the detrimental treatment of women in general. There is a concern as well about the misogynist lyrics in some rap, which are seen as promoting abusive treatment of women. Most music videos with violence have an attractive role model perpetrating that violence, leading to the belief that this is acceptable behavior. Music videos also reinforce inaccurate stereotypes of violent black males and vulnerable white females (Rich et al. 1998).

Computer and Video Games

After a child becomes inured to passively experienced violent imagery on television and videotapes, the next step is active participation in the violence through video games. There are benefits of video games, such as improved hand-eye coordination, relaxation, and the ability to support rehabilitative services in some populations. We know less about the effects of video games than we do about the effects of television (Strasburger 1995). However, these games have become progressively more realistic since their introduction in the early 1970s. Furthermore, the player's point of view in the game has advanced from a third-person to a first-person perspective. This helps make the game a more effective "killing simulator," with frequent repetitions and accompanying positive reinforcement, similar to training methods used for law enforcement and military personnel. In contrast to what is found in military training, however, players of video games are always rewarded for shooting; the failure to shoot is never the correct option (Grossman and DeGaetano 1999).

Boys average about 4 hours weekly playing violent video games, and girls average about 2 hours weekly. Additional time is spent on nonviolent games (Dill and Dill 1998). Most children find the games habit-forming, often playing longer than they had initially intended (Griffiths and Hunt 1995). Video games have more impact than television because of several factors. These include the fact that video games are more interactive, requiring violent actions from the individual playing them. These violent actions are justified, either to complete a mission or in self-defense. There are additional direct rewards for violent behaviors in the form of points and increasing levels of accomplishment. As the goal of the game is often to encourage aggressive actions, there are no realistic consequences for violent behavior in the more violent video games. Empathy toward others may be discouraged in games that frame other individuals as targets instead of as people. Violent video games often promote stereotyped images of women as helpless and/or objects for violent victimization. Finally, video games utilize several means of teaching simultaneously: modeling, practice, and reinforcement, as well as associating violence with fun. Virtual reality games are a more extreme form of the same problem (Dill and Dill 1998; Griffiths and Hunt 1995). Both boys and girls experience an increase in aggression and/or violence as a result of observing or playing virtual reality or video games. The increase is greater with virtual reality games (Dill and Dill 1998).

Internet

The Internet is used for many purposes, including communication (through e-mail, bulletin boards, and chat rooms), education (surfing for research or current news), and fun (such as multiplayer games). Although there is useful material available for all ages, violent, hate-oriented material may be accessed either purposefully or by accident, when sites are accessed while conducting a search.

Web sites may be established by actual hate groups or by individuals. Many are aimed directly at children. They may have violently racist or religiously intolerant jokes or cartoons, videos, or sexually related material ("163 and Counting," 1998). The ease of reaching thousands of people through this medium provides a means of recruitment not previously available. In the past, recruitment generally targeted teens who were isolated, not attending school, or on the streets for some reason. Through the Internet, smarter, younger, more affluent, and less marginalized youths are targeted. Some are merely bored and looking for something new. They are more vulnerable to indoctrination at younger ages ("A Skinhead's Story," 1998). In 1998 there were 537 hate groups in existence in the United States ("Hate Group Count Tops 500," 1999). This number rose to 602 in 2000 ("Hate Group Numbers Rise," 2001). In 1998, 254 hate sites based in the United States could be found on the Internet ("Hate Group Count Tops 500," 1999). In 2001, 366 U.S.-based hate sites were identified ("Hate Group Numbers Rise," 2001). Many of these sites describe or condone violence. All are accessible to children and adolescents searching the Internet.

Cumulative Effects

The greater the number of violent stressful events that a juvenile is exposed to, the more frequently aggression will be seen in the future (Attar et al. 1994). The greater the amount of personal experience with violence, the more hopeless the juvenile will feel, likely resulting in the expectation of an early and/or violent death for him- or herself (DuRant et al. 1995; Hinton-Nelson et al. 1996). There may also be an interactive effect between physical abuse by either parent and exposure to television (Heath et al. 1989).

The combination of media violence, community violence, and physical violence within the home is a trio of mutually reinforcing factors, each enhancing the effect of the others and increasing the likelihood of aggression and violence in the viewer or player of video games. Children who are abused watch more television and prefer more violent shows than others do; ultimately, they may commit more violent crimes in later life (Josephson 1995). The more exposed an adolescent is to violence, the more likely he is to carry a weapon or become a perpetrator of violence (Strasburger and Donnerstein 1999). These factors combine with numerous other biological, psychological, and social factors (see Chapter 25, "Overview of Juvenile Law"). Recent exposure to violence contributes 24% of the factors that influence whether the person will become violent. Five percent is affected by parental monitoring, and between 5% and 15% is from media violence (Singer et al. 1999; Strasburger and Donnerstein 1999).

PSYCHOSOCIAL EFFECTS: A DEVELOPMENTAL PERSPECTIVE

Developmental Symptoms

Psychological symptoms that may be experienced by children or adolescents who are affected by witnessing violence on an acute or chronic basis are most effectively considered on a developmental basis. In this way, we can more clearly understand the differences in presentation—depression may present differently in a 6-year-old than in a 16-year-old. Some symptoms are seen regardless of age. Anyone exposed to violence may experience symptoms of anxiety or withdrawal, have sleep or appetite disturbances, or have somatic complaints (Pynoos 1993).

As infants are in the process of becoming attuned to the world outside the mother's uterus, their developmental tasks include making their needs known—to receive food, sleep, and grow while developing trust in caretakers. Developmental symptoms seen in infants are disturbances of global functioning (Zeanah and Scheeringa 1997). These may include excessive crying, eating, or sleeping, failure to thrive, increased irritability, and, as the child grows older, fear of being alone. Toddlers are learning to explore their environment and control their impulses, including aggression. Their symptoms will be disruptions in these tasks, with disturbances in autonomy, motor activity, and aggression (Osofsky and Fenichel 1994).

Preschoolers acquire skills such as language and control of bowel and bladder. These skills can be lost through regression as a result of exposure to violence (Drell et al. 1993). They may also experience delays in acquiring new skills or reenact traumatic experiences in their play. School-age children may also be delayed in acquiring new skills; this may present as a learning difficulty. A further developmental task is the consolidation of social skills; with its disruption we may see an impairment in developing interpersonal relationships. Adolescents are more likely to experience substance abuse and/or indiscriminate sexual or other high-risk or delinquent behaviors, some of which may reenact the trauma. There may be an increase in hostility or premature closure of identity formation (Gabarino et al. 1992).

Academic performance can be affected for multiple reasons. A child may be distracted by intrusive thoughts of the violence that he or she has witnessed. Some children have learned to use dissociation to isolate experiences as a defense mechanism against traumatic or violent incidents. These children may dissociate in school, disrupting the learning process. Children whose sleep is disturbed due to violent activities in the household or neighborhood may not be able to learn during the day simply because they are too tired (Osofsky et al. 1993). Finally, children may have difficulty concentrating because they are in a state of constant physiological arousal from experiencing a persistent fear state (see Chapter 19, "Neurodevelopmental Impact of Violence in Childhood").

Not all children experience problems in academic functioning. Some children, in order to avoid preoccupation with violence at home or in the neighborhood, focus all of their energies on school and do exceptionally well. Unfortunately, this may lead parents, teachers, and helping professionals to mistakenly conclude that the trauma is not affecting the child.

Psychiatric Syndromes

As noted above, there are multiple emotional and behavioral symptoms that can result from witnessing chronic violence in its multiple forms. Similarly, multiple psychiatric disorders may be seen, including posttraumatic stress disorder, generalized anxiety disorder, conduct disorder, attachment disorders of infancy, adjustment disorders, conversion disorder, somatization disorder, brief psychotic episode, or dissociative disorder. Posttraumatic stress disorder and other symptoms in response to trauma can be seen after school shootings (Schwarz and Kowalski 1991).

Compared with natural disasters and accidents (such as car accidents and fires with personal injury), intentional events (such as kidnapping, murder, and war) result in more severe symptoms of posttraumatic stress disorder (American Psychiatric Association 2000). This is related to the fact that intentional cruelty and evil disrupt one's ability to trust others (Gabarino et al. 1992). Most studies show that proximity to the traumatic experience contributes to the severity of symptoms (Nader et al. 1990; Schwarz and Kowalski 1991).

PROTECTIVE FACTORS

Not all children who are exposed to violence develop symptoms. Only 3% to 10% of the population is predisposed to violence when frustrated (Pennell and Browne 1999). Up to 80% of children exposed to significant stressors do not sustain developmental damage (Gabarino et al. 1992; Richters and Martinez 1993b). A child can tolerate one or two risk factors before suffering damage to emotional development. The accumulation of multiple risk factors without offsetting protective factors results in behavioral and emotional problems (Gabarino et al. 1992).

A child has individual protective factors that assist in preventing developmental damage. These include early bonding between the child and his or her parents, relationships that promote social development, and the presence of a consistent caring adult (who may be someone not involved in the early bonding relationships). It is helpful if the child is raised in an environment that promotes emotional development, including the verbalization of feelings. The child who also utilizes all supports available through the school and attends religious services has a stronger sense of having a purpose in life. The age of the child at the time of exposure can be a protective factor—the older she is, the less likely that there will be a significant effect. Resilient children have one or more close friends, enjoy school, and may have a particular teacher who serves as a positive role model. These children have an enduring sense of their own personal control and an ability to make some sense of the chaos surrounding them. In addition, these children find support in community programs that guide parents in enhancing the parent-child relationship (Anthony and Cohler 1987; Gabarino et al. 1992).

The resilient family also has protective characteristics that can help prevent violence. The most resilient families earn more money, utilize a solid support network, which includes religious institutions, and are active in their schools. These families also utilize the resourcefulness of their children when they bring home information about potential supports. They move to better neighborhoods when they can. These families are able to manage intense emotions without the use of violence. They see the protection of their children as their most important task (McManus 1995). The stability and safety of the child's household is a significant protective factor itself (Richters and Martinez 1993b).

ASSESSMENT OF EXPOSURE TO VIOLENCE

When does exposure to violence become a concern? This must be answered on an individual basis for each young person we encounter. We cannot answer this question fully unless we have information about the child or adolescent's exposure to violence. This information can then be assessed in the context of the child's behavior, the

TABLE 21–2. Taking a media history

What channels do you watch on television? What are your favorite shows?
What kind of movies do you like? What are your favorites?
How long do you watch television daily?
Who watches television with you?
What kind of music do you listen to? Who are your favorite groups?
What are the house rules about television, video games, and music?
Do you surf the Internet? What do you do there?

Source. Adapted from American Medical Association 1996; Strasburger and Donnerstein 1999.

remainder of his or her history, and the potential interactions of the varied aspects of that history. The evaluation of all children and adolescents should include questions about their exposure to violence (Freeman et al. 1993; Pittel 1996; Singer et al. 1995). Children should be asked if there are fights, shootings, or stabbings in their neighborhoods. It is useful to know if the child has ever seen anyone beaten up or hurt in a fight or if the child has ever seen anyone who has been shot. If the answer is yes to any of these questions, it then becomes helpful to ask about the child's relationship to the individual, and if the event was only seen briefly or watched at length. Any affirmative answers should be followed up with appropriate questions regarding affective reactions (Pittel 1996).

Media history screening questions are listed in Table 21–2. The child and adolescent psychiatrist should learn what kinds of television shows and movies are watched and with whom. Similarly, asking what kinds of music and the favorite artists that the youth listens to most often gathers important baseline information. How much time the child or adolescent spends on the computer and the Internet and in what kinds of computer activities the juvenile engages can be equally enlightening. This information may serve to inform the parent (if present during that portion of the interview) as well as the psychiatrist.

INTERVENTIONS AND PREVENTION

No single agency can prevent violence. Because the causes of violence are multifactorial, means of prevention and intervention must be multifocal. Parents, health care providers, child advocates, public agencies (law enforcement and government), and the media must all accept responsibility.

Interventions

With exposure to community violence, the reestablishment of routine and a sense of order is the first intervention. There are established treatments for posttraumatic stress disorder and other sequelae of childhood trauma that are beyond the scope of this chapter. School programs can help process any ongoing trauma through discussion groups, thus fostering resiliency. Children who cope well with ongoing trauma clearly utilize their school as a refuge. Early intervention programs are unquestionably useful when the child has other supports in the family and community. Media education can also occur in the schools, reinforcing lessons that are ideally taught at home and that could also be disseminated in public service announcements (Strasburger and Donnerstein 1999).

For media violence, interventions are listed in Table 21–3. Clear communication about the parent's opinion of media violence is imperative, serving both to filter and interpret information and to educate the child or adolescent (Grossman and DeGaetano 1999; Strasburger and Donnerstein 1999). Changing the channel, with an explanation, from an inappropriate show can have a powerful modeling effect for children and adolescents. Children whose parents are involved in their television choices are less likely to choose to watch inappropriate shows (Mediascope, Inc. 1996a).

Similarly, parents should be aware of what video and computer games are being played, what music is being listened to, and what Web sites are frequented, establishing expectations of what is considered appropriate and inappropriate. Parents should try out video games and refuse to purchase violent ones (Funk and Buchman 1995; Grossman and DeGaetano 1999). Regarding music, the parent can discuss the realistic versus the unrealistic nature of the videos, including any negatively stereotyped portrayals of gender or ethnic groups in videos (American Academy of Pediatrics 1999a). The discussion of the use of special effects and production techniques used to make media more compelling helps give children the necessary tools to question what they see.

The clinician can use the opportunity of an evaluation to educate the parent about the potential effects of media violence on the child. Parents should be encouraged to be actively involved in their children's media decisions. Media literacy information should be provided to parents to help them with this endeavor. In the advocacy role, the clinician can also communicate with television and motion picture production companies, legislative bodies, and government agencies regarding the negative effects of media violence (Strasburger and Donnerstein 1999).

TABLE 21–3. Media violence interventions for parents

Watch TV and play video games with your children.
Consider the child's developmental level when making media decisions.
Consider the context of any violence when making media decisions.
Be aware of content of media used by children in and out of the home.
Clearly communicate your opinion of media violence.
Discuss permanent effects of real-life violence.
Teach that violence is violence, whether used by the hero or by the villain.

Source. Adapted from Federman 1998; Grossman and DeGaetano 1999; Murray 1997; National Association for the Education of Young Children 1990; Strasburger and Donnerstein 1999; Voojis and van der Voort 1993; Wilson et al. 1996.

Prevention

Teaching children about violence in the media is a process. It is most important to protect the youngest children (those under 8) from violence, because their neurological systems are still developing. They have not yet acquired the ability to develop insight into their reactions to the violence, to verbalize them, or to self-soothe; they should not see sensational violence (see Table 21–1). Given the violent scenes and discussions that are part of day-to-day living, preschoolers should not watch the news. By age 11 or 12 the child's language skills and thinking processes are adequate to watch news shows directed toward middle schoolers. Generally, only teens and high school students have achieved the developmental tasks necessary to adequately process the news (Grossman and DeGaetano 1999).

In the prevention of media violence, a plan involving no more than 2 hours daily of total screen time, including time spent watching television, videotapes, playing video and computer games and surfing the Internet has been recommended, with no screen time for children under age 2 (American Academy of Pediatrics 1999a). The use of filtering or blocking software when surfing the Internet is another protective mechanism that is available (American Academy of Pediatrics 1999b). Children and adolescents will benefit from realizing that television, videotapes, and video games are not a right, but a privilege (Funk and Buchman 1995). Homework is to be completed before screen time. This is particularly important if there are learning or behavior problems, because in these cases overexposure to television and video games is even more problematic (Grossman and DeGaetano 1999).

Further research into the effects of violence in the media will hopefully reproduce but also expand previous findings. The entertainment and news media, as well as the people and agencies who are involved in the regulation of the industry, must commit to more responsible portrayals of the human condition (Strasburger and Donnerstein 1999). Without this, our society can only become more affected and more violent. Ultimately, only combined action by parents, child advocates, government, and the entertainment industry will help reverse the current tide of violence in the airwaves and cyberspace and decrease violence in the communities.

REFERENCES

163 and counting…hate groups find home on the Net. Intelligence Project of the Southern Poverty Law Center. Intelligence Report, Issue 89, Winter 1998, pp 24–25

Almqvist K, Brandell-Forsberg M: Iranian refugee children in Sweden: effects of organized violence and forced migration on preschool children. Am J Orthopsychiatry 65:225–237, 1995

American Academy of Pediatrics Committee on Communications: Media violence. Pediatrics 95:949–951, 1995

American Academy of Pediatrics: Understanding the impact of media on children and teens, 1999a [http://www.aap.org/family/mediaimpact.htm]

American Academy of Pediatrics: The Internet and your family, 1999b [http://www.aap.org/family/interfamily.htm]

American Medical Association: Physician Guide to Media Violence. Chicago, IL, American Medical Association, 1996

American Psychiatric Association: Diagnostic and Statistical Manual of Mental Disorders, 4th Edition, Text Revision. Washington, DC, American Psychiatric Association, 2000

Anthony E, Cohler B (eds): The Invulnerable Child. New York, Guilford, 1987

A skinhead's story—an interview with a former racist. Intelligence Project of the Southern Poverty Law Center. Intelligence Report, Issue 89, Winter 1998, pp 21–23

Attar BK, Guerra NG, Tolan PH: Neighborhood disadvantage, stressful life events and adjustment in urban elementary-school children. J Clin Child Psychol 23:391–400, 1994

Bell CC: Community violence: causes, prevention, and intervention. J Natl Med Assoc 89:657–662, 1997

Cloud J: What can the schools do? Time, May 3, 1999, pp 38–40

Comstock G, Strasburger VC: Deceptive appearances: television violence and aggressive behavior—an introduction. J Adolesc Health 11:31–44, 1990

Cooley-Quille MR, Turner SM, Beidel D: Emotional impact of children's exposure to community violence: a preliminary study. J Am Acad Child Adolesc Psychiatry 34:1362–1368, 1995

Davidson J, Smith R: Traumatic experiences in psychiatric outpatients. J Trauma Stress 3:459–475, 1990

Dill KE, Dill JC: Video game violence: a review of the empirical literature. Aggression and Violent Behavior 3:407–428, 1998

Drell M, Siegel C, Gaensbauer T: Posttraumatic stress disorder, in Handbook of Infant Mental Health. Edited by Zeanah C. New York, Guilford, 1993, pp 291–304

DuRant RH, Getts A, Cadenhead C, et al: Exposure to violence and victimization and depression, hopelessness and purpose in life among adolescents living in and around public housing. J Dev Behav Pediatr 16:233–237, 1995

DuRant RH, Rich M, Emans SJ, et al: Violence and weapon carrying in music videos. Arch Pediatr Adolesc Med 151:443–448, 1997

Eron LD, Huesmann LR: The control of aggressive behavior by changes in attitudes, values, and the conditions of learning, in Advances in the Study of Aggression. Edited by Blanchard RJ, Blanchard DC. Orlando, FL, Academic Press, 1984, pp 139–171

Federman J (ed): National Television Violence Study, Vol 2: Executive Summary. Santa Barbara, CA, The Center for Communication and Social Policy, University of California, Santa Barbara, 1997

Federman J (ed): National Television Violence Study, Vol 3: Executive Summary. Santa Barbara, CA, The Center for Communication and Social Policy, University of California, Santa Barbara, 1998

Fick AC, Osofsky JD, Lewis ML: Perceptions of violence: children, parents, and police officers, in Children in a Violent Society. Edited by Osofsky JD. New York, Guilford, 1997, pp 261–276

Freeman LN, Mokros H, Poznanski EO: Violent events reported by normal urban school-aged children: characteristics and depression correlates. J Am Acad Child Adolesc Psychiatry 32:419–423, 1993

Funk JB, Buchman DD: Videogame controversies. Pediatr Ann 24:91–94, 1995

Gabarino J, Dubrow N, Kostelny K, et al: Children in Danger: Coping With the Consequences of Community Violence. San Francisco, CA, Jossey-Bass, 1992

Gadow KD, Sprafkin J: Television "violence" and children with emotional and behavioral disorders. Journal of Emotional and Behavioral Disorders 1:54–63, 1993

Gerbner G, Signorielli N: Violence Profile, 1967 Through 1988–89: Enduring Patterns. Philadelphia, PA, University of Pennsylvania, Annenberg School of Communication, 1990

Griffiths MD, Hunt N: Computer game playing in adolescence: prevalence and demographic indicators. Journal of Community and Applied Social Psychology 5:189–193, 1995

Gröer M, Howell M: Autonomic and cardiovascular responses of preschool children to television programs. Journal of Child and Adolescent Psychiatric and Mental Health Nursing 3:134–138, 1990

Grossman D, DeGaetano G: Stop Teaching Our Kids to Kill. New York, Crown, 1999

Hate group count tops 500; number of Internet sites soars. Southern Poverty Law Center Report, March 1999, pp 1, 3

Hate group numbers rise. Southern Poverty Law Center Report, May 2001, p 3

Healy JM: Understanding TV's effects on the developing brain, 1998 [http://www.aap.org/advocacy/chm98nws.htm]

Heath L, Bresolin LB, Rinaldi RC: Effects of media violence on children—a review of the literature. Arch Gen Psychiatry 46:376–379, 1989

Hickey G: No fear, no life expectancy on city streets. Richmond Times–Dispatch, January 5, 1998, pp A1, A6

Hill HM: Urban violence—reclaiming childhood for children at risk. Violence Update, December 1994, Vol 5, No 4, pp 1, 2, 4, 10

Hill HM: The impact of community violence on young children: strategies of intervention. Paper presented at the Second National Conference of Children and Violence, Houston, TX, November 1995

Hinton-Nelson MD, Roberts MC, Snyder CR: Early adolescents exposed to violence: hope and vulnerability to victimization. Am J Orthopsychiatry 66:346–353, 1996

Iwao S, Pool IS, Hagiwara S: Japanese and U.S. media: some cross-cultural insights into TV violence. Journal of Communication 31:28–36, 1981

Jenkins EJ, Bell CC: Exposure and response to community violence among children and adolescents, in Children in a Violent Society. Edited by Osofsky JD. New York, Guilford, 1997, pp 9–31

Josephson W: Television Violence: A Review of the Effects on Children of Different Ages. Ottawa, ON, Heritage Canada, 1995

Kostelny K, Gabarino J: Coping with the consequences of living in danger: the case of Palestinian children and youth. International Journal of Behavioral Development 17:595–611, 1994

McManus PT: Resiliency in the African-American family. Paper presented at the Second National Conference on Children and Violence, Houston, TX, November 1995

Mediascope, Inc: Summary of Findings and Recommendations: National Television Violence Study Executive Summary 1994–1995. Studio City, CA, Mediascope, Inc, 1996a, pp viii–xiii

Mediascope, Inc: Television violence and its context: a content analysis, 1994–95: National Television Violence Study Executive Summary 1994–1995. Studio City, CA, Mediascope, Inc, 1996b, pp 3–7

Molitor F, Hirsch KW: Children's toleration of real-life aggression after exposure to media violence: a replication of the Drabman and Thomas studies. Child Study Journal 24:191–207, 1994

Murray JP: Media violence and youth, in Children in a Violent Society. Edited by Osofsky JD. New York, Guilford, 1997, pp 72–96

Nader K, Pynoos RS, Fairbanks L, et al: Childhood PTSD reactions one year after a sniper attack. Am J Psychiatry 147:1526–1530, 1990

National Association for the Education of Young Children: National Association for the Education of Young Children Position Statement on Media Violence in Children's Lives. Young Children 45(5):18–21, 1990

Osofsky J: The effects of exposure to violence on young children. Am Psychol 50:782–788, 1995

Osofsky J, Fenichel E (eds): Caring for Infants and Toddlers in Violent Environments: Hurt, Healing and Hope. Arlington, VA, Zero to Three/National Center for Clinical Infant Programs, 1994

Osofsky JD, Wewers S, Hann DM, et al: Chronic community violence: what is happening to our children? Psychiatry 56:36–45, 1993

Pennell AE, Browne KD: Film violence and young offenders. Aggression and Violent Behavior 4:13–28, 1999

Perry DG, Bussey K: Self-reinforcement in high and low aggressive boys following acts of aggression. Child Dev 48:653–657, 1977

Phillips DP, Carstensen LL: Clustering of teenage suicides after television news stories about suicide. N Engl J Med 315:685–689, 1986

Pittel EM: How to take a violence history: guidelines for interviewing youth at risk for violence. AACAP News 27(5):9–12, September/October 1996

Pynoos RS: Traumatic stress and developmental psychopathology in children and adolescents, in The American Psychiatric Press Review of Psychiatry, Vol 12. Edited by Oldham JM, Riba MB, Tasman A. Washington, DC, American Psychiatric Press, 1993, pp 205–238

Rich M, Woods ER, Goodman E, et al: Aggressors or victims: gender and race in music video violence. Pediatrics 101:669–674, 1998

Richters JE, Martinez P: The NIMH community violence project, I: children as victims of and witnesses to violence. Psychiatry 56:7–21, 1993a

Richters JE, Martinez P: Violent communities, family choices, and children's chances: an algorithm for improving the odds. Dev Psychopathol 5:609–627, 1993b

Rosenthal R: Media violence, antisocial behavior and the social consequences of small effects. Journal of Social Issues 42:141–154, 1986

Sack WH, Clarke G, Him C, et al: A 6-year follow-up study of Cambodian refugee adolescents traumatized as children. J Am Acad Child Adolesc Psychiatry 32:431–437, 1993

Schwarz ED, Kowalski JM: Malignant memories: PTSD in children and adolescents after a school shooting. J Am Acad Child Adolesc Psychiatry 30:936–944, 1991

Singer MI, Anglin TM, Song L, et al: Adolescents exposure to violence and associated symptoms of psychological trauma. JAMA 273:477–482, 1995

Singer MI, Miller DB, Guo S, et al: Contributors to violent behavior among elementary and middle school children. Pediatrics 104:878–884, 1999

Strasburger VC: Adolescents and the Media—Medical and Psychological Impact. Thousand Oaks, CA, Sage, 1995

Strasburger VC, Donnerstein E: Review article: children, adolescents, and the media: issues and solutions. Pediatrics 103:129–139, 1999

Tepperman J: Toxic lessons: what do children learn from media violence? January-February 1997 [http://www.4children.org/news/1-97toxl.html. Accessed November 14, 2000]

Voojis MW, van der Voort THA: Learning about television violence: the impact of a critical viewing curriculum on children's attitudinal judgments of crime series. Journal of Research and Development in Education 26:133–142, 1993

Vos Post J: Open questions on the correlation between television and violence, 1995 [www.magicdragon.com/EmeraldCity/Nonfiction/Socphil.html]

Weine S, Becker DF, McGlashan TH, et al: Adolescent survivors of "ethnic cleansing": observations on the first year in America. J Am Acad Child Adolesc Psychiatry 34:1153–1159, 1995

Williams TM: The Impact of Television: A Natural Experiment in Three Communities. New York, Academic Press, 1986

Wilson BJ, Kunkel D, Linz D, et al: Violence in television programming overall: University of California, Santa Barbara Study: National Television Violence Study Executive Summary 1994–1995. Studio City, CA, Mediascope Press, 1996, pp 8–30

Zeanah CH, Scheeringa MS: The experience and effects of violence in infancy, in Children in a Violent Society. Edited by Osofsky JD. New York, Guilford, 1997 pp 97–123

CHAPTER 22

Children's Access to Weapons

Peter Ash, M.D.

Case Example 1

Michael is being evaluated for depression and suicidal ideation. He reports that he doesn't own a gun, but his father collects guns. "Dad keeps the guns locked up. He thinks I don't know where the key is. Hah!"

Case Example 2

Henry, age 15 (aka Shooter, "'cause I shoot my mouth off"), has been arrested for aggravated assault, which he denies committing, arising out of an incident in a club parking lot where another youth was shot. He is being evaluated at the request of his defense attorney in preparation for a hearing on waiving jurisdiction to an adult court.

After being told that a report will be sent to the defense attorney, Henry tells the evaluator that he was given his first gun at age 12 by a gang leader and told to "take care of myself." He reports that now he seldom carries a weapon when selling drugs because, "If they know you're packing, they'll shoot first." He says he takes a gun to school, but he "hides it out in the bushes" because the school has implemented a policy mandating mesh book bags and metal detectors. He sometimes carries a gun other places "to feel safe." He carries a gun "to the club...because that's where the trouble is." He has witnessed three shootings, including one in which the victim died. He denies ever firing a gun "except the two times I shot back," and he denies any intent to shoot anyone else.

LEGAL ISSUES

The federal Youth Handgun Safety Act (1996) made it unlawful for any person to provide a handgun to a juve-

nile (someone younger than age 18 years) and made it unlawful for a juvenile to possess a handgun, with very limited exceptions. At the time of its passage, most states already had similar laws in place. Federal law and most states do allow parents to give their child a rifle for purposes of hunting or target shooting.

Because handgun ownership by minors is already illegal, the heated public debate on gun control tends to touch on juvenile issues via regulations on adults who provide minors with access. Weapons other than firearms are considerably less restricted, although weapon carrying is often regulated by type (laws against switchblades, for example) or by site (such as restrictions involving airports and schools).

A few states have passed "safe storage" laws, which make gun owners criminally liable if someone is injured because a child gains unsupervised access to a gun. Such laws appear to reduce unintentional deaths of children but do not appear to show significant declines in adolescent suicide and homicide (Cummings et al. 1997).

Another area that has been considered has to do with regulations that would require safety devices to make guns unusable by inappropriate persons. For example, there have been proposals for built-in trigger locks (to prevent a small child who happened upon a loaded gun from being able to fire it) and for so-called smart guns, which would register (through hand identification or responding to a separate releasing device worn by the owner, such as a special glove or magnet) who was holding the gun and only fire if held by the owner. Such technologies are still in their infancy and not widely implemented.

STATISTICS AND DEVELOPMENTAL ISSUES

Guns as Risk Factors

Guns are very common in American culture: there are about 200 million guns in the United States, nearly one for every man, woman, and child, and about a third of those weapons are handguns (Wright 1995). Surveys suggest that slightly less than half the households in the United States contain a gun (U.S. Bureau of Census 1996), a rate that has stayed fairly constant for about 40 years.

Youths have considerable access to these weapons. Between 1985 and 1994, the risk of dying from a firearm injury more than doubled for youths ages 15 to 19 years (National Center for Injury Prevention and Control 1996), an increase that came to be seen as a public health emergency. In the period since 1994, these rates have been dropping. The increase in adolescent homicide rates from the mid-1980s through 1994 has been largely attributed to increasing gun carrying by adolescents (Dahlberg 1998; Fingerhut et al. 1998). In 1997, about a third of high school boys reported carrying a weapon in the previous 30 days, and of those, about a third carried a gun (Brener et al. 1999). Boys were seven to eight times more likely than girls to carry a gun (Brener et al. 1999). Ash and colleagues (1996) found that among incarcerated delinquent juveniles, almost all the boys owned a handgun, and half the girls did. Although violence among youth has been falling since 1994, homicide remains the second leading cause of death among adolescents.

Guns are a risk factor for psychiatric difficulties aside from homicide. The presence of a handgun in the home has been shown to double the risk of adolescent suicide (Brent et al. 1991). Three-quarters of youths who shoot themselves do so with a gun they or a relative own (Grossman et al. 1999). For many youths who live in high-crime areas, witnessing of violence is all too common, with consequent anxiety and posttraumatic stress disorder (PTSD). The recent rash of highly publicized school shootings has increased the anxiety of many students. In the mid 1990s, more than 7% of a nationally representative sample of high school students reported being assaulted with a weapon at school, a rate that has remained fairly constant despite a decrease in reported gun carrying by students over the same period (Brener et al. 1999).

Why Adolescents Own Guns

Research suggests there are two primary reasons youths own guns: to hunt (rifles) and to help them feel safe (handguns). Few adolescents initially obtain a gun to assist them in committing a crime (Ash et al. 1996; Sheley and Wright 1993). Owning a gun for hunting usually implies a rifle rather than a handgun and is more common outside urban areas, whereas owning a handgun to feel safe is more common a reason in urban areas, although still prevalent in nonurban areas (Sadowski et al. 1989). Weapons obtained for hunting are seldom used in crimes because a rifle is difficult to conceal.

Obtaining Guns

It appears that most youths who will obtain a gun first do so in early adolescence (Ash et al. 1996; Brener et al. 1999; Sadowski et al. 1989). The majority of these youths receive their first gun passively: someone gives it to them, whether it be a parent giving his or her child a hunting rifle or a peer giving a friend a handgun "for protection." Relatively few youths actively obtain (buy, borrow, or steal) their first gun in response to being threatened. In middle to late adolescence, youths tend to obtain additional handguns more actively, by buying them on the street or from an adult who is willing to buy one legally and sell it to them, through borrowing (surprisingly common), or by stealing. What is striking about these adolescents obtaining guns is the diversity of methods employed (typical of unregulated markets) and how they will often own a succession of guns—passing, loaning, or selling their weapons to other youths.

Carrying Handguns

The major risk for handguns is not that the youth owns a gun, but that he (usually) carries it with him and can then impulsively use it during a confrontation. The bulk of research on which youths will carry a handgun has not focused on personality variables but on demographic and epidemiological variables, and it has found that socioeconomic and environmental characteristics (e.g., level of neighborhood crime) are most predictive. Among personality characteristics, the likelihood of carrying a handgun has also been associated with risk taking, depression, stress, and quick temper (Simon et al. 1998).

CLINICAL EVALUATION

Indications for Asking About Weapons

There are three main components of a weapons history that are useful to ask about in any clinical evaluation: history of weapon-related trauma, access to weapons, and ownership of a firearm. More detailed questions about these issues are indicated if the clinician suspects particular clinical problems or obtains a positive response to screening questions. Questions about weapon-related trauma are particularly important in assessing anxiety disorders, especially PTSD; access to weapons is particularly relevant when assessing depression and risk factors for suicide; and all three components are relevant when assessing severe conduct disorder or delinquency. Although especially important in adolescence, the relevant components should be addressed in all youths who present with one of those three conditions. More rare, but certainly deserving of a careful examination of weapons history, are those youths who report thoughts about wanting to hurt others but have no history of delinquent behavior.

Trauma

Even without a history of trauma, does the youth worry about weapon-related trauma? The most common concerns here have to do with worry that the youth will be shot at school, that he or she lives in a dangerous neighborhood, or that a parent will use a weapon, most commonly when there is a history of parental substance abuse and/or spousal abuse. What is the history of victimization by weapons? How often has the youth been shot at? Seen someone else shot? Lost friends or family members by shootings? Youths who live in high-crime areas are frequently traumatized as bystanders or victims, and membership in a delinquent peer group greatly elevates this risk. In response to such trauma, did the youth think about getting a gun? If so, did he or she actually get one? Why or why not? When youths are asked how else they might feel safe, they are typically unable to identify viable options.

Access to Weapons

Are there guns in the home? How are they stored? Does the youth have access? Could he or she get access? Has the youth fired a gun? Does he or she own a gun?

Weapon Ownership History

Obtaining the first weapon.   Most youths who obtain guns do so in early adolescence. Youths who hunt often receive rifles as gifts in early adolescence, and the gun industry commonly advertises rifles to early adolescents' parents as a rite-of-passage gift. Ash et al. (1996) found that among juvenile delinquents who ever obtained a weapon, more than half did so by age 14, even though they tended to use them in offenses in mid-adolescence. More than half of juvenile delinquents obtained their first handgun passively, either by being given the handgun

or by coming across it accidentally, either at home or during a burglary or auto theft. If a youth has a weapon, the interviewer should ask about the feelings and reasons involved in obtaining it.

Obtaining subsequent weapons.   How many other guns has the youth owned? Although first guns are often obtained passively, subsequent weapons are often obtained more actively. Peer group influences are important, and the youth should be asked how many of his or her friends own or carry guns. Delinquent juveniles report obtaining guns easily by buying them on the street, finding adults (often drug users) to buy a gun for them, borrowing guns from others, or stealing them. Also, it is important to ask how often the youth has sold or loaned a gun to others.

Development of gun carrying.   Few youths who own a gun decide to give it up, but the frequency with which they carry the weapon in public varies widely. Much weapon use is impulsive: the explosion in youth homicide rates does not appear to reflect an increase in the number of violent episodes—what has increased is the deadliness of the violence. It is important to ask how frequently and under what circumstances a youth carries a weapon and what factors have influenced changes in the carrying pattern. Only a very small minority of juveniles carry a handgun most of the time. For many, gun carrying is intermittent and situation-specific. Social situations that involve other youths who are thought to carry guns are especially high risk. In high-crime areas, students are not very likely to take guns into schools because many schools have implemented intensive gun surveillance techniques, such as mesh book bags, weapon detectors, and locker checks, but students may hide the gun near the school and pick it up when they leave. Drug-dealing youths often carry weapons for protection, but some make the strategic decision not to out of fear of being shot preemptively because the attacker believes the dealer has a gun. How does the youth feel when carrying a weapon? Many report high levels of anxiety about being caught, and this anxiety can be used therapeutically to discourage future carrying. The stereotype that boys carry guns to feel "macho" appears to apply only to a minority of delinquent youths. The more often a youth carries a gun, the higher the risk that he will use it.

Intent to use.   Does the youth plan his or her weapon use? Is there a pattern of escalating threats, gun carrying, or planning violence? Does he or she have suicidal intent? Hold a grudge? Stated intent to use a weapon generally represents a psychiatric emergency requiring hospitalization on grounds of dangerousness.

Interventions

1. *Need to intervene immediately.* If the youth has access to weapons and is at high risk for using them, the clinician will need to act to remove that access or hospitalize the youth. There are a number of ways to remove access, depending on the situation. In the case of guns in the home, negotiating with the parents to make the home safe is often required (but see the "Pitfalls" section, which follows). Occasionally, if a youth is in therapy, the therapist may have the youth give him or her the weapon to hold. Many therapists, however, will not feel comfortable about this or may not have a place to store the weapon securely. If the gun has been stolen, the therapist may be liable for receiving stolen property. Also, in the case of handguns, the therapist must remember that returning the handgun to the minor is illegal.

2. *Promoting a rational assessment of the risks of carrying weapons.* Most handgun-carrying youths are already anxious about carrying weapons, and such anxiety can be used to motivate the exploration of a more adaptive solution. The therapist can point out the risks of carrying, help bring the underlying anxiety about personal safety into clearer focus where it can be addressed, and discuss alternative strategies for being safe.

3. *Prevention.* The prevention of youth firearm violence is currently a major public health issue that is being addressed from a multitude of perspectives, including prevention of suicide (see Youth Suicide by Firearms Task Force 1998), violence prevention (see Group for the Advancement of Psychiatry 1999), and by law enforcement (see Bureau of Alcohol, Tobacco, and Firearms 1999).

PITFALLS

Evaluator's Attitudes About Guns

Many psychiatrists have very limited experience with guns, find them frightening, or may be strong advocates of gun control. As such, they often have limited empathy with the enjoyment that guns provide to a very large segment of the population. Clinicians often have to work with parents to limit their children's access to weapons. Most of these parents own guns for hunting, but some own them for protection; they often feel fairly comfortable around guns. It is important to realize that for the vast majority of adult gun owners, gun ownership is important, and they are often quite sensitive and react negatively to what they perceive as a knee-jerk gun control advocate's view of themselves as a danger to society. Brent et al. (2000) found that only about one-quarter of parents were compliant with a recommendation to remove guns from the home. Working with such parents to limit gun access is a delicate task requiring an appreciation of the importance guns represent for the adults. In a similar vein, negotiating with a depressed child to give up a rifle he enjoys hunting with or with a frightened student who feels society has failed to protect her, and therefore has little claim on stopping her from protecting herself, requires a clear-sighted appreciation of the value the child places on possessing the weapon.

Underreporting Based on Concern About Confidentiality

Without the protection of confidentiality, many youths will be reluctant to report accurate histories of their gun ownership out of concern that such reports might get them into further trouble or have other consequences they wish to avoid. Yet confidentiality can rarely be promised. In a clinical situation, issues about gun ownership may cause the clinician to be concerned about safety issues, and the clinician may feel obligated to intervene actively, either to prevent harm to the youth or harm to another. Such interventions may include telling parents of the risk, hospitalization or civil commitment, or giving a *Tarasoff* warning, depending on the particulars of the situation.

In a forensic evaluation, the youth is advised at the outset of the limits of confidentiality, and the usual benefit of disclosure that is present in a clinical situation—that the youth may receive treatment—is less often present. In an evaluation for waiver to adult court (e.g., Case Example 2), an extended history of gun ownership or use may tilt the scales toward the youth being tried as an adult. Because it is illegal for a minor to own a handgun, it is important that the evaluator not obtain sufficiently detailed information that would constitute a criminal confession or lead the police to be able to obtain evidence that could be used to convict without making sure that the youth is clear about his Miranda rights and the way the information is likely to be used. Psychiatric interviews are not police interrogations. More generic information ("I owned three guns and shot at five different guys") may tend to make the youth look antisocial, but it is unlikely to lead to prosecution. The psychiatrist should focus primarily on the thoughts and feelings that went with the gun-related behaviors, a focus that can often be maintained without the youth incriminating himself or herself.

Overreporting to "Impress" the Examiner

Whereas many clinicians are concerned that youths will want to appear "macho" and overreport heavy involvement with guns, the literature suggests that this is relatively uncommon, although there are obvious validity problems. Interviewer characteristics are no doubt important: the naive interviewer who gives wide-eyed reactions ("Really? You own *eight* guns?") or who is clearly unfamiliar with the ways of the street invites false-positive responses, as does the interviewer who uses leading questions. If the evaluator suspects overreporting, questions that almost always deserve negative answers, even from juvenile delinquents with considerable gun experience, can be used: "How often have you bought a handgun?…Borrowed a gun?…Rented a gun?" (Renting guns is very rare; buying or borrowing guns is common.) Or: "How many machine guns have you owned?" (Youth ownership of machine guns is extremely rare, with the occasional exception of a gang member who is associated with adult organized crime.)

CASE EXAMPLE EPILOGUES

Case Example 1

Michael was assessed as being moderately depressed, and in that context, his access to his father's gun collection was quite worrisome. The therapist shared some of his concern with Michael, and asked how Michael would feel about the clinician advising the father to remove the guns from the house until Michael felt better. Michael said, "He won't do it, but you can tell him." The clinician was prepared to advise the father even if Michael objected. When the father was told, he agreed to move his collection to a relative's house where there were no children. Michael was impressed that "he cares enough about me to do that."

Case Example 2

Henry elaborated his history of a pattern of predictably carrying a handgun to social events and was assessed as being at significant risk for future violent confrontations. In addition, on inquiring further into Henry's reactions to witnessing shootings, the evaluator elicited clear symptoms that met criteria for PTSD. However, the evaluator could not conclude that treating Henry's PTSD would significantly reduce his being a threat to others. In the view of Henry's defense attorney, the need for treatment of PTSD did not outweigh the attorney's expectation that the chronic gun carrying would cause the judge to see his client as a career criminal. The attorney decided to bury the expert's report and retain another expert "after I have a talk with that young man [his client]."

ACTION GUIDELINES

A. For all youths, screen for
   1. History of weapon-related trauma
   2. Access to weapons
   3. Ownership of a weapon
   4. Homicidal and suicidal ideation

B. For suspected diagnoses
   1. Anxiety disorder and/or PTSD: inquire about weapon-related trauma to self or if witnessed
   2. Depression: assess availability of firearm in the home as a risk factor for suicide
   3. Conduct disorder: take detailed weapons history

C. Obtain a weapons history
   1. Use of weapons other than firearms
   2. Has the youth ever owned a weapon? If yes, assess
      a. Rifles only for recreation or owned a handgun
      b. Obtaining first weapon: passive versus active, reasons, circumstances
      c. The extent to which members of peer group own and carry weapons
      d. Obtaining other weapons: types of weapons, methods of obtaining
      e. Current frequency of handgun carrying; if youth is carrying a handgun in public, obtain history of how carrying developed
      f. History of threatening with or firing the gun
      g. Future intent to use

REFERENCES

Ash P, Kellermann AL, Fuqua-Whitley D, et al: Gun acquisition and use by juvenile offenders. JAMA 275:1754–1758, 1996

Brener ND, Simon TR, Krug EG, et al: Recent trends in violence-related behaviors among high school students in the United States. JAMA 282:440–446, 1999

Brent DA, Perper JA, Allman CJ, et al: The presence and accessibility of firearms in the homes of adolescent suicides: a case-control study. JAMA 266:2989–2995, 1991

Brent DA, Baugher M, Birmaher B, et al: Compliance with recommendations to remove firearms in families participating in a clinical trial for adolescent depression. J Am Acad Child Adolesc Psychiatry 39:1220–1226, 2000

Bureau of Alcohol, Tobacco, and Firearms: Youth Crime Gun Interdiction Initiative. Washington, DC, U.S. Government Printing Office, 1999

Cummings P, Grossman DC, Rivara FP, et al: State gun safe storage laws and child mortality due to firearms. JAMA 278:1084–1086, 1997

Dahlberg LL: Youth violence in the United States: major trends, risk factors, and prevention approaches. Am J Prev Med 14:259–272, 1998

Fingerhut LA, Ingram DD, Feldman JJ: Homicide rates among US teenagers and young adults: differences by mechanism, level of urbanization, race, and sex, 1987 through 1995. JAMA 280:423–427, 1998

Grossman DC, Reay DT, Baker SA: Self-inflicted and unintentional firearm injuries among children and adolescents: the source of the firearm. Arch Pediatr Adolesc Med 153:875–878, 1999

Group for the Advancement of Psychiatry: Violent behavior in children and youth: preventive intervention from a psychiatric perspective. J Am Acad Child Adolesc Psychiatry 38:235–241, 1999

National Center for Injury Prevention and Control: National Summary of Injury Mortality Data, 1987–1994. Atlanta, GA, Centers for Disease Control and Prevention, 1996

Sadowski LS, Cairns RB, Earp JA: Firearm ownership among nonurban adolescents. American Journal of Diseases of Children 143:1410–1413, 1989

Sheley JF, Wright JD: Gun acquisition and possession in selected juvenile samples. Washington, DC, National Institute of Justice, Office of Juvenile Justice and Delinquency Prevention: Research in Brief, 1993

Simon TRP, Richardson JLD, Dent CWP, et al: Prospective psychosocial, interpersonal, and behavioral predictors of handgun carrying among adolescents. Am J Public Health 88:960–963, 1998

U.S. Bureau of the Census: Statistical Abstract of the United States: 1996. Washington, DC, U.S. Government Printing Office, 1996

Wright JD: Ten essential observations on guns in America. Society 32:63–68, 1995

Youth Suicide by Firearms Task Force: Consensus statement on youth suicide by firearms. Archives of Suicide Research 4:89–94, 1998

Youth Handgun Safety Act, 18 USC § 922(x), (1996)

CHAPTER 23

Risk Assessment of Violence in Youths

Diane H. Schetky, M.D.

Case Example 1

Ethan is an 8-year-old boy from a rural community who lives in a shared custody arrangement with his parents. He presented with a 4-year history of fire setting, which culminated with him burning down a barn using a magnifying glass. He is an engaging, articulate, and well-mannered boy who is conflicted about his fire setting. He tells the child psychiatrist, Dr. Kovak, that he hears voices telling him "do it, do it" and that his fire setting is often triggered by seeing explosions or fire on TV. His draws a picture of a volcano erupting but maintains control over his impulses during play. His parents are very concerned and agree to take turns bringing him to weekly treatment in the nearest town, which is 2 hours away.

Case Example 2

Sixteen-year-old Sam is referred to Dr. Chu for a violence assessment by the director of special education at his school, who had a "spooky" feeling about Sam even though Sam has never actually threatened anyone. In addition, Sam has learning problems involving expressive language, and for the past year he has rarely attended school. His mother, who is schizophrenic, accompanies him to the evaluation and seems quite preoccupied with violence by her ex-husband. She relates that Sam has lost interest in school, neglects his hygiene, is a loner, is moody, and is still very angry about his parents' divorce.

Sam, is a tall, lanky, apathetic adolescent who smiles inappropriately. He has no interest in school or work but does like to read horror stories. He denies hallucinations, and his speech is well organized. He shares troubling persistent thoughts, which he has had for the past few years, that involve killing various people he knows, including his father and stepmother. He reports that the thoughts are becoming more extreme, that he is fantasizing about how he

might attack people at school, and that he fears that one of these days he will act on his anger. He shows little empathy. He has no concerns about going to prison if he acts on his thoughts and speculates that he might have more friends there than he does in school. He shows little insight and does not think he needs therapy.

Case Example 3

Jason, a biracial 14-year-old, is serving time in the detention center for probation violation, which includes smoking pot, stealing from a relative to support his drug habit, and truancy from school. A court-ordered evaluation is requested and will be used in sentencing. The case is assigned to Dr. Freedman, who is doing a court rotation as part of her child psychiatry training. Jason lives with his single mother, a recovering alcoholic, who admits she has no control over him and often knows nothing of his whereabouts. She is a poor historian and doesn't remember much about Jason's life during the years when she was drinking. Jason's father is serving time in prison and has had little contact with him.

Jason deems the evaluation a waste of time and thinks his behavior is no big deal. He is disheveled in his appearance and has a crude self-inflicted tattoo on his forearm that says "life sucks." His manner with Dr. Freedman is angry and disrespectful. She perseveres and informs him that the evaluation, which is court ordered, will be used in sentencing. He tells her he has no use for the authorities and just wants people to get off his back. She empathizes with his plight and learns that Jason has no use for school, either, and that he has been suspended several times for violent behavior toward other kids. On probing further, she learns that from an early age he was "dissed" because of his dark skin and called "retard" because he was in special education. He tells her that he decided he would get more respect if he acted tough, and so he joined a gang and began terrorizing other kids. For the most part, his peers have left him alone.

Jason speaks with much bravado about how tough he is and shows no concern for his victims, whom he figures "deserve what they get." She learns that he was severely beaten by one of his mother's many boyfriends as a child and that he has been cruel to animals. He denies suicidal ideation. He doesn't see his violence as a problem, has limited insight, and attributes his behavior to "a short fuse." His one goal in life is to become a member of the Hell's Angels motorcycle club.

OVERVIEW OF YOUTH VIOLENCE

Requests for risk assessments occur commonly as part of school or agency consultations or in forensic presentencing evaluations that are designed to help the courts decide on appropriate dispositions. In addition, concerns about potential for violence arise in the course of psychotherapy and making decisions about admitting patients to or discharging patients from hospitals. This chapter briefly reviews some of the literature on youth violence in order to assist the clinician in evaluating youths for potential for violence. Some of the studies reviewed refer to delinquency and antisocial behavior rather than to just aggression, and the two categories often overlap. Treatment and legal issues will be dealt with in subsequent chapters in Parts V, "Juvenile Offenders," and VI, "Legal Issues," of this volume.

Prevalence

Violence may involve physically aggressive behavior toward others, self, or objects or may be limited to verbal abuse or threatening with a weapon. Violent youths are a heterogeneous population, and the causes of their violence are multifaceted. One in seven juvenile arrests in 1995 was for a crime involving violence or the threat of violence, and 25% of juveniles in custody in 1995 were held for violent crimes. In addition, many youths engage in violent or threatening behavior that does not result in arrest. Between 1988 and 1994, youth violence increased by 61% and arrests of juveniles for homicides increased by 90% (Snyder and Sickmund 1995). Perpetrators of violence are younger than in the past, and their crimes are more likely to be lethal. This alarming rise in violence has been attributed to the ready availability of handguns and drugs. Between 1987 and 1993, the juvenile homicide rate involving firearms increased by 182% (Sickmund et al. 1997). Homicides by juveniles peaked in 1994, when

juveniles were implicated in about 2,300, or 16% of all, homicides (Office of Juvenile Justice and Delinquency Prevention 1998).

Between 1987 and 1994, the arrest rate for female juvenile violent crime more than doubled, whereas the rate for males increased only by two-thirds. Even though the rate of juvenile violent crime has declined, the female rate remains 85% above the 1987 rate. However, the number of juvenile females charged with homicide has remained low and constant at about 130 females per year. Female gang membership also remains low, having risen from about 6% of gang membership in 1992 to 10% in 1995 (Snyder and Sickmund 1999).

Youths now commit more violence per capita than adults, although 70% of violent offenses are committed by only 20% of delinquent youths. This is particularly true of gangs. Nationwide, violent juvenile crime has been declining over the past few years, and rates are now at a 10-year low. Fewer youths are carrying weapons and engaging in fighting. However, given the growth of the adolescent population, we can expect to see more juvenile crime in the years to come. Youthful offenders are more likely than adults to exhibit violence as part of a group and much of youth violence occurs in the context of interpersonal relationships. One-third of high school students engage in abusive behaviors, and boys and girls are equally abusive when it comes to emotional abuse. Research suggests that bullying and trading insults constitutes ominous "entry-level" abuse that tends to escalate. In the past, this sort of behavior was often overlooked by school personnel, who viewed it as normal behavior and minimized its impact on other students. However, studies have shown that there is much truth to the saying "bully by 8, behind bars by 28."

The United States has the unenviable distinction of having the highest per capita rate of homicide in the world for youths, as well as for adults. In the late 1980s, the homicide rate for males ages 15–20 was 21.9 per 100,000. In contrast, the next highest rate among 22 developed countries was 5.0 for Scotland (Fingerhut and Kleinman 1990). Homicide is now the leading cause of death among black males ages 15–24 years, and 92% of juvenile homicide victims were murdered by persons of their own race (Snyder and Sickmund 1999). Although the number of homicides committed by black youths is dropping sharply, accounting for much of the recent decline in youth homicide rates, the rate for white youths remains flat (Office of Juvenile Justice and Delinquency Prevention 1998). Most victims of homicides committed by juveniles are male, and 30% are younger than age 18. Slightly more victims are white than are black. In 1995, the juvenile homicide rate declined by 17%; nearly all of this decline was in homicides involving firearms. Homicide rates vary greatly from state to state, with the highest rates occurring in California and Texas and the lowest rates in Minnesota and Massachusetts.

In recent years, there has been concern about school-associated deaths, most of which have been caused by firearms (Kachur et al. 1996). In the past, such violence was viewed as an urban phenomenon, to which many people turned their backs. In the mid- and late 1990s, a wave of school killings occurred in rural and suburban America, places previously considered safe, which alarmed the public and gave rise to concerns about school safety. In spite of the publicity given to these killings, schools remain basically safe places. Children are actually safer inside schools than outside, with only 12% of violent crimes against children and 1% of juvenile homicides and suicides occurring inside schools (Kachur et al. 1996). Violent crimes committed by juveniles are most likely to occur in the 4 hours after school and in early evening hours.

In addition to mortality related to violence, we need to be concerned with violence-related injuries and their cumulative cost to society, which in 1993 ran about 4 billion dollars (Mandel et al. 1993). There is also an enormous emotional toll related to the impact of witnessing violence and to traumatic bereavement. Among inner-city adolescents, 80% have witnessed assault and almost 25% have seen someone murdered (Schwab-Stone et al. 1999). Exposure to violence is associated with the development of both internalizing and externalizing behaviors that feed the cycle of violence.

Categories of Youth Violence

Aggressive behavior often occurs in the context of a conduct disorder. DSM-IV-TR classifies conduct disorders by whether they are childhood- or adolescent-onset type and specifies severity as well (American Psychiatric Association 2000). A different approach, based on animal models of aggression, classifies aggression as impulsive or predatory (Vitiello and Stroff 1997). Impulsive aggression is often associated with affective arousal but not necessarily with persistent antisocial behavior and is characterized by high levels of autonomic arousal. It may be associated with low levels of serotonergic activity (Brown et al. 1979) or with damage to frontal or temporal lobes. Individuals who manifest predatory aggression, in contrast, show low levels of arousal, and their aggression is usually premeditated and a means toward achieving their goals, which are often antisocial. These distinctions have important implications for treatment.

Yet another way to look at aggression has to do with its course across the life span. Moffitt (1993) has proposed the categories of Life-Course-Persistent antisocial behavior versus Adolescent-Limited antisocial behavior. Tolan and Guerra (1994) categorize youth violence as either situational, relationship, predatory, or psychopathological. Most youth violence falls in the first two categories, with violence occurring within the context of interpersonal relationships, and only about 5% of youth violence falls in the category of predatory aggression. It is estimated that about 5% of boys show stable antisocial behavior with onset in their preschool years. Moffitt (1993) notes that a wave of adolescents will join this group and engage in similar types of antisocial behavior, which renders the two groups indistinguishable by type of crime committed alone.

Benedek and Cornell (1989) developed typologies of youths who commit homicide. In their study of 72 incarcerated youths, they found that 42% of homicides occurred in the context of conflict, 51% in the context of committing a crime, and only 7% were psychotic. Those adolescents who killed in the course of a crime were more likely to have delinquent backgrounds and to kill strangers. In contrast, conflict-related homicides often involved victims who were friends or family. They noted that adolescents who committed conflict-related homicide had relatively less troubled backgrounds than those in the crime-related category, and they speculate that these adolescents might be more amenable to treatment.

Myers and Scott (1998) studied 18 male adolescents who had committed homicide and found that 72% had murdered in the course of committing a crime and 28% during interpersonal conflict. In contrast to Benedek and Cornell (1989), they found that 98% of their subjects had experienced one or more psychotic symptoms, most commonly paranoid ideation. These symptoms were much more common in the homicide group than in controls consisting of adolescents with conduct disorder on an inpatient psychiatric unit, only 27% of whom reported psychotic symptoms. Myers and Scott noted that those in the homicide group, despite having long-standing and conspicuous emotional and behavioral problems that preceded their crimes, had not received any mental health interventions. High rates of psychotic symptoms among juvenile murderers have also been reported by Lewis et al. (1988).

Developmental Issues

In most children, aggression begins in the first year of life. It peaks in the second year of life, at which point it is reported in 80% of toddlers, and is greater in those children with siblings (Tremblay et al. 1999). The development of language helps toddlers find other outlets for their anger and frustrations, and most children begin to internalize controls around this age. Children who fail to learn to inhibit aggression in the preschool years may go on to exhibit chronic physical aggression and difficulty curbing it in later years (Tremblay et al. 1999).

Difficult temperament in infancy has been linked to later conduct problems. A prospective study of such children conducted in Australia found that aggression emerges when difficulties in infancy interact with negative maternal perceptions of the child and a stressful environment. The authors note that parents of aggressive and/or hyperactive children may perceive them as being unrewarding and stressful, which may in turn lead to a dysfunctional mother-child relationship (Samson et al. 1993). Early intervention in these cases is recommended to help parents avoid negative coercive cycles and learn more positive interactions with their children.

The role of attachment problems in crime and violent behaviors is discussed at length by Fonagy and colleagues (1997) and Meloy (1992). Absent or insecure attachments are thought to be risk factors for aggressive and disruptive behaviors in childhood and later life. Disorganized attachment appears to have the worst outcome in terms of vulnerability to becoming violent. Disruptive behaviors often reflect on less than optimal parenting and may be a cry for attention and limits. Absence of attachment may lead to poor internalization of parental controls and values and character traits that predispose to violence. These authors note that failure to attach to parents may be transferred to institutions and figures of authority, who may become targets of antisocial behavior.

The development of empathy is an important factor that inhibits aggression and promotes prosocial behavior. The capacity for empathy, which usually develops between ages 4 and 7, involves the ability to discriminate the perspective and role of another person and the ability to respond emotionally (Feshbach 1975). Boys who are highly empathic are less aggressive than those who are deficient in empathy, and many studies show a relationship between antisocial behavior and significant delays or arrest in the development of empathy (Ellis 1982; Lee and Prentice 1988). As a result of delays in moral and cognitive development, many delinquents operate at a preconventional level and are deficient in their abilities for reciprocal role taking (Jurkovic and Prentice 1977).

The developmental tasks of adolescence include separation-individuation, establishing gender identity, auton-

omy, and a future orientation. Peer groups weigh heavily in this process and may be beneficial, or they may steer youths into activities they might not consider on their own. Adolescents may engage in risk-taking behavior and experiment with new behaviors as part of finding out who they are; this may sometimes involve aggressive or antisocial activities. Puberty may further fuel aggressive instincts, and some males may attempt to define their masculinity through the use of aggression. Adolescents, like younger children, are influenced by media violence, over which parents have less control.

In addition to peer pressure and media violence, adolescents may be witness to street violence, have less parental supervision, and have more access to means of violence. Weapons or cars in the hands of adolescents using alcohol are a potentially lethal combination.

Violence may hold a particular allure for teens who are having difficulty negotiating the tasks of adolescence. They may see it as a means of getting respect from peers, fending off bullies, dominating or getting one's way, taking a stance against authorities, or assuming adult status. Teens and children who lack social and cognitive skills may turn to violence as a means of resolving conflict. Unfortunately, this message is reinforced over and over again in the media. Violence may also be a means of warding off shame and of identifying with the aggressor rather than being a helpless victim.

Biological Factors

Studies linking testosterone to aggression in males have been done almost exclusively with adult subjects. A study of typical Swedish adolescent boys found an association between self-reports of physical and verbal aggression and low frustration tolerance with higher plasma testosterone levels (Olweus et al. 1980). Late menarche in girls has been correlated with low risk for conduct problems, and girls with early onset-menarche appear to be more susceptible to the influence of older peers (Caspi and Moffitt 1991).

Recent studies have looked at the role of serotonin in aggression in children and found a correlation between low central serotonin transmission and aggression in children and adolescents (Halperin et al. 1994; Kruesi et al. 1992). Primate studies have also found a correlation between low 5-hydroxyindoleacetic acid (5-HIAA) and increased dysregulation and social aggression (Higley et al. 1996). Pine et al. (1996) found an association between low levels of serotonin and harsh parent-child interaction. It has yet to be resolved whether serotonin dysfunction is a shared family trait or whether it results from family dysfunction. Autonomic arousal may be predictive of which antisocial adolescents go on to become adult criminals. As noted above, several studies have shown that persons with antisocial behavior show less autonomic and cortical arousal than do control subjects who are not antisocial. McBurnett et al. (2000) found that low cortisol levels were associated with persistence and early onset of aggression; they concluded that low hypothalamic-pituitary-adrenal axis activity is a correlate of severe and persistent aggression in male children and adolescents. Another study found that cortisol levels in adolescent girls with conduct disorder were significantly lower than levels in age-matched controls (Pajer et al. 2001). A prospective study of antisocial adolescents who desisted from crime found that they had higher levels of arousal than a group of adolescents who persisted with antisocial behavior (Raine et al. 1995; also see Chapter 19, "Neurodevelopmental Impact of Violence in Childhood").

Violence and Mental Illness

The relationship between violence and mental illness has not been extensively studied in teens. A recent study by the MacArthur Foundation (Steadman et al. 1998) cast doubt on the long held assumption that persons diagnosed with mental illness are at greater risk for violence. This study of adults released from mental institutions found that they were at no greater risk for violence, when compared to control subjects in their communities, unless they had substance abuse problems in addition to mental illness, in which case the risk exceeded that for controls. Noncompliance with medication has also been found to be a risk factor for violence among those people diagnosed with serious mental illness (Torrey 1994).

Many authors have noted the association between attention-deficit/hyperactivity disorder (ADHD) and conduct disorders (Barkley et al. 1990; Loeber et al. 1995; Manuzza et al. 1998), and Robins (1978) found that 55% of children with ADHD have antisocial personality disorder as adults, often in association with substance abuse problems. Research suggests that aggressive-type ADHD may be associated with antisocial familial factors and psychosocial disadvantage. Pure ADHD children with or without cognitive problems tend to do well if they have stable, caring families (Loney et al. 1981). Defiance has also been seen as a developmental precursor of conduct disorder (Lahey et al. 1992; Loeber et al. 2000; Satterfield et al. 1994).

Poor academic performance has been thought to contribute to low self-esteem and indirectly to acting-out behaviors. In a critical review, Cornwall and Bawden (1992) concluded that data suggest that reading disabilities, per se, do not cause aggressive behavior but that reading disabilities may worsen preexisting aggressive behavior. When one looks at IQ scores alone, several studies have found that sociopaths tend to score higher on performance than on verbal scales of the Wechsler Intelligence Scales for Children (WISC) and the Wechsler Adult Intelligence Scales (WAIS) (Quay 1987). Walsh and Beyer (1986) found that adolescents with discrepancies of 15 points or more showed significantly higher levels of antisocial behavior and tended to begin their antisocial behavior at earlier ages than did delinquents with lower discrepancies between performance and verbal scores.

Both victimization and witnessing violence have been shown to lead to increased aggressive behavior (Meloy et al. 2001). Posttraumatic stress disorder is prevalent among delinquent youths, and the heightened arousal, hypervigilance, and irritability that accompany this condition may contribute to excessive aggression and may be mistaken for ADHD. Other conditions associated with increased likelihood of assaultive behavior in children and adolescents include schizophrenia or psychotic symptoms, mental retardation, and traumatic brain injury.

Alcohol use and abuse is commonly found in association with aggressive behavior. It may potentiate aggression by reducing inhibition, by acting as a stimulant, and by altering judgment and impulse control. Most studies linking substance abuse to crime have been conducted with adults. The few studies conducted with adolescents have shown contradictory findings regarding the association between alcohol and violence or criminal behavior (Carpenter et al. 1988; Dawkins 1997; Elliot et al. 1989; Huizinga 1986; Meyers et al. 1998; White et al. 1993).

Many studies have implicated prefrontal lobe dysfunction as a factor contributing to antisocial behavior (Pennington and Ozonoffs 1996; Satterfield and Schell 1984; Scarpa and Raine 1997). Certainly, deficits in this area can be expected to contribute to impulsivity, mood instability, difficulty in delaying gratification, solving problems, and learning from experience. Neurological impairment is likely to be associated with persistent violence, and many studies show that a disproportionate percentage of repeat offenders have some evidence of brain dysfunction.

An adoptee study of Danish cohorts found higher-than-expected recidivistic nonviolent criminal behavior in male adoptees whose birth parents had criminal involvement or mental disorder (Moffitt 1987). However, the same study found no significant links for rates of violence. Lyons et al. (1995), in a large twin study, concluded that shared family environment was an important factor in childhood antisocial behavior and that genetic causal factors were more pronounced for adult than for juvenile antisocial traits. The interesting question of whether the juvenile courts should address the matter of genetics and culpability is discussed by Kovnick (1999). Should courts decide to give more weight to the role of genetic factors in crime, ethical issues will arise concerning dispositional alternatives, eugenics, how much weight should be given to a particular gene, and whether blaming genes will result in less effort being put into preventative programs.

Demographic and Other Factors

Poverty, low socioeconomic status, low age of mother at time of birth, low birthweight, and maternal smoking during pregnancy have been found to contribute to the onset of conduct disorder (Loeber et al. 1995; Sampson and Lauritsen 1994; Virkkunen et al. 1996; Weissman et al. 1999; Zingraff et al. 1993). Arseneault and colleagues (2000) found that adolescent boys with minor physical anomalies, particularly of the mouth, were at risk for violent delinquency. The authors commented that insults during specific phases of gestation may cause atypical brain development as well as physical anomalies. Furthermore, they noted that the anomalies may interfere with behavior regulation, feeding, communication, and social development. Arseneault et al. failed to find any interaction between the anomalies and family adversity in terms of predicting violent delinquency. A 31-year follow-up study of a large 1966 birth cohort in Finland found that being an only child increased the crude odds ratio for committing a violent crime later in life 1.8-fold. When only-child status was combined with perinatal risk factors (low birthweight, preterm birth, perinatal brain injury, or maternal smoking), the odds ratio was 4.4-fold and it rose to 8.8-fold when an absent father was added. The authors speculated that only children may miss out on the positive effect of siblings in social learning and that single mothers may have difficulty contributing to their children's sense of justice. Arseneault and colleagues also noted that absent fathers might have antisocial personality disorders and that genetics could be influencing the conduct of their offspring (Kemppainen et al. 2001).

Economic and racial inequality and population density have also been implicated as causes of violence. Scott (1999) discussed gang participation as a risk factor for violence, noting that gangs are no longer exclusively urban or male phenomena. Typically, gang violence relates to territory disputes or competition for status. Violence may be vindictively directed toward other gangs or toward one's own gang members who fail to show dis-

respect toward rival gangs. Gang presence in schools is reported to be increasing and with it victimizations of students (Snyder and Sickmund 1999).

Negative behavior by parents toward adolescents, authoritarian parenting style, and lack of parental involvement have been implicated in the etiology of antisocial behavior and violent behavior (Farrington 1989; Reiss et al. 1995). Childhood maltreatment is a well-known risk factor for violent behavior (Loeber et al. 1995), as is witnessing domestic abuse (see Chapter 20, "Domestic Abuse as a Risk Factor for Children and Youth"); it is also a substantial risk factor for dating violence (Wolfe et al. 2001). The role of abuse in contributing to difficulty with affect regulation was reviewed by Cicchetti and Toth (1995) and is also covered in Chapter 19 ("Neurodevelopmental Impact of Violence in Childhood"). The role of the media in promoting violence is addressed in Chapter 21 ("Effects of Witnessing Violence on Children and Adolescents").

Life Course

According to self-reports, youth violence peaks at age 17 in males. Property crimes peak in teen years, then drop off, whereas family violence increases with age (Gottfredson and Hirschi 1986). Most studies agree that antisocial behavior is usually established by late adolescence and that it is unusual for it to begin after that.

Loeber (1982) found that first arrest before age 11 was an important predictor of long-term adult offending. Various other researchers confirm that the onset of conduct disorder prior to age 10 carries a much worse prognosis than adolescent-onset conduct problems (Hinshaw 1994; Kratzer and Hodgins 1997; Loeber and Stouthamer-Loeber 1987; Moffitt 1993; Steiner et al. 1997). Most adolescents do not persist with aggressive antisocial behavior, and Robins (1978) found that fewer that 50% of adolescents with severe antisocial behavior became antisocial adults. A significant number of children with conduct disorders will have either a criminal record or mental disorder by age 30 and will be at increased risk for death before age 30 (Kratzer and Hodgins 1997).

Moffitt (1993) developed criteria to help differentiate the two groups. Those youths with adequate attachments, first police contact after age 13, and guilt and awareness of harmful effects of their behavior fare best and were categorized as Adolescent-Limited antisocial youths. Their delinquent behavior is marked by inconsistency and instability and may be influenced by what she calls "social mimicry" of more delinquent peers. They tend to have a greater repertoire of prosocial skills than the early-onset delinquents. In contrast, those youths who had behavior problems in childhood, ADHD, oppositional defiant disorder, cognitive deficits, poor attachments, predatory offenses, and low guilt fell into the category of Life-Course-Persistent antisocial youths. Moffitt further delineates how restricted behavioral repertoires among Life-Course-Persistent antisocial youths lock them into their antisocial behavior along with the reciprocal interactions between personality traits and environment.

Kratzer and Hodgins (1999) tested Moffitt's theory regarding age-related patterns of offending and did a prospective longitudinal study of a large cohort of Swedish male and female offenders. In contrast to Moffitt, they found that female offenders were more likely to begin their criminal careers as adults. Early-onset offenders, both male and female, committed more different types of crimes and Kratzer and Hodgins concluded that early-onset offenders were more violent than adolescent or adult-onset offenders.

A subgroup of children with conduct disorders with severe behavior patterns corresponds more closely to adult psychopathy. Notable features of these children are the presence of a callous- unemotional interpersonal style and high rates of conduct problems, in addition to oppositional defiant disorder or conduct disorder. It is speculated that it is these traits that account for persistence of antisocial behavior in early-onset conduct disorder (Christian et al. 1997). Interestingly, children with high intelligence fared better in this study, but only in the absence of parents with antisocial personality disorder. Satterfield et al. (1994) found that boys with ADHD who had high defiance scores were at greater risk for later antisocial behavior. Tremblay et al. (1994) found that impulsivity was the best predictor of early-onset, stable, highly delinquent behavior and that impulsivity and novelty-seeking personalities often overlap with ADHD, as has been confirmed in other studies. Similar findings were reported by White et al. (1994), who found that impulsivity strongly differentiated stable serious delinquents from other delinquents in early adolescence.

A Canadian study suggests that girls with medium to high ratings of disruptive behaviors in elementary school are likely to have conduct disorder diagnoses in adolescence (Cote et al. 2001). Little research has been done on the outcome of antisocial adolescent girls. The number of violent crimes committed by girls is increasing, particularly among blacks. The crime rate in adulthood for delinquent girls ranges between 25% and 46% in most studies (Pajer 1998). As with boys, the diagnosis of conduct disorder in girls has predictive value for the development of antisocial personality disorder and increases the likelihood that they will not complete high school, and girls with delinquency plus mental problems have the worst outcome in terms of coping with adult life (Werner and Smith 1992).

LEGAL ISSUES

Duty to Protect Under Tarasoff

The 1976 case of *Tarasoff v. Regents* established that a therapist has a duty to *protect* third parties who are *foreseeably* endangered by their patients. The therapist is expected to take *reasonable* steps to warn the intended victim of the danger, such as notifying police, admitting the patient to a hospital, increasing frequency of appointments, adjusting medication, or alerting the patient's family. If in doubt, the therapist should seek consultation. The decision to notify an intended victim violates patient confidentiality and should only be made after carefully weighing the history and mental status of the patient. There is no duty to warn at-large in the absence of an identified victim under *Tarasoff*. However, clinicians could be held liable for failing to detain a violent patient. Not all states have *Tarasoff* laws, but some states may have similar case law in effect.

Commitment

The decision to commit a patient requires balancing individual rights to liberty, privacy, and autonomy against the protection of society. In addition, the patient must meet the threshold for involuntary commitment, which under *Addington v. Texas* (1979) requires clear and convincing evidence that a patient is both mentally ill and dangerous. These issues are covered in more detail in Chapter 31, "Psychiatric Commitment of Children and Adolescents." In every case, the clinician needs to consider the least-restrictive alternative. For instance, an angry, abusive, oppositional, acting-out teen may not be manageable in a public school setting but might well respond to the limits of a day treatment center and not require hospitalization.

RISK ASSESSMENT

Clinicians have a poor track record when it comes to making long-term predictions of violence. Much of the early research in this area, which is reviewed by Otto (1992), failed to take into account different types of violence and the degree of confidence on the part of the clinician. McNeil et al. (1998) found that when predicting short-term risk of violence among inpatients, a high degree of confidence regarding the potential of a patient becoming violent correlated with subsequent violence. Lidz et al. (1993) studied predictions of violence by psychiatrists seeing patients in an emergency room and found that overall accuracy was only 53%. There was a tendency to underestimate violence among women, who actually had a higher number of violent incidents than men. Others have found that psychiatrists tend to overestimate the likelihood of danger. To date, there is very little research on predicting violence in children and adolescents.

Dangerousness is not a clinical diagnosis but rather a judgment based on social policy that has implications for loss of liberty. As noted by Resnick (1995), if in doubt, the legal system acquits, whereas the medical system is likely to admit. Psychiatrists are often asked by the courts or others to predict violence when in fact they are ill equipped to do so. At best, they can offer risk assessments for the likelihood of imminent danger based upon 1) risk factors, 2) type of violence, and 3) the risk level, which changes over time. Factors to take into consideration in making such assessments include history of violent behavior, including frequency, magnitude, context of violence, psychiatric diagnosis, and the nature of the violent fantasies and threats. Predatory aggression needs to be differentiated from affective aggression, and it is more difficult to predict and treat.

Psychiatric conditions that may carry an increased risk for violence include borderline, antisocial, paranoid, and narcissistic personality disorders, disruptive disorders, mental retardation, certain organic conditions, schizophrenia, delusional disorders (particularly those involving perceived threats), and mania or jealousy. Paranoid symptoms may be associated with transient violence, whereas violence associated with organic impairment is likely to be more persistent. Violence may also occur in profoundly depressed patients, as is seen in murder-suicides and those who strike out in despair, and in dissociative disorders. Patients who have been victimized in the past may be prone to acting on well-rehearsed fantasies for defending themselves in event of actual or perceived assault.

A large meta-study sponsored by the Office of Juvenile Justice Prevention found that the best predictor of violent or serious delinquency in the 6- to 11-year age group was serious delinquency and the best predictor of future violence in this age group was substance abuse. The authors concluded that risk for violence is compounded by numerous risk factors and that the larger the number of risk factors a youth has, the greater the risk of violence (Hawkins et al. 2000).

Factors that might mitigate against violence also need to be considered. These might include a responsible family capable of close supervision, a good therapeutic relationship and willingness to comply with treatment recommendations, absence of prior history of violence, good reality testing, ego strengths, and feeling conflicted over violent thoughts.

CLINICAL ISSUES

The Clinician's Safety

Assaults by patients on psychiatrists have been well documented, and approximately 40% of psychiatrists will be attacked by a patient in their lifetime (Tardiff 1996). Psychiatric residents and inexperienced clinicians seem to be at particular risk, as are psychiatric staff working on inpatient units, understaffed units, and in emergency rooms. Women in positions of authority appear to be at equal risk for assaults as their male colleagues. Among child inpatients, boys are more likely than girls to be assaultive, particularly if they have been diagnosed with conduct disorder. The clinician may be unaware of the diagnosis when he or she first approaches a new patient, and basic precautions should be taken if working in a high-risk environment. The physical location and layout of the interviewing room should be assessed. Are there security personnel nearby? If not, does an alert system exist, such as panic buttons, phone codes, or radio devices? Is the room free from objects that could easily be used as weapons (e.g., lightweight furniture, heavy-duty staplers, medical equipment such as test tubes, syringes, etc.)? Is the room large enough so that the clinician does not intrude upon the patient's personal space? Is there a policy in place for handling out of control patients? If concerned about personal safety, consider whether it is wise to position oneself between the patient and the door; in some instances one might choose to keep the door ajar or open. If assessing a potentially violent child, it is prudent to remove personal effects (e.g., jewelry, eyeglasses) or curios in the office that the child might demolish or use as weapons. Having a parent nearby may help with setting limits and is useful in the event that the interview needs to be prematurely terminated.

If the clinician has the benefit of knowing ahead of time about a history of violence or vindictive behavior, he might think twice about doing a forensic evaluation on such a patient in his or her private office. For instance, if evaluating a parent for termination of parental rights, he might opt to see him or her in the offices of Protective Services. In one such case, the parent of a child in custody had threatened to blow up the local Department of Child Protective Services and was no longer allowed on their premises. The author ended up evaluating him and his wife in the living room of their home with a police officer sitting in the adjacent kitchen.

Measures should be taken to not provoke volatile patients. These include speaking softly, not demeaning or threatening the patient in any way, empathic listening, and monitoring one's body language as well as the patient's. Defensive postures, such as standing above the patient or with arms crossed, should be avoided. It is useful to address the patient by name, establish verbal contact, and try to talk down a patient who is threatening violence. Limits should be gently but firmly set, and giving limited choices may be effective. Arguments and promises should be avoided, and it may even be useful to agree that it is all right to disagree. If a patient arrives for an appointment intoxicated, the appointment should be rescheduled. Physical defense maneuvers are beyond the scope of this chapter but are covered by Tardiff (1996).

Issues of Consent and Confidentiality

As discussed in Chapter 4, "Introduction to Forensic Evaluations," it is important that the person being assessed be aware of whom the examiner is working for, the purpose of the evaluation, and the limited confidentiality of the examination. Even when patients are so informed, they may lose sight of this in the course of the evaluation, particularly if the psychiatrist is empathic, and they may need to be reminded of these issues.

Taking a Violence History

In years past, child and adolescent psychiatrists were loath to inquire about violent tendencies in children. In part, this may have been related to the wish to believe in the innocence of youth, but it was also linked to the fact that few knew what to do with the information they might receive. This situation has changed as a result of the increased prevalence of youth violence, greater awareness of posttraumatic stress disorder, and a litigious climate in which clinicians may be held liable for violent acts committed by their patients. Most clinicians now almost routinely inquire about victimization and violent tendencies, at least in their adolescent and adult patients. It is also important to explore exposure to violence as a witness or bystander (Pittel 1998).

Questions about violent thoughts should include their chronicity, intensity, and whether or not they are escalating. Patients with mental illness may be more likely to act upon violent fantasies of long-standing duration because they serve as well-rehearsed scenarios (Steadman et al. 1998). Delusions most commonly involve thoughts of persecution or mind/body control and are fluid over time. Delusions should be explored, particularly those involving thought control override, such as beliefs that people are spying on them or controlling their thoughts. Some delusions in schizophrenic patients may actually mitigate against violence if they lead to social isolation. On the other hand, paranoid delusions, when combined with substance abuse, increase the potential for violence (Steadman 1998). The research on the association between command hallucinations and violence remains scant and methodologically weak (Rudnick 1999). Many schizophrenic patients are able to ignore command hallucinations; however, patients who recognize these voices are more likely to respond to them than those who do not (Junginger 1995).

Additional helpful factors to know in assessing imminent danger include the degree to which a patient's violent thoughts are ego-dystonic, the patient's capacity for empathy and self-control, whether substance abuse is involved, and whether the patient has access to weapons. Resnick (1995) reminds us that the only difference between assault and homicide is the lethality of the weapon used. Does the patient have a specific plan? If so, how well thought out is it, and is there an intended victim? What has stopped him from acting on it, and does he have concerns about consequences of his violence either to himself or others?

Many victims of violence or sexual abuse, particularly males, may become perpetrators of violence, hence the need to inquire about these tendencies. A patient is likely to be more forthcoming about these matters if the clinician maintains a nonjudgmental stance and monitors his body language. Questions about violence might include asking what was the most violent act he ever committed? How did he feel about what he did? What makes him angry and does he have any nonviolent means of resolving conflict? Is he able to walk away from a potential fight? What is his capacity for empathy with the victim? If he is homicidal, does he have a plan and a means or carrying it out? Has he considered the consequences to himself, and are they deterrents? When appropriate, the clinician should ask about date violence or participation in gang violence.

Additional questions might include asking about role models for violence within their home. What is their

TABLE 23–1.   Risk assessment of violence in youths

1. Past history of violence toward self, others, objects, or animals and fire setting
2. Bullying or early-onset conduct disorder
3. Witnessing violence or victimization
4. Severity, frequency, and chronicity of violence
5. Context: predatory or affective
6. Attachment and empathy
7. Intent, formulation, and means
8. Comorbid risk factors—psychosis, conduct disorder, ADHD, organicity, substance abuse
9. Peer and media influences
10. Degree of conflict and willingness to seek and use help
11. Ego strengths
12. Support systems and role models at home

exposure to media violence and video games? How do they feel about it, and have they become habituated to it? Frequency and precipitants of violent acts should be explored and a determination made as to whether violence is predatory or affective.

Taking a weapons history is covered in Chapter 22, "Children's Access to Weapons," and is discussed by Pittel (1998). Similar inquiries should be made about substance abuse, sexual history, gang membership, and any criminal involvement, and age of onset and frequency of these activities. Head trauma may be common in children who engage in risk-taking behavior or come from abusive backgrounds. Academic history may provide clues to comorbid problems with learning or conduct problems.

Family history of substance abuse or domestic violence, antisocial behavior, and child abuse should be obtained from the child, when appropriate, and from parents as well. Factors to be reviewed in assessing the risk of violence are summarized in Table 23–1.

Interviewing

Location of the Interview

Privacy is helpful but not always possible when interviewing incarcerated youths. Lockups may be noisy, and interview rooms are usually designed for observation. Youths may be in shackles or handcuffs, which are both uncomfortable and humiliating. In some instances, the examiner may request that they be removed. Forensic examiners need to come to terms with their own discomfort in such facilities. The risk of harm coming to them may be decreased with incarcerated youths, as security is nearby and factors contributing to their violence (i.e., interpersonal conflict, substance abuse, or predatory behavior) are usually not an issue with the forensic evaluator in a structured environment.

Establishing an Alliance

Establishing an alliance may be difficult with teens who have antiauthority attitudes. Treating them with respect and giving them choices may enlist their cooperation. Humor may be used to dispel anxiety and resistance. Taciturn or oppositional children and adolescents and those with poor verbal skills may often be drawn out with use of drawings or games. Exploration of violent fantasies may be done through drawings, which may be particularly helpful for youths with poor verbal skills. With younger children, play will reveal a great deal about patterns of aggression and whether their anger is diffuse or focused on one person. Repetitive scenarios of aggression or victimization may suggest posttraumatic stress disorder. Children and adolescents who do not wish to talk may sometimes be willing to share their poetry or short stories. Written work may also suggest learning disabilities.

Physical Appearance

Physical appearance provides clues to mental status and diagnoses. Tattoos are rampant in antisocial populations and can provide road maps to the chronology of conduct problems. Tattoos in teens are usually crude and self-inflicted, as one must be 18 to frequent a tattoo parlor. Swastikas and other symbols cry out hatred and alienation, "love" written on the knuckles of one hand and "hate" on the other may speaks of ambivalence, and a teddy bear hidden on the calf of one incarcerated delinquent spoke of his need for a transitional object. Tattoos may provide clues to gang activity (e.g., one youth had tattooed his forearm with "UGT," which stood for Underground Thugs, in large letters). Hairstyle, body piercings, scars from fights, child abuse, or self abuse, and logos on T-shirts are also fertile fields of inquiry. Body posture may suggest defeat and despair or convey the bravado of a defiant youth. If acute intoxication is suspected, physical signs consistent with this, such as dilated pupils, dysarthria, incoordination, flushing, and perspiring, should be noted.

Mental Status Examination

A formal mental status examination is useful for assessing cognitive deficits, level of intellectual functioning, and screening for psychosis or organicity. Questions about judgment are often very revealing. Thoughts of suicide or homicide should always be explored in this population.

Malingering

If a youth is being charged with a crime and faces possible incarceration, the possibility of malingering should be considered. Malingering involves deliberately faking symptoms of an illness for personal gain, and it differs from factitious disorders in that the goal is external rather than the wish to be in the patient role. A youth in detention might fake mental illness in hopes that she will be sent to a mental hospital instead of a correctional facility. Some teens, on the other hand, may exaggerate their bad behavior in order to impress peers and would rather be seen as bad than as mad in order to avoid psychiatric hospitalization. Facial expressions and presence or absence of eye contact are not reliable clues for detecting lies. Clues to malingered mental illness include inconsistencies in history, symptoms, and presentation, a tendency to call attention to their symptoms, and stereotypical presentations of what they know about certain disorders. There is likely to be a disparity between what they report in the way of symptoms and what the evaluator observes. Suspicions should also be aroused by reports of hallucinations without delusions, hallucinations that are present all the time, and those that consist only of indistinct voices. Malingerers usually have difficulty faking the negative symptoms and more subtle signs of schizophrenia.

Budding psychopaths are skilled at manipulating and conning, and there is no reason why they should treat forensic evaluators any differently than other persons in their lives. They may entice sympathies, be persuasive in their protestations of innocence, portray themselves as victimized or misunderstood, or feign remorse.

The Meaning of Violence

Efforts should be made to explore the meaning of violence in the patient's life and development and try to reach a psychodynamic formulation. Violence may be a way of trying to rectify underlying issues of shame. Self-esteem is often fragile in this population, and narcissistic injury may trigger violent outbursts. Violence may be viewed as a way of resolving hopelessness and despair and assuming control over their lives. As noted by Malmquist (1996), homicide may represent misplaced aggression and become a paradoxical alternative to suicide. Suicidal ideation and affective disorder should always be explored in this population, along with violence potential and substance abuse. Youths with features of borderline personality disorder may resort to violence as a means of handling rejection or loss. Delinquents who are unable to relate their feeling s regarding commission of violent acts are of concern and at risk for repeating these acts.

The clinician needs to ferret out comorbid psychiatric disorders and determine if there are treatable conditions underlying aggressive behavior and what strengths there are with which to work.

Corroboration

Forensic reports are much stronger when they include a broad database. In assessing violence, this might include observations from family, school personnel, physicians, therapists, staff in hospitals or youth detention facilities when relevant, and police records. This is particularly important when assessing conditions such as posttraumatic stress disorder, which are primarily subjective. Psychological testing is useful in confirming diagnoses and ruling out malingering.

Interventions

As noted above, Table 23–1 summarizes risk factors to be considered in assessing the imminent risk to others and the likelihood of repeated violence in a youth. The examiner's report to the court should specify what sort of facility, program, and intervention the youth requires. Recommendations should be feasible, and it is often useful to have a backup plan (see Table 23–2). Table 23–3 covers issues to be considered in making a decision to discharge. Pressures to discharge patients prematurely from psychiatric hospitals are common under managed care; should this occur, the clinician should file an appeal if she believes that discharging a youth entails too much risk. She has an ethical duty to continue care whether or not the insurance company is willing to pay for it if the youth is still in crisis.

TABLE 23–2.   Decisions about dispositional options for outpatients

1. What are the diagnoses, and what is the risk for imminent violence?
2. Does the youth require hospitalization?
3. Are *Tarasoff* warnings indicated?
4. Is a consultation and/or a second opinion indicated?
5. Can the youth's violent tendencies be managed outside a hospital?
6. If so, are resources available and feasible?
7. Is there a stable family to support outpatient recommendations?
8. Does the youth have access to weapons?
9. Will substance abuse preclude outpatient treatment?
10. Is the youth willing to comply with outpatient treatment?
11. Is medication likely to help?
12. If no mental illness is present, what other resources should be recommended to deal with the youth's violent behavior?

TABLE 23–3.   Deciding when it is safe to discharge a violent patient

1. Has the underlying problem that brought the patient into the hospital been treated?
2. Are problems with violence related to alcohol or drugs? If so, is outpatient treatment feasible and is the patient willing to address substance abuse issues?
3. Have other comorbid conditions been addressed?
4. Does the patient show some understanding of what triggered his or her violence and has he or she developed coping skills for dealing with anger?
5. Will the youth be returning to a delinquent peer group?
6. Is there a stable family?
7. Have weapons been removed from the youth's home?
8. Is there an appropriate school setting for the youth? Have special education needs been addressed?

PITFALLS

Countertransference

Countertransference may operate in a variety of ways in forensic evaluations. The clinician may pull back out of fear and be so detached as to have difficulty relating to the patient. Prior personal experience with trauma may make it difficult to hear accounts of violence. Judgmental attitudes may also interfere with the evaluation. On the other hand, adolescents may be compelling and elicit the clinician's sympathies regarding their abusive pasts to the point where the clinician is too sympathetic and forgiving and loses objectivity and sight of the purpose of the evaluation.

Role Confusion

The risk of wearing two hats has been repeated throughout this text. Clinicians must be clear with themselves and patients as to whether their roles are therapeutic or forensic. The forensic evaluator must resist the temptation to be therapeutic rather than focus on gathering and interpreting data in order to address the legal issues at hand.

Denial

It is easy to minimize the potential for violence, particularly if one likes or identifies with a patient. Denial may result from not taking an adequate violence history and may also stem from clinicians' discomfort with vivid descriptions of violent thoughts and actions.

Gullibility

It is easy to be taken in by adolescents, and the possibility of malingering or faking bad or good must always be considered. Corroborative evidence serves as a good check and balance in this regard. Staff who work daily with patients may be in a better position to detect malingering as they see patients at multiple points in time in a variety of circumstances and are more aware of manipulative behavior.

False Confessions

The clinician should bear in mind that younger children and some adolescents may be highly suggestible, as was discussed in Chapter 14 ("Reliability and Suggestibility of Children's Statements"). In forensic settings, children may confess to crimes they did not commit, particularly if questioning is coercive or highly suggestible or they feel intimidated by the examiner. They also may fail to appreciate the consequences of making a false confession.

Inadequate Assessment

Considering the stakes of potential loss of liberty through incarceration or hospitalization and the risk of harm to others, great care needs to be taken in both making assessments of violence and gathering as much information as possible and from a variety of sources.

The Limits of Prediction

Long-range predictions about violence should be avoided. The clinician is on firmer territory if she restricts herself to risk assessment for imminent harm.

CASE EXAMPLE EPILOGUES

Case Example 1

Dr. Kovak feels hopeful about this case based on a stable home environment, commitment and cooperation from the parents, Ethan's young age, his eagerness for help, and conflict about his behavior. Nonetheless, she is concerned about his entrenched and escalating pattern of fire setting and the limited fire-fighting equipment in his small community. Ethan begins to recognize that his fire setting is often triggered by anger with his mother and her perceived role in the divorce, which he has had difficulty verbalizing. Therapy allows him to redirect his anger and learn cognitive skills to deal with his impulse to start fires. He starts to realize that setting fires does not make his anger go away and only makes him feel worse. After a few months of therapy, his drawings are more contained, his schoolwork and self-esteem improve, and he is much better able to verbalize his feelings with his parents. There are no further incidents of fire setting.

Case Example 2

Dr. Chu views Sam as a fairly disturbed young man who is schizoid, alienated, and learning disabled and who has poor social skills and little empathy. Sam's increasing retreat into fantasy, constricted lifestyle, and family history raise concerns about a thought disorder. He appears to be ill equipped to deal with the many traumas he has endured in his life, and there is little in the way of family support. Dr. Chu suspects that beneath Sam's rage there is depression. He concludes that Sam would pose some risk to students and faculty were he to return to school and that, if he did return, he would most likely meet with failure both academically and socially, which might set him back even further. Recommendations are made for psychological testing to rule out a thought disorder, medication evaluation, therapy, and a day treatment program. In addition, it is suggested that his mother try to curb his exposure to media violence and remove weapons from the home.

Dr. Chu ponders whether he has a duty to protect under *Tarasoff*. His client, in this case, is the school, not Sam. Sam is aware that a report will be released to the school. In as much as Sam has identified some potential victims, Dr. Chu decides to share information regarding Sam's homicidal thoughts with the school and with his parents. In addition, keeping him out of school, providing treatment, and transferring him to a secure and therapeutic setting will offer further protection to possible victims.

Case Example 3

Dr. Freedman feels a bit overwhelmed with the diagnostic possibilities and decides to request school records and get psychological testing to help her clarify the nature of Jason's learning problems, the possibility of attention-deficit/hyperactivity disorder, and to help rule out organicity. She feels more certain about her diagnoses of substance abuse and a conduct disorder, most likely oppositional defiant disorder. Even though Jason shows some antisocial features, she avoids diagnosing him with a personality disorder given his young age, but she is concerned by the early onset of his aggressive behavior and his callousness. In hindsight, she realizes she probably should have probed further for symptoms of posttraumatic stress disorder and depression.

She is guarded about his prognosis. Jason's only allegiances are to fellow gang members, his identity seems rooted in his antisocial behavior, and he is impulsive, has poor role models and no supports to speak of, and may be cognitively disabled. Chronic marijuana use has further limited his adolescent development and coping skills and has perhaps contributed to his apathy. His early history of bullying and violence suggests that he is likely to continue with his violent behavior. She recommends, pending results of psychological testing, that he be sent to a secure correctional facility that will be able to meet his needs for special education, possible vocational training, and help with cognitive and social skills, anger management, and substance abuse. A trial of medication might be helpful, depending on results of testing.

ACTION GUIDELINES

A. Be aware of risk factors and do not shy away from taking violence and substance abuse histories.

B. Look for treatable disorders that may be comorbid with conduct disorders.

C. Adhere to ethical and legal obligations.

D. Seek consultation when in doubt.

E. Limit predictions to short-term risk assessments.

REFERENCES

Addington v Texas, 441 US 418 (1979)

American Psychiatric Association: Diagnostic and Statistical Manual of Mental Disorders, 4th Edition, Text Revision. Washington, DC, American Psychiatric Association, 2000

Arseneault L, Tremblay R, Boulerice B, et al: Minor physical anomalies and family adversity as risk factors for violent delinquency in adolescence. Am J Psychiatry 157:917–923, 2000

Barkley R, Fischer M, Edelbrock C, et al: The adolescent outcome of hyperactive children diagnosed by research criteria: an 8 year prospective follow-up study. J Am Acad Child Adolesc Psychiatry 29:546–557, 1990

Benedek E, Cornell D: Juvenile Homicide. Washington, DC, American Psychiatric Press, 1989

Brown D, Goodman F, Ballenger J, et al: Aggression in humans: correlates with cerebrospinal fluid amine metabolites. Psychiatry Res 1:131–139, 1979

Carpenter A, Glassner B, Johnson D, et al: Kids, Drugs, and Crime. Lexington, MA, Lexington Books, 1988

Caspi A, Moffitt T: Individual differences are accentuated during periods of social change: the sample case of girls at puberty. J Pers Soc Psychol 61:157–168, 1991

Christian R, Frick P, Hill N, et al: Psychopathy and conduct problems in children: implications for subtyping children with conduct problems. J Am Acad Child Adolesc Psychiatry 36(2):233–241, 1997

Cicchetti D, Toth S: A developmental psychopathology perspective on child abuse and neglect. J Am Acad Child Adolesc Psychiatry 43:541–565, 1995

Cornwall A, Bawden H: Reading disabilities and aggression: a critical review. J Learn Disabil 25:281–288, 1992

Cote A, Zoccolillo M, Tremblay R, et al: Predicting girl's conduct disorder in adolescence from childhood trajectories of disruptive behaviors. J Am Acad Child Adolesc Psychiatry 40:678–684, 2001

Dawkins M: Drug use and violent crime among delinquents. Adolescence 32(126):396–405, 1997

Elliott D, Huizinga D, Menard S: Multiple problem youth: delinquency, substance abuse, and mental health problems. New York, Springer-Verlag, 1989

Ellis P: Empathy: a factor in antisocial behavior. J Abnorm Child Psychol 10:123–134, 1982

Farrington D: Early predictors of adolescent aggression and adult violence. Violence Vict 4:79–100, 1989

Feshbach N: Empathy in children: some theoretical and empirical considerations. The Counseling Psychologist 5(2):25–30, 1975

Fingerhut L, Kleinman J: International and interstate comparisons among young males. JAMA 263:3292–3295, 1990

Fonagy P, Target M, Steele M, et al: The development of violence and crime as it relates to security of attachment, in Children in a Violent Society. Edited by Osofsky J. New York, Guilford, 1997, pp 150–170

Gottfredson M, Hirschi T: The value would appear to be zero: an essay on career criminals, criminal careers, selective incapacitation, cohort studies, and related topics. Criminology 24:213–234, 1986

Halperin J, Vanshdeep A, Silver L, et al: Serotonergic function in aggressive and nonaggressive boys with attention deficit hyperactivity disorder. Am J Psychiatry 151:243–248, 1994

Hawkins D, Herrnkohl D, Farrington P, et al: Predictors of violent or serious delinquency by age group: a comparative ranking. Juvenile Justice Bulletin (Washington, DC), April 2000 [http://www.ncjrs.org/html/ojjdp/jjbul2000_04_5/pag4.html]

Higley J, Mehlman P, Poland R: CSF testosterone and 5-HIAA correlates with different types of aggressive behavior. Biol Psychiatry 40:1067–1082, 1996

Hinshaw S: Conduct disorder in childhood: conceptualization, diagnosis, comorbidity, and risk status for antisocial functioning in adulthood, in Experimental Personality and Psychopathology Research. Edited by Fowles DC, Stoker P, Goodman S. New York, Springer, 1994, pp 3–44

Huizinga D: The relationship between delinquent and drug use behaviors in national sample of youths, in Crime Rates Among Drug Abusing Offenders. Edited by Johnson B, Wish E. New York, Interdisciplinary Research Center, Narcotic and Drug Research, Inc, 1986, pp 145–194

Junginger K: Command hallucinations and the prediction of dangerousness. Psychiatr Serv 46:911–914, 1995

Jurkovic G, Prentice N: Relations of moral and cognitive development to dimensions of juvenile delinquency. J Abnorm Psychol 86:414–420, 1977

Kachur A, Stennies G, Powell K, et al: School associated violent deaths in the United States 1992–94. JAMA 275:1729–1733, 1996

Kemppainen L, Jokelainen J, Jarvelin M, et al: The one-child family and violent criminality: a 31-year follow-up study of the northern Finland 1966 birth cohort. Am J Psychiatry 158:960–962, 2001

Kovnick K: Juvenile culpability and genetics, in Genetics and Criminality: The Potential Misuse of Scientific Information in Court. Edited by Botkin J, McMahon W, Francis L. Washington, DC, American Psychological Association, 1999, pp 211–223

Kratzer L, Hodgins A: Adult outcomes of child conduct problems: a cohort study. J Abnorm Child Psychol 25(1):65–81, 1997

Kratzer L, Hodgins S: A typology of offenders: a test of Moffitt's theory among males and females from childhood to age 30. Criminal Behavior and Mental Health 9:57–73, 1999

Kruesi M, Hibbs E, Zahn T, et al: A 2 year prospective follow up study of children and adolescents with disruptive behavior disorders. Arch Gen Psychiatry 49:429–435, 1992

Lahey B, Loeber R, Quay H, et al: Oppositional defiant and conduct disorders: issues to be resolved for DSM-IV. J Am Acad Child Adolesc Psychiatry 31:529–546, 1992

Lee M, Prentice M: Interrelations of empathy, cognition, and moral reasoning with dimensions of juvenile delinquency. J Abnorm Child Psychol 16:127–139, 1988

Lewis D, Pincus J, Bard B, et al: Neuropsychiatric, psychoeducational, and family characteristics of 14 juveniles condemned to death in the United States. Am J Psychiatry 145:584–589, 1988

Lidz C, Mulvey E, Gardner W: The accuracy of predictions of violence to others. JAMA 269:1007–1011, 1993

Loeber R: The stability of antisocial and delinquent child behavior: a review. Child Dev 53:1431–1446, 1982

Loeber R, Stouthamer-Loeber M: Prediction, in Handbook of Juvenile Delinquency. Edited by Quay H. New York, Wiley, 1987, pp 225–282

Loeber R, Green S, Keenan K, et al: Which boys will fare worse: early predictors of the onset of conduct disorder in a six year longitudinal study. J Am Acad Child Adolesc Psychiatry 34:499–509, 1995

Loeber R, Burke J, Lahey B, et al: Oppositional defiant and conduct disorder: a review of the past 10 years, part I. J Am Acad Child Adolesc Psychiatry 39:1468–1484, 2000

Loney J, Kramer J, Milich RS: The hyperactive child grows up: predictors of symptoms, delinquency and achievement at follow-up, in Psychosocial Aspects of Drug Treatment for Hyperactivity. Edited by Gadow KD, Loney K. Boulder, CO, Westview Press, 1981, pp 381–416

Lyons M, True W, Eisen S, et al: Differential heritability of adult and juvenile antisocial traits. Arch Gen Psychiatry 52:906–915, 1995

Malmquist C: Homicide: A Psychiatric Perspective. Washington, DC, American Psychiatric Press, 1996

Mandel M, Magnusson P, Ellis J, et al: The economics of crime. Business Week, December 13, 1993, pp 72–81

Manuzza S, Klein R, Bessler A, et al: Adult psychiatric status of hyperactive boys grown up. Am J Psychiatry 155:493–498, 1998

McNeil D, Sanberg D, Binder R: The relationship between confidence and accuracy in clinical assessment of psychiatric patients: potential for violence. Law Hum Behav 22(6): 655–669, 1998

Meloy R: Violent Attachments. Northvale, NJ, Jason Aronson, 1992

Meloy R, Hempel A, Mohandie K, et al: Offender and offense characteristics of a nonrandom sample of adolescent mass murderers. J Am Acad Child Adolesc Psychiatry 40:719–128, 2001

Meyers M, Stewart D, Brown S: Progression from conduct disorder to antisocial personality disorder following treatment for adolescent substance abuse. Am J Psychiatry 155:479–485, 1998

Moffitt T: Parental mental disorder and offspring criminal behavior: an adoption study. Psychiatry 50:346–360, 1987

Moffitt T: Adolescent-limited and life-course-persistent antisocial behavior: a developmental taxonomy. Psychol Rev 100:674–701, 1993

Myers W, Scott K: Psychotic and conduct disorder symptoms in juvenile murderers. Homicide Studies 2(2):160–175, 1998

Office of Juvenile Justice and Delinquency Prevention Statistical Briefing Book Online, 1998 [http://ojjdp.ncjrs.org/ojstatbb/qa048.html]

Olweus D, Mattsson A, Schalling D: Testosterone, aggression, physical and personality dimensions in normal adolescent males. Psychosom Med 42(2):253–269, 1980

Otto R: Prediction of dangerous behavior: a review and analysis of "second-generation" research. Forensic Reports 5:103–133, 1992

Pajer A: What happens to "bad girls?": a review of the adult outcomes of antisocial adolescent girls. Am J Psychiatry 155: 862–870, 1998

Pennington B, Ozonoffs S: Executive functions and developmental psychopathology. J Child Psychol Psychiatry 37: 51–87, 1996

Pine D, Wasserman G, Coplan R, et al: Platelet serotonin 2A receptor characteristics and parenting factors for boys at risk for delinquency. Am J Psychiatry 153:538–544, 1996

Pittel E: How to take a violence history: J Am Acad Child Adolesc Psychiatry 37:1100–1102, 1998

Pollock V, Briere J, Schneider M, et al: Childhood antecedents of antisocial behavior: parental alcoholism and physical abusiveness. Am J Psychiatry 147:1290–1293, 1990

Quay H: Intelligence, in Handbook of Juvenile Delinquency. Edited by Quay H. New York, Wiley, 1987

Raine A, Venebles P, Williams M: High autonomic arousal and electrodermal orienting at age 15 years as protective factors against criminal behavior at age 29 years. Am J Psychiatry 152:1595–1600, 1995

Reiss R, Hetherington E, Plomin R, et al: Genetic questions for environmental studies: differential parenting and psychopathology in adolescence. Arch Gen Psychiatry 52:925–936, 1995

Resnick P: Forensic Psychiatry Review Course. Seattle, WA, American Academy of Psychiatry and Law, 1995

Robins L: Sturdy childhood predictors of adult antisocial behavior: replications from longitudinal studies. Psychol Med 8:611–622, 1978

Rudnick A: Relation between command hallucinations and dangerous behavior. J Am Acad Psychiatry Law 27:253–258, 1999

Sampson T, Lauritsen J: Violent victimization and offending: individual-, situational-, and community-level risk factors, in Understanding and Preventing Violence, Vol 3: Social Influences. Edited by Reiss A, Roth J, Miczek K. Washington, DC, National Academy Press, 1994, pp 1–114

Samson A, Smart D, Prior M, et al: Precursors of hyperactivity and aggression. J Am Acad Child Adolesc Psychiatry 32:1207–1216, 1993

Satterfield JH, Schell A: Childhood brain function differences in delinquent and non-delinquent hyperactive boys. Electroencephalogr Clin Neurophysiol 57:199–207, 1984

Satterfield J, Swanson J, Schell A, et al: Prediction of antisocial behavior in attention-deficit hyperactivity disorder boys from aggression/defiance scores. J Am Acad Child Adolesc Psychiatry 33:185–190, 1994

Scarpa A, Raine A: Biology of wickedness. Psychiatric Annals 27:624–629, 1997

Schwab-Stone M, Chen A, Greenberger W, et al: No safe haven, II: the effects of violence exposure on urban youth. J Am Acad Child Adolesc Psychiatry 38:359–367, 1999

Scott C: Juvenile violence. Psychiatr Clin North Am 22:71–83, 1999

Sickmund M, Snyder H, Poe-Yamagata E: Juvenile offenders and victims: 1997 update on violence. Washington, DC, Office of Juvenile Justice and Delinquency Prevention, 1997

Snyder H, Sickmund M: Juvenile Offenders and Victims: A National Report (Document NCI-153569). Washington, DC, U.S. Department of Justice, Office of Juvenile Justice and Delinquency Prevention, 1995

Snyder M, Sickmund M: Juvenile Offenders and Victims: 1999 National Report. Washington, DC, U.S. Department of Justice, Office of Juvenile Justice and Delinquency Prevention, 1999

Steadman H, Mulvey E, Monahan J, et al: Violence by people discharged from acute psychiatric inpatient facilities and by others in the same neighborhood. Arch Gen Psychiatry 44:393–401, 1998

Steiner H, Williams S, Benton-Hardy L, et al: Violent crime paths in incarcerated juveniles: psychological, environmental, and biological factors, in The Biosocial Bases of Violence. Edited by Raine A, Farrington D, Brenna R, et al. New York, Plenum, 1997, pp 325–328

Tarasoff v Regents, 17 Cal 3d 425, 551 P2d 334, 131 Cal Rptr 14 (1974)

Tardiff K: Assessment and Management of Violent Patients. Washington, DC, American Psychiatric Press, 1996

Tolan P, Guerra N: What Works in Reducing Adolescent Violence: An Empirical Review of the Field. Boulder, CO, Center for the Study and Prevention of Violence, 1994

Torrey EF: Violent behavior by individuals with serious mental illness. Hospital and Community Psychiatry 45:653–662, 1994

Tremblay R, Pihl R, Vitaro R, et al: Predicting early onset of male antisocial behavior from preschool behavior. Arch Gen Psychiatry 51:732–738, 1994

Tremblay R, Japel C, Perusee D, et al: The search for the age of 'onset' of physical aggression: Rousseau and Bandura revisited. Criminal Behavior and Mental Health 9:8–23, 1999

U.S. Department of Justice: Early Warning Timely Response, A Guide to Safe Schools [http://www.air.org/cecp/actionguide]

Virkkunen M, Eggert M, Rawlings R, et al: A prospective follow-up study of alcoholic violent offenders and fire setters. Arch Gen Psychiatry 53:523–529, 1996

Vitiello B, Stroff D: Subtypes of aggression and their relevance to child psychiatry. J Am Acad Child Adolesc Psychiatry 36:307–315, 1997

Walsh A, Beyer A: Wechsler performance–verbal discrepancy and antisocial behavior J Soc Psychol 126(3):419–420, 1986

Weissman M, Warner V, Wickramaraatne P, et al: Maternal smoking during pregnancy and psychopathology in offspring followed to adulthood. J Am Acad Child Adolesc Psychiatry 38(7):892–899, 1999

Werner E, Smith R: Overcoming the Odds: High Risk Children From Birth to Adulthood. Ithaca, NY, Cornell University Press, 1992

White H, Brick J, Hansel S: A longitudinal investigation of alcohol use and aggression in adolescence. J Stud Alcohol (suppl 11):62–77, 1993

White J, Moffitt T, Caspi A: Measuring impulsivity and examining its relationship to delinquency. J Abnorm Psychol 103(2):192–205, 1994

Wolfe D, Scott K, Wekerle C, et al: Child maltreatment: risk of adjustment problems and dating violence in adolescence. J Am Acad Child Adolesc Psychiatry 40:282–289, 2001

Zingraff M, Leiter J, Myer K: Child maltreatment and youthful problem behavior. Criminology 31:173–202, 1993

CHAPTER 24

Prevention of Youth Violence

Dewey G. Cornell, Ph.D.

Case Example

The conflict between two rival groups of teenage girls escalated dramatically over a period of weeks. Minor incidents, such as a humorous remark that was taken as an insult and joking criticism of unfashionable clothing, were followed by increasingly malicious rumors ("her boyfriend cheats on her," "her baby has AIDS") and then threatening remarks ("I'm gonna whip her good"). One night the girls confronted one another on a downtown street and harsh words erupted into a brawl that had to be broken up by the police. One girl was cut with a knife, so her friends vowed revenge.

The conflict expanded when friends of the girls felt compelled to choose sides, and some of the rivals' boyfriends also became involved. The boys introduced guns into the dispute, and a shooting incident at a late-night dance aroused public concern and brought official attention to the problem. Nevertheless, police patrols and juvenile court hearings did little to lessen the feud. Many fearful students refused to attend school or venture to the local mall, while other students reportedly began carrying weapons in anticipation of the need to defend themselves. Faced with growing tension among students at school, along with dozens of calls from worried parents, the local school principal observed, "I knew I had a problem and I knew I needed help."

LIABILITY ISSUES

Violence prevention may seem antithetical to the work of a forensic clinician, who so often deals with an apprehended offender in the aftermath of a violent crime. Nevertheless, knowledge of prevention methods is informative to forensic practice in several respects. Forensic clinicians often consult at juvenile detention facilities and correctional centers; others may advise schools and youth service agencies on programs for at-risk youth. Even in forensic evaluations, experts who provide input into dispositional and sentencing decisions should have an up-to-date understanding of prevention research findings and the effectiveness of current prevention practices. More generally, knowledge gained from prevention research aids in understanding the etiology of violence, which in turn undergirds all efforts to explain criminal behavior and assist the court in determining matters ranging from criminal responsibility to future dangerousness.

Liability is perhaps the most pervasive legal issue in the prevention field. Clinicians are familiar with the hazards of professional liability for violence committed by their patients, and there is an available literature on risk management and *Tarasoff* liability (Monahan 1993; VandeCreek and Knapp 1993), but other forms of liability must be considered. Increasingly, institutions, industries, and even parents face potential lawsuits associated with the violence committed by youth. Forensic clinicians may become involved as consultants to assist in risk management prior to violence or as investigating experts in a lawsuit after violence has occurred.

Lawsuits have been aimed at the entertainment industry for products that allegedly encourage or contribute to violent behavior, such as lyrics that may promote suicide, movies that depict shooting up a classroom, and video games that may teach marksmanship and desensitize youth to violence. Such suits raise scientific questions about the state of knowledge concerning the influence of media violence on behavior, as well as legal questions about the scope of liability for industry products that might be provocatively labeled "social toxins"

(Garbarino 1995). Gun manufacturers and distributors are also vulnerable to lawsuits for their role in making guns and ammunition available to children. For example, in one lawsuit known to the author, a discount store settled a lawsuit involving sale of bullets to a juvenile. The juvenile used the ammunition to load a gun and shoot a deliveryman during a robbery.

Schools are subject to lawsuits if they do not take appropriate steps to protect students from the threat of violence. Although previous court decisions have tended to minimize the obligation of public schools to take action when students have been harmed (for example, see *DeShaney v. Winnebago County Dept. of Social Services* 1989), in *Davis v. Monroe County Board of Education* (1999), the U.S. Supreme Court found a school board liable for failing to take appropriate action in the case of a student who repeatedly and severely sexually harassed a classmate. The *Davis* decision could be applied more generally to cases in which one student repeatedly and severely bullies or injures another.

School officials need guidance on appropriate steps to take when a student threatens violence or injures someone; increasingly, school psychologists are asked to evaluate potentially dangerous youth, and administrators must decide when to remove a student from school. This difficult problem is further complicated when the student has legal status as disabled due to emotional disturbance or some other disabling condition. Federal law places strict limitations on the actions schools can take to discipline such students, particularly when the student's behavior can be attributed to the disabling condition (Mazin et al. 1998).

Moreover, as schools adopt security measures, such as hiring security officers and installing metal detectors and video monitors, they set a standard that may leave less secure schools vulnerable to claims of being negligent. The prevailing standards for school security are rapidly being increased (Cornell 1998). On the other hand, schools can be sued for taking actions that are deemed excessively restrictive or infringing on students' rights, such as conducting unwarranted searches or imposing unreasonable dress codes (Mazin et al. 1998). Schools must protect the due process rights of students accused or suspected of illegal behavior (National School Safety Center 1995).

Independent studies of school shootings by the Federal Bureau of Investigation (FBI) (O'Toole 2000) and the U.S. Secret Service (Reddy et al. 2001) have concluded that schools should not attempt to profile potentially violent students because such methods are so unlikely to be successful and will result in high rates of false-positive identification. Instead, schools should adopt a threat assessment approach, a more comprehensive process of evaluating individuals who have made threats of violence, taking into account the nature and circumstances of the threat. Threat assessment attempts to manage the risk of violence through individualized intervention plans. For example, the evaluator may determine that the student needs treatment for depression, protection from bullying, or family counseling. In only the most extreme cases does threat assessment lead to law enforcement investigation and legal consequences.

PREVENTION

Prevention efforts can take many forms and be undertaken at many stages—ranging from primary prevention programs in early childhood broadly aimed at strengthening healthy family functioning and improving social competence to secondary programs for youth in the early stages of delinquency to tertiary prevention in the form of institutional treatment for serious juvenile offenders intended to reduce criminal recidivism. Unfortunately, effective prevention is exceedingly difficult to demonstrate. Prevention failures are readily identified when a crime is committed, but successful cases go unreported; the causal link between the prevention program and an individual nonviolent outcome is never certain. Only controlled outcome studies, preferably using an experimental design with random group assignment, can offer scientifically convincing evidence of program effects.

Early studies of delinquency prevention and intervention programs found little evidence of success—generating the widely held view that "nothing works" (Elliott 1997). However, more recent reviews of literature and the U.S. Surgeon General's report on youth violence (U.S. Department of Health and Human Services 2001) refute this pessimistic conclusion. There is now a large body of evidence supporting the effectiveness of many different prevention and intervention approaches (Elliott 1997; Lipsey and Wilson 1998; Sherman et al. 1997; U.S. Department of Health and Human Services 2001). Although many programs that are untested, or that have been tested and found wanting, remain in place, administrators and practitioners now have many viable options to consider in designing violence prevention programs for their communities, schools, or agencies.

This chapter presents a selective overview intended to demonstrate the range and variety of effective youth violence prevention strategies currently available. None of the programs described here are without practical and methodological limitations, and claims of effectiveness must be qualified in many respects; for example, a good prevention program probably reduces violence by about 25%—an impact that is meaningful and cost-effective, but which leaves a great deal of room for improvement (Elliott 1997; Lipsey and Wilson 1998). Nevertheless, the overall message of this chapter is positive and even optimistic: In the past decade, knowledge concerning youth violence prevention has surged forward, and forensic clinicians should incorporate this knowledge into their thinking and practice.

Conflict Resolution

Conflict resolution is the practice of settling disputes by engaging the parties in a problem-solving process in which the disputants collaboratively determine their own solution (Bodine and Crawford 1998). Conflict resolution differs from the more conventional practice of relying on third parties or authorities to arbitrate disputes. In complex cases, mediators may guide the disputants through the negotiation process but refrain from assuming the role of arbitrator or decision maker.

Clearly, conflict resolution is not appropriate in all cases and requires cooperation of both parties; nevertheless, conflict resolution programs can be an effective intervention in schools and other institutions. One potential advantage of conflict resolution is that it results in solutions that are acceptable to both parties so that the conflict is more decisively concluded, thereby reducing the risk of renewed conflict later on. Conflict resolution also teaches the participants skills that they can use in conflictual situations in which authorities are not available to intervene.

Less serious disputes can be resolved by peers trained in methods of conflict resolution. Even primary school students can learn to mediate peer conflicts using structured methods such as the "Teaching Students to Be Peacemakers" program (Johnson and Johnson 1995a). It is remarkable to observe a mediation team of two 7-year-olds guide two of their classmates through a 10-minute conflict mediation process that successfully resolves their dispute. Controlled outcome studies (Johnson and Johnson 1995b) demonstrate that students can learn conflict resolution skills and apply them to actual conflicts in both school and family settings. This program substantially reduced classroom behavior problems and improved academic achievement.

Social Competence and Problem Solving

Children as young as age 4 can be taught to solve interpersonal problems in an empathic and considerate man-

ner. Social competence generally refers to the ability to get along with others and cope with problems effectively and so is broader in scope and more foundational in purpose than conflict resolution. There are several well-designed and rigorously evaluated programs that teach social competence (Caplan et al. 1992; Greenberg et al. 1995) in school settings. One of the best-known programs, Interpersonal Cognitive Problem Solving (ICPS, also known as "I Can Problem Solve") teaches children to identify problems, recognize the feelings and perspectives of others, consider the consequences of alternative solutions, and then choose the best course of action (Shure 1992, 1996). Numerous evaluations, including multiyear follow-up studies, document that training improves children's behavior and generalizes across classroom, home, and peer situations (Shure 1997).

Another well-validated program, the Primary Mental Health Prevention (PMHP) project (Cowen et al. 1996) provides carefully supervised, paraprofessional counseling for children with emotional or behavioral problems. There are specialized components to teach social problem solving, assist children with divorced parents, facilitate peer relationships, and encourage cooperative learning (the "Study Buddy" program). PMHP has a dissemination and training program that has established programs in hundreds of school districts nationwide.

Bullying Reduction

Bullying is so well known as a common childhood experience that it may be minimized or overlooked as a serious problem. Yet studies (Kochenderfer and Ladd 1996; Olweus 1993) indicate that victims of bullying suffer from a wide range of problems, from acute distress and anxiety to impaired concentration and poor academic achievement. Over time, victims can develop poor self-concepts, experience psychosomatic symptoms, and become school-avoidant. Long-term effects of bullying can include depression and poor self-esteem in adulthood. In Norway, nationwide efforts to reduce bullying were triggered by the suicide of three 10- to 14-year-old boys who had been chronically bullied by peers (Olweus 1993). Disturbingly, many of the youth involved in the highly publicized series of school shootings in the United States were reported to have been victims of bullying (Gabel 1999).

Children who bully their peers often engage in other forms of aggressive and antisocial behavior, including truancy, vandalism, theft, and substance use (Olweus 1993). In adulthood, former bullies are four times more likely to engage in serious criminal activity (Olweus 1993).

The prevalence of bullying is usually assessed by self-report surveys, although varying definitions and methods produce somewhat differing results. A nationally representative study of 15,686 students in grades 6–10 (Nansel et al. 2001) found that 30% of students reported moderate or frequent involvement as bullies or victims. Approximately 13% of the boys and 5% of the girls reported being bullied on a weekly basis. Victimization generally declines with age, although the numbers of youth who acknowledge bullying others peak in the middle school years (Nolin et al. 1996; Olweus and Limber 1999).

Bullying can be substantially reduced through systematic school-based programs. Olweus (1993) developed and implemented a landmark program that cut bullying in Norway by approximately 50%. His work has lead to the development of a model program that has been successfully used in Germany, England, and the United States in elementary, middle, and junior high schools (Olweus and Limber 1999). In addition to reducing the frequency of bullying behavior, bullying programs have other positive effects on the school climate, such as improving classroom discipline and enhancing student attitudes toward school.

There are generally four phases to a bullying reduction program. In the assessment phase, school officials review their policies and practices and gather information about the nature and extent of bullying behaviors at school. An anonymous student survey is often a critical source of information and also provides baseline data that can be used to assess program effectiveness. In the training phase, the school holds a series of meetings, conferences, or assemblies to provide students, teachers, and parents with information about bullying. The purpose of the training phase is to increase awareness of bullying as a problem and to generate schoolwide commitment to no longer tolerate or overlook it. Students and parents are made aware of school policies against bullying and are advised how to respond to bullying behaviors. Students who do not engage in bullying nevertheless may encourage bullying as bystanders who observe or reinforce the bully's performance.

During the subsequent implementation phase, which continues through the school year, school staff enforce policies against bullying and provide social skills training programs and other individually appropriate services for students identified as bullies. In addition, there are individual or group counseling services for students who have been victims of bullying. In the fourth phase, school officials evaluate the effectiveness of their efforts, using student survey data and other sources of information and make plans for the program's operation the following school year.

Supervised Recreation

The peak times for juvenile crime occur during the hours immediately after school (Snyder et al. 1997). The level of juvenile offenses at 3 P.M. on school days is more than three times greater than at noon or midnight. These observations alone indicate that many youth are not adequately supervised after school and suggest that after-school basketball is a more promising prevention strategy than midnight basketball.

Several controlled studies have found that well-supervised after-school recreation programs substantially reduce juvenile crime, drug use, and vandalism. A Canadian study (Jones and Offord 1989) of an intensive after-school program (using sports, music, dancing, and scouting) demonstrated a 75% reduction in juvenile arrests, while arrests at a comparison site rose 67%. A study by the U.S. Office of Substance Abuse Prevention of the effect of Boys and Girls Clubs of America (BGCA) recreational centers on public housing developments reported 22% lower levels of drug activity and increased levels of parent involvement at sites with BGCA centers compared with control sites without these centers (Schinke et al. 1992). A rigorously designed 3-year longitudinal study of 16 BGCA clubs in eight states (St. Pierre et al. 1997) also found reductions in alcohol and drug use, particularly in clubs that included active parent involvement. The BGCA has more than 1,700 affiliated clubs serving over 2.2 million children (Bureau of Justice Assistance 1995).

Mentoring

Many adolescents today lack parental role models. The proportion of births in the United States by unmarried mothers has grown from just 6% in 1960 to more than 32% in 1995 (U.S. Bureau of the Census 1998). Approximately 28% of adolescents in the United States live without one or both parents; among incarcerated juvenile offenders, the rate is much higher: 70% for boys and 59% for girls (Cornell et al. 1999). In this context, it is not surprising that mentoring has grown increasingly popular as a means of preventing delinquent behavior. Although parental absence has psychological, social, and economic consequences that cannot be remedied by mentors, most children respond enthusiastically to the prospect of individual attention from a caring adult.

The primary evidence in support of mentoring is an evaluation of the Big Brothers Big Sisters of America conducted by Public/Private Ventures (McGill 1997; Tierney and Grossman 1995). In a controlled experimental study, 959 youth ages 10 to 16 from eight cities were randomly assigned a mentor or placed in a wait-list control group. After 18 months, mentored youth were 46% less likely than control youth to initiate drug use, 27% less likely to initiate alcohol use, and 32% less likely to hit someone. The study also reported improved relationships with other adults and peers and 52% less truancy.

The results of the Big Brothers Big Sisters evaluation provide impressive evidence in support of mentoring, but they do not necessarily generalize to the many different sorts of activities and adult-youth relationships currently described as mentoring. The Big Brothers Big Sisters program has a more structured program than many other mentoring efforts (McGill 1997). Volunteer mentors are screened, trained, and then supervised by case managers. Mentors typically meet with their "little sibling" an average of three to four hours weekly throughout the year. There is no specific set of activities for the mentor pairs; instead, there is an emphasis on befriending the youth and engaging in fun activities that build a positive relationship (McGill 1997).

Mentoring can be challenging work, and as many as one-half of mentoring efforts may end prematurely because one or both parties decide to discontinue the relationship (Morrow and Styles 1995). A qualitative study (Morrow and Styles 1995) of successful and unsuccessful mentoring relationships suggested that mentors who emphasize the patient development of a friendly, supportive relationship are more likely to be successful than mentors who take a more prescriptive approach or set specific expectations for the youth, such as improving grades or changing behavior. Successful mentors were more likely to spend time listening rather than making judgments or lecturing their little siblings.

Child and Family Programs

Primary prevention efforts aimed at preschool children can have substantial benefits for families and the quality of a child's social and academic adjustment (Tremblay and Craig 1995). The Perry Preschool Project found that children randomly assigned to a preschool and home visit program not only did better in school than control children but also had fewer arrests as juveniles and adults (Berreuta-Clement et al. 1985). One strength of the Perry Preschool Project was its emphasis on facilitating parental involvement in children's academic and social development. The RAND report "Investing in Our Children: What We Know and Don't Know About the Costs and Benefits of Early Childhood Interventions" (Karoly et al. 1998) distinguished between the weak evidence supporting many programs and strong evidence in support of several programs that have verifiable, long-term benefits.

For school-age children already exhibiting disruptive or disobedient behavior, secondary prevention in the form of parent education can be highly effective (Brestan and Eyberg 1998). Parent management training for aggressive children improves children's behavior and is a cost-effective means of preventing future crime (Greenwood et al. 1998). Among the well-validated approaches to parent education are the following:

- The Parent Management Training for Conduct Disordered Children, developed by Patterson (Patterson et al. 1992) at the University of Oregon Social Learning Center, helps parents recognize discipline strategies that unwittingly promote antisocial behavior and teaches them more effective alternatives.
- The Barkley Parent Training Program uses an explicit manual to teach a 10-step model to parents of children with severe behavior problems (Barkley 1997).
- The Parenting Program for Young Children (Webster-Stratton 1998) is a 24-week program delivered to groups of parents in 2-hour weekly meetings using video vignettes to demonstrate positive parenting techniques.
- Family and Schools Together (FAST) is a comprehensive program that incorporates parent training and home visits along with school-based efforts to improve the social skills and academic performance of elementary school children (Conduct Problems Prevention Research Group 1992; McDonald et al. 1997).

For delinquent youth, family therapy can be a useful form of tertiary prevention. Functional family therapy (Alexander and Parsons 1982) makes use of cognitive and behavioral methods to improve family relationships and increase reciprocity and cooperation among family members. Outcome studies demonstrated that functional family therapy improved family relationships and reduced recidivism among adolescents referred by juvenile court for offenses such as truancy, theft, and unmanageable behavior (Klein et al. 1977).

Multisystemic therapy (Henggeler et al. 1998) is one of the most cost-effective and powerful treatments for serious juvenile offenders and their families. In controlled outcome studies, multisystemic therapy was superior to standard treatments for chronic juvenile offenders, inner-city at-risk youth, families in which child abuse occurs, and other traditionally difficult populations. A hallmark of the multisystemic approach is the therapist's role as a problem solver who works closely with parents to identify and remedy problems in a wide variety of areas, ranging from a child's school attendance to marital discord. Typically, therapists begin treatment by visiting the family several times a week for sessions ranging from 15 to 90 minutes and gradually taper contacts over a 4- to 6-month period. Therapists make flexible use of family therapy, parent education, and cognitive-behavioral techniques to improve family relationships, strengthen parental authority and effectiveness, and modify children's behavior.

PITFALLS

One of the most common pitfalls in the prevention field is the adoption of unvalidated programs. All too often programs are selected based on theoretically or philosophically appealing features in the absence of objective evidence of program effectiveness. Once programs are implemented, it becomes extremely difficult to criticize them or make substantial changes. Objective evaluations of popular programs, such as Intensive Supervised Probation (MacKenzie 1997; Petersilia and Turner 1993) and boot camps (Cowles et al. 1995; MacKenzie and Souryal 1994), have produced disappointing results that proponents have been unwilling to accept (see review in Chapter 26, "Assessment and Treatment of Juvenile Offenders").

Drug Education

Drug education programs typically involve school-based instruction about the negative effects of alcohol and drug use, accompanied by efforts to encourage responsible decision making. No prevention program is more popular, or more controversial, than Drug Abuse Resistance Education (D.A.R.E.). D.A.R.E. began in 1983 as a collaborative effort between the Los Angeles Police Department and the Los Angeles Unified School District and has been adopted in over 70% of the nation's school districts, as well as in 44 foreign countries ("Truth and D.A.R.E.," 1996). The original core curriculum was designed for uniformed police officers to teach a specific drug prevention curriculum to students in their last (fifth or sixth) grade of elementary school, although there are D.A.R.E. programs for other grade levels that are less widely used.

In 1994, Ringwalt and colleagues released an evaluation of the D.A.R.E. program based on a meta-analysis of eight methodologically rigorous studies involving 9,300 students from 215 schools. All eight studies assessed students before and after completion of the core D.A.R.E. curriculum and included control groups of students not receiving D.A.R.E. The results indicated that D.A.R.E. was most effective at increasing knowledge about drug

use and in improving social skills. There was a small improvement in attitudes toward police, attitudes about drug use, and self-esteem. Unfortunately, however, the effect size for reported drug and alcohol use was not statistically significant. These results helped generate a storm of criticism and an often contentious debate concerning the merits of D.A.R.E. Some researchers and reporters who presented unfavorable findings about D.A.R.E.'s effectiveness were the recipients of harsh criticism and even harassment (Glass 1998; Rosenbaum and Hanson 1998).

In defense of D.A.R.E., one limitation of most outcomes studies was that they examined drug and alcohol use shortly after completion of D.A.R.E., when students are 11 or 12 years old and the baseline rates of drug use are so low that the effects of D.A.R.E. might not be evident. To overcome this limitation, Rosenbaum and Hanson (1998) reported results of a 6-year longitudinal study of 1,798 students from 36 schools. This methodologically rigorous study employed randomized control groups and corrected for many statistical and methodological problems of previous studies. There were expectations that this study would salvage D.A.R.E.'s reputation and demonstrate conclusively that it was effective. Unfortunately, this study again found that D.A.R.E. did not reduce drug use, and in suburban schools, D.A.R.E. was associated with a 3%–5% increase in drug use. A 10-year follow-up study again found D.A.R.E. to be ineffective (Lynam et al. 1999).

To its credit, D.A.R.E. has made changes to its curriculum and focused more efforts on older students who are most likely to use drugs. Recently, D.A.R.E. advocates and critics have met to discuss constructive methods of improving D.A.R.E. and resolving some of the controversial questions about D.A.R.E.'s effectiveness (William Modzeleski, personal communication, February 1999).

Educators are well advised not to fashion their own alternatives to D.A.R.E., since many non–D.A.R.E. drug education programs are either ineffective or worse and have the unintended effect of *increasing* drug use (Rosenbaum and Hanson 1998).

There is, however, evidence that some drug education programs are effective. Interactive programs that emphasize interpersonal skills to counter peer pressure and use a participatory teaching approach are more effective than programs that rely on moral exhortation, fear arousal, or self-esteem building (Gottfredson 1997; Ringwalt et al. 1994). Life Skills Training (Botvin 1998) is one of the most effective and well-documented drug education programs. Unlike D.A.R.E., Life Skills Training is taught by teachers in the sixth or seventh grade, with 15 sessions in the first year and booster sessions the following 2 years. The program emphasizes self-management and social skills, as well as skills specifically related to dealing with peer pressure to use drugs. Outcomes averaged from a dozen studies indicate that Life Skills Training reduces tobacco, alcohol, and marijuana use 50%–75% and that treatment effects are sustained 6 years later.

Program Integrity

Even when a prevention approach has been adequately validated, it may not be faithfully implemented in each new setting. No program is immune to inadequate institutional support, insufficient funding, poorly trained staff, or failure to adhere to program standards. For example, the success of the mentoring program conducted by the Big Brothers Big Sisters of America does not guarantee that all mentoring programs will be effective, particularly when mentors are not carefully selected, trained, and supervised. Studies show that program integrity is critical to effective prevention (Lipsey and Wilson 1998). The well-validated multisystemic therapy approach is demonstrably less effective when therapists fail to adhere to its core treatment principles and guidelines (Henggeler et al. 1997). Boys and Girls Clubs of America centers are much more effective when the staff is well trained and motivated to fully implement a standard educational program (Pope et al. 1995).

CASE EXAMPLE EPILOGUE

The school principal began by contacting the local social services agency, police department, and juvenile court authorities in order to develop a coordinated community response. A comprehensive plan was developed, which included 1) conflict mediation with the rival groups, 2) individual educational and social service plans to meet the needs of specific group members, 3) a schoolwide violence prevention program, and 4) expanded after-school programs.

First, a team of professional mediators met with the girls individually and convinced them to attend a day-long mediation session at a neutral, secure site. With gentle guidance and minimal direction from the mediators, the girls listened and spoke in turn. For hours the girls aired their grievances, unraveled rumors, and clarified misunderstandings. At an appropriate time, the mediators advised the girls that they could devise their own plan for ending the feud, but they were careful not to take sides or make specific suggestions. It is critical to this form of mediation that solutions are devised by the opposing parties rather than imposed from an outside authority. In this way the girls decided to "squash" their dispute and settled on terms for reconciliation.

Second, school and community professionals met with individual girls and their parents to devise educational and social service plans. Several of the girls qualified for special education services, while others enrolled in vocational or job placement programs. One young woman needed parent support services and child care arrangements for her infant son. Most of the girls received some form of individual and/or family therapy. In several cases, the resolution of juvenile charges was linked to treatment compliance and school attendance.

The school principal met with a group of student leaders and encouraged their efforts to form an antiviolence organization that initiated a nonviolence campaign in the school. Several hundred students signed a pledge not to engage in fights and to support nonviolent means of resolving conflict. School discipline policies were revised, penalties for fighting were stiffened, and school security was enhanced with the addition of a school resource officer provided by the local police department. The school psychologist established a therapeutic group for at-risk students that emphasized anger control and conflict resolution training.

The city council agreed to provide space for a nonprofit organization to establish an after-school recreational program. The program was well staffed and included services to encourage homework completion and school attendance. The previously existing mentoring program was expanded and revamped to emphasize more training and supervision of mentors.

To the surprise and relief of authorities, the girls ended their dispute and engaged in no further acts of aggression or violence toward one another. After 2 years, the agreement was still being honored, and some of previous rivals had become friends. Two of the girls obtained high school equivalency diplomas and all of the others graduated with their classmates. The school recorded a marked decline in fights, discipline referrals, and suspensions.

ACTION GUIDELINES

Forensic experts consistently deal with a highly skewed sample of the youth offender population—the most serious crimes committed by the most troubled and perplexing youth. There may be little occasion to study successful outcomes; follow-up information becomes available primarily when a youth is arrested for another crime. Contrary to common perceptions about the chronicity and intractability of juvenile offenses, most youth never return to juvenile court after their first referral (Snyder and Sickmund 1995), and many if not most aggressive youth desist in their aggressive behavior as they mature

(Loeber and Stouthamer-Loeber 1998). Yet such commonplace positive outcomes are far removed from the experiential knowledge base of the forensic clinician, who encounters only those cases in which prevention efforts have failed. Knowledge of effective, research-validated prevention strategies can deepen the clinician's understanding of violence and broaden his or her expertise as a consultant and advocate. Forensic clinicians must strive to remain current in the field.

In the days of patent medicine, consumers had little basis for choosing treatments beyond the product's superficial appeal and the persuasiveness of its salesmen. Controlled outcome studies and outcome evidence were largely unavailable so that effective treatments went unrecognized or unused. In the violence prevention field today, there are numerous appealing, but scientifically nonvalidated, approaches that divert limited resources from the implementation of sounder strategies and more defensible methods. The need for further research and further improvement in youth violence prevention notwithstanding, there has been substantial progress in efforts to develop effective programs and strategies. Forensic clinicians can play an important role in advancing the field of violence prevention by educating policy makers and practitioners about the availability of a wide array of effective methods for preventing youth violence and by emphasizing the necessity of rigorous program implementation followed by objective evaluation of program outcomes.

The U.S. Department of Education (1998) developed four principles of effectiveness to guide the development and implementation of drug and violence prevention programs using funds from the Safe and Drug Free-Schools and Communities Act. Summarized here, the principles require that all Title IV–funded prevention programs

1. Be based on a thorough assessment of objective data about the drug and violence problems in the school or community served
2. Be devised to attain a clearly defined set of measurable goals and objectives
3. Be designed and implemented based on research evidence that the strategies used prevent or reduce drug use, violence, or disruptive behavior among youth
4. Undergo periodic outcome evaluations to determine progress in achieving its goals and objectives, and to modify and improve its programs and refine its goals and objectives as appropriate.

These principles could well be applied to any violence prevention effort.

REFERENCES

Alexander JF, Parsons BV: Functional Family Therapy. Monterey, CA, Brooks/Cole, 1982

Barkley RA: Defiant Children: A Clinician's Manual for Assessment and Parent Training. New York, Guilford, 1997

Berreuta-Clement JR, Schweinhart LJ, Barnett WS, et al: Changed Lives: The Effects of the Perry Preschool Program on Youths Through Age 19. Ypsilanti, MI, High Scope Press, 1985

Bodine RJ, Crawford DK: The Handbook of Conflict Resolution Education: A Guide to Building Quality Programs in Schools. San Francisco, CA, Jossey-Bass, 1998

Botvin GJ: Life Skills Training. Boulder, CO, Institute of Behavioral Science, University of Colorado, 1998

Brestan EV, Eyberg SM: Effective psychosocial treatments of conduct-disordered children and adolescents: 29 Years, 82 Studies, and 5272 Kids. J Clin Child Psychol 27:180–189, 1998

Bureau of Justice Assistance: Boys and Girls (BandG) Clubs of America. Bureau of Justice Assistance Fact Sheet. Washington, DC, U.S. Department of Justice, 1995

Caplan M, Weissberg RP, Grober JS, et al: Social competence promotion with inner-city and suburban young adolescents: effects on social adjustment and alcohol use. J Consult Clin Psychol 60:56–63, 1992

Conduct Problems Prevention Research Group: A developmental and clinical model for the prevention of conduct disorder: the FAST Track Program. Dev Psychopathol 4:509–527, 1992

Cornell DG: Designing Safer Schools for Virginia: A Guide to Keeping Students Safe From Violence. Charlottesville, VA, Thomas Jefferson Center for Educational Design, 1998

Cornell DG, Loper AB, Atkinson A, et al: Youth Violence Prevention in Virginia: A Needs Assessment. Richmond, VA, Virginia Department of Health, 1999

Cowen EL, Hightower AD, Pedro-Carroll JL, et al: School-Based Prevention for Children at Risk: The Primary Mental Health Project. Washington, DC, American Psychological Association, 1996

Cowles EL, Castellano TC, Gransky LA: "Boot Camp" Drug Treatment and Aftercare Interventions: An Evaluation Review (National Institute of Justice Research Report). Washington, DC, National Institute of Justice, 1995

Davis v Monroe County Board of Education, 119 SCt 1661 (1999)

DeShaney v Winnebago County Dept of Social Services, 489 US 189 (1989)

Elliott DS: Editor's introduction, in Blueprints for Violence Prevention. Series edited by Elliott DS. Boulder, CO, Institute of Behavioral Science, University of Colorado, 1997, pp xi–xxiii

Gabel E: Patterns of violence. Time, May 31, 1999, pp 36–37

Garbarino J: Raising Children in a Socially Toxic Environment. San Francisco, CA, Jossey-Bass, 1995

Glass S: Truth and D.A.R.E.: the nation's most prestigious drug prevention program for kids is a failure: why don't you know this? Rolling Stone, March 5, 1998, pp 42–43

Greenberg MT, Kusche CA, Cook ET, et al: Promoting emotional competence in school-aged children: the effects of the PATHS curriculum. Dev Psychopathol 7:117–136, 1995

Greenwood PW, Model KE, Rydell CP, et al: Diverting children from a life of crime: measuring costs and benefits (Document No MR-699-1-UCB/RC/IF). Santa Monica, CA, RAND, 1998

Gottfredson DC: School-based crime prevention (chapter 5), in Preventing Crime: What Works, What Doesn't, What's Promising: A Report to the United States Congress. Edited by Sherman LW, Gottfredson DC, MacKenzie D, et al. Washington, DC, U.S. Department of Justice, Office of Justice Programs, National Institute of Justice, 1997

Henggeler SW, Melton GB, Brondino MJ, et al: Multisystemic therapy with violent and chronic juvenile offenders and their families: the role of treatment fidelity in successful dissemination. J Consult Clin Psychol 65:821–833, 1997

Henggeler SW, Schoenwald SK, Borduin CM, et al: Multisystemic Treatment of Antisocial Behavior in Children and Adolescents. New York, Guilford, 1998

Johnson DW, Johnson RT: Teaching Students to Be Peacemakers, 3rd Edition. Edina, MN, Interaction Book, 1995a

Johnson DW, Johnson RT: Teaching students to be peacemakers: results of five years of research. Peace and Conflict: Journal of Peace Psychology 4:417–438, 1995b

Jones MB, Offord DR: Reduction of anti-social behavior in poor children by non-school skill development. J Child Psychol Psychiatry 30:737–750, 1989

Karoly LA, Greenwood SM, Everingham JH, et al: Investing in our children: what we know and don't know about the cost and benefits of early childhood interventions (Document No MR-898-TCWF). Santa Monica, CA, RAND, 1998

Klein NC, Alexander JF, Parsons BV: Impact of family systems intervention on recidivism and sibling delinquency: a model of primary prevention and program evaluation. J Consult Clin Psychol 45:469–474, 1977

Kochenderfer BJ, Ladd GW: Peer victimization: cause or consequence of school maladjustment. Child Dev 67:1305–1317, 1996

Lipsey MW, Wilson DB: Effective intervention for serious juvenile offenders: synthesis of research, in Serious and Violent Juvenile Offenders: Risk Factors and Successful Interventions. Edited by Loeber R, Farrington DP. Thousand Oaks, CA, Sage, 1998, pp 313–345

Loeber R, Stouthamer-Loeber M: Development of juvenile aggression and violence: some common misconceptions and controversies. Am Psychol 53:242–259, 1998

Lynam DR, Milich R, Zimmerman R, et al: Project DARE: no effects at 10-year follow-up. J Consult Clin Psychol 67:590–593, 1999

MacKenzie DL: Criminal justice and crime prevention (chapter 9), in Preventing Crime: What Works, What Doesn't, What's Promising: A Report to the United States Congress. Edited by Sherman LW, Gottfredson D, MacKenzie DL, et al. Washington, DC, National Institute of Justice, 1997

MacKenzie DL, Souryal C: Multisite Evaluation of Shock Incarceration. Washington, DC, National Institute of Justice, 1994

Mazin LE, Hestand JT, Koester RE: An Educator's Legal Guide to Stress-Free Discipline and School Safety. Bloomington, IA, National Education Service, 1998

McDonald L, Billingham S, Conrad T, et al: Families and Schools Together (FAST). Families in Society 78:140–155, 1997

McGill D: Big Brothers/Big Sisters of America. Boulder, CO, Institute of Behavioral Science, University of Colorado, 1997

Monahan J: Limiting therapist exposure to Tarasoff liability: guidelines for risk containment. Am Psychol 48: 242–250, 1993

Morrow KV, Styles MB: Building Relationships With Youth in Program Settings: a study of Big Brothers/Big Sisters. Philadelphia, PA, Public/Private Ventures, 1995

Nansel TR, Overpeck M, Pilla RS, et al: Bullying behaviors among US youth: prevalence and association with psychosocial adjustment. JAMA 285:2094–2100, 2001

National School Safety Center: Student Searches and the Law. Malibu, CA, National School Safety Center, 1995

Nolin MJ, Davies E, Chandler K: Student victimization at school. Journal of School Health 66:216–226, 1996

Olweus D: Bullying at School: What We Know and What We Can Do. Oxford, England, Blackwell, 1993

Olweus D, Limber S: Bullying Prevention Program. Boulder, CO, Institute of Behavioral Science, University of Colorado, 1999

O'Toole ME: The school shooter: a threat assessment perspective. Quantico, VA, National Center for the Analysis of Violent Crime, Federal Bureau of Investigation, 2000

Patterson GR, Reid JB, Dishion TJ: Antisocial Boys: A Social Interactional Approach. Eugene, OR, Castalia, 1992

Petersilia J, Turner S: Evaluating Intensive Supervision Probation/Parole: Results of a Nationwide Experiment. Washington, DC, National Institute of Justice, 1993

Pope CE, Lovell R, Bynum T, et al: Evaluation of Boys and Girls Clubs in Public Housing. Washington, DC, U.S. Department of Justice, Office of Justice Programs, National Institute of Justice, 1995

Reddy M, Borum R, Vossekuil B, et al: Evaluating risk for targeted violence in schools: comparing risk assessment, threat assessment, and other approaches. Psychology in the Schools 38:157–172, 2001

Ringwalt C, Greene J, Ennett S, et al: Past and Future Directions of the DARE Program: An Evaluation Review: Draft Final Report (Award #91-DD-CX-K053). Washington, DC, National Institute of Justice, 1994

Rosenbaum D, Hanson GS: Assessing the effects of school-based drug education: a six-year multi-level analysis of project D.A.R.E. Journal of Research in Crime and Delinquency 35:381–412, 1998

Schinke SP, Orlandi MA, Cole KC: Boys and Girls Clubs in public housing developments: prevention services for youth at risk. Journal of Community Psychology (OSAP special issue):118–128, 1992

Sherman LW, Gottfredson D, MacKenzie D, et al: Preventing Crime: What Works, What Doesn't, What's Promising: A Report to the United States Congress. Washington, DC, National Institute of Justice, 1997

Shure MB: I Can Problem Solve (ICPS): An Interpersonal Cognitive Problem-Solving Program. Champaign, IL, Research Press, 1992

Shure MB: Raising a Thinking Child: Help Your Young Child to Resolve Everyday Conflicts and Get Along With Others. New York, Pocket Books, 1996

Shure MB: Interpersonal Cognitive Problem Solving: primary prevention of early high-risk behaviors in the preschool and primary years, in Primary Prevention Works. Edited by Albee GW, Gullotta TP. Thousand Oaks, CA, Sage, 1997, pp 167–188

Snyder HN, Sickmund M: Juvenile Offenders and Victims: A National Report. Washington, DC, Office of Juvenile Justice and Delinquency Prevention, 1995

Snyder HN, Sickmund M, Poe-Yamagata E: Juvenile Offenders and Victims: 1997 Update on Violence. Washington, DC, Office of Juvenile Justice and Delinquency Prevention, 1997

St. Pierre IL, Mark MM, Kaltreider DL, et al: Involving parents of high-risk youth in drug prevention: a three-year longitudinal study in Boys and Girls Clubs. Journal of Early Adolescence 17:21–50, 1997

Tierney JP, Grossman JB: Making a Difference: An Impact Study of Big Brothers/Big Sisters. Philadelphia, PA, Public/Private Ventures, 1995

Tremblay R, Craig W: Developmental crime prevention, in Building a Safer Society, Vol 19: Crime and Justice. Edited by Tonry M, Farrington D. Chicago, IL, University of Chicago Press, 1995, pp 151–236

Truth and D.A.R.E.: Washington cities shelve anti-drug curriculum. Law Enforcement News, November 30, 1996 [http://www.lib.jjay.cuny.edu/len/96/30nov/html/5.html]

U.S. Bureau of the Census: Statistical Abstracts of the United States: 1998, 118th Edition. Washington, DC, U.S. Bureau of the Census, 1998

U.S. Department of Education: Notice of Final Principles of Effectiveness. Federal Register 63(104):29901–29906, 1998

U.S. Department of Health and Human Services: Youth Violence: A Report of the Surgeon General. Rockville, MD, U.S. Department of Health and Human Services, 2001 [http://www.surgeongeneral.gov/library/youthviolence/]

VandeCreek L, Knapp S: Tarasoff and Beyond: Legal and Clinical Considerations in Treatment of Life-Endangering Patients, Revised Edition. Sarasota, FL, Professional Resource Exchange, 1993

Webster-Stratton C: Preventing conduct problems in Head Start children: strengthening parenting competencies. J Consult Clin Psychol 66:715–730, 1998

SUGGESTED READINGS

Current information on prevention strategies and programs is readily available via the Internet:

Center for the Study and Prevention of Violence: www.colorado.edu/cspv

National Crime Prevention Council Online Resource Center: www.ncpc.org

National Resource Center for Safe Schools: www.safetyzone.org

National School Safety Center: www.nssci.org

PAVNET Online: Partnerships Against Violence Network: www.pavnet.org

Virginia Youth Violence Project: youthviolence.edschool.virginia.edu

PART V

Juvenile Offenders

Juvenile law differs in content and application from the law affecting adults. In Chapter 25, Dr. Malmquist alerts the reader to these differences and their importance and provides a useful synopsis of the evolution of laws pertaining to juveniles. Drs. DePrato and Hammer discuss a variety of program options for juvenile offenders and provide some badly needed evidence-based data on what programs appear to be most effective for this population in Chapter 26.

Dr. Shaw writes about an especially problematic type of youthful offender, the sexually aggressive youth, and shares with the reader his extensive experience working with this population. Unfortunately, we know that many youthful sexual offenders become adult sexual predators. His chapter (Chapter 27) provides hope

regarding improved techniques for early detection and intervention.

Dr. Scott addresses the waiver of juveniles to adult court, an issue that has recently received much press, in Chapter 28. As politicians, educators, criminologists, and the public debate solutions to a high-profile problem, forensic clinicians may provide knowledgeable consultation in this arena. Finally, in Chapter 29, Drs. Voigt, Heisel, and Benedek examine issues of competency and insanity/criminal responsibility in the juvenile offender. These are areas in which many child and adolescent forensic examiners lack experience, but ones in which potentially they have much to offer. It is hoped that this chapter will allow them to feel more comfortable doing these evaluations.

CHAPTER 25

Overview of Juvenile Law

Carl P. Malmquist, M.D., M.S.

The story of juvenile law at the beginning of the twenty-first century is contained in the vicissitudes of the juvenile court throughout the twentieth century. The changes that have occurred need to be seen in the context of the origin of a special court for children and what the situation was before that time. Changing norms and views about juveniles operated to culminate in several landmark legal decisions in the latter part of the twentieth century. Since Illinois created the first juvenile court in 1899, the juvenile justice system has been under siege with arguments about its mission and whether it is possible to achieve its goals. From the initial emphasis on pursuing "the best interests of the child," critics have argued for such changes as lowering the age of juvenile jurisdiction significantly, abandoning a rehabilitative focus, and abolishing the juvenile court system itself, except perhaps for preadolescent age groups (Ainsworth 1991).

PRECURSORS TO JUVENILE LAW

In the colonial United States, as an English colony and following English law, children were basically viewed the same as adults for legal purposes of attaining criminal status. Someone who violated the law was viewed as having exercised a free choice in so doing. This meant that the person had supposedly made a rational choice to pursue a particular action. The choice was viewed as one based on pursuing personal benefit so as to optimize pleasures or economic interests. There were a few exceptions, such as a child less than 7 years of age not being held criminally responsible, which harked back to Roman law. Under the common law a child between the ages of 7 and 14 was presumed responsible, but it was a rebuttable presumption that had to be proven in court. After age 14, no distinction from the adult population was made.

In this confused situation, in which all ages were mixed both at trial and after conviction, it was apparent that many of the minors were in court for diverse reasons; these varied from homicide to being a neglected or dependent child. Hence, what first began to change in the course of the nineteenth century was a growing concern about wayward children and their disposition after a finding of guilt. This represented a shift from the idea of family being the primary mode of social control exerted over juveniles, as exemplified in colonial times where the father had absolute control (and responsibility) over the family members and their misbehavior. In the 1641 Massachusetts Body of Liberties, children who disobeyed their parents were actually subject to the death penalty (Hawes 1971). The first legal changes occurred in the form of creating separate institutions where juveniles could be housed separately from their fellow adult prisoners.

One of these early developments was the Houses of Refuge, first created in New York in 1825. The thinking behind them was quite similar to contemporary thinking—that exposure of juveniles to adults in the same penal facilities would have a corrupting effect on them. The idea behind removing juvenile offenders from prisons was to instill middle-class norms in them, such as neatness, punctuality, and dedication to work. The implicit belief was that if such behaviors could be inculcated in the juvenile, a future life of crime would be avoided. What quickly happened was a mingling of juveniles who had committed crimes with other juveniles who were simply homeless or destitute. This approach basically created a mechanism of social control without any legality beyond the aspirations of those who had created these institutions.

Early legal challenges arose from different ends of the spectrum. In a Pennsylvania case, *Commonwealth v. M'Keagy* (1831), a father had placed his son in the Philadelphia House of Refuge on the basis of his being an idle and disorderly person. Because no crime had been committed and the family was not poor, the placement was rejected. A few years later, the opposite situation arose when a father attempted via habeas corpus to gain the release of his daughter. The parent was asserting a violation of his parental rights for control, but the court took the view that the child "has been snatched from a course which must have ended in confirmed depravity" (*ex parte Crouse* 1838).

The idea of *parens patriae* was injected into the Crouse case as the state being the guardian of its children and if necessary supplanting the actual parents. This concept would permeate the unfolding of state intervention thereafter. It had come from English courts, which gave the right to the monarch to protect people who did not have full legal capacity, and it allowed chancery courts to oversee dependent and neglected children. The United States courts went one step further to include alleged delinquent children. In time the Houses of Refuge were superseded by the emergence of state reformatories for juveniles. As the nineteenth century progressed, the history of these institutions became that of repeated scandals, abusive physical discipline, overcrowding, and an emphasis on order and regimentation (Miller and Ohlin 1985). Over time they became custodial institutions rather than rehabilitative ones, and eventually state or municipal governments took over their administration.

One more major antecedent to the emergence of the juvenile court itself as a separate legal institution was what historians call the Progressive Era (1880–1920). It was a time of major social and industrial change, with an increase in concentrated wealth and accompanying concerns about protecting private property and maintaining law and order. In the second half of the nineteenth century, a reform group referred to as the Child Savers had arisen; they believed that churches had to do more for the urban poor. They were critical of the Houses of Refuge for not reaching enough children and believed the solution was to emphasize family life. Part of their mission was to "place out" poor and vagrant children in farm families in the West, thinking this would reform wayward youth (Krisberg and Austin 1993). This corresponded to a growing skepticism about the effectiveness of reform schools in controlling delinquent behavior. Yet, the Progressive movement had a basic belief that government action would benefit children and solve the increasing number of social problems.

A variety of laws were enacted on that basis. Compulsory education, and regulation of child labor, were thus enacted with the idea that they would strengthen family life and in that way promote better child development and control over delinquency (Sutton 1988). It is out of this background that the juvenile court system and juvenile law emerged.

THE EMERGENCE OF THE JUVENILE COURT

The preceding historical and cultural developments coalesced with some other factors to give rise to the first juvenile court, in Illinois. It happened that most of the early institutions in Illinois had been destroyed by fire, with the result that large numbers of juveniles were simply being housed in the county jail with adults. A group of wealthy reformers from the upper classes mounted a campaign to do something. They recruited other groups to get behind them, and a draft of a juvenile court act was the result (Krisberg and Austin 1993). Whereas some interpret this as a benevolent intervention, others have seen this intervention as a middle- and upper-class action to control the increasing numbers of immigrant and poor children (Platt 1969). The reformers were seen as women from those social classes that had achieved power and who thought their mission was to rescue American youths. Their ideas were intended to restore the authority of parents, emphasize the role of women in the home, obtain proper training for youths, and save children from the immorality of life on the streets.

Parallel to this social ferment, there were also new ideas about human behavior. The classical school of criminology, with its emphasis on people simply choosing to violate the law, was being superseded by a positivistic view that was looking for causal factors operating in criminal behavior. Diverse social factors that operated to promote antisocial acts were proposed, and these factors were to be identified by a scientific methodology. The methodology could involve biological, neuropsychiatric, social, or economic factors. It was a paradigm shift to look for causes, and it fit into the agenda of what a new institution, such as the juvenile court, was supposed to do. The focus was to shift from the act to the actor in a quest for understanding, which could then give rise to the correct preventive and treatment strategies.

From this orientation came the "rehabilitative ideal," with new approaches administered through the courts of probation, parole with supervision, and indeterminate sentencing; these all fit in with the idea of what a juvenile court would achieve with minors. Because decisions and interventions were all to be done on the basis of the best interests of the child, no need to inquire about the rights of juvenile defendants was seen. It was to be done for the juveniles' own good, but society would also benefit thereby. Part of the trade-off was that the juvenile was not to be seen as convicted of a crime but simply adjudicated delinquent. As a consequence, adjudications of juveniles in the juvenile court were not to be used as prior convictions if the individual later ended up in an adult criminal court.

The idea soon spread to almost all states. By 1912, 22 states had established juvenile courts, and by 1925, only 2 states had not (Krisberg and Austin 1993). The additional courts were patterned closely after the Illinois statute. The courtrooms were to be informal, hearings were to be private, records were to be kept confidential, proceedings were classified as civil and not criminal, and the court was given great discretion in determining dispositions. These innovations were a product of the view that individualized justice demanded that the court needed such wide latitude to rehabilitate juveniles. What also emerged from the child-saving aspect was the expansion, not only beyond possible criminal behavior and into delinquency per se, but into a wide variety of situations and statuses for children. Thus, dependency and neglect cases came under the jurisdiction of the juvenile court (later renamed CHINS/PINS for "children/persons in need of supervision"). In time a broader variety of misbehaving children and status offenses were also encompassed under juvenile law to prevent dissolute living.

As part of this approach, because the issue was not to prove that a criminal act had been committed but rather to intervene for the sake of the child's best interests, there would not be a requirement for lawyers. A legal scholar saw juvenile court judges being actively hostile to the presence of lawyers in the juvenile courts, even in delinquency proceedings (Feld 1993). Although there would be a court hearing, it would be a civil and not a criminal proceeding, and therefore it was argued that the constitutional standards used in adult criminal courts would not be needed. If the juvenile was to be confined with a loss of liberty, an indeterminate amount of time might be needed since the confinement was not to be viewed as a punishment but part of a rehabilitative process. The "habits of legality" would thus be bypassed (Allen 1996). There was even an ideal that the judges in

juvenile courts would have a wide background in the social and behavioral sciences in contrast to the usual legal education. To accompany this changed legal atmosphere, there was to be an array of experts for the court to call upon, such as probation officers, pediatricians, and mental health experts.

Three by-products arose from this system. One was not to focus on the offense itself, as the juvenile was to be assessed in terms of both the sociocultural milieu in which he or she operated and his or her personality. A result of this might be that a minor offense could lead to a major intervention. The second by-product was the subjective assessment carried out by the judge. The perception of the judge in each case was to operate apart from the rule of law. This would then become the key ingredient for the outcome of the case. Third, because attorneys were not viewed as essential in this process, there were no juries, and questionable rules of evidence were employed, it was never clear whether the proceedings were to be viewed primarily as legal, quasi-legal, administrative, or simply a welfare intervention on a *parens patriae* basis.

THE PERIOD UP TO THE 1960S

Until the 1960s the framework as outlined above regarding the juvenile law processes and law remained with very little change. What is interesting is that even from the early years of the juvenile court, questions were raised about the functioning of the court. In 1911 and 1912 there were exposés about the actual conditions and operations of the juvenile court (Ryerson 1978). By the 1920s, volunteers had been replaced by social workers, who initially gave the court a social agency perspective. Depending on the juvenile court in question, the orientation could be psychoanalytic, biological, or that of some other therapeutic orientation.

Beginning in the 1930s, the treatment focus began to shift from the individual juvenile to broader social factors operating in the life of the juvenile. Sometimes broad factors, such as poverty, inequality, or racism, began to be considered. In other juvenile courts the influence of the peer group began to be emphasized. In yet others, there was a circling back to the early days, with a new look at family influences and the failure of socialization processes, such as in schools (Empey and Stafford 1991). Juvenile reform schools, with various names attached to them, were present in all states as an option for legal disposition. Legal challenges seemed dormant, but the failure of the juvenile court movement to reach its objectives was setting the stage for what would emerge in the 1960s: a series of legal challenges that would change the course of juvenile law.

Many questions had arisen: Was it desirable to withhold certain constitutional rights from juveniles? What was the basis for not affording certain due process rights to juveniles? Was there such a thing as individualized treatment being provided to juveniles in the system? One problem that was uncovered was the merging of dependent and neglected children with alleged delinquents, who needed separate processing and disposition. More specifically, the processes of adjudication of delinquency, which could lead to a loss of liberty, were seen as needing procedural safeguards, which were lacking.

KEY CASES

Between 1966 and 1975, five key cases involving the juvenile court were decided by the U.S. Supreme Court. These have sometimes been referred to as beginning the process of "criminalizing" the juvenile court. They did not criminalize it entirely, but they did change the procedures significantly. The changes were in a direction that sharply emphasized the rights of juveniles caught up in the processes of adjudication of delinquency in which they could lose their liberty. As such, the changes were revolutionary.

The first case, in 1966, was *Kent v. United States*, which required due process rights for juveniles for the first time. The issue centered on the due process rights of a juvenile involved in the waiver process to adult court. Kent was a 16-year-old charged with three counts each of housebreaking and robbery and two counts of rape. He first admitted these offenses, and others as well, during interrogation. It is not known at what point his mother was informed of his arrest, but on the second day of his detention it was noted that she retained a lawyer for him. A waiver hearing was scheduled in the juvenile court. Defense counsel submitted an affidavit from a psychiatrist stating that Kent needed psychiatric hospitalization. The juvenile court judge did not rule on the motions of Kent's lawyer or discuss the case with Kent or his parents. The court made no findings, nor were any reasons given for the certification to adult court. Reports from the juvenile court staff and the probation officer that the juvenile's mental state was deteriorating were ignored. An order was entered simply waiving the juvenile to the adult court for trial. Kent was then indicted in adult court on eight counts, found guilty, and sentenced to 30 to 90 years in prison.

On appeal to the U.S. Supreme Court, it was noted that the parents had not been notified in time, that the interrogation and detention took place without the parents or a lawyer being present, and that basic rights, such as the right to remain silent and to counsel, had not been communicated. The Supreme Court held that the procedures followed had been inadequate and that the juvenile had the right to a waiver hearing. At such a hearing the juvenile would be present, and the judge had to provide reasons for the waiver. An appendix to the opinion gave eight criteria for the juvenile courts to consider in deciding the issue of waiver. A famous quote from Justice Abe Fortas concluded that "the child receives the worst of both worlds: that he gets neither the protection accorded to adults nor the solicitous care and regenerative treatment postulated for children."

In 1975 another case arose involving judicial waiver. In *Breed v. Jones*, a 17-year-old was first adjudicated delinquent in the juvenile court for committing an armed robbery. After the adjudication but before a disposition took place, a fitness hearing was held, but the court then found the juvenile was not amenable to the juvenile court processes and waived the case to adult court. Jones was then convicted of first-degree robbery in adult court.

The issue in this case was whether double jeopardy had occurred, because at the time of being adjudicated a delinquent, the juvenile had been put in jeopardy. The U.S. Supreme Court held there was double jeopardy and that for a waiver to occur to adult court, the case had to be transferred before adjudication took place. As Chief Justice Burger stated, "We believe it is simply too late in the day to conclude that a juvenile is not put in jeopardy at a proceeding whose object is to determine whether he has committed acts that violate a criminal law and whose potential consequences include both the stigma inherent in such a determination and the deprivation of liberty for many years" (*Breed v. Jones* 1975).

In re Gault (1967) went to the heart of several due process issues that had not been granted juveniles. The case focused on the due process rights of a juvenile in the juvenile court process who could lose his freedom by way of being incapacitated in an institution. Gerald Gault was a 15-year-old charged with "lewd phone calls," described as being of the "irritatingly offensive, adolescent, sex variety." A petition simply alleged that Gault was a delinquent minor in need of care and custody. The complaint had been lodged by a woman neighbor who never appeared at the hearing. The judge made some inquiries of the boy, whose answers seemed to incriminate him, although there was no sworn testimony and no transcript of proceedings. Gault was not assisted by an attorney or advised of his right to one. At the conclusion of the hearing Gault was committed as a juvenile delinquent to the State Industrial School until age 21.

Because Arizona law did not permit appeals in juvenile cases, a writ of habeas corpus was filed with the Supreme Court of Arizona. The superior court dismissed the writ, and the Supreme Court of Arizona then affirmed this ruling. On appeal the U.S. Supreme Court reversed the Arizona court, and for the first time certain due process rights enjoyed by adults were granted to juveniles in the juvenile court facing the possibility of incarceration. These were 1) notice of the charges, 2) right to counsel, 3) right of confrontation and cross-examination, and 4) privilege against self-incrimination. Two other areas of rights were not granted in the Gault case: the right to a transcript of the proceedings, and the right to appellate review. The court indicated that "unbridled discretion, however benevolently motivated, is frequently a poor substitute for principle and procedure" and "the condition of being a boy does not justify a kangaroo court."

The U.S. Supreme Court seemed to be trying to salvage the legality of the juvenile court system despite this ruling. It pointed out that the decision should not impair the procedures for processing and treating juveniles. Thus, a footnote stated the decision did not apply to preadjudication or postadjudication treatment of juveniles. Several questions were still left unanswered.

The next question to come up before the U.S. Supreme Court regarding juveniles was the standard of proof to be used in determining delinquency. *In re Winship* (1970) dealt with this issue in a New York case in which a 12-year-old was sent to a state training school for taking $112 from a woman's purse. The standard of "preponderance of the evidence," in contrast to the adult standard of "beyond a reasonable doubt," was used. This standard, under the New York Family Court Act, was the lowest needed. The U.S. Supreme Court reversed the New York Court of Appeals in holding that juveniles are entitled to proof beyond reasonable doubt when they are charged with violating a criminal law. In this case the juvenile judge had acknowledged that the juvenile was convicted by the preponderance of the evidence standard but that he would not have been convicted by a standard of beyond a reasonable doubt. The standard of evidence to be used in adjudicating delinquency for violating a law was to be the same standard used in adult criminal courts. The standard conveys the degree of confidence expected for adjudication, because the evidence often proposed is assailable under a lower standard.

A remaining issue dealt with the right to a jury trial. The issue was whether the due process clause of the Fourteenth Amendment guaranteeing a jury trial applied to juveniles at the adjudicatory stage. In *McKeiver v. Pennsylvania* (1971) the U.S. Supreme Court held that it was not a constitutional requirement. The court expressed concern that such a full adversarial process would put an end to the informal, protective proceedings in juvenile court. It noted that a jury is not a necessary part of every criminal proceeding. The jury was not seen as strengthening the fact-finding function. Justice Blackmun was reluctant to say that the juvenile court does not yet still hold out some promise. If an individual judge wanted to use an advisory jury or a particular state wished to adopt a jury trial requirement, that would be possible. However, it was just not seen as constitutionally mandated.

The issue of jury trials will continue to arise in state courts. A North Carolina case which arose before McKeiver involved 45 African American juveniles ages 11 to 15 years who, along with some adults, were protesting school assignments and a new school's construction (*In re Barbara Burrus* 1969). The charges involved impeding traffic, and a consolidated hearing was held. Each juvenile requested a jury trial, which was denied, and the juveniles were placed on probation. Requests for jury trials may emerge in various state courts, with the judge deciding the issue on a case-by-case basis unless there is some state statute controlling the matter.

CONTINUING ISSUES IN JUVENILE LAW

Bail for juveniles is a continuing and unresolved issue. The initial problem is that in the early case of *ex parte Crouse* (1838), the U.S. Supreme Court held that the Bill of Rights did not apply to minors. Hence, arguments under the Eighth Amendment as to whether bail is excessive left matters to the state courts regarding bail for juveniles. The outcome has been diverse. The operating presumption has been that releasing juveniles to their parents secures their future appearance at a juvenile court hearing. However, this approach may be changing by way of juvenile judges using bail as a means of keeping a youth detained; such an approach actually amounts to a form of preventive detention. Hawaii, Kentucky, Oregon, and Utah prohibit bail; Arkansas, Colorado, Connecticut, Georgia, Massachusetts, Nebraska, Oklahoma, South Dakota, and West Virginia permit bail (Bartollas and Miller 1998). Similar to adult criminal courts, some juvenile courts are releasing juveniles on their own personal recognizance or under the supervision of a third party.

The specific question of preventive detention of juveniles was heard in the U.S. Supreme Court in the case of *Schall v. Martin* (1984). Pretrial detention is seen as justified for those who might run away and/or commit another offense. In *Schall*, a class action constitutional challenge to the New York Family Court Act was made on the basis that the act permitted detention without due process. The federal district court and court of appeals struck down the act, but they were reversed by the U.S. Supreme Court, which held that the statute served a legitimate state objective of protecting juveniles and society from the hazards of pretrial crime.

Greg Martin was a 14-year-old who allegedly hit a youth on the head with a loaded gun and stole his jacket and sneakers. When he was arrested, the gun was in his possession. The incident occurred at 11:30 P.M., and Martin then lied to the police about where and with whom he lived. He was detained for 15 days between the initial hearing and the completion of the fact-finding hearing. At that time he was adjudicated delinquent and given 2 years probation.

The entire prevention schema raises several controversial issues:

1. What are the time limits for detaining a juvenile?
2. What types of facilities are permitted for a juvenile under such detention?
3. Most juveniles are put in preventive detention on the premise that they might commit an offense. The majority opinion in *Schall v. Martin* was that "from a legal point of view there is nothing inherently unattainable about a prediction of future criminal conduct." Although this may be a valid legal position, it does not square with the actual predictive abilities of those who work in the social or behavioral sciences.
4. From the vantage point of the juvenile, preventive detention is experienced as a punishment even though it is not treated legally as such but only viewed as a confinement prior to adjudication.

As a result of the criminalization of many processes of the juvenile court, issues arose in the juvenile setting similar to those in adult criminal courts involving the police. The Fourth Amendment's prohibition against unauthorized searches and seizures is one such area. In 1961 the Supreme Court affirmed such rights for adults (*Mapp v. Ohio*). This meant that evidence could not be seized without probable cause and without a proper search warrant. In 1967 the Court applied the rule to juveniles as well unless they had consented to a search or were caught in the act (*State v. Lowry*). A prime area in which these issues are being played out is in the schools.

The presence of weapons or drugs within schools raises many issues involving searches. The searches may involve student lockers, athletic lockers, video cameras, breathalyzers, use of dogs to detect the presence of drugs, and so on.

In *New Jersey v. T.L.O.* (1985), a high school teacher discovered two girls smoking in a school lavatory. They were taken to the assistant principal, at which point one girl admitted violating a school rule but T.L.O., age 14, did not. The assistant principal demanded to see her purse, opened it, and found a pack of cigarettes and cigarette rolling papers, which made him suspicious of drug use. Proceeding further, he found a small amount of marijuana, a pipe, empty plastic bags, a substantial quantity of one-dollar bills, an index card that listed students who owed T.L.O. money, and two letters that implicated her in marijuana dealing. The police were notified, and T.L.O. then confessed to selling marijuana at school.

In the juvenile court the contention was that the Fourth Amendment had been violated in the search of T.L.O.'s purse, as well as in her confession, which was allegedly tainted by the unlawful search. The juvenile court denied the motion to suppress on the basis that the school official had a "reasonable suspicion" that a crime had been committed or that there were needs to maintain school discipline or policies. The Supreme Court of New Jersey reversed, but the U.S. Supreme Court was satisfied that the search did not violate the Fourth Amendment and reversed. The principle upholding such searches was based on the reasonableness of the search, its scope, the age of the student, and her behavior at the time. In essence it meant that, if these conditions were met, a search warrant or having probable cause were not necessary. The balancing test applied by the U.S. Supreme Court meant that the students' expectations of privacy were to give way to the need for school discipline.

A host of related issues from the area of adult criminal procedure get raised in the context of juvenile law as well. These will simply be noted here, as many of these issues are being raised in different jurisdictions through the country. Thus, the ability of a parent to waive certain procedural rights of their juvenile offspring comes under scrutiny. The requirement for a notice of a hearing in writing as provided in *Gault* is one area. Endless variations can occur, such as what constitutes an adequate notice to the minor *and* parents, parents who are separated or divorced, and so on.

Confessions by juveniles touch on many controversial areas. Even before *Gault*, the Supreme Court had held that police interrogation might be excessive. In *Haley v. Ohio* (1948), a 15-year-old had confessed after 5 hours of questioning by several police officers, which was seen as excessive. In *Gallegos v. Colorado* (1962) there was no evidence of prolonged questioning but rather a 5-day detention period during which time Gallegos's mother tried unsuccessfully to see him and he was cut off from seeing an attorney or adult advisory. The Supreme Court held that a lawyer, adult relative, or friend could have given this 14-year-old the protection that his immaturity could not. To convict him by means of his confession was viewed as treating him as though he had no constitutional rights.

Related issues involve the requirement of some states for a parental presence during interrogation, confessions to probation officers, and the limits of interrogation under *Miranda v. Arizona* (1966). For example, if a minor asks for a lawyer, must the questioning stop? What if the parent so asks but the minor does not? If the juvenile asks for some other adult that they have had a special relationship with, such as a therapist, is the questioning supposed to stop? A 16-year-old implicated in a murder was given a Miranda warning but he then asked to see his probation officer, which was denied. The question was whether this was on the same level as a request for an attorney. After the denial, he talked to the police and implicated himself in the murder (*Fare v. Michael C* 1979). In this case the Supreme Court, in a 5 to 4 decision, held that the request to see a probation officer was not in effect a request to see an attorney.

Many of these issues relate to juveniles waiving their constitutional rights. Supposedly a right can be waived if it is done voluntarily, knowingly, and intelligently. Yet for juveniles the question regards their capacity to waive their rights by these criteria. Grisso's (1981) study, which revealed that almost all 14-year-olds and one-half of 15- and 16-year-olds did not understand the importance of their Miranda rights, is relevant. Although they might have voluntarily waived their rights, the question is how knowingly it was done. The question of fingerprinting juveniles raises many issues of a similar type, as does participating in police lineups and agreeing to have their photographs taken.

Issues pertaining to competency to participate in various stages of juvenile proceedings, as well as to raise an insanity defense, are relevant in this context as well and are covered in Chapter 30, "Legal Issues in the Treatment of Minors."

Finally, the question of capital punishment for juveniles who committed the offense in question while a juvenile, but then were certified to adult court, found guilty, and sentenced to execution arose. Given that the juveniles were tried as adults, should the punishment imposed on them be the same as for someone who was an adult at the time of committing the act? *Thompson*

v. Oklahoma (1988) decided that executing a defendant who was 15 at the time of the offense would violate the Eighth Amendment's prohibition against cruel and unusual punishment. The following year, the U.S. Supreme Court decided that a juvenile who was 16 at the time of the offense and pled guilty to first-degree murder could be executed (*Missouri v. Wilkins* 1989), as could a 17-year-old involved at that age in a rape and murder (*Stanford v. Kentucky* 1989).

THE FUTURE OF JUVENILE LAW

Shifts in juvenile jurisprudence are governed by changing social policy as well as appellate decisions affecting substantive and procedural issues. If the age of juvenile jurisdiction is lowered and certification made easier, many of the more violent juveniles are removed from the system. On the opposite end, if status offenses are removed as well, another sizable group is removed from juvenile jurisdiction. The reigning phrase continues to be the "amenability to treatment" so that a juvenile could be detained and/or punished within the confines of the juvenile system in hopes that a noncriminal adult will be the eventual result. Unless the system of juvenile law is to be merged entirely into criminal law (except for preadolescents), individualized assessment will always continue to play a role. Tension occurs when serious offenses occur with the recurring question of dangerousness. Zimring (1998b) contrasts the attributes favorable for juvenile retention (while noting overlap): amenability to treatment, immaturity, lack of commitment to criminal values, changeability, accepting of help, offense typical for developmental phase, acceptance of responsibility, and nondangerousness. Tension continues throughout the juvenile justice system regarding focusing on the acts in question versus the actors in terms of their personalities and social backgrounds.

One paradox is that the most serious legal offenses are not necessarily committed by the most mature juveniles. In fact, the most violent acts seem to be committed by juveniles who are immature, poorly educated, and have less comprehension of how the broader world functions. The complexity of the situation is seen if we move beyond the simple appellation of "serious violence."

Consider that 95% of juvenile violence involves aggravated assaults, robberies, and assaults (Federal Bureau of Investigation 1998). Zimring (1998a) conceptualizes vertical and horizontal discriminations for offenses. Thus, a juvenile legal system would first need to assess which types of attacks and robberies rank high priority. Legal classifications themselves operate in part, such as homicides being vertically higher than assaults. Horizontal discriminations assess specifics of the individual act. For example, if a street shooting gets a high penal priority, what should the relative penalties be for the following accomplices: a juvenile who drove the car to the scene, a juvenile who bought the gun, and another who had knowledge about the pending assault but kept silent. No juvenile law or sentencing grid alone can sort out the culpability of such actors.

The increase in homicides by juveniles reveals two more areas that continue to operate in a state of ambivalence and confusion. The lack of regulation of firearms will simply be noted. However, a similar lack of clarity in principles operates with juvenile homicide itself. The practice is simply to focus on the age for certification to adult courts, with the accompanying assumption that once certified, justice has been accomplished. What may push the system into an appraisal are younger perpetrators of serious violence whose age demands a deeper assessment of what set of principles should operate (Howell 1997).

REFERENCES

Ainsworth JE: Re-imaging childhood and reconstructing the legal order: the case for abolishing the juvenile court. North Carolina Law Review 69:1083–1133, 1991

Allen FA: The Habits of Legality. New York, Oxford University Press, 1996

Bartollas C, Miller SJ: Juvenile Justice in America, 2nd Edition. Upper Saddle River, NJ, Prentice Hall, 1998

Breed v Jones, 421 US 519 (1975)

Commonwealth v M'Keagy (PA 1831)

Empey LT, Stafford MC: American Delinquency: Its Meaning and Construction, 3rd Edition. Belmont, CA, Wadsworth, 1991

Ex parte Crouse, 4 Wharton 9 (PA 1838)

Fare v Michael C, 442 US 707 (1979)

Federal Bureau of Investigation: Crime in the United States: Uniform Crime Reports, 1997. Washington, DC, U.S. Government Printing Office, 1998

Feld BD: Justice for Children. Boston, MA, Northeastern University Press, 1993

Gallegos v Colorado, 370 US 49 (1962)

Grisso T: Juveniles Waiver of Rights: Legal and Psychological Competence. New York, Plenum, 1981

Haley v Ohio, 332 US 596 (1948)

Hawes JM: Children in Urban Society: Juvenile Delinquency in Nineteenth-Century America. New York, Oxford University Press, 1971

Howell JC: Juvenile Justice and Youth Crime. Thousand Oaks, CA, Sage, 1997

In re Barbara Burrus, 275 NC 517 (1969)

In re Gault, 387 US 1 (1967)

In re Winship, 397 US 358 (1970)

Kent v United States, 383 US 541 (1966)

Krisberg B, Austin JF: Reinventing Juvenile Justice. Newbury Park, CA, Sage, 1993

Mapp v Ohio, 367 US 643 (1961)

McKeiver v Pennsylvania, 403 US 528 (1971)

Miller A, Ohlin L: Delinquency and Community. Beverly Hills, CA, Sage, 1985

Miranda v Arizona, 384 US 436 (1966)

Missouri v Wilkins, 492 US 361 (1989)

New Jersey v T.L.O., 469 US 325 (1985)

Platt AM: The Child Savers. Chicago, IL, University of Chicago Press, 1969

Ryerson E: The Best Laid Plans: America's Juvenile Court Experiment. New York, Hill & Want, 1978

Schall v Martin 104 S Ct 2403 (1984)

Stanford v Kentucky, 402 US 361 (1989)

State v Lowry, 95 J Super 307, 230 A2d 907 (1967)

Sutton JR: Stubborn Children: Controlling Delinquency in the United States, 1640–1981. Berkeley, CA, University of California Press, 1988

Thompson v Oklahoma, 487 US 815 (1988)

Zimring FE: American Youth Violence. New York, Oxford University Press, 1998a

Zimring FE: The jurisprudence of youth violence, in Youth Violence. Edited by Tonry M, Moore MH. Chicago, IL, University of Chicago Press, 1998b, pp 476–501

CHAPTER 26

Assessment and Treatment of Juvenile Offenders

Debra K. DePrato, M.D.
Jill Hayes Hammer, Ph.D.

Case Example 1

Tasha, a 14-year-old girl, was adjudicated as a delinquent on charges of simple kidnapping and unauthorized use of a vehicle. While waiting in the car for her mother, who was in a store, Tasha drove away with her 4-year-old sister, who was asleep in the front seat. Tasha was sentenced to 5 years at a "training school," but was released into an intensive aftercare program after serving 1 year. She has a history of physical and sexual abuse, maternal neglect and abandonment, running away, precocious sexual behavior, truancy, cruelty to animals, and fire setting. She was diagnosed as a child with schizoaffective disorder by a mental health center psychiatrist.

Case Example 2

Greg, a 15-year-old boy, presented to the emergency room with a gunshot wound to his leg. He apathetically reported that late that evening, while riding his bike with friends, someone fired a stray bullet, accidentally hitting him. Greg's mother was concerned that he uses drugs. His parents were never married. During their sporadic and volatile 5-year relationship, the father was abusive to both her and Greg. His father has been in prison for the past 8 years.

The extended family, however, is supportive and active in a local church. Greg's mother earned her high school equivalency diploma; however, she was laid off from her job more than a year ago. Lack of finances led to their living in an increasingly violent neighborhood. About 2 years ago, on entering middle school, Greg began failing subjects and skipping school; he was recently expelled for the remainder of the school year. Prior to expulsion, he was referred to

the juvenile court. The emergency room doctor has now referred Greg to your clinic for a psychiatric evaluation and treatment plan.

The current juvenile justice system grew from rehabilitative goals envisioned in the closing years of the nineteenth century. Whereas children were previously treated as little adults and subjected to the same criminal justice penalties as adults, a growing awareness of the need for treatment and protection for minors turned the states toward assuming a parental role (i.e., *parens patriae*) in dealing with juvenile offenders. Even a new argot evolved—"taken into custody" replaced "arrest;" "trial" became "hearing;" "conviction" was now "adjudication," "sentence," or "disposition." Juvenile "delinquents" were no longer sent to prison; instead, they were remanded to reformatories or trade schools. Early reformers created the Illinois Juvenile Court Act, which established the first juvenile code in 1899, with emphasis on rehabilitation.

In the United States juvenile justice system, a child can commit two categories of offenses: delinquency offenses and status offenses. *Delinquent*, a legal term, means that a child has been found guilty of at least one crime that, if committed by an adult, could be punishable by law (e.g., theft, rape). Truancy, ungovernability, and running away are considered status offenses. As noted in Chapter 25, "Overview of Juvenile Law," *In re Gault* (1967) ruled that delinquent offenders were to be afforded the same due process rights as an adult charged with a crime with the exception of jury trial. Prior to

Gault, all offenders (status and delinquent) were treated equally and were offered no legal protections. The Juvenile Justice and Delinquency Act of 1974 provided status offenders with protection from the harshest form of punishment—incarceration in juvenile correctional facilities. In order to continue receiving federal funding, states could no longer lock up status offenders in training facilities. Response to the new restrictions resulted in rapid growth of community-based treatment programs and the child mental health movement.

Once a youth is charged as delinquent, he or she may enter a diversion program, be adjudicated and receive probation, or sent to a secure training school or a juvenile rehabilitation and correctional facility. Some researchers suggest that by grouping deviant youths together, unforeseen negative side effects may occur (Arnold and Hughes 1999). Social learning theory (i.e., Albert Bandura's research, wherein he showed that children learn through observation) indicates that training schools tend to train additional deviance rather than prosocial behaviors.

RISK AND PROTECTIVE FACTORS FOR CHRONIC JUVENILE DELINQUENCY

Attempts to predict who will and will not commit juvenile crime have been inaccurate, producing many false positives. Using only base rates of delinquency in a given population would likely provide more accurate findings. Nevertheless, identification of the risk factors associated with chronic delinquency can highlight relationships among developmental disorders, family status, and patterns of crime and recidivism. Such identification allows for prevention and intervention, hopefully producing a more favorable outcome—less crime—for those at risk and for the general population. Risk factors of future delinquency are well researched and generally can be grouped into genetic, individual, family, community, peer, and school risk factors (Steiner and the Work Group on Quality Issues 1997). Table 26–1 lists the risk factors that appear consistently as correlates of antisocial behavior.

Researchers have suggested that delinquency is positively correlated with a number of risk factors. Risk factors are mediated, however, by protective factors, which appear to act as a shield from future delinquency. Prosocial peer relationships, high intelligence, clear standards for behavior, good academic achievement, fast autonomic conditioning, organized recreational activities, attachment to parents, school, and teachers, as well as a

TABLE 26–1. Risk factors associated with delinquent behavior

Individual
Low intelligence; cognitive, learning, and language problems
Poor impulse control
Not taking responsibility for behavior
Admiration for antisocial behavior
Perception of others as hostile
Early onset of delinquency
Child working more than 20 hours per week
Poor social skills

Family
Poverty
Low education levels
Conflict and hostility at home
Ineffective parental discipline and monitoring
Physical/sexual abuse
Familial substance abuse and psychiatric problems
Parental criminal history
Lack of warmth and affection between parents and child

Peers
Association with delinquent youth
Association with youth who use drugs or alcohol
Membership in gangs

School
Poor achievement/grades
Falling behind same-age peers
Sense of isolation or prejudice from peers
Poor attendance

Community
Availability of drugs and weapons
Poor support network
Isolation from neighbors
Living in "dangerous" neighborhoods
Frequent family moves

positive response to authority are all reported to be protective factors (Browning et al. 1999; Hoge et al. 1996). The influence of risk and protective factors changes at different developmental levels. Peer influence to a preschool youngster is much less important than it is to an adolescent, and parental influence on an adolescent is less important than it is to a preschooler. Therefore, diagnosticians need to carefully assess what risk and protective factors are more salient given a child's developmental stage.

Less is known about the development of delinquency in females than in males. Risk factors for female delinquency may be more prevalent (Henggeler et al. 1987), as female offenders are more likely to have experienced physical abuse (80%) or sexual abuse/sexual assault (70% versus 32% in boys; Janus et al. 1987). Females are twice as likely as males to be diagnosed with comorbid emotional disorders, but they are less likely to get treatment (Offord et al. 1991). Along the same lines, males are more likely to externalize their emotional difficulties through acting out and criminality, whereas females are more likely to develop internalizing disorders. However, the long-term consequences of a conduct disorder in females may be more severe than that seen in males (Zoccolillo and Rogers 1991).

DELINQUENCY AND MENTAL DISORDERS

Numerous studies have described the prevalence of a given disorder in juvenile offenders. These studies, however, often yield different rates. Possible reasons for these discrepancies include different 1) methodologies, 2) ways of diagnosing mental illness in delinquents, and 3) populations. Table 26–2 lists the prevalence rates of psychiatric disorders among juvenile delinquents.

When the prevalence of disorders in the incarcerated juvenile population was compared with that of juveniles in the general population, it was concluded that incarcerated delinquents had twice the overall rate of mental disorders, with anxiety disorders being 1.5 times more prevalent, mood disorders being 3 times more prevalent, and substance abuse disorders being 14 times more prevalent (Eppright et al. 1993; Hollander and Turner 1985; Marsteller et al. 1997; McManus et al. 1984; Mezzich 1990; Zagar et al. 1989). Interestingly, behavior disorders were no more common among the incarcerated delinquent population than in the general population. Females differ from their male cohorts with regard to psychiatric diagnosis in that they are more likely to be diagnosed with anxiety and mood disorders, whereas males more often meet diagnostic criteria for disruptive behavior disorders and substance use disorders (Zoccolillo and Rogers 1991).

ASSESSMENT ISSUES SPECIFIC TO JUVENILE DELINQUENCY

A thorough and accurate assessment of a delinquent is key to adequately addressing the treatment needs of the child and his or her family. The assessment must target all the risk and protective factors for both the delinquent and his or her environment and identify those factors in

TABLE 26–2.   Prevalence of psychiatric disorders among juvenile delinquents

Psychiatric disorder	Percentage meeting diagnostic criteria
No diagnosis	0–7
Adjustment disorder	17
Anxiety disorder	29.7
Attention-deficit/hyperactivity disorder	9–46
Borderline intelligence	14–55
Conduct disorder	28.5–98
Oppositional defiant disorder	1–12.9
Impulse-control disorder	6
Learning disorders	22
Mental retardation	4–19
Bipolar disorder	12.7
Dysthymia	18.3
Major depressive disorder	1
Any personality disorder	18–75
Schizophrenia and other psychotic disorders	3–63
Any substance abuse	20–29.5

Source.   Percentages were acquired from the following articles: Eppright et al. 1993; Hollander and Turner 1985; Marsteller et al. 1997; McManus et al. 1984; Mezzich 1990; Zagar et al. 1989.

which a treatment intervention is possible and realistic. Knowledge of the literature in this area is essential, as well as an understanding of which treatments work with this population and which do not.

The results of the clinician's evaluation and treatment recommendations have serious implications for the child's life. An adequate evaluation will direct treatment to reduce risk factors while enhancing protective factors, thus minimizing the possibility of the youth's further involvement in delinquent activities. Inadequate evaluation and treatment will have little impact upon the juvenile's situation and often leads to treatment failure, resulting in serious legal consequences for the youth, such as incarceration.

The typical assessment of a juvenile delinquent occurs following adjudication and before sentencing. The judge, attorneys, and/or probation and parole officers often desire an assessment to aid in the disposition of the case and to address specific treatment recommendations. The questions often asked by referral sources include how to best protect the community from the child, the child's risk of re-arrest, identification of a mental disorder(s), types of treatment recommended and their availability, and the least restrictive environment necessary. To answer these questions, clinicians must approach the evaluation with a broad ecological perspective, including

TABLE 26–3.   Assessment guidelines

1. Understand the legal question at hand.
2. Review the legal records, such as previous charges, victim's statements, police report of the current delinquent charge, and behavioral reports from detention center.
3. Gather all pertinent records, including medical, mental health, and school records of the child and, if indicated, those of the primary guardian(s).
4. The clinical interview of the child must specifically address the functioning of the child in the family, the functioning of the child at school, the peer group of the child, the neighborhood where the child resides, a thorough mental status examination assessing all cognitive domains, premorbid functioning prior to the delinquent act, past legal history, acute or chronic stressors in the child's life, a weapons and violence history, substance use, sexual or physical abuse, medical problems, and prosocial skills.
5. The clinical interview must include the primary caretakers of the child, specifically addressing their style of parenting, evidence of a mental disorder or substance abuse disorder that interferes with parenting, ability to interact successfully with the child's environment (such as school and peer group), the family's support system, and the strengths of the family system.
6. Collateral interviews should be conducted with individuals familiar with the child, such as a current treatment provider, teacher, probation officer, detention staff, and so on.
7. Psychological assessment is indicated for educational purposes, and to "develop a full picture of a juvenile's learning style with the juvenile's emotional development and behavior" (Melton et al. 1997, p. 436).

a thorough investigation of the juvenile's behavior in the home, school, workplace, and neighborhood (Melton et al. 1997). The evaluation should address the child's functioning in the environment in which he or she lives, as well as the primary caretaker's ability to effectively parent across a variety of settings, including home and school. By assessing the child within the system in which he or she lives, one can correctly identify areas for needed intervention and the strengths of the child and family that will prompt success of treatment. Refer to Table 26–3 for guidelines for assessing juvenile delinquents.

JUVENILE JUSTICE MODELS

Identification of factors that contribute to chronic delinquency and factors protecting from delinquency, if incorporated into treatment models, may produce programs with improved outcomes for delinquent youths.

Youths can be involved in treatment at different points in the court process: preadjudication in diversion programs, while on probation and living in the community, when placed out of the home in a more restrictive environment, and following incarceration if on parole or in an aftercare program.

Diversion Programs

Diversion of juvenile offenders from the juvenile justice system evolved in the 1970s, based on the belief that penetration into the juvenile justice system is more harmful than beneficial; the two main reasons being that involvement in the juvenile justice system gives the

child a delinquent self-image, and that it stigmatizes the child in the opinion of others (such as teachers, parents, officers) (Lundman 1993). Diversion programs defer the child's adjudication so that the child's charge will be dropped if he or she successfully completes treatment. It can be argued that diversion programs revert juvenile offenders to a pre-*Gault* status, in that they have no legal representation or trial, and many of these children's charges would be dismissed had they gone to trial.

Lundman's review of the major diversion programs and research efforts since the 1970s reveals several points. Many diversion programs include greater numbers of referrals of juveniles for lesser charges, thereby "net widening," or adding children to the juvenile justice system who would not otherwise be included. In the late 1970s, the Office of Juvenile Justice and Delinquency Prevention (OJJDP) funded four jurisdictions for experimentally designed diversion projects in which offenders would have otherwise penetrated further into the system due to their current delinquent charge. Types of treatment involved individual and family therapy, and educational, employment, and recreational interventions. Three groups were compared: those released without services, those given diversion services, and those who had further involvement in the juvenile justice system. Re-arrest rates of the three control groups, 6 and 12 months posttreatment, showed no significant differences. Another study, the Adolescent Diversion Project, revealed that community-based diversion interventions produced lower delinquency rates than did return-to-court intake (i.e., those children who did not receive services but were remanded to court). Taken together, "diversion of juveniles accused of status and property crimes is at least as effective as further penetration into the justice system" (Lundman 1993).

Juvenile Drug Court

One of the newest forms of diversion for juvenile offenders is the juvenile drug court, patterned upon the adult drug court model. Juvenile drug courts are diversionary for first-time juvenile offenders charged with a drug-related offense. Drug courts are modeled after the Miami drug court, created in Dade County in 1989 to address the overwhelming growth of drug-related criminal caseloads and the potential impact on public safety (Goldkamp 1994). As described by Goldkamp, the Miami drug court model features a courtroom-based team approach combined with outpatient drug treatment. One year of involvement is required, and adult defendants proceed through phases (detoxification, counseling, educational/vocational assessment and training, and graduation). Outcomes in the Miami drug court revealed promising criminal justice and safety implications. Drug court defendants had a somewhat lower rate of recidivism, and, if rearrested, averaged two to three times longer to first rearrest. Defendants who self-reported the highest rates of drug abuse had the poorest outcomes. One side effect of frequent court appearances was the increased failure-to-appear rate. It was noted that as defendants are supervised more closely, their violations are noticed more frequently than when they are on standard probation. A treatment approach based on an addiction model with relapse expected is extremely important so that the program does not become overly punitive, resulting in higher rates of incarceration. Among the most critical policy decisions in establishing a drug court were those of target population and volume (Goldkamp 1994).

Correctional- and Institutional-Based Programs

About 53% of adjudicated juvenile delinquents are given probation, and 28% are placed outside the home. Corrections-based programs can be effective in reducing recidivism, according to recent meta-analyses (Andrews et al. 1990; Lipton and Pearson 1996), as long as specific principles are followed throughout incarceration.

In general, OJJDP noted that treatment programs must share these principles:

- Target specific characteristics and problems of offenders that can be changed in treatment and that are predictive of future criminality.
- Implement known treatment methods for participating offenders, and use proven therapeutic techniques with educated, experienced staff.

- Allow adequate duration of program time for desired outcome.
- Offer the most intensive programming for offenders with the highest risk of recidivism.
- Utilize individualized cognitive and behavioral treatment methods that maximize positive reinforcement for prosocial behavior.

Foster and Group Homes

Group home treatment of status and delinquent offenders dates back to the early 1900s in Chicago and New York. The program caught on nationally in the 1960s and 1970s (Piper and Warner 1980; Weber 1981). Group homes typically house from 4 to 12 adolescents. Children generally reside in a family-type setting with houseparents (foster families, trained individuals or couples, counselors, or caseworkers). Residents are usually enrolled in community public schools, may earn the privilege of regular visits with their families on weekends, may hold part-time jobs, and may even enjoy some independent personal time (Krueger and Hansen 1987). Children may benefit from individual and/or family therapy, as well as from behavior management plans (i.e., token economy systems). Group homes are typically cost-effective and provide an alternative to incarceration (Haghighi and Lopez 1993). Specialized services and schools within an institution are not necessary, as community resources are available.

Alternative Programs

Boot camps.   Since 1983, juvenile justice agencies and police jurisdictions in many states have established both juvenile and adult boot camps. The premise of these programs is to shock delinquents into not offending through placing them in a 90- to 180-day military-style program involving work, exercise, and strict requirements that the rules of the program must be followed (Burns and Vito 1995; Freeman 1993; Greenwood 1996; Jones and Ross 1997; MacKenzie 1990; MacKenzie and Parent 1992). In addition to treatment components similar to other programs (e.g., education), boot camps emphasize moral development through instruction in responsibility for one's behavior, involvement in group-related activities, and development of and commitment to a value system (Freeman 1993; Fullard 1998).

Boot camps are reported to cost less than incarceration (if they reduce confinement), although researchers have generally shown that boot camps are ineffective at reducing recidivism and have relatively high dropout rates; however, they do influence moral development

(Freeman 1993; MacKenzie 1991; MacKenzie et al. 1995). The above studies investigated the effects of boot camp programs on adults; it is suggested that the effectiveness of programs targeted at juvenile offenders be reported.

Wilderness programs.   Removing seriously delinquent youths from their environments and placing them with peers and program staff in a remote location (e.g., mountains, desert) that requires teamwork, support, and goal-setting to "survive" is touted by some as effective in reducing recidivism (Greenwood and Turner 1987), though others had less positive findings (Castellano and Soderstrom 1992; Deschenes and Greenwood 1998).

Scared Straight.   The assumption in Scared Straight programs is that juvenile offenders who are brought to prisons and exposed to prison life through lectures, tours, and scare tactics by adult prisoners would fear prison life because of the severe punishment and therefore act in a law-abiding manner (Lundman 1993). Rigorous research studies have proven, however, that Scared Straight does not reduce recidivism and may actually be harmful (Finckenauer 1982; Lundman 1993; Michigan Department of Corrections 1967, as reported in Lundman 1993; Orchowsky and Taylor 1981).

Aftercare and Reintegrative Confinement

Effectively transitioning juvenile offenders from incarceration back into the community is critical, especially as numbers of incarcerated juveniles increase and institutions become overcrowded and expensive. In addition, long-term incarceration of juvenile offenders has not been shown to result in reduction of juvenile arrests after release. According to Altschuler and colleagues (1999), reintegrative confinement emphasizes

- Preparing confined offenders for reentry into the specific communities to which they will return
- Making the needed arrangements and linkages with agencies and individuals in the offender's community in direct relation to known risk and protective factors
- Ensuring the delivery of required services and supervision after discharge

Three OJJDP-funded integrative release/aftercare programs had different results; however, commonalties and recommendations for reform were noted by OJJDP:

1. Aftercare must be community-based and in a continuum to parallel programs within the correctional institution (i.e., the institution must design services to prepare youths to reintegrate into their communities, with aftercare to follow).
2. Aftercare must be sufficiently funded for adequate numbers of well-trained, well-supervised staff who can respond to issues of family, education, drug abuse, and employment upon the juvenile's return to the community.
3. Formal assessment must occur in order to identify high-risk offenders who require this level of intensive services and supervision.
4. Reduced caseload sizes, greater contact by staff, and clear planning for positive long-term impact are necessary along with a graduated response regarding sanctions (so that the process is not overly punitive while providing greater supervision).

TREATMENT MODELS

Different types of treatment are offered as part of court-related programs for delinquent and status offending youth. Treatment prognosis of behavior-disordered and antisocial youths was considered dismal, yet recent treatment models have shown more successful outcomes. Reviews of delinquency literature of the 1970s gave no indication that treatment worked (Henggeler 1989). Previous forms of treatment focused on a small part of the delinquent's behavior; treatment was office-based, often inaccessible, and disregarded environmental factors leading to out-of-home placements (Henggeler 1994). System design and agency interaction often led to fragmented services with lack of coordination of care. Regarding mild forms of antisocial behavior, Kazdin (1995) noted promising treatment with behavioral parent training, cognitive-behavioral therapy, and functional family therapy. Structured skill-oriented treatments described by Lipsey (1992) revealed improvement in delinquents in general. MultiSystemic Therapy (MST; Borduin and Henggeler 1990) has shown improved outcomes for serious and violent juvenile offenders and substance-abusing youths. Individual treatment has not been shown to prevent or improve juvenile delinquency in real-world settings (Lundman 1993) and was not designed for antisocial youths. Family preservation alone has shown no long-term improvement in outcomes for children versus traditional office-based services. Up to 50% of youths who are hospitalized are admitted for behavioral disorders; even though no studies show that hospitalization is more beneficial than long-term community-based treatments, and youths with antisocial and family pathology show the least benefit (Henggeler 1994).

Comorbid conditions must be thoroughly assessed and treated. Treatment with medication alone does not adequately treat psychopathology. Medication management is an adjunct to treatment and is more useful in crisis management and short-term interventions (Steiner and the Work Group on Quality Issues 1997). Medications may include antidepressants, lithium, anticonvulsants, and propranolol, although no outcome studies have been performed to show efficacy. Attention-deficit/hyperactivity disorder (ADHD) is the best case for medication management, as it is highly correlated with the later onset of conduct disorder (Foley et al. 1996); effective treatment of ADHD may prevent the onset of conduct disorder.

Most treatment programs do not improve delinquency for two reasons. Antisocial behavior is caused by many factors and involves all aspects of the child's life, and interventions must target the correlates of antisocial behavior (Henggeler et al. 1994).

Family Therapy

A literature review by Chamberlain and Rosicky (1995) looked at the various forms of family therapy and their outcomes for treatment (1989–1994). In general, the results of their study reviewed three major categories: 1) Social Learning Family Therapy (SLFT), designed to alter dysfunctional patterns of parent-child interactions by building parental skills; 2) Structural Family Therapy (SFT), designed to alter family systems related to poor organization, cohesion, and structure; and 3) Multi-target Ecological Treatment (MET), designed for multistressed families combining approaches of SLFT and SFT.

Compared with individual treatment, SLFT showed long-term improvement up to 1 year after treatment (Bank et al. 1991). In comparing parent groups, adolescent groups, and combined parent and adolescent groups, parent groups showed significantly improved family functioning 1 year after treatment. SFT, when combined with therapeutic foster care versus residential care, showed significantly decreased rates of later hospitalization and incarceration and was more cost-effective. MET is usefully implemented via therapeutic foster care and via family preservation, is less costly than other out-of-home placements or hospitalization, and shows improved treatment outcomes.

Poor response to family therapy in general was related to three factors:

1. *Attrition*—Families who dropped out tended to be in lower socioeconomic classes (SECs), had mothers who were depressed, were agency referred, and had more severe conduct problems in the identified child.
2. *Family stress and lack of social support*—The probability of poor treatment outcome increases as SEC gets lower and social isolation increases. Stress can be alleviated somewhat by social support, thereby enhancing effectiveness of treatment.
3. *Child variables*—In general, family therapy is more effective for younger children and for teenagers with conduct problems.

In summary, family therapy is a useful mode of treatment; however, results from clinic studies were less positive than those from research-based therapy studies. Earlier intervention, service delivery in the community, and agency coordination may further improve family therapy outcomes.

Group Therapy

There is growing evidence that grouping delinquent and antisocial youths together for group treatment purposes may produce a negative effect (Arnold and Hughes 1999). The literature shows little evidence of long-term improvement in youths after treatment in groups (Beelmann et al. 1994). There is a strong association between delinquent youths and their peer group. There is some evidence that first-time offenders become worse when grouped with other children with more serious behavior problems (Fo and O'Donnell 1975), in that a delinquent peer group is a risk factor for chronic delinquency. Arnold and Hughes (1999) noted that "homogeneous group treatment of delinquent or at-risk youth opens up the possibility for reinforcement of deviant values, affiliation with peers who model antisocial behavior and values, increased opportunities for criminal activity, [and] stronger identification with a delinquent subculture" (p. 110). Group therapy is often offered in correctional settings; however, better outcomes were noted when family therapy was utilized. More research studying the positive and negative outcomes must be performed in this area.

MultiSystemic Therapy

"MultiSystemic Therapy was developed to address major limitations of existing mental health services for juvenile offenders and has received the most empirical support as an effective treatment for serious and violent criminal behavior in adolescents" (Borduin 1999, p. 243). MultiSystemic Therapy (MST) is designed to influence the known correlates and causes of serious antisocial behavior in a social-ecological framework. MST interventions target identified child and family problems within and between multiple systems in which family members are embedded, and such interventions are delivered in the natural environment (home, school, neighborhood). Goals of MST are to give parents the skills to address the current and future problems of the identified child as well as other children in the family and to empower adolescents to cope with family and environmental problems. MST utilizes strategies from multiple forms of therapy to affect the risk factors of each identified family and child. All treatment is individualized, goal-directed, flexible, and the responsibility of the provider. Barriers to parenting, such as untreated mental illness, substance abuse, lack of knowledge, and lack of social supports, are targeted in treatment.

Interventions with the child include increasing prosocial activities with mainstream peer groups while decreasing involvement with antisocial youth, addressing issues of academic performance, and increasing social skills. MST emphasizes assessment and utilization of strengths in the child and family to promote positive change.

MST is an "in-community" treatment, so that the youth and family learn successful skills to negotiate the environment in which they live. This treatment is conducted by a master's-level therapist for 4 to 8 families over a 3- to 5-month course of treatment. A treatment team provides supervision, and special training in MST is required.

On a systems level, MST provides an alternative to incarceration or out-of-home placement. For MST to be successful, the service organization must be committed to its success and the program must collaborate effectively with other agencies such as school, the courts, probation, and social services. MST has been shown to be successful in a number of offender groups: general delinquents, violent and/or chronic delinquents, and substance users and abusers. MST is being researched in pregnant and postpartum substance abusers, early adolescent violent offenders, and child and adolescent sex offenders. MST is cost-effective and produced improved treatment outcomes when compared with out-of-home placement and incarceration.

In 1990, it was noted that the knowledge of substance abuse treatment for adolescents was poor. No research looked at the outcomes for inpatient, day treatment, or residential care for adolescent users, and there was little research on outpatient care. Etiological factors for substance abuse are much like those for antisocial youth involving individual, family, peer, and school factors. MST resulted in youths with fewer arrests, less reported drug use, and fewer days in out-of-home placement at 6 months posttreatment.

Teaching-Family Group Home

In the Teaching-Family Group Home (TFGH) model, a married couple (called "teaching parents") receives training and supervision in behavior management, skills teaching, motivation, and other concepts. They generally staff a single-family house (although campus-based programs exist), where 6 or so delinquent adolescents between the ages of 12 and 17 reside for an average of 6 to 12 months. An array of services is offered to the residents, including individualized behavior change programs, individual therapy, and family therapy. Each child also participates in daily meetings where rules, rule infractions, and consequences for such infractions are determined (Bedlington et al. 1988; Braukmann and Wolf 1987; Braukmann et al. 1985).

The rates of criminal offenses and the percentage of youths involved in criminal activities declined significantly during TFGH residency. However, TFGH residents fared no better posttreatment than control subjects in group homes did on these variables. Researchers pointed out that many of the natural families of the delinquent youths were mentally ill and were resistant to treatment. They further related that recidivism was not unlikely after the youths returned to live with the same families that initially contributed, at least in part, to their delinquent behavior.

Treatment Foster Care

Supervision (Sampson and Laub 1993), consistent disciplining (Capaldi et al. 1997), and adult support and mentoring (Werner and Smith 1982) may hinder a trajectory toward future delinquency. Patricia Chamberlain (1998) proposed Treatment Foster Care (TFC) to fulfill these variables, whereby a delinquent youth is placed in a family home with no other, or only one other, child. The foster parent receives didactic and experiential training. Additionally, the foster parent consults daily with case managers or former TFC parents, and a case manager is available for crisis intervention 24 hours a day. Weekly meetings are held to review the youth's progress in his or her individualized program. Interpersonal skills training and prosocial activities are emphasized for the resident. Individual, family, and psychiatric treatments are available. Family therapy is aimed at teaching the biological parents effective behavior management strategies and eliminating obstructions to competent parenting. A school-home note system is also used to promote communication between caregivers and teachers. The youngster is consistently monitored initially, with no unsupervised time in the community. As the youth progresses, more independence is gained. On leaving TFC, the youth is returned home, and aftercare groups and on-call case managers are available to the family for 6 months following release (Chamberlain and Reid 1998; Chamberlain et al. 1996). TFC is reported to be effective for youths with emotional and behavior difficulties (Moore and Chamberlain 1994), and studies are under way with young children (ages 3–7 years) and with adolescent girls.

In several outcome studies, Chamberlain and colleagues compared TFC with other group home care, enhanced treatment services, and assessment only (Chamberlain 1990; Chamberlain and Reid 1998). They found that there was a significant negative correlation between the number of days in TFC care and the number of days of later incarceration. Youths involved in TFC had significantly fewer arrests than youths in other group home settings, and significantly fewer youths in TFC went on to offend again. Additionally, Chamberlain indicated that TFC youths were more likely to complete the program than youths in other group home programs, as the latter were three times more likely to run away or be expelled from the program.

PITFALLS

Inadequate Assessment

To best plan intervention and treatment for a juvenile offender, a thorough assessment must be performed. Knowledge of the literature regarding risk and protective factors is essential so that assessment of these factors is included as part of the evaluation of the child and family. In addition, information beyond that provided by the child and guardian is necessary in order to assess the child's and family's functioning within their environment and to assess credibility. After gathering and assimilating the data, a treatment plan targeting the child's needs and promoting the child's and family's strengths can be made.

Assuming All Court-Related Treatments Are "Equal"

Outcomes of models of treatment vary widely, and many have no data available. There are juvenile justice models that are not actually treatment but are court-related models that attempt to keep children out of the formal court process. Treatment offered within these programs, such as diversion, can range from no treatment to multiple therapeutic interventions. Correctional institutions offer treatment involving different methods, such as medication, group therapy, family therapy, or individual

therapy. The evaluator must be knowledgeable about the treatment of juvenile offenders, and which treatment programs are efficacious for the individual offender. The evaluator must be able to recommend a treatment plan that is both realistic and useful. Many children are involved in treatment that has little chance of decreasing recidivism. Unfortunately, these children are seen as treatment failures when they relapse into delinquent behavior and receive more punitive sanctions. Frequently, in diversion and aftercare programs, increased supervision and lack of appropriate treatment set the stage for more frequent sanctions.

Lack of Outcome Studies

Treatment providers for juvenile offenders, no matter where they practice—from hospitals to outpatient clinics to correctional institutions—should be aware of their own outcomes regarding recidivism for their patients. It is imperative that those who render treatment be competent in this area of practice by staying current with the literature on treatments that have positive outcomes, using models that have therapeutic success, and attempting to monitor their own outcomes, at least with regard to recidivism rates.

CASE EXAMPLE EPILOGUES

Case Example I

After release from the correctional institution, Tasha returned to live with her mother and was placed in an intensive aftercare program while on parole. Two months later, Tasha violated her parole by not meeting with her parole officer. Unfortunately, Tasha's stay in corrections and her aftercare program did not prepare her for reintegration back into her own community. Group therapy with her counterparts was the only treatment offered at the training school. During aftercare, Tasha continued group therapy and received increased supervision. Tasha and her mother both acquired skills necessary to decrease Tasha's chance of recidivism. An evidence-based treatment plan, addressing risk and protective factors with regard to parenting, school, community, and peer difficulties, was needed to rehabilitate Tasha and reduce her chances of recidivism. MST or TFC would have been appropriate options.

Case Example 2

In this case, the child psychiatrist needs to consider the context of the evaluation. The court has not ordered this assessment, so the typical limits of confidentiality apply. That is, without consent from Greg's mother, one cannot inform the court or probation officer of Greg's involvement in this incident. Assessment revealed a number of risk factors for delinquency including a deviant peer group, possible drug use, access to weapons, poor parenting skills, physical abuse, parental arrest, parental discord, low parental income, living in a dangerous neighborhood, underachievement in school, and truancy. Protective factors were identified as good premorbid functioning and involvement in positive social activities. It is necessary to gather more information about Greg's treatment history (what has helped and what has not), interview other family members, and investigate what treatment options may be available through social services. A tentative treatment plan would involve minimizing Greg's involvement with the deviant peer group while maximizing involvement with a prosocial peer group and parent training.

ACTION GUIDELINES

Understand the Legal Context of the Evaluation

The mental health professional should understand the context in which he or she is to perform the evaluation. Is it prior to adjudication as part of a diversion program, so that the juvenile must waive confidentiality and agree to treatment in order to participate? Is it following adjudication of a charge, and the court has ordered the evaluation for dispositional recommendations? Is it after the youth is incarcerated, and an aftercare plan is being formulated for reintegration into the community as a high-risk offender? The context of the evaluation is extremely important so that the professional can competently provide the recommendations most suited for the individual child's needs with the goal of decreased recidivism.

Performance of a Thorough Assessment and Treatment Plan

A thorough assessment, which evaluates the child and family in the context of the environment in which they live, is necessary. For the child to be successful, he or she will need to be able to negotiate within his or her community. Primary caretakers must be able to function effectively in their parental role. The evaluator must assess all of the causes of the antisocial behavior.

Promotion of Evidence-Based Treatment

Treatment outcomes of juvenile offenders range from positive outcomes to no change to increased recidivism rates. Mental health providers need to understand, uti-

lize, and promote those treatment programs for juvenile offenders that actually improve the child's and family's functioning and decrease recidivism rates. Referral sources should inquire regarding outcome data for programs, and more treatment providers should implement basic outcome data to monitor the effectiveness of their treatment. This information will ultimately improve the quality of care rendered to juvenile offenders by increasing our knowledge base of what actually works, and in what context.

Promote Agency Collaboration

For ultimate treatment success, service organizations working with juvenile offenders must effectively communicate, collaborate, and plan. These include agencies such as the court system, probation, corrections, social services, mental health, developmental disabilities, substance abuse, and the school system. Service agencies often have inadequate lines of communication and frequently fight over "who this child belongs to," leaving services fragmented. Few forensic evaluators know even their local programs in depth. In order to serve the community best, while saving resources, agencies must work more closely in developing a continuum of care.

REFERENCES

Altschuler DM, Armstrong TL, MacKenzie DL: Reintegration, supervised release, and intensive aftercare (juvenile justice bulletin NCJ 175715). Washington, DC, Office of Juvenile Justice and Delinquency Prevention, U.S. Department of Justice, 1999

Andrews DA, Zinger I, Hoge RD, et al: Does correctional treatment work? a clinically relevant and psychologically informed meta-analysis. Criminology 28(3):369–404, 1990

Arnold ME, Hughes JN: First do no harm: adverse effects of grouping deviant youth for skills training. Journal of School Psychology 37(1):99–115, 1999

Bank L, Marlowe JH, Reid JB, et al: A comparative evaluation of parent-training interventions for chronic delinquents. J Abnorm Child Psychol 19:15–33, 1991

Bedlington MM, Braukmann CJ, Ramp KA, et al: A comparison of treatment environments in community-based group homes for adolescent offenders. Criminal Justice and Behavior 154(3): 349–363, 1988

Beelmann A, Pfingsten U, Losel F: Effects of training social competence in children: a meta-analysis of recent evaluation studies. J Clin Child Psychol 23:260–271, 1994

Borduin CM: Multisystemic treatment of criminality and violence in adolescents. J Am Acad Child Adolesc Psychiatry 38:242–249, 1999

Borduin CM, Henggeler SW: A multisystemic approach to the treatment of serious delinquent behavior, in Behavior Disorders of Adolescence: Research, Intervention, and Policy in Clinical and School Settings. Edited by McMahon RJ, Peters RDV. New York, Plenum, 1990, pp 63–80

Braukmann CJ, Wolf MM: Behaviorally based group homes for juvenile offenders, in Behavioral Approaches to Crime and Delinquency: A Handbook of Application, Research, and Concepts. Edited by Morris EK, Braukmann CJ. New York, Plenum, 1987, pp 135–159

Braukmann CJ, Bedlington MM, Belden BD, et al: Effects of community-based group-home treatment programs on male juvenile offenders' use and abuse of drugs and alcohol. Am J Drug Alcohol Abuse 11(3–4):249–278, 1985

Browning K, Thornberry TP, Porter PK: Highlights of findings from the Rochester Youth Development Study (fact sheet #99103). Washington, DC, Office of Juvenile Justice and Delinquency Prevention, U.S. Department of Justice, 1999

Burns JC, Vito GF: An impact analysis of the Alabama boot camp program. Federal Probation 59(1):63–67, 1995

Capaldi DM, Chamberlain P, Patterson GR: Ineffective discipline and conduct problems in males: association, late adolescent outcomes, and prevention. Aggression and Violent Behavior 2(4):343–353, 1997

Castellano T, Soderstrom I: Therapeutic wilderness programs and juvenile recidivism: a program evaluation. Journal of Offender Rehabilitation 17(3–4):19–26, 1992

Chamberlain P: Comparative evaluation of specialized foster care for seriously delinquent youths: a first step. Community Alternatives: International Journal of Family Care 13(2):21–36, 1990

Chamberlain P: Treatment foster care (juvenile justice bulletin NCJ 173421). Washington, DC, Office of Juvenile Justice and Delinquency Prevention, U.S. Department of Justice, 1998

Chamberlain P, Reid JB: Comparison of two community alternatives to incarceration for chronic juvenile offenders. J Consult Clin Psychol 66:624–633, 1998

Chamberlain P, Rosicky JG: The effectiveness of family therapy in the treatment of adolescents with conduct disorders and delinquency. J Marital Fam Ther 21:441–459, 1995

Chamberlain P, Ray J, Moore KJ: Characteristics of residential care for adolescent offenders: a comparison of assumptions and practices in two models. Journal of Child and Family Studies 5(3):285–297, 1996

Deschenes EP, Greenwood PW: Alternative placements for juvenile offenders: results from the Nokomis Challenge Program. Journal of Research in Crime and Delinquency 35(3):267–294, 1998

Eppright TD, Kashani JH, Robison BD, et al: Comorbidity of conduct disorder and personality disorders in an incarcerated juvenile population. Am J Psychiatry 150:1233–1236, 1993

Finckenauer JO: Scared Straight and the Panacea Phenomenon. Englewood Cliffs, NJ, Prentice-Hall, 1982

Fo WSO, O'Donnell CR: The buddy system: effect of community intervention on delinquent offenses. Behavior Therapy 6:522–524, 1975

Foley HA, Carlton CO, Howell RJ: The relationship of attention deficit hyperactivity disorder and conduct disorder to juvenile delinquency: legal implications. Bulletin of the American Academy of Psychiatry and the Law 24(3):333–345, 1996

Freeman LW: Boot camp and inmate moral development: no significant effect. Journal of Offender Rehabilitation 19(3/4):123–127, 1993

Fullard DA: A New York City version of correctional boot camp: an overview. Federal Probation 62(1):62–67, 1998

Goldkamp JS: Miami's treatment drug court for felony defendants: some implications of assessment findings. The Prison Journal 73(2):110–166, 1994

Greenwood PW: Responding to juvenile crime: lessons learned. Future Child 6(3):75–85, 1996

Greenwood PW, Turner S: Evaluation of the Paint Creek Center: a residential program for serious delinquents. Criminology 31(2):263–279, 1987

Haghighi B, Lopez A: Success/failure of group home treatment programs for juveniles. Federal Probation 57(3):53–58, 1993

Henggeler SW: Delinquency in Adolescence. Newbury Park, CA, Sage, 1989

Henggeler SW: A consensus: conclusion of the APA Task Force Report on innovative models of mental health services for children, adolescents, and their families. J Clin Child Psychol 23 (suppl):3–6, 1994

Henggeler SW, Edwards JE, Bourdoin CM: The family relations of female juvenile delinquents. J Abnorm Child Psychol 15:199–209, 1987

Henggeler SW, Schoenwald SK, Pickrel SG, et al: The contribution of treatment outcome research to the reform of children's mental health services: multisystemic therapy as an example. Journal of Mental Health Administration 21(3):229–239, 1994

Hoge RD, Andrews DA, Leschied AW: An investigation of risk and protective factors in a sample of youthful offenders. J Child Psychol Psychiatry 37(4):419–424, 1996

Hollander HE, Turner FD: Characteristics of incarcerated delinquents: relationship between developmental disorder, environmental and family factors, and patterns of offense and recidivism. Journal of the American Academy of Child Psychiatry 24:221–226, 1985

In re Gault, 387 US 1 (1967)

Janus M, McCormack A, Burgess AW, et al: Adolescent Runaways: Causes and Consequences. Lexington, MA, Lexington Books, 1987

Jones M, Ross DL: Is less better? boot camp, regular probation and rearrest in North Carolina. American Journal of Criminal Justice 21(2):147–161, 1997

Kazdin AE: Conduct Disorders in Childhood and Adolescence, 2nd Edition. Thousand Oaks, CA, Sage, 1995

Krueger R, Hansen JC: Self-concept changes during youth-home placement of adolescents. Adolescence 22(86):385–392, 1987

Lipsey M: The effect of treatment on juvenile delinquents: results from meta-analysis, in Psychology and Law, International Perspectives. Edited by Loesel F, Bender D. Berlin, Germany, Walter De Gruyter, 1992, pp 131–143

Lipton D, Pearson FS: The CDATE Project: reviewing research on the effectiveness of treatment programs for adult and juvenile offenders. Paper presented at the annual meeting of the American Society of Criminology, Chicago, IL, November 1996

Lundman RJ: Prevention and Control of Juvenile Delinquency, 2nd Edition. New York, Oxford University Press, 1993

MacKenzie DL: Boot camp prisons: components, evaluations, and empirical issues. Federal Probation 54(3):44–52, 1990

MacKenzie DL: The parole performance of offenders released from shock incarceration (boot camp prisons): a survival time analysis. Journal of Quantitative Criminology 7(3): 213–236, 1991

MacKenzie DL, Parent DG: Boot camp prisons for young offenders, in Smart Sentencing: The Emergence of Intermediate Sanctions. Edited by Byrne JM, Lurigio AJ, Petersilia J. London, Sage, 1992, pp 103–119

MacKenzie DL, Brame R, McDowall D, et al: Boot camp prisons and recidivism in eight states. Criminology 33(3):327–357, 1995

Marsteller FA, Brogan D, Smith I, et al: The prevalence of psychiatric disorders among juveniles admitted to regional youth detention centers operated by the Georgia Department of Juvenile Justice, Atlanta, GA, Technical Report, 1997

McManus M, Alessi NE, Grapentin WL, et al: Psychiatric disturbance in serious delinquents. Journal of the American Academy of Child Psychiatry 23:602–615, 1984

Melton GB, Petrila J, Poythress NG, et al: Psychological Evaluations for the Courts, 2nd Edition. New York, Guilford, 1997

Mezzich AC: Diagnostic formulations for violent delinquent adolescents. Journal of Psychiatry and Law 18(1):165–190, 1990

Moore KJ, Chamberlain P: Treatment foster care: toward development of community-based models for adolescents with severe emotional and behavioral disorders. Journal of Emotional and Behavioral Disorders 2(1):22–30, 1994

Offord DR, Boyle MH, Racine YA: The epidemiology of antisocial behavior in childhood and adolescence, in The Development and Treatment of Childhood Aggression. Edited by Pepler DJ, Rubin KH. Hillsdale, NJ, Lawrence Erlbaum, 1991, pp 31–54

Orchowsky S, Taylor K: The insiders juvenile crime prevention program: an assessment of a juvenile awareness program. Richmond, VA, Research and Reporting Unit, Division of Program Development and Evaluation, Virginia Department of Corrections, 1981

Piper E, Warner JR Jr: Group homes for problem youth: retrospect and prospects. Child and Youth Services 3(3/4):1–12, 1980

Sampson RJ, Laub JH: Crime in the Making: Pathways and Turning Points Through Life. Cambridge, MA, Harvard University Press, 1993

Steiner H and the Work Group on Quality Issues: Practice parameters for the assessment and treatment of children and adolescents with conduct disorder. J Am Acad Child Adolesc Psychiatry 36 (10 suppl):122S–139S, 1997

Weber RJ: Group homes in the 1980s. Washington, DC, National Center for the Assessment of Alternatives to Juvenile Justice Processing, National Institute of Justice, 1981

Werner EE, Smith RS: Vulnerable but Invincible: A Study of Resilient Children. New York, McGraw-Hill, 1982

Zagar R, Arbit J, Hughes JR, et al: Developmental and disruptive behavior disorders among delinquents. J Am Acad Child Adolesc Psychiatry 28:437–440, 1989

Zoccolillo M, Rogers K: Characteristics and outcome of hospitalized adolescent girls with conduct disorder. J Am Acad Child Adolesc Psychiatry 30:973–981, 1991

CHAPTER 27

Sexually Aggressive Youth

Jon A. Shaw, M.D.

Case Example 1

George, a 14-year-old boy, was brought in for treatment after anally sodomizing two younger boys and tying one up with ropes and sticking a knife to his throat. He showed little remorse, regret, or victim empathy. He had a history of sexually victimizing other boys. In his therapy he would reveal and openly acknowledge "violent sexual fantasies." He described how he "seeks out" little boys, wishes to "trap them," and wants "to have control over them." He spoke of the pleasure he derived from having the "power to make anybody I want do anything I want." He enjoyed his victims being "scared, shaking, and cooperative." He coerced them by threatening to cut off their penises or shoot them in the head.

He had a history of aggressive and impulsive behavior and had been called a bully. He reportedly "sexualized" everybody. He grabbed the breasts of his 60-year-old grandmother, and there was a history of sexually touching younger children. When asked about his feelings while sexually molesting children, he responded, "My mother did this to me and I decided I will do it to them." He reported that in his family, "We would have sex together." He claimed that since about age 5 years, "We would have sex with each other, Mom, Dad, sister, and me." There was a long history of physical abuse, neglect, and abandonment. His mother was sent to jail for sexually molesting his sister. He was ordered into foster care when he was age 7 "based on abandonment and a history of being exposed to deviant sexual behavior." His school and academic record was characterized by behavior problems and poor academic performance in spite of good intelligence.

He recalls how from age 4 to age 7 his mother would come home drunk and make him sleep with her, forcing him down upon her, coercing him to have oral sex with her, and laying on top of him trying to get him to stick his penis into her. He described these experiences without affect, minimizing their importance. He spoke of "enjoying the scary moment." It was only with continuing therapy that he began to talk about feeling trapped, his repugnance to her drunken breath, her threats to deprive him of food, her slapping him, and her vague threats to castrate him. The mother had a history of being sexually abused by her own father. He stated that he had a "big problem...if I don't get help I will be doing these things to kids the same that they did to me, get arrested...maybe the electric chair."

Case Example 2

Tony, a 12-year-old boy, was referred to treatment after being apprehended for sexual assault. He presented with a history of breaking and entering 10 times during the previous year. Although it was initially thought that this was for the purpose of stealing, it became apparent that it was motivated by a wish to molest women as they slept. He would peep through the windows, spying on a woman until she went to sleep; he would then sneak into her room and proceed to uncover her and begin to sexually touch her. He had been caught four times for this behavior and had been placed in juvenile detention each time for short periods with no change in his criminal behavior. He reported that since the age of 11 he felt a compulsion to observe women, ages 20–30 years, through windows as they were undressing or taking a shower. As this compulsion became stronger, it became associated with the wish to break into the house in order to sexually touch the women. He had the fantasy that the women would wake up and want to have sex with him. He did not understand the nature of this compulsion and was initially very vague when talking about his sexual activities. Tony reports that in kindergarten he was instructed by his teacher to sit under her desk and stroke her legs repetitively, and he recalled moments of sexual arousal and excitement.

On admission to the residential treatment center Tony was found to be very depressed and suicidal, with symptoms of insomnia, psychomotor retardation, appetite disturbance, and self-recrimination.

Case Example 3

Jorge, a 13-year-old youth, was brought into treatment after repetitively sexually abusing his 7-year-old sister by forcing her to fellate him and vaginally penetrating her. He showed little remorse or regret. In spite of her protestations and crying, he would persist in his behavior. His family minimized the behavior, noting that he was just being a boy. In the course of therapy, he described his masturbatory fantasy, which graphically illustrates how one's own sexual victimization gets played over and over again in sexual offending behavior.

He reports the fantasy as "I walk into a small room, there is a girl, 10 to 11 years of age. She is sitting and writing at a desk. I look around to see if there is anybody around. I look twice. I scream at her to stand up. She looks scared and helpless. She is terrified. I tear off her dress. I begin to fondle her. She fights back. I overpower her. I feel strong. I force her to suck my penis. I stick my penis in her vagina. I interrupt the fantasy. I try to intervene. Suddenly the image turns into my father. I remember my father coming into my room. It is a small room. He begins to fondle me, touching my penis. I remember he tore off my clothes and made me suck his penis and he stuck his penis into my anus. I felt powerless and afraid. I don't like to feel powerless. It's when I feel powerless that I begin to imagine raping a girl. When I tear off her dress I feel in control." He describes being powerless as meaning, "I can't control other people." Further discussion led to his remembering the sexual excitation, the erection he felt when his father abused him. He had two feelings. He felt scared, helpless and terrified but he also had the feeling of sexual excitement. He didn't understand why he was sexually aroused. He felt guilty about the sexual excitement.

The majority of adult sex offenders will commit their first act of sexual aggression before age 18 years. Studies of juvenile sex offenders indicate that the majority commit their first sexual offense before age 15 and not infrequently before age 12. There is increasing awareness that children under age 12 may be sexually aggressive toward other children.

Sexually aggressive acts perpetrated by youths have become increasingly common. Sexual assault is one of the fastest growing crimes in the United States. Whereas adolescents (ages 15–18 years) make up only 6% of the population of the United States, they commit 25% of the index crimes, such as arson, homicide, manslaughter, robbery, aggravated assault, and burglary (Siegel and Senna 1988). Forcible rapes by juveniles have increased

20% (Office of Juvenile Justice and Delinquency Prevention 1995). The highest risk for the initiation of serious violent behavior occurs between ages 15 and 16 years (Elliott 1994b). In Elliott's (1994a, 1994b) longitudinal study of a national probability sample of 1,725 youths (ages 11–17 years), he found that the prevalence of serious violent offenses, such as rape, that involved causing some injury or use of a weapon peaked at age 17 years for males and ages 15 and 16 years for females. It is generally estimated that 20% of all rapes and 30% to 50% of all child molestations are perpetrated by male adolescents (Disher et al. 1982).

Ageton (1983) concluded from a probability sample of male adolescents ages 13–19 years that the rate of sexual assault per 100,000 adolescent males ranged from 5% to 16%. A survey of high school students revealed that 20% had been involved in forcing sex upon another person and that 60% of the boys found it acceptable in one or more situations for a boy to force sex on a girl (Davis et al. 1993). Ryan and colleagues (1996), in their national survey of 1,600 sexually abusive youths, reported that they came from all racial, economic, ethnic, and religious backgrounds and generally mirrored the population. They ranged in age from 5 to 21 years, with a modal age of 14 years, and were predominantly male. Whereas the majority of juvenile sexual offenders are adolescents, there is increasing concern about sexually aggressive and exploitative behaviors in prepubescent and latency-age children (Araji 1997; Gil and Johnson 1993).

DEFINITIONS

Terms such as sexual aggression, sexually abusive behavior, sexual offense, sexual offender, paraphilia, rape, and sexual harassment refer to the various dimensions of sexual exploitation.

Sexual aggression invariably involves the use of threat, intimidation, exploitation of authority, or force with the aim of imposing one's sexual will on a nonconsenting person for the purpose of personal gratification that may or may not be predominantly sexual in nature.

Sexually abusive behavior is defined as "any sexual behavior which occurs 1) without consent, 2) without equality, or 3) as a result of coercion" (National Task Force on Juvenile Sex Offending 1993). In this context the following clarifications have been offered. *Consent* is defined as implying agreement encompassing the following: 1) an understanding of what is proposed, 2) knowledge of societal standards for what is being proposed, 3) awareness of potential consequences and alternatives,

4) assumption that agreement or disagreement will be respected equally, 5) voluntary decision, and 6) mental competence. *Equality* is "two participants operating with same level of power in a relationship, neither being controlled or coerced by the other." *Coercion* is defined as "exploitation of authority, use of bribes, threats of force, or intimidation to gain cooperation or compliance" (National Task Force on Juvenile Sex Offending 1993).

A *sexual offender* is an individual who has committed an act of sexual aggression that has "breached societal norms and moral codes, violated federal, state, municipal law, statute or ordinance and which usually but not necessarily results in physical or psychological harm to the victim" (National Task Force on Juvenile Sex Offending 1993). Generally the term *sexual offender* refers to an individual who 1) has been convicted of committing a sex crime in violation of the state or federal laws, 2) has been awarded deferred adjudication for a sex crime under state or federal laws, 3) admits to having violated state and federal laws with regard to sexual misconduct, or 4) evidences a paraphilia (American Psychiatric Association 1994).

Paraphilia refers to "recurrent, intense sexually arousing fantasies, sexual urges, or behaviors generally involving 1) nonhuman objects, 2) the suffering or humiliation of oneself or one's partner, or 3) children or other nonconsenting persons that occur over a period of at least 6 months" (American Psychiatric Association 2000). In order for a youth to be given a diagnosis of a pedophilia, he must be at least age 16 years and at least 5 years older than the victim.

Rape has been defined as an act, "to seize or take by force for sexual gratification" (National Task Force on Juvenile Sex Offending 1993). The concept of rape has been broadened to encompass a more generic sexual assault against others and may include any criminal sexual assault, heterosexual or homosexual, which involves the use of force.

Sexual harassment has been defined as the "unwelcome sexual attention which may consist of sexual overtures, requests, advances and verbal or physical contact of a sexual nature" (Equal Employment Opportunity Commission, Title VII, 1980)

PSYCHIATRIC LEGAL ISSUES

Waiver

Society is increasingly demanding that juveniles be held more accountable for their criminal acts. A number of states have passed legislation redefining the spectrum of crimes and the minimum age at which juveniles may be referred to the adult court. In some states there are no age restrictions for trying a juvenile in the adult court if the crime is perceived as particularly violent or heinous. Although sexual crimes vary in severity and offenders vary as to amenability to treatment, there is a readiness in some jurisdictions to waive all juvenile sexual offenders to the adult court. Waiver of juveniles into the adult court system leads to penalties reserved for adult criminals, may lead to incarceration with adults, decreases the probability of appropriate treatment, and lessens the probability of parole.

Competency

With the increasing readiness to waive juveniles to the adult court, there are increasing concerns regarding competency of juveniles to stand trial in the adult court system. Cognitive, moral, and personality development are still in the process of evolving during the juvenile years. The trend toward trying juveniles in adult courts raises a number of questions. Among them are questions regarding the juvenile's capacity to understand the legal case against him, his ability to meaningfully consult with his attorney, and his judgment in making responsible decisions regarding his defense. This is particularly relevant with juvenile sex offenders, who often are comorbid for learning and academic-related problems and not infrequently may manifest intellectual deficits.

Record Confidentiality

The clinical records of juveniles referred for clinical assessment of alleged sexual crimes and those in treatment may be made public. The clinician should explain his role to the juvenile and his family and the limits of confidentiality prior to the clinical interview and before administering assessment instruments. Clinicians who do not inform their clients of the risk of disclosure may themselves be vulnerable to civil suit. Paradoxically, whereas disclosure may enhance the possibility of being judged amenable to treatment, it may increase the severity of further legal consequences if further information is uncovered regarding the nature and severity of the sexually aggressive acts. It is generally advisable to conduct the clinical assessment following adjudication with the intent of determining amenability to treatment, required level of care, and estimated risk of recidivism.

Community Notification and Registration Requirements

The Violent Crime Control and Law Enforcement Act of 1994 (P.L. 103-322, September 13, 1994) mandated that states establish registries for individuals convicted of sexual crimes. "Megan's Law" (P.L. 104-145, May 17, 1996), the 1996 amendment to the law, requires state and law enforcement agencies to release relevant information regarding dangerous sexual offenders in order to protect the community. Presently, convicted sexual offenders are required to register under this law and to notify local enforcement agencies of change of address. A number of states have sexual offender registration laws that apply to juveniles, and that number is likely to increase as more states pass legislation in compliance with federal guidelines.

Assessment of the Risk of Recidivism

Clinicians are being asked with increasing frequency by the courts to determine the risk of further sexual offenses. These assessments may be utilized to make dispositional decisions regarding when a sexual offender may be released to the public. As there are risk factors that have been associated with increased dangerousness, this presently remains a clinical judgment; there are no empirically validated objective measures that have proven to be predictive.

CLINICAL ISSUES

The Profile of Sexually Aggressive Youth

Juvenile sex offenders are a heterogeneous population. The overwhelming majority are male. They are represented in every socioeconomic class and every racial, ethnic, religious, and cultural group. Psychosocial and clinical features frequently found in the history of juvenile sex aggressors include 1) impaired social and interpersonal skills, 2) prior delinquent behavior, 3) impulsivity, 4) academic difficulties, 5) family instability, 6) family violence, 7) abuse and neglect, and 8) psychopathology.

There are essentially four kinds of sexual offenders: 1) the offender with a true paraphilia and a well-established deviant sexual arousal pattern, 2) the antisocial youth whose sexual offending behavior is but one facet of his opportunistic exploitation of others, 3) the juvenile compromised by a psychiatric or neurobiological disorder such that he is unable to regulate and modulate his impulses, and 4) the youth whose impaired social and interpersonal skills result in his turning to younger children for sexual gratification, which is unavailable from his peer groups. Most juvenile sexual offenders combine various features of each.

The Spectrum of Sexual Offenses

Sexual offending behavior ranges from sexual behavior without physical contact (e.g., obscene phone calls, exhibitionism, voyeurism, lewd photographs) to varying degrees of child molestation involving direct sexual contact (e.g., frottage, fondling, digital penetration, fellatio, sodomy, and various other sexually aggressive acts). There is a considerable range of diversity and severity of sexual offending behavior. In some instances the sexual offending behavior may be related to social and emotional immaturity, curiosity, and experimentation. In others the sexually aggressive acts are but one facet of a pattern of aggressive and violent acts against others or a manifestation of severe emotional, behavioral, and developmental psychopathology.

The most common sexual crimes are those associated with indecent liberties or sexual touching. A national survey of sexually aggressive youths ages 5 to 21 years from a diversity of outpatient and residential programs found that 68% of the sexual offenses involved penetration and/or oral-genital behavior (i.e., vaginal or anal penetration without oral-genital contact, 35%; oral-genital contact, 15%; penetration and oral-genital contact, 18%) (Ryan et al. 1996). The typical juvenile sex offender younger than age 18 has committed eight to nine sexual offenses with six to eight victims.

Victim Profile

The victims of juvenile sex offenders are younger children. Ninety percent of sexual abuse victims are between the ages of 3 and 16. The majority of the victims are younger than age 9, and approximately 25% to 40% are younger than age 6. Most victims of male sex offenders are females. Adolescent sex offenders commit most of the sexual assaults against boys. Boys, when victimized, tend to be younger than their female counterparts.

The Role of Coercion

It is generally recognized that even though juveniles usually employ coercion in the process of committing sexual offenses, they are less likely to harm their victims when compared with adult sex offenders. The coercion is usually expressed as bribery, intimidation, threats of harm or violent injury, physical force, and, rarely, the use of a weapon. Most victims report higher levels of coercion and force than is self-reported by offenders. Fehrenbach and colleagues (1986) found that 22% of the offenders continued their sexually aggressive acts even when the victims expressed "hurt or fear."

The Role of Sexual Victimization

Sexual behavior is commonly affected by a history of sexual victimization. There is evidence of increased reports of sexual victimization in the history of sexual abusers. Boys and girls exposed to sexual abuse and deviant sexual experiences are at risk for early erotization and precocious sexualization. Sexually abused boys are more likely to be sexually aroused at the time of sexual victimization and to subsequently exhibit more sexual behaviors as compared with sexually abused girls.

Reports of sexual victimization in the history of adolescent sex offenders vary from 19% to 82%. Boys and girls who have been sexually victimized may experience their first sexual arousal during the victimization. The victims of sexual abuse may internalize the aggressive and erotic facets of the sexual experiences into preferred patterns of deviant sexual gratification through a process of social learning, imitation, modeling, and identifying pathways. Boys who have been sexually abused often demonstrate higher rates of aggression, impulsivity, sexual preoccupations and sexually inappropriate behaviors. They tend to have an earlier onset of sexual offending behavior, to have more victims, and to manifest greater psychopathology and interpersonal problems. The younger the child when he commits his first sexual offense, the more likely that the child has been sexually victimized. The factors related to the sexual abuse experience and that are thought to increase the risk for inappropriate sexual behaviors are sexual arousal at the time of the sexual abuse, uncertainty and confusion about sexual identity, compensatory hypermasculinity, and a readiness to reenact the sexually victimizing experience.

As important as sexual victimization is in the history of juvenile sexual abusers, it is not exculpatory. Most victims of sexual abuse do not grow up to be abusers. As a form of child maltreatment, it is only one of a number of critical factors that may contribute to the risk of becoming sexually abusive. Nevertheless it is essential to understand the role of sexual victimization in the patterning of sexual offending behavior and as a critical factor in the planning of therapeutic interventions.

Psychopathology

Sexually aggressive behavior is associated with a matrix of behavioral, emotional, and developmental problems. Juvenile sexual offenders manifest a range of psychopathological and personality disturbances. Comparisons of delinquent juveniles whose violence is nonsexual and those who are nonviolent have generally found few significant differences between the groups. Compared with non–sexually abusive delinquents and conduct-disordered youths, sexually aggressive youths are twice as likely to have been sexually abused and to perform less well on academic achievement tests (Lewis et al. 1979; Shaw et al. 1993).

Psychiatric comorbidity has been found in approximately 60%–90% of adolescent sexual abusers. The most prevalent comorbid psychiatric disorders are conduct disorder, 45%–80%; mood disorders, 35%–50%; anxiety disorders, 30%–50%; substance abuse, 20%–30%; and attention-deficit/hyperactivity disorder, 10%–20% (Becker et al. 1986, 1991; Kavoussi et al. 1988; Shaw 1999; Shaw et al. 1993). The younger the child when he committed his first sexual offense, the higher the number of coexisting psychiatric diagnoses (Shaw et al. 1996).

Juvenile sexual offenders often manifest severe personality traits that include narcissistic, borderline, conduct-disordered, and antisocial behaviors. The younger the age at onset of sexual offending behavior and the younger the adolescent was at the time of his own sexual victimization, the more likely he is to exhibit personality trait disturbances. The high prevalence of narcissistic and borderline psychopathology among sex offenders is consistent with histories of severe emotional, physical, and sexual abuse. Sexual offending behavior is strongly linked to core antisocial psychopathology with severe character disturbances.

Delinquency

Sexual offending behavior is often one facet of a long and sometimes multifaceted history of delinquent behavior. The great majority of sexually aggressive youths have a history of prior nonsexual delinquent behavior ranging from cruelty to animals, vandalism, and theft to aggravated assault. Twenty-five percent have committed three or more nonsexual criminal offenses. Rape is often the final step in an escalating sequence of violent criminal activity. It is evident that there is a subset of sexually aggressive offenders characterized by core antisocial features in which the sexual aggression is only one facet of a lifestyle in which the individual opportunistically exploits others for personal gain.

Family and Social Environment

Most juvenile sex offenders live at home when committing their sexual offenses. The family environment is frequently characterized by family conflict, poor family cohesion, family instability, family dysfunction, exposure to violence, harsh, inconsistent parenting, and physical and sexual maltreatment. Juvenile sex offenders usually manifest impaired social and interpersonal skills. Two-thirds have been described as socially isolated, one-third do not have any friends, and approximately one-half are reported to be loners. There is some evidence that juvenile sex offenders unable to relate to their own peer group may turn to younger children for the gratifications denied to them by their own peer group.

School and Academic Problems

Juvenile sex offenders usually present with a history of academic and school-based behavior problems such as learning problems, learning disabilities, and truancy. They generally perform less well on tests of academic skills and are below grade level in such tasks as reading and arithmetic. Not infrequently, there are learning deficiencies and vulnerabilities associated with neurobiological and cognitive impairments that have often compromised the juvenile's capacity to do well in school and to assimilate and integrate complex social information.

The Female Juvenile Sex Aggressor

There have been few studies of female sexual aggression. Anderson (1996) surveyed young college women and found that 29% had engaged in sexual coercion (verbal pressure, lying, threatening to end a relationship); 21% had committed sexual abuse (sex with a minor 5 or more years younger, use of position of power and authority); and 43% reported initiating sexual contact by using sexually aggressive strategies. In a study by Mathews et al. (1997), female juvenile aggressors were more likely than a matched group of male juvenile sexual offenders to have been sexually abused at a younger age (50%–95%) and to have had multiple abusers and are three times more likely to have been sexually abused by a female. Studies of juvenile sexual aggressors indicate they are most likely to commit their sexual offenses while baby-sitting.

The Developmentally Disabled Juvenile Sexual Aggressor

There is some suggestion that developmental disabilities are overrepresented in juvenile sex offenders. The prevalence of sexual offending behavior is at least as common if not more common in the developmentally disabled population. Low verbal IQ has been correlated with sexually inappropriate behavior (McCurry et al. 1998). The clinical characteristics, spectrum of sexual offenses, and victim profiles of developmentally disabled sex offenders are not demonstratively different from those of non–developmentally disabled sex offenders.

CLINICAL ASSESSMENT

The American Academy of Child and Adolescent Psychiatry has published "Practice Parameters for the Assessment and Treatment of Children and Adolescents Who Are Sexually Abusive of Others" (American Academy of Child and Adolescent Psychiatry 1999). These guidelines describe how clinical assessment should be conducted.

Review of Records

Important sources of information include medical and psychological reports, police and offense reports, victim statements, protective services reports, and probation reports. The collateral information should be obtained before the individual interview; otherwise, one is left relatively unprepared to deal with the offender's normal proclivity to minimize and deny.

Clinical Interview

The cornerstone of assessment and evaluation of the sexual abuser is an extensive and comprehensive individual clinical interview. Major issues to be addressed follow.

Minimization and Denial

The clinician should assess the sexual aggressor's capacity for cooperation, honesty, and forthrightness, and his acceptance of responsibility for his sexual offense as well as his sense of remorse and regret. It is known that half of all juvenile sexual offenders will deny the sexual offending behavior at the time of referral and that this denial is usually supported by the offender's family. Only one in five will accept full responsibility for the sexual offense. Most sexually aggressive youths exhibit little empathy or remorse, and one-third will blame the victims, stating that the victim consented to the sexual activity in spite of all evidence to the contrary. It will be necessary to confront minimization, denial, and omissions of important information.

The Nature of the Sexually Aggressive Behavior

It is often a difficult task to explicate and uncover the details of the sexually abusive behavior. Because specific laws have been transgressed, the offender is often less than forthcoming. Issues of shame, guilt, and fear of punishment impede disclosure. Most offenders are not motivated to disclose the circumstances of their sexually aggressive behavior until they are confronted or fear the consequences if they do not talk.

The clinician attempts to answer a number of questions regarding the sexually aggressive episode: Was the sexually aggressive act planned or impulsive? What was the relationship with the victim, the age difference between perpetrator and victim, and the precipitating factors that led to the sexually aggressive behavior? What was there about the victim that attracted the perpetrator? What is the nature of the sexually aggressive offense(s), the frequency and duration of the sexually aggressive behavior, and the characteristics of the coercive behavior? How did the sexual offender attempt to avoid detection? What is the juvenile's understanding of the effects of his sexual behavior on the victim, the consequences of his behavior, and his insight into the wrongfulness of his sexual behavior?

Sexual History

The interviewer should assess the child's sexual knowledge and education, sexual development, and sexual experiences. The clinician will need to explore the history of sexually aggressive behaviors, including previous incidents of sexual abusive behavior; the pattern and spectrum of previously committed sexually aggressive acts; the victim profile; the internal and external triggers that preceded the sexually aggressive behavior; the role of aggression and sadism in the sexual offense; the need to dominate, control, and humiliate the victim; the erotization of the aggression; the history of sexual victimization, physical abuse, and emotional neglect; the history of exposure to inappropriate and sexually explicit behavior; and the history of prior non–sexually delinquent behavior.

Developmental and Psychosocial History

Other areas of the assessment process are those associated with a comprehensive developmental history: family history of psychiatric disorder, the nature of the pregnancy, perinatal history, developmental milestones, family relationships, early identifying models, capacity for relationships, school experiences, social skills, substance abuse, and prior medical and psychiatric history. The family assessment provides an opportunity to understand the early developmental and environmental context within which the sexual abuser developed.

Legal History

Is there a history of arrests, convictions, incarcerations, use of weapons, or cruelty to animals?

Medical and Psychiatric History

It is important to obtain a comprehensive medical and psychiatric history, with specific attention to sexually transmitted diseases, HIV infection, psychopathology, and psychiatric comorbidity.

School and Academic History

A specific area of concern is the evaluation of intellectual capacities and academic performance. Information is obtained from the school and from formal psychoeducational and psychological assessments.

Mental Status Examination

A comprehensive mental status examination is carried out to assess the presence of psychopathology, personality disturbances, organicity, and substance abuse and to acquire an understanding of adaptive, coping, and defensive strategies. Suicidal thoughts and risk should be assessed specifically. Apprehension by judicial authority and the associated shame of exposure, embarrassment, stigmatization, fear of punishment, and incarceration are risk factors for suicidal behavior.

Psychological Testing

There are no specific empirical measures or psychometric tests that can identify, diagnose, or classify sexual abusers. Psychological tests are used adjunctively as part of an overall comprehensive evaluation to understand the personality, motivations, ego strengths, intelligence, defense and coping strategies, psychopathology, sexual knowledge, and sexual behaviors of the offender. Neuropsychological testing and psychoeducational assessment may be required when one suspects neurologically based deficits and/or learning disabilities. Measures of learning are an essential part of the assessment procedure. When indicated, family assessment measures may be administered to more fully unravel family dynamics and family process.

Phallometric Assessment

Phallometric assessment of sexual arousal in response to depictions of children is usually reserved for the most severe and recidivist sexual aggressors. This procedure has generally been used with caution with minors due to the lack of empirical studies, problems of obtaining informed consent, and a reluctance to expose children and adolescents to further sexual stimulation through the portrayal of deviant sexual activities. Caution should be employed in the use of phallometric measures, as there are maturational and developmental factors that may affect the patterns of sexual arousal and erectile measures (Kaemingk et al. 1995).

Evaluation of Dangerousness

An essential element in treatment planning is the evaluation of the severity of the sexual offending behavior and the risk of recurrence of sexual offending behavior. Because the majority of juvenile sex offenders have a prior history of nonsexual delinquent acts, the clinician is concerned about recidivism not only for the sexual offenses but also for nonsexual delinquent acts. There is evidence that the recidivism rate is higher for nonsexual delinquent acts than it is for the sexual offenses. Considerations in evaluating the risk of further sexual offenses include the frequency and diversity of the sexual offenses; the severity of the aggressive and/or sadistic behavior; the premedition or impulsivity of the sexual offending behavior; psychopathology; neurological impairment; prior antisocial or violent behavior; motivation for treatment; intelligence; psychological mindedness; capacity for empathy; and family, community, and social support systems.

PITFALLS

Lack of Information

The readiness of the sexual offender to minimize and deny his sexually aggressive behavior, the frequency and severity of his sexually aggressive acts, and his reluctance to discuss his inner sexual life, sexual fantasies, and deviant sexual arousal patterns and motivations may lead to only a superficial knowledge base on which to consolidate clinical judgment and recommendations.

Focusing the Clinical Assessment Exclusively on the Sexually Aggressive Acts

The proclivity to focus only on the sexually aggressive acts may preclude a careful assessment of the comorbid psychiatric, neurological, and psychological conditions that may have contributed significantly to the sexual offender's behavior.

Countertransference

The readiness to experience a spectrum of feelings, ranging from forgiveness and expiation (associated with unrealistic fantasies of rescue) to horror and disgust, may compromise an intellectually honest and comprehensive evaluation regarding amenability to treatment.

CASE EXAMPLE EPILOGUES

Case Example 1

George remained generally unresponsive to treatment within a residential setting for adolescent sex offenders and was subsequently transferred to another residential program for continuing therapy.

Case Example 2

Tony responded well to a therapeutic residential program for adolescent sex offenders. He subsequently attended a public school during the daytime and was slowly integrated back into the home environment, where he made a good adjustment with continuing outpatient supportive therapy.

Case Example 3

Jorge was able with some insight to evolve some empathy, not only for his own victimization but also for his sexual victims, and he subsequently showed a good response and was reintegrated back into his family.

REFERENCES

Ageton SS: Sexual Assault Among Adolescents. Lexington, MA, Lexington Books, 1983

American Academy of Child and Adolescent Psychiatry: Practice parameters for the assessment and treatment of children and adolescents who are sexually abusive of others. 38 (12 suppl):55S–76S, 1999

American Psychiatric Association: Diagnostic and Statistical Manual of Mental Disorders, 4th Edition, Text Revision. Washington, DC, American Psychiatric Association, 2000

Anderson PB: Correlates of college women's self-reports of heterosexual aggression. Sex Abuse 8(2):121–133, 1996

Araji SK: Sexually Aggressive Children. Thousand Oaks, CA, Sage, 1997

Becker J, Cunningham-Rathner J, Chaplain M: Adolescent sex offenders. Journal of Interpersonal Violence 1:431–445, 1986

Becker JV, Kaplan MS, Tenke CE, et al: The incidence of depressive symptomatology in juvenile sex offenders with a history of abuse. Child Abuse Negl 15:531–536, 1991

Davis TC, Peck GQ, Storment JM: Acquaintance rape and the high school student. J Adolesc Health 14:220–224, 1993

Disher RW, Wenet GA, Paperney DM, et al: Adolescent sexual offense behavior: the role of the physician. Journal of Adolescent Health Care 2:279–286, 1982

Elliott DS: The developmental course of sexual and non-sexual violence: results from a national longitudinal study. Paper presented at the annual meeting of the American Association for the Treatment of Sexual Abusers, San Francisco, CA, January 1994a

Elliott DS: Youth Violence: An Overview (pamphlet; F-693). Boulder, CO, The Center for the Study and Prevention of Violence, University of Colorado Boulder Institute for Behavioral Sciences, 1994b

Equal Employment Opportunity Commission: Title VII Guidelines on Sexual Harassment (Rules and Regulations, 74676–74677). Federal Register 45:219, 1980

Fehrenbach PA, Smith W, Monastersky C, et al: Adolescent sex offenders: offender and offense characteristics. Am J Orthopsychiatry 56:225–233, 1986

Gil E, Johnson TC: Sexualized Children: Assessment and Treatment of Sexualized Children and Children Who Molest. Rockville, MD, Launch Press, 1993

Kaemingk KL, Koselka M, Becker JV, et al: Age and adolescent sexual arousal. Sex Abuse 7(4):249–257, 1995

Kavoussi RJ, Kaplan M, Becker JV: Psychiatric diagnoses in adolescent sex offenders. J Am Acad Child Adolesc Psychiatry 27:241–243, 1988

Lewis DO, Shankok SS, Pincus JH: Juvenile male sexual assaulters. Am J Psychiatry 136 (suppl 9):1194–1196, 1979

Mathews R, Hunter JA, Vuz J: Juvenile female sexual offenders: clinical characteristics and treatment issues. Sex Abuse 9:187–199, 1997

McCurry C, McClellan J, Adams J, et al: Sexual behavior associated with low verbal IQ in severe mental illness. Ment Retard 36:23–30, 1998

Megan's Law, Pub L 104-145, May 17, 1996, 110 Stat 1345

Office of Juvenile Justice and Delinquency Prevention: Juvenile Offenders and Victims: A Focus on Violence (Summary; NCJ 153570). U.S. Department of Justice, Office of Justice Programs, 1995

National Task Force on Juvenile Sex Offending: Revised Report. Juvenile and Family Court Journal 44 (suppl 4):3–108, 1993

Ryan G, Miyoshi TJ, Metzner JL, et al: Trends in a national sample of sexually abusive youths. J Am Acad Child Adolesc Psychiatry 34 (suppl 1):17–25, 1996

Shaw JA: Male adolescent sex offenders, in Sexual Aggression. Edited by Shaw JA. Washington, DC, American Psychiatric Press, 1999, pp 169–194

Shaw JA, Campo-Bowen AE, Applegate B, et al: Young boys who commit serious sex offenses: demographics, psychometrics and phenomenology. Bulletin of the American Academy of Psychiatry and the Law 21:399–408, 1993

Shaw JA, Applegate B, Rothe E: Psychopathology and personality disorders in adolescent sex offenders. American Journal of Forensic Psychiatry 17(4):19–38, 1996

Siegel LJ, Senna JJ: Juvenile Delinquency, 3rd Edition. San Francisco, CA, West Publishing, 1988

Violent Crime Control and Law Enforcement Act of 1994, Pub L 103-322, September 13, 1994, 108 Stat 1796

CHAPTER 28

Juvenile Waivers to Adult Court

Charles L. Scott, M.D.

Case Example 1

Joe, a 15-year-old male, is facing a complaint of first-degree murder. At the time of the crime, Joe was smoking PCP (angel dust) and feeling like a "zombie." As Joe walked down the street eating a piece of pizza, he saw a young woman (unknown to him) in a car. He decided to steal the car. When the woman told him, "you don't want this old car," Joe pulled out a handgun and shot her in the face. Joe told the evaluating psychiatrist that the victim deserved to die because she waited too long to hand over her keys.

At age 8, Joe was placed in a foster home after child protective services substantiated charges of severe physical abuse and neglect. At age 9, he was discovered drowning the foster family's cat in the bathtub. He had severe violent outbursts and was aggressive toward foster family members. A pediatrician diagnosed him with attention-deficit/hyperactivity disorder. Joe was prescribed methylphenidate (a stimulant), without benefit. By age 11, he was placed in a group home, where he assaulted staff and peers and ran away on two different occasions. Two years later, he was hospitalized on an inpatient psychiatric unit for 4 weeks after he started a fire in the group home. He was diagnosed with conduct disorder and dysthymic disorder. He was prescribed fluoxetine (an antidepressant) and valproic acid (a mood stabilizer sometimes used to treat aggression) with no change in his behavior noted.

Three weeks after being placed in a secure treatment facility, Joe ran away and joined a street gang. He began smoking marijuana and crack cocaine daily. He sold crack cocaine to make money. At age 14 he was detained in juvenile hall after he was caught stealing a car. Two weeks later he escaped while being interviewed by a social worker. He returned to the streets and began using PCP in addition to marijuana and cocaine. Five days after his escape, he shot the victim. Within hours after stealing her car, he was apprehended and taken to juvenile hall. While in juvenile hall detention, he found a mop handle, which he shoved in the mouth of a peer who had teased him.

Case Example 2

Cindy is a 15-year-old girl facing a complaint of first-degree murder of a 16-year-old male classmate named Simon. Witnesses reported that Simon and Cindy were sitting in different areas of the school cafeteria during the lunch hour. After Simon smiled and waved at Cindy from his table, she pulled a sharp knife out of her purse and walked over to Simon, whereupon she stabbed him in the chest. She returned to her table and resumed eating her lunch.

Cindy reported to the evaluating psychiatrist that she did not mean to harm Simon and only meant to "scare him" so that he would stop teasing her. She appeared very distant when talking about the event, expressed no remorse, and stated that it was an "accident." Student witnesses reported that Simon never teased Cindy and was very friendly and outgoing to all students. Cindy had no prior involvement with juvenile hall or police authorities and had no prior psychiatric history or drug or alcohol history. She was an above-average student in regular classes. Teachers and peers described her as quiet and withdrawn, with poor verbal skills. On the Minnesota Multiphasic Personality Inventory—Adolescent (Butcher and Williams 2000), she had elevated scores on the scales of paranoia, schizophrenia, and social introversion. While detained in juvenile hall, she was aloof and quiet, though compliant with rules. Interviews with her parents indicated that she was a reclusive child who chronically misinterpreted the actions of others.

In 1998, law enforcement agencies in the United States made an estimated 2.6 million arrests of persons younger than age 18 years. Although the arrest rate for juvenile crime has dropped since the peak year of 1994 (Snyder 1999), the American public has become skeptical regarding the ability of juvenile courts to rehabilitate wayward youths. In response, most jurisdictions have adopted a "get tough" attitude toward juveniles, highlighted by the phrase: "If you do the crime, you do the time." Increasing legal mechanisms have arisen to waive (also known as *transfer*) juveniles to adult criminal court. In those transfers that involve an actual hearing, the mental health professional's evaluation plays a significant role in the juvenile court's decision.

PSYCHIATRIC LEGAL ISSUES

Traditionally, the most common mechanism for transferring a juvenile from juvenile (civil) court to adult (criminal) court involves a juvenile court transfer hearing. Here, a juvenile court judge decides whether a youth is waived to adult court based on the information presented. This process is also known as a *judicial* or *discretionary* waiver. In reaction to public frustration with juvenile violence, additional mechanisms have been put in place and have played increasingly significant roles in juveniles being tried as adults. Because of the differences in these mechanisms, they will be reviewed individually.

Judicial Waiver

In the 46 states with a judicial waiver mechanism, a juvenile court judge decides whether to transfer the youth to adult criminal court for prosecution. Depending on the jurisdiction, a judicial waiver is also referred to as a *discretionary waiver, certification, bind-over, transfer, decline,* or *remand hearing.* Although the state prosecutor normally initiates the request for a judicial waiver, a juvenile or his or her parents may request a waiver in several states (Snyder and Sickmund 1995).

Between 1987 and 1994, the number of juvenile cases judicially waived to adult court increased by nearly 75%. After peaking in 1994, a downward trend developed, with a nearly 30% decline noted between 1994 and 1997. Of the cases judicially waived to adult court in 1997, those youths who had committed an offense against property were about as likely to be transferred to adult court as those youths involved in an offense against a person. Offenses against people make up the largest share of waived caseload for black youths, whereas white youths are more commonly judicially waived for offenses against property. African Americans are more commonly judicially waived than youths of other racial backgrounds,

and the number of black youths being judicially waived to adult court has increased at rates greater than that for white youths (Puzzanchera 2000). No one reason has been cited to explain this disparity, although research examining the possibility of racial bias throughout the juvenile justice system is ongoing.

In 30 states, probable cause that the juvenile actually committed the offense must be established before a judicial waiver hearing occurs. Three states do not require a probable cause determination but do require the court to consider the "prosecutorial merit" when making a waiver determination. In the District of Columbia and Maryland, the juvenile's guilt is assumed for the purposes of a waiver determination (Griffin et al. 1998).

In all states, a discretionary waiver requires a hearing in juvenile court at which information regarding the juvenile is presented to the judge. At this hearing, the prosecutor bears the burden of proof, except in those states that designate special circumstances under which this burden may be shifted to the youth (also called presumptive waiver). The majority of states have established the burden of proof standard at the discretionary waiver hearing as "a preponderance of the evidence" (approximately 51% or greater). A few states use the higher "clear and convincing" standard (between 70% and 80%) when deciding whether to transfer the juvenile to adult court. In seven states, once a case is sent to criminal court, the criminal court holds jurisdiction over any lesser offenses in addition to the more serious offense that triggered the transfer. Many states set a minimum age for a youth to be considered for a discretionary transfer. For example, in Vermont a 10-year-old child charged with murder or certain offenses against persons or property may be tried as an adult after a judicial waiver hearing. In at least 17 states, once a juvenile has reached a certain age, he may be judicially transferred to adult court for any offense determination (Griffin et al. 1998).

There are no nationally mandated criteria for judges to consider when deciding whether to transfer a juvenile to criminal court. The majority of states adopt (in various degrees) criteria delineated by the U.S. Supreme Court in the 1966 case of *Kent v. United States.* This case was the first U.S. Supreme Court case involving juvenile court proceedings. Morris Kent was a 16-year-old boy charged with several counts of robbery and rape. Despite a motion for a waiver hearing by Kent's attorney, the juvenile judge waived Kent to adult court without a hearing. Kent argued that the waiver was invalid and sought to have the criminal indictment dismissed on the grounds that the judge had not made a full investigation before waiving him to criminal court. The U.S. Supreme Court held that the failure to provide a hearing violated Kent's Fourteenth Amendment right to due process. The Court held that before a juvenile could be sent by a judge to adult court, the juvenile was entitled to a hearing, access by counsel to records involved in the waiver, and a written statement by the judge outlining reasons for the waiver. In an appendix to its opinion, the Court listed eight "determinative factors" to be used by the judge in deciding whether to judicially waive a youth. These factors included 1) the seriousness of the offense, 2) the violence of the offense, 3) whether the offense was against person or property, 4) whether probable cause existed, 5) the desirability of trying the whole case in one court, 6) the juvenile's personal circumstances, 7) the juvenile's prior criminal record, and 8) the likelihood of rehabilitation (*Kent v. United States* 1966). Most state statutes on judicial waiver incorporate aspects of these factors into two broad categories: a juvenile's risk for future dangerousness and a juvenile's amenability to treatment. In addition, some state statutes consider what is in the best interests of the child and the best interests of the community. Oregon is unique in focusing on whether the juvenile has the capacity "to appreciate the nature and quality of [his or her] conduct" as part of its judicial waiver evaluation determination (Griffin et al. 1998).

Mandatory Waiver

In a mandatory waiver, the state statute requires that juveniles of a specified minimum age who commit a particular offense be sent to adult court. Unlike in judicial waiver hearings, the roles of the juvenile court and mental health expert are very limited. In general, the court typically verifies that the statutory requirements of the mandatory waiver are met and issues the necessary transfer order. Mandatory waiver also differs from statutory exclusion waivers (see the following section). In statutory exclusion waivers, juveniles (accused of specified crimes) go directly to adult court, with the juvenile court having no role in the case. Fourteen states have a mandatory waiver provision. The North Carolina statute has set its minimum age for mandatory transfer at 13, the youngest age of any state (Griffin et al. 1998).

Statutory Exclusion Waiver

A statutory exclusion waiver (sometimes called *automatic transfer*) removes certain age, offense, and prior record categories from the juvenile court's jurisdiction. In the 28 states with this provision, any youth that matches a specified category is excluded from being defined as a "child" for juvenile court jurisdictional purposes. Under this mechanism, the individual begins his or her proceedings in adult, not juvenile, court. State statutes vary as to the criteria used to establish a statutory exclusion. For example, in New Mexico only first-degree murders committed by a youth age 15 or older are excluded from juvenile court. Mississippi, in contrast, statutorily excludes all felonies committed by individuals 17 or older from juvenile court. In Wisconsin, all youths age 10 or older charged with murder begin their legal proceedings in adult criminal court (Griffin et al. 1998).

Several concerns have been voiced regarding statutory exclusion policies (Kruh and Brodsky 1997). First, although incarceration is generally more expensive than juvenile court treatment programs (Tate et al. 1995), statutory exclusion bypasses consideration for treatment in the juvenile justice system. Second, statutory exclusions place juveniles with no prior delinquency petitions or exposure to treatment efforts directly into adult court (Gillespie and Norman 1984). Third, criminal justice statistics indicate that the majority of juvenile violence is committed by a small subset of chronic juvenile offenders and that many violent youth "grow out" of their violent behavior (Wolfgang et al. 1972). Critics of statutory exclusions argue that statutory exclusions fail to consider the uniqueness of each child and thereby risk unnecessary and inappropriate management of the youth in adult criminal courts. Critics have nicknamed this approach "Justice on Autopilot."

Presumptive Waiver

In a presumptive waiver, the juvenile (rather than the state) bears the burden of proving that he or she should not be sent to adult court. In the 15 states with this provision, the waiver to criminal court is presumed appropriate, although this presumption may be rebutted. If the juvenile meets specified age or offense criteria, then he must demonstrate that he is amenable to treatment within the juvenile court jurisdiction. In four states, the youth must prove by "clear and convincing" evidence (between 70% and 80% proof) that the waiver to adult court is not justified. Criteria establishing a presumptive waiver vary between states. Some states highlight a youth's prior offense history, whereas other states emphasize the youth's age or current offense. Alaska is the only state that presumes children younger than age 14 charged with a violent offense are unamenable to treatment (Griffin et al. 1998).

Direct File Waiver

In those states with a waiver provision known as direct file, the prosecutor is granted the authority to file the case in juvenile or criminal court. Because outcomes for juveniles charged with the same offense vary based on the prosecutor in their jurisdiction, this approach has been nicknamed "Justice by Geography." In direct file provisions, both juvenile and adult courts have the power to hear cases involving certain offenses, a process known as *concurrent jurisdiction*. The criteria established by the 15 states with this mechanism vary widely. Guidelines include age of offender, type of offense, and the extent of the juvenile's past offense history. Arkansas permits the prosecutor to file a case involving a youth charged with soliciting a minor to join a street gang directly to criminal court. In Florida, if the youth is age 16 or older, the prosecutor can file misdemeanor charges in adult court for prosecution (Griffin et al. 1998). Although there are no current national statistics on the number of juvenile cases filed directly into criminal court, there is growing evidence that prosecutorial files will eventually outnumber judicial waivers (Snyder and Sickmund 1995).

Critics of the direct file mechanism express concern that prosecutors have no special training in making reasoned transfer decisions (Kruh and Brodsky 1997). A case study in Chicago determined that attorneys ignored established transfer criteria and tried juveniles as adults in situations involving a public outcry regarding the offense or in "companion cases" in which two juveniles with substantially different prior records were both tried in adult court (Keiter 1973).

Reverse Waiver

The term *reverse waiver* refers to those instances when a juvenile's case is initially filed in criminal court, with subsequent transfer to juvenile court. When deciding whether to return the juvenile to juvenile court, the adult court usually examines characteristics of the particular youth and community protection interests. In six states, a reverse waiver can occur even when a juvenile court judge has already held a transfer hearing that resulted in the youth being sent to adult court. In these cases, a return of the case to juvenile court is available only if the juvenile court's decision was "substantially groundless" or if other "exceptional circumstances" can be shown (Griffin et al. 1998).

Once an Adult, Always an Adult Waiver

Thirty-one states have this special waiver category for juveniles. Under this principle, once a youth has been sent to adult court, the youth faces criminal prosecution in adult court for all subsequent offenses. In the majority of states, this provision applies only to those youths convicted of an offense in adult court. However, in Califor-

nia, a charge against a juvenile may be filed directly in adult court even if no conviction followed the original transfer. In Mississippi, no conviction on the first adult court–prosecuted offense is required if the juvenile is subsequently accused of a felony (Griffin et al. 1998).

CONDUCTING WAIVER EVALUATIONS

The judicial waiver hearing represents the waiver process most likely to involve a mental health professional. Prior to beginning the evaluation, the clinician should request a copy of his or her state's statute governing this issue. In addition to conducting interviews of the juvenile and pertinent family members, collateral records should be reviewed. These include medical and mental health records, school reports, probation reports, rap sheets, police reports, juvenile hall records, and the results of a general screening measure for intelligence. It is important to explain to the juvenile and family the purpose and scope of the evaluation with particular attention to the lack of confidentiality in this setting (Quinn 1992).

Because discretionary waivers require evaluation of risk for future dangerousness and amenability to treatment, these areas are reviewed in detail in the following sections.

Assessment of Future Dangerousness

A mental health professional's ability to predict future violent behavior over an extended period of time has realistic limitations. When conducting an assessment regarding a juvenile's future dangerousness, the clinician outlines past and current risk factors associated with increased rates of violence. As with adults, one of the most important factors in determining a juvenile's risk for future violence is a past history of violence. Certain demographic factors are associated with increased rates of violence among juveniles. Male juveniles are arrested for violent offenses six times more often than female juveniles (Poe-Yamagata and Butts 1996). After age 13, the rate of homicide increases sharply during each year of adolescence until age 18 (Federal Bureau of Investigation 1993). The age of the youth at the time that he or she commits the first violent act helps determine the risk for further violent behavior. Nearly half of those youths who commit a serious violent offense prior to age 11 continue to perform violent acts into their 20s (Elliott 1994). The greater the number of incidents, types, and circumstances of a youth's illegal behavior, the higher the risk of future criminal behavior (Robins and Ratcliff 1980; Snyder and Sickmund 1995). Additional information to assess potential dangerousness includes exposure to violence within the family, carrying of weapons, and participation in gangs (Scott 1999).

There are no specific psychological tests or measures that can accurately predict whether a juvenile will demonstrate violent behavior in the future. Tests that are frequently used to assess mental and personality disorders in this population include the Minnesota Multiphasic Personality Inventory—Adolescent (Butcher and Williams 2000), the Millon Adolescent Clinical Inventory (Millon 1993), and the Child Behavior Checklist (Achenbach and Edelbrock 1993; Grisso 1998). The Hare Psychopathy Checklist—Youth Version (Forth and Mailloux 2000) is currently being studied to determine its predictive validity for violence recidivism among juveniles.

Assessment of Amenability to Treatment

Most state statutes require an evaluation to determine if the youth is not amenable to treatment or rehabilitation. State statutes' definitions of amenability are often vague, with little or no specification regarding how much success in which areas is considered sufficient (Barnum 1987). In general, amenability to treatment focuses on the likelihood that treatment interventions will successfully rehabilitate the youth in his or her remaining time under the juvenile court's jurisdiction. Many state statutes instruct the court to consider the likelihood of rehabilitation through resources available in the community. In other jurisdictions, lack of resources is not justification for deciding that the youth is not amenable to treatment (Grisso 1998).

Several steps are important in assessing a youth's amenability to treatment. First, the clinician should determine the presence, if any, of a psychiatric diagnosis. When reviewing previous treatment, the evaluator should carefully examine the accuracy of any previous diagnosis. Second, the clinician should review types and efficacy of provided treatment. Various interventions include pharmacotherapy, individual psychotherapies, cognitive-behavioral therapy, family therapy, group therapy, inpatient hospital milieu therapy, drug and alcohol treatment, residential placement, vocational rehabilitation, special education interventions, treatment for sex offenders, boot camps, work programs, and response to incarceration. When assessing the adequacy of pharmacotherapy, important factors include the appropriateness of the medication as well as duration and adequacy of dosing. Although the clinician may determine that lost treatment opportunities have occurred in the past, the focus

for the transfer evaluation remains on the youth's current likelihood of treatment response.

Third, the evaluator should assess the individual's motivation for treatment and past history of treatment compliance. Evidence of previous poor motivation includes frequently missed scheduled appointments, noncompliance with medication, refusal to participate in individual or group therapy, and recurrent running away from court-ordered placement. One potential indicator for current motivation for treatment is the juvenile's willingness to "admit the crime." However, the examiner must consider the possibility that a juvenile's denial regarding his or her alleged offenses may be appropriately self-protective—to prevent statements in the transfer evaluation from being used at a later hearing to convict. To help clarify this issue, the evaluator can examine how much the juvenile uses denial in areas that are unrelated to the specific offense (Barnum 1987).

Finally, conclusions regarding the likelihood that a youth will benefit from treatment must include statements regarding how much time is necessary for the treatment to be effective. For older adolescents, effective treatment may not be possible if only a short period of time remains before the juvenile court's jurisdiction ends (Barnum 1987).

WRITING THE PSYCHIATRIC EVALUATION REPORT IN JUDICIAL WAIVERS

In the report prepared for the waiver hearing, the evaluator should include a statement of nonconfidentiality, the referral question, and an outline of the sources of information and should provide a thorough description of the youth's personal background. Areas to review include current problems, social and developmental history, attachment history, educational background, psychiatric history and treatment, family history, drug and alcohol history, occupational history, involvement with the juvenile justice system, a thorough mental status examination, and a discussion of psychiatric diagnoses. Good and poor prognostic indicators regarding a youth's risk for future dangerousness and amenability to treatment should be outlined.

Because a waiver hearing may result in the juvenile being tried in adult court, the report should address the juvenile's competency to stand trial in adult court (Benedek 1985). Juvenile defendants are generally presumed competent to stand trial. Approximately half the states have recognized the right of juveniles to be competent to participate in juvenile proceedings. Only Virginia mandates an evaluation of a juvenile's competency to stand trial when considering a waiver to adult court. Most other states require a competency to stand trial evaluation if the juvenile's competency is in question (Grisso 1998). Particular attention should be given to a juvenile's competency when the juvenile is younger than age 12, has a previous diagnosis of mental illness, mental retardation, borderline intellectual functioning, or learning disability, or demonstrates problems with memory or reality orientation (Grisso et al. 1987). In addition, some juveniles may be deemed incompetent due to developmental immaturity. In this situation, the youth may gain competence with the passage of time. No clear national legal guidelines exist on managing the juvenile who is incompetent secondary to developmental immaturity rather than a mental illness or defect. Theoretically, judges have the option of keeping the youth under the jurisdiction of juvenile court, dismissing the charges, or postponing the trial until the youth achieves greater maturity (Grisso 1998).

The clinician should also report whether or not the juvenile can give an account of his or her actions related to the alleged offense. The relationship of mental health symptoms to the juvenile's actions is important to review in a general manner. The inclusion of specific details of the offense, particularly those that are incriminating, should be avoided, as the transfer hearing occurs prior to the actual adjudication of the offense (Quinn 1992).

SUMMARY

Those juveniles who are transferred to adult court face significantly different consequences than those who remain in the juvenile justice system. In the adult criminal justice system, a juvenile faces loss of anonymity, potential life imprisonment, and the possibility of the death penalty if age 16 or older. Juveniles who are transferred to adult court are more likely to be incarcerated and have higher rates of recidivism. However, the relative effectiveness of juvenile and adult court dispositions is uncertain due to the inadequacy of research designs (Loeber and Farrington 1998).

As illustrated by the case examples (see Case Example Epilogues, which follow), juveniles facing identical complaints may have dramatically different profiles. At the waiver hearing, the evaluator illustrates to the court the uniqueness of each youth. As society develops new mechanisms to automatically place juveniles in criminal court, judicial waiver hearings are becoming increasingly less common. Nevertheless, their continued existence remains important. The waiver hearing itself symbolizes the competing arguments society poses regarding the management of delinquent youth. This continued dilemma represents a choice between the hope for rehabilitation or the acceptance of failure.

CASE EXAMPLE EPILOGUES

Case Example 1

The court-appointed psychiatrist diagnosed Joe with conduct disorder, severe; cannabis dependence; cocaine abuse; and PCP abuse. Identified risk factors for future violence included a lengthy past history and range of aggression beginning in early childhood, using and selling drugs, affiliation with street gangs, continued violence in a locked setting, and familiarity with firearms combined with a comfortable willingness to use them. Joe's prognosis for amenability to treatment was considered poor due to his previous treatment failures and frequent escapes from secure settings. Substance abuse treatment was felt unlikely to ameliorate his violent behavior as his violence predated his use of drugs and continued when abstinent. After a judicial waiver hearing, Joe was transferred to adult criminal court, where he was found guilty and sentenced to life in prison.

Case Example 2

A review of Cindy's record showed no previous history of violent or aggressive behavior. A psychiatric evaluation revealed a gradual decline in functioning with increasing social isolation, paranoia, and a delusional belief that students were laughing at her hair. While in juvenile hall, Cindy was started on a low dose of an antipsychotic with a decrease in her suspiciousness of others. After the court-appointed psychiatrist's report described her history and likely amenability to treatment, the prosecutor removed the petition for a waiver hearing.

REFERENCES

Achenbach TM, Edelbrock CS: Manual for Child Behavior Checklist and Revised Child Behavior Profile. Burlington, VT, University of Vermont, Department of Psychiatry, 1993

Barnum R: Child psychiatry and the law—clinical evaluation of juvenile delinquents facing transfer to adult court. J Am Acad Child Adolesc Psychiatry 26:922–925, 1987

Benedek EP: Waiver of juveniles to adult court, in Emerging Issues in Child Psychiatry and the Law. Edited by Schetky DH, Benedek EP. New York, Brunner/Mazel, 1985, pp 180–190

Butcher JN, Williams CL: Essentials of MMPI-Z and MMPI-A Interpretation, 2nd Edition. Minneapolis, MN, University of Minnesota Press, 2000

Edens JF, Skeem JL, Cruise KR, et al: Assessment of "juvenile psychopathy" and its association with violence. Behav Sci Law 19:53–80, 2001

Elliott D: National Youth Survey (United States): Wave V, 1980 (Computer File), ICPSR version. Boulder, CO, University of Colorado, Behavioral Research Institute (producer), 1988. Ann Arbor, MI, Inter-university Consortium for Political and Social Research (distributor), 1994

Federal Bureau of Investigation: Supplementary Homicide Reports 1976–1991 (machine-readable data files), 1993

Forth AE, Mailloux DL: Psychopathy in youth: what do we know? in The Clinical and Forensic Assessment of Psychopathy. Edited by Gacono CB. Mahwah, NJ, Lawrence Erlbaum, 2000, pp 25–54

Gillespie LK, Norman MD: Does certification mean prison: some preliminary findings from Utah. Juvenile and Family Court Journal 35:23–35, 1984

Griffin P, Torbet P, Szymanski L: Trying juveniles as adults in criminal court: an analysis of state transfer provisions. Washington, DC, Office of Juvenile Justice and Delinquency Prevention, 1998

Grisso T: Forensic Evaluation of Juveniles. Sarasota, FL, Professional Resource Press, 1998

Grisso T, Miller M, Sales B: Competency to stand trial in juvenile court. Int J Law Psychiatry 10:1–20, 1987

Keiter RB: Criminal or delinquent? a study of juvenile cases transferred to the criminal court. Crime and Delinquency 19:528–538, 1973

Kent v United States, 383 US 541 (1966)

Kruh IP, Brodsky SL: Clinical evaluations for transfer of juveniles to criminal court: current practices and future research. Behav Sci Law 15:151–165, 1997

Loeber R, Farrington DP: Serious and Violent Juvenile Offenders: Risk Factors and Successful Interventions. Thousand Oaks, CA, Sage, 1998

Millon T: Millon Adolescent Clinical Inventory Manual. Minneapolis, MN, National Computer Systems, 1993

Poe-Yamagata EP, Butts JA: Female offenders in the juvenile justice system: statistics summary. Washington, DC, Office of Juvenile Justice and Delinquency Prevention, 1996

Puzzanchera CM: Delinquency cases waived to criminal court, 1988–1997 (fact sheet #02). Washington, DC, Office of Juvenile Justice and Delinquency Prevention, 2000

Quinn KM: Waiver or transfer to adult court, in Handbook of Psychiatric Practice in the Juvenile Court. Work group chaired by Kalogerakis MG. Washington, DC, American Psychiatric Association, 1992, pp 79–85

Robins LN, Ratcliff KS: Childhood conduct disorders and later arrest, in The Social Consequences of Psychiatric Illness. Edited by Robins LN, Clayton PJ, Wing JK. New York, Brunner/Mazel, 1980, pp 248–263

Scott CL: Juvenile violence. Psychiatr Clin North Am 22:71–83, 1999

Snyder H: Juvenile arrests, 1998 (juvenile justice bulletin NCJ 179064). Washington, DC, Office of Juvenile Justice and Delinquency Prevention, 1999

Snyder HN, Sickmund M: Juvenile offenders and victims: a national report. Washington, DC, Office of Juvenile Justice and Delinquency Prevention, 1995

Tate DC, Reppucci ND, Mulvey EP: Violent juvenile delinquents: treatment effectiveness and implications for future action. Am Psychol 50:777–781, 1995

Wolfgang M, Figlio R, Sellin T: Delinquency in a Birth Cohort. Chicago, IL, University of Chicago Press, 1972

CHAPTER 29

State-of-Mind Assessments

Competency and Criminal Responsibility

C. J. Voigt, M.D.

Diane E. Heisel, M.D.

Elissa P. Benedek, M.D.

Case Example 1

Bob, a 15-year-old high school student, is facing a charge of first-degree murder in the death of his mother. On the day of the murder, his father returned home from work and discovered his wife stabbed to death. He then called police and, against their advice, searched the home. He found his son hiding in the basement, reading the Bible and chanting, "Kill the Devil." When police arrived, Bob appeared unaware of their presence and continued his chanting, despite their attempts at questioning him regarding his mother's death. Secondary to his bizarre presentation, he was transported to the local hospital. After a medical workup, Bob was admitted to the hospital's psychiatric unit for further evaluation and treatment.

During his hospitalization, Bob professed an unwavering belief in witchcraft. He told his clinician that he listened to music every day and that the music had directed him to kill his mother. He had resisted harming her for some time, but on the day of the offense, there were a variety of signs that he believed were clear indications that he must kill his mother. He stated he knew she was an agent of Satan and that she would ultimately seduce him if he did not kill her. He went into the kitchen, obtained a knife, and stabbed her to death when he found her in the living room.

Bob's father described him as becoming progressively withdrawn and apathetic over the past few months, frequently secluding himself in his room. He had stopped seeing his friends, and his school attendance was sporadic. He had not been eating, claiming his mother had poisoned his food. Teachers described a similar withdrawn, distracted presentation.

Case Example 2

Alex, a 16-year-old boy, was charged with first-degree murder in the death of his 14-year-old brother, Michael. On the day of the incident, his mother came home from work and found Michael in the bedroom, unresponsive in a pool of blood. A metal pipe and knife were on the carpet next to him. He appeared to have been stabbed several times in the chest and hit on the head with the pipe. Alex was also in the bedroom, attempting to arouse Michael and attending to his own minor lacerations.

When questioned by police, Alex stated that he and his brother had been attacked by two intruders, whom he recognized as schoolmates who had teased them and picked fights with them in the past. Alex's parents were unaware of any problems with others at school. His mother claimed the only fighting she knew of was "between the boys," which she viewed as normal sibling behavior. His teachers stated that Alex had many friends at school. They were also unaware of any rivalries at school. Due to the lack of evidence of an intruder and the inconsistencies in his account, the police began to suspect that Alex might have been his brother's assailant. He was eventually charged. Questions of competency and criminal responsibility were raised by his attorney, and evaluations were ordered by the court.

Case Example 3

Mary, a 16-year-old honor student, was charged with first-degree murder in the death of her boyfriend, Sam. The previous month, Mary's parents had ended their 20-year marriage after a 2-year bitter legal battle. Over the last year, Mary's friends and teachers noted a change in her behavior: she was frequently truant from school and her grades began to fall. Rumors circulated that Mary was drinking and "had taken up with an older man." Mary told her friends, "He's the one for me. I want to be with him forever." Several weeks prior to the murder, Mary's drinking became more noticeable. Her friends suspected that her boyfriend had "dumped her" for someone else.

On the night of the murder, Mary drank half a bottle of wine and two beers. Later that evening, she took her father's gun and decided to confront Sam. Arriving at his apartment, Mary found Sam and his new girlfriend. She fired six shots at the couple, fatally wounding Sam. Mary fled the scene but was eventually questioned by police and charged with first-degree murder. Mary's attorney requested competency, criminal responsibility, and diminished capacity evaluations. The forensic examiner recommended that Mary be found competent and criminally responsible. Diminished capacity was addressed separately.

The arrest rate of juvenile offenders who commit violent crimes decreased by 36% between 1994 and 1999 (Snyder 2000). However, in the 14 years preceding this decrease, the arrest rate had increased by 60%, and the number of juveniles arrested on a charge of murder had doubled (Puzzanchera 1998). As a result of this dramatic increase in adolescent violence and the ongoing media attention given to this problem, many states have passed "get tough on juvenile crime" legislation, reexamining how juveniles may be held accountable for their actions. Therefore, an increasing number of juvenile offenders are becoming involved with the criminal justice system, prompting more frequent state-of-mind assessments.

PSYCHIATRIC LEGAL EXAMPLES

Competency to Stand Trial

The concept of competency to stand trial is deeply rooted in the traditions of English common law and has been described as having both ritual and fairness functions. Court procedure requires a plea from an accused person. Early on, courts recognized "that certain lunatics or deaf mutes could not plead because of their affliction or disability" (Schetky and Benedek 1991), and provisions other than trial were developed for such persons.

Additionally, it has long been held that it is necessary for a criminal defendant to present his or her case in court and that it is unfair to try an individual whose mental disturbance or youth prevents such participation in his or her own defense. In contemporary criminal law, the function or role of competency to stand trial has been described as continuing the tradition of preserving both ritual and fairness in trial proceedings, including 1) safeguarding of the accuracy of the criminal adjudication, 2) guaranteeing a fair trial, 3) preserving the integrity and dignity of the legal process, and 4) ensuring that defendants found guilty understand why they are being punished.

The modern standard for competency to stand trial was contained in the 1960 U.S. Supreme Court decision in *Dusky v. United States*, wherein the court defined the test for competency as "whether a defendant has sufficient present ability to consult with his lawyer within a reasonable decree of rational understanding and whether he has a rational as well as factual understanding of the proceedings against him." The language in *Dusky*, with its emphasis on a defendant's cognitive capacities ("rational as well as factual understanding") and communicative abilities ("ability to consult with his lawyer"), has become the minimal constitutional requirement for competency to stand trial.

Historically, the question of competency to stand trial was raised primarily with adult offenders. In the early 1990s, the U.S. Department of Justice reported an alarming increase in violent crime committed by juveniles. State legislatures responded to this increase in youth violence by revising state laws dealing with the age at which a juvenile offender could be waived to adult criminal court. As a result, the frequency with which the concept of competency to stand trail must be considered in the juvenile population is on the rise. Nationwide, forensic examiners report an increase in requests for evaluation.

The influx of juvenile cases has not only stressed the overcrowded criminal court system but has also caused conflict within the departments of the legal system itself. In August 1999, the Michigan Court of Appeals began to hear arguments on whether juveniles who were convicted of violent crimes in the adult court must serve adult prison sentences. The 1996 Michigan Juvenile Justice Reform Legislation allows for automatic waiver of juveniles charged with specific crimes (Clark 1996). These crimes include the following:

1. Arson of a dwelling
2. Assault with intent to murder
3. Assault with intent to maim

4. Attempted murder
5. Conspiracy to commit murder
6. Solicitation to commit murder
7. First-degree murder
8. Second-degree murder
9. Kidnapping
10. First-degree criminal sexual conduct
11. Armed robbery
12. Carjacking
13. Manufacture, sale, delivery, or possession of 650 grams or more of a controlled substance

The American Civil Liberties Union and the Criminal Defense Attorneys of Michigan filed briefs with the court of appeals regarding the constitutionality of the legislation. The Michigan Prosecutors Association filed a brief in support of it. Three judges from Oakland and Wayne Counties refused to sentence four juvenile defendants who had been found guilty of robbery, first-degree murder, and rape until this question was settled. The challenge was unsuccessful; the Michigan Court of Appeals upheld 1996 Michigan Juvenile Justice Reform Legislation as constitutional.

Evaluation

Over the past three decades, a number of evaluation models have been developed to aid the forensic examiner with regard to whether a defendant is competent to stand trial. These include the following.

Competency screening instruments. Competency screening instruments are assessments given to defendants to determine if the question of competency is relevant and whether further evaluation is warranted. A comprehensive discussion and comparison of the following instruments has been provided by Melton et al. (1997):

1. The Competency Screening Test (CST)—a 22-item sentence completion test
2. The Georgia Court Competency Test (GCCT)
   a. GCCT—consists of six categories with a total of 17 questions focusing on general knowledge, specific legal knowledge, and courtroom layout
   b. GCCT-MSH (Georgia Court Competency Test–Mississippi State Hospital)—expands the initial GCCT to 21 items; additional questions test a defendant's familiarity with legal counsel and courtroom etiquette.
3. The Competency Checklist provides a review of three essential areas: comprehension of court pro-

ceedings, ability to advise counsel, and susceptibility to decompensation while awaiting or standing trial.
4. The Competency Assessment Interview (CAI) identifies 13 areas of functioning relevant to the role of a criminal defendant.
5. The Interdisciplinary Fitness Interview (IFI) is administered by a mental health professional and an attorney. Four items are relevant to competency, and 11 items test possible psychopathology.
6. The Computer Assisted Competence Assessment Tool (CACAT) contains 272 questions on legal knowledge, social history, and psychological functioning. Questions are multiple choice, yes or no, or true or false responses, summarized by a computer-generated narrative.
7. The MacArthur Competence Assessment Tool—Criminal Adjudication (Mac CAT-CA) uses a highly structured format that questions a defendant's ability to understand his or her present legal situation, think rationally, and appreciate abstract as well as specific knowledge pertaining to the case.
8. The Competency Assessment for Standing Trial for Defendants With Mental Retardation (CAST-MR) was specifically developed for the evaluation of mentally retarded individuals. The CAST-MR consists of three sections with a total of 50 questions.
   a. Section I—Multiple-choice questions testing basic legal knowledge
   b. Section II—Multiple-choice questions testing the ability to assist legal counsel (Sections I and II require a fourth-grade reading level)
   c. Section III—Oral questions testing fundamental understanding of the case

The above-mentioned competency testing instruments were developed to evaluate adult defendants and therefore must be adapted for use in the child/adolescent population.

In order to obtain the relevant information necessary to formulate an opinion, it is essential that the psychiatrist enter into the evaluation with a framework around which questions may be based. One of the most commonly used assessment instruments is the CAI, developed by Dr. A. Louis McGarry in 1973. This assessment tool addresses 13 areas of functioning as follows:

1. Appraisal of available legal defenses
2. Level of unmanageable behavior
3. Quality of relating to the attorney
4. Planning of legal strategy
5. Appraisal of role of defense counsel, prosecuting attorney, judge, jury, defendant, witness

6. Understanding of court procedure
7. Appreciation of charges
8. Appreciation of range and nature of possible penalties
9. Appraisal of likely outcome
10. Capacity to disclose to attorney available pertinent facts surrounding the offense
11. Capacity to realistically challenge prosecution witnesses
12. Capacity to testify relevantly
13. Self-defeating versus self-serving motivation

When assessing a youth for competency to stand trial, the examiner must provide the court with an evaluation of the juvenile's abilities as they pertain to the legal question. Dr. Thomas Grisso has added additional structure to the functional areas identified by McGarry in the CAI by grouping them into four categories of abilities as follows (Grisso 1998a):

1. Understanding of charges and potential consequences
2. Understanding of the trial process
3. Capacity to participate with attorney in a defense
4. Potential for courtroom participation

Although an assessment instrument may help provide structure to an interview, it does not cover all the information one needs in formulating an opinion. A thorough clinical evaluation, including mental status examination, psychological testing, and a review of the records, continues to be an integral part of the evaluation. Specific assessment of the defendant's ability to be educated about the pertinent legal issues is also necessary.

No strict protocol exists for a competency evaluation of a juvenile, but adherence to certain standards will facilitate a thorough examination prior to interviewing the defendant. As in all forensic evaluations, the psychiatrist must begin by examining potential conflicts of interest and issues of bias before deciding to consider a referral. The psychiatrist must then clarify what he or she can and cannot do, set reasonable timelines, and, if applicable, establish method of payment and fees with the referring party.

Once a referral is accepted, it is critical to review as much background material as possible, including police reports, treatment records, and other relevant documents. A referral for a competency evaluation may come from the defense attorney or from the court. If the court requests the competency evaluation, the name of the juvenile's attorney should be provided. If it is not, the name should be obtained from the court and the defense attorney contacted regarding the upcoming

evaluation of his or her client. This gives the psychiatrist the opportunity to obtain additional information needed for a complete evaluation. The wording of the order (the referral question) should be reviewed to guarantee that the examiner has an understanding of why the court is referring the juvenile for evaluation. If the psychiatrist has any concerns about this matter, the court should be contacted for further clarification. At the onset of the interview, the juvenile should be informed of the limits of privilege and confidentiality. The examiner must make sure these concepts are understood by having the juvenile explain them in his or her own words.

In writing a report, it is important to keep in mind the purpose of the evaluation: to address a legal question, rather than patient relief. Because it will be sent to non–mental health professionals, one should avoid the use of psychiatric jargon. The goal is to present a comprehensive evaluation regarding the issues before the court. Information necessary to provide a foundation for your opinion must be included; however, one should not go beyond the question asked. The following items should always be included in addition to pertinent clinical information: the type of order and applicable statutes, a section identifying all sources of information used (medical records, school records, police reports, phone calls, and ancillary interviews), a section addressing the limits on confidentiality discussed and consents obtained, and a summary of findings as well as a discussion of legal questions with recommendations.

Competency to Waive Miranda Rights

Whereas competency to stand trial is the most common competency referral in the evaluation of the juvenile, another is competency to waive Miranda rights. The landmark decision of the U.S. Supreme Court in *Miranda v. Arizona* (1966) affirmed and defined important rights of adult criminal suspects. If confessions made are to be used as evidence at trial, they must be made with the suspect's knowledge that they have the right to avoid self-incrimination (Fifth Amendment) and the right to advice of counsel (Fourteenth Amendment). These rights must be understood and acknowledged prior to or during any legal proceeding while in custody, such as police questioning. A defendant's confession cannot be used against him if it is found that he could not have waived the above rights "voluntarily, knowingly, and intelligently." The U.S. Supreme Court extended the Constitutional rights of adults to juveniles at all stages of the delinquency proceedings in *Kent v. United States* (1966) and *In re Gault* (1967).

The question of whether juveniles were competent to waive these rights was outlined in *People v. Lara* (1967), elaborated in *West v. United States* (1968), and affirmed in *Fare v. Michael C* (1979). These cases highlighted the issue that a juvenile's waiver of rights would require a more thorough examination and special considerations not usually raised in adult cases. The validity of the juvenile's waiver cannot be based on any single factor, such as age, IQ, or developmental status. It must be decided in light of the *totality of circumstances*, incorporating both features of the situation in which the confession was made and characteristics of the individual that contribute to his or her ability to understand and apply the Miranda warnings.

The significance of these rights is even greater today with the advent of increased transfer to the adult courts and the more serious consequences of conviction. The determination of whether or not a minor has knowingly and intelligently waived his or her rights depends on a number of issues and circumstances that must be reconstructed, as this is generally a retrospective evaluation.

Aspects of the situation to consider include length of detention; time of day; condition of surroundings; attempts at or perception of intimidation or coercion; presence of a parent, guardian, or "interested adult"; support and guidance available; how warning is given; style of questioning; and documentation of waiver. Characteristics of the individual to be considered include: age, intelligence, level of education, functional abilities, developmental level, and prior experience with the law.

Dr. Thomas Grisso (1998b), in collaboration with the National Institute of Mental Health, developed four standardized tools to assess both an individual's comprehension and an individual's appreciation of the Miranda warning in the context of the case against her. They are the Comprehension of Miranda Rights, Comprehension of Miranda Rights—Recognition, Comprehension of Miranda Vocabulary, and the Function of Rights in Interrogation.

The general issues involved in accepting a referral, conducting an evaluation, and writing a report have already been discussed in the preceding text. Specific sections discussing the juvenile's ability or inability to understand the Miranda warning, reasons for any deficits discovered, information obtained regarding the circumstances of the police encounter, disclosure of rights, and individual's response should also be addressed in the report.

Competency to Be Executed

In 1986, the U.S. Supreme Court decided in *Ford v. Wainwright* that an incompetent defendant could not be executed. Although competency to be executed was not defined, Justice Powell in a concurring opinion suggested that the Eighth Amendment "forbids the execution only of those who are unaware of the punishment that they are about to suffer and why they are to suffer it." However, the issue of whether a state can involuntarily medicate an individual sentenced to death in order to make him competent to be executed is still undecided.

The constitutionality of the juvenile death penalty was addressed in the 1988 *Thompson v. Oklahoma* decision. The U.S. Supreme Court held that execution of an offender age 15 or younger at the time of the crime is unconstitutional. The following year, in *Stanford v. Kentucky* (1989), the U.S. Supreme Court held that the Eighth Amendment does not prohibit the death penalty for crimes committed at age 16 or 17, regardless of statutory provisions (Streib 1999).

Currently, 38 states and the federal government have death penalty statutes. Of these 39 jurisdictions, 15 states have chosen age 18 (at the time of the crime) as the minimum age, 4 states use age 17, and the remaining 20 states use age 16. As of June 1999, there are 4 female and 66 male inmates on death row for crimes committed when they were 16 or 17 years of age. They are incarcerated in 16 different states and have been on death row from a few months to over 20 years. Approximately one-third of these individuals are confined in Texas. Between 1973 and June 1999, 13 males were executed for crimes committed as a juvenile. These executions have taken place in Texas, South Carolina, Louisiana, Missouri, Georgia, Virginia, and Oklahoma; thus far, only one of the individuals was 16 at the time of his offense.

Insanity Defense and Criminal Responsibility

Insanity is a legal term that denotes a mental state that is sufficiently disordered or incapacitated so as to relieve a defendant of blameworthiness or criminal responsibility for an offense. The definition of insanity varies in different states, but nearly all require a similar quality of cognitive or volitional impairment induced by serious mental disorders (Favole 1983). The intent of the insanity defense is to protect against the conviction and punishment of those who cannot legally be held accountable for their behavior. The courts reason that a defendant who was so psychologically disturbed or intellectually deficient at the time of an alleged offense (as to be considered insane) lacks the moral guilt or criminal intent (*mens rea*) that is necessary for criminal liability. Traditionally, in common law the finding of guilt requires evidence that the defendant has committed an act and has possessed a certain guilty state of mind or intention.

The standards of legal insanity have developed from the 1843 trial of Daniel M'Naughten, who was accused of killing the secretary to the prime minister of Great Britain. M'Naughten was ultimately acquitted as insane. The court's decision so angered Queen Victoria that she ordered her Law Lords to reexamine the standards by which a defendant could be found insane. The Lords recommended the standard as "to establish a defense on the ground of insanity, it must be clearly proved that at the time of the committing of the act, the party accused was laboring under such a defect of reason, from the disease of the mind, as not to know the nature and quality of the act he was doing, or if he did know it, that he did not know he was doing what was wrong" (Miller 1994). This standard has been called the "right/wrong test" (M'Naughten's Rule 1843), and it requires complete noncomprehension of behavior.

The M'Naughten standard was supplemented in many jurisdictions by language intended to broaden the scope of insanity to include conditions characterized by impairment in affective control or volitional control. These so-called irresistible impulse rules applied in situations in which a defendant apparently knew right from wrong (was not cognitively disturbed) but lacked sufficient capacity as a result of mental disease or defect to refrain from committing an act. The irresistible impulse standard has been difficult to distinguish from an unresisted impulse. The American Psychiatric Association position statement on the insanity defense noted, "The line between an irresistible impulse and an impulse unresisted is probably no sharper than the line between twilight and dusk" (American Psychiatric Association 1982). This concept has been difficult to operationalize in terms that are useful and convincing to a judge or a jury. There have been several efforts to eliminate the irresistible impulse portion of the insanity defense, including the Durham rule (*Durham v. United States* 1954), which also eliminated the cognitive and volitional components of the M'Naughten standard and offered instead a "product test," allowing a finding of not guilty by reason of insanity if the accused's unlawful act "was the product of a mental disease or defect." This was designed to allow greater latitude and scope to psychiatric testimony; however, this was never widely accepted outside the District of Columbia and was ultimately rejected there in 1972.

The current standard for an insanity defense is the language in the American Law Institute (ALI) test: "A person is not responsible for criminal conduct if at the time of such conduct as a result of mental disease or defect he lacks substantial capacity either to appreciate

the criminality (wrongfulness) of his conduct or to conform his conduct to the requirements of the law" (Schetky and Benedek 1991, p. 221). This standard was adopted in the majority of federal jurisdictions and a significant number of states. The ALI test excludes mental disease or defect manifested only by repeated antisocial or otherwise abnormal behavior. Following the trial of John Hinckley Jr. (who attempted to assassinate President Reagan), in which he was found not guilty by reason of insanity, a modified ALI standard was developed and endorsed by the American Bar Association and the American Psychiatric Association. This modification eliminated the volitional component, thus narrowing the context in which the insanity defense may be used. It was passed by Congress in 1984 and limited the federal test for criminal responsibility to include only a defendant who as a result of severe mental disease or defect was unable to appreciate the nature and quality or wrongfulness of his acts.

Regarding the juvenile offender, the ALI test is the most applicable; however, the insanity defense is rarely raised in the juvenile court system. Two possible explanations for this may be 1) the major mental disorders that typically provide the basis for the insanity defense in adult cases (such as psychotic disorders) may be less frequently diagnosed in juveniles; and 2) historically, the juvenile justice system was created for rehabilitative or treatment purposes rather than punishment. However, as the number of violent crimes committed by juvenile offenders increased, punishment played more of a role in the juvenile court. Courts have been forced to consider the issue of legal insanity, and most have ruled that this defense should be considered as an option. Grisso (1998c) states: "Most clinicians in juvenile forensic work have never been asked to perform an insanity evaluation for juvenile court." However, as the number of juveniles being waived into the adult court system for serious offenses increases, it is likely there will be an attempt to consider the insanity defense in a larger number of juvenile offenders.

Guidelines for evaluating an adolescent for the insanity defense do not differ from those for an adult. The evaluation should consist of a comprehensive psychiatric assessment plus information pertaining to how the juvenile was functioning at the time of the alleged crime. This would include reviewing allowable records (medical, psychiatric, school, and legal), police reports, information from third parties (parents, friends, or significant other[s]) and obtaining the juvenile's version of the alleged crime.

The Infancy Defense

The infancy defense refers to a concept that underage youths are not criminally responsible for their acts. It has its roots in English common law rules for criminal capacity. Those rules presumed that a youth younger than age 7 years was incapable of being held criminally responsible. Between ages 7 and 14 was the zone of presumptive incapacity—the burden being on the government to prove capacity beyond a reasonable doubt if it wished to prosecute. Fourteen became the age of adulthood for purposes of criminal responsibility (Fitch 1989).

With the establishment of the juvenile court in 1899 and its emphasis on treatment rather than punishment, the status of the common law rules became uncertain. They were frequently rejected, as their purpose was to insulate young children from the criminal justice system, a role that the creation of the juvenile justice system fulfilled. Therefore, courts as a general rule have rejected the infancy defense.

With the current trends of states trying juveniles as adults at earlier ages than previously and the increasing number of criminal cases appearing in the juvenile court, this defense should again be considered. States differ considerably, some allowing adult sanctions for children of any age; therefore, it is imperative that one consult state law when determining local standards (Shepherd 1999).

The infancy defense is distinguished from the defense of criminal responsibility in that in the infancy defense a showing of developmental immaturity is commonly asserted rather than mental illness.

Diminished Capacity

Diminished capacity is an affirmative defense based on the defendant's mental state at the time of the crime; it still results in criminal conviction, but with mitigation of the sentence. Although definitions differ among jurisdictions, diminished capacity generally implies that the defendant's capacity to form the requisite intent (*mens rea*) required for certain events is somehow affected or diminished. However, the mental incapacity of the youngster is not so severe as to lead to an insanity defense. It may be a mental or emotional disturbance or intoxication that interferes with the defendant's capacity to form intent. It is based on the difference between general- and specific-intent crimes. A successful diminished capacity defense can reduce a specific-intent crime to a lesser included general-intent offense (e.g., reduction of first-degree homicide to manslaughter). If no lesser offense exists, it can theoretically result in acquittal.

However, this rarely occurs. The doctrine of diminished capacity remains controversial. It is most often used when an adolescent is intoxicated. Defendants' attorneys will postulate a defense to show that despite the fact the defendant committed the crime, he or she did not intend to do so.

Guilty but Mentally Ill

Guilty but mentally ill statutes have been enacted in 12 states (Alaska, Delaware, Georgia, Illinois, Indiana, Kentucky, Michigan, New Mexico, Pennsylvania, South Carolina, South Dakota, and Utah) as an alternative to a finding of insanity. Michigan originated the defense in 1975 in an attempt to allow alternatives to a finding of insanity. The guilty but mentally ill verdict implies that the defendant has been found guilty of an offense and also met statutory criteria to be considered mentally ill but not legally insane. The mental illness is generally not connected to the crime. This verdict has been criticized because although it clearly labels the offender mentally ill, it does not guarantee treatment under the law, nor does it appear that the population using the verdict is any more likely than the general population to receive treatment. Additionally, the creation of this verdict as an alternative to not guilty by reason of insanity has done very little to affect the number of not guilty by reason of insanity findings. Again, one must consult state law regarding applicable standards.

SUMMARY

In November 1999, national headlines featured a 13-year-old male found guilty of second-degree murder in Michigan. He was 11 years old at the time of the crime. The media extensively covered his trial, because he was the youngest child charged with first-degree murder in the nation. His picture appeared on *Betraying the Young*, an Amnesty International publication (1998).

Reports of adolescent violence continue to be headline news and the subject of prime-time television programming. The public is both fascinated and horrified by the details. Society, in an attempt to deal with youth violence, has taken a "get tough on juvenile crime" stance, resulting in an increasing number of youths entering the criminal justice system. Examiners in the forensic area are being forced to sort out multiple complex issues involved in the evaluation of younger children. Because current statutory definitions were developed for adult offenders, simply applying the standards to juveniles without a developmental context is inadequate. One must always consider the court's question within the context of a comprehensive child and adolescent evaluation.

PITFALLS

Conflict of Interest

When performing any type of forensic evaluation, the psychiatrist must keep in mind at all times his or her role in the process. Examiners must always be aware that bias may exist, and in order to minimize this potential, it is recommended that they never allow themselves to be in the dual roles of examiner and therapist. There may also be a temptation to be sympathetic to the side of the case that has retained your services. It is imperative that your guidelines and the freedom to form your own opinion be discussed with the referring attorney prior to the evaluation.

Knowledge of the Law

The law with regard to legal insanity, competency, diminished capacity, and guilty but mentally ill differs in each of the states. Knowledge of the applicable statutes in case law is necessary. The referring attorney may serve as a resource regarding the important issues in a particular case. Conversely, although the psychiatrist may know certain areas of law better than a novice attorney and, therefore, also serve as a reference for him or her, the ultimate responsibility for the legal issues in any situation lies with the attorney and the court system.

Seduction

When a child or adolescent is charged with a serious crime, it is often a high-profile case. Before agreeing to participate in such an evaluation, it is critical for the psychiatrist to examine his or her motivation, therefore minimizing the possibility of being seduced by the notoriety of the case.

Malingering

Secondary to the severity of the consequences a defendant may face if found guilty of the alleged crime, it is important to always consider the possibility of malingered mental illness.

CASE EXAMPLE EPILOGUES

Case Example 1

Secondary to his irrational mental state, Bob's attorney requested a competency evaluation. He was recommended incompetent to stand trial by the forensic examiner, and this recommendation was accepted by the court. Bob was then transferred to a forensic hospital for further evaluation and treatment. He continued to profess that he heard the voice of the Devil demanding he behave in a certain manner. He maintained that it was Satan he had killed and would frequently ask that he be allowed to speak with his mother. When visited by his attorney, he was unable to demonstrate any rational understanding of the legal situation or his involvement in the alleged crime. With therapy and neuroleptic medication, Bob was restored to competency within the period of time allowed by the court. He was subsequently evaluated for criminal responsibility, recommended exculpable, and adjudicated legally insane (i.e., mentally ill and unable to appreciate the wrongfulness of his conduct or conform his conduct to the requirements of the law). Bob was then rehospitalized and treated in a forensic hospital. Once it was felt that he was no longer a danger to himself or others, he was placed in the community, followed by a psychiatrist, and treated with supportive psychotherapy and neuroleptic medication.

Case Example 2

During the competency evaluation, Alex reported auditory and visual hallucinations that began several days prior to the homicide. He described "Evil Guy," a little green man who stood on his finger and told him to do "bad things," such as smoke dope, drink, and kill his brother. Alex claimed that the voices were outside his head and bothered him constantly. He said he was powerless to disobey them and had no strategies to diminish them. Alex claimed a minimal understanding of his legal situation and talked to examiners in a childlike manner. For example, when asked what might happen if he were convicted of a homicide, he said, "They will probably send me to summer camp; then my mother would come and get me."

Alex was admitted to a psychiatric hospital for further evaluation. He continued to claim that "Evil Guy" disturbed him on the unit. However, staff observed that Alex showed no unusual behavior, nor did he appear to be distracted by internal stimuli. Over time, as he became more comfortable with his surroundings, it was noted that although he claimed no understanding of his crime and potential outcome, he engaged in conversation with peers regarding his "legal trouble" and its possible consequences. No medication was prescribed, and he improved over the course of his hospitalization.

Alex had been tested in an outpatient setting prior to the offense. On a Wechsler Intelligence Scale for Children—Revised (WISC-R), he obtained a full-scale IQ of 118, placing him in the high-average range of intellectual functioning. On the Minnesota Multiphasic Personality Inventory (MMPI), his clinical scores were all within the average range. During hospitalization, he was retested. He refused to answer many of the WISC-R questions that he had answered as an outpatient. His MMPI profile was invalid, with extreme elevation on all clinical scales.

Clinicians concluded after lengthy psychological testing and clinical evaluation that Alex was competent. He was malingering and did not meet criteria for legal insanity. However, an outside clinician unaware of the insanity statute recommended that Alex be considered legally insane because of the bizarre nature of the crime. The examiner's recommendation was based on Alex's demeanor and his account of the event. He did not question whether Alex's report of the event may have been self-serving. A jury, using the definition of legal insanity, found that he did not meet the statutory requirements. He was found guilty and is presently serving a 25-year prison term for second-degree murder.

Case Example 3

Mary's attorney, in an attempt to have her first-degree murder charge (a specific-intent crime) reduced to manslaughter (a lesser included general-intent crime), considered using a diminished capacity defense. As is often the case in most states, voluntary intoxication did not meet the statutory guidelines for a diminished capacity defense. Therefore, the approach was unsuccessful. Mary was ultimately charged with first-degree murder in the death of her boyfriend.

REFERENCES

American Psychiatric Association: Statement on the Insanity Defense. Washington, DC, American Psychiatric Association, 1982

Amnesty International: Betraying the young: human rights violations against children in the U.S. justice system. AI Index: AMR 51/57/98, November 1998 [http://www.amnesty.org]

Clark P: 1996 Juvenile Justice Reform Legislation. Criminal Defense Newsletter 19 (9–10), June–July 1996. Detroit, MI, State Appellate Defender Office, 1996 [http://www.sado.org/]

Durham v United States, 94 US App DC 228, 214 F2d 862 (1954)

Dusky v United States, 362 US 402 (1960)

Fare v Michael C, 442 US 707 (1979)

Favole R: Mental disability in the American criminal process: four issue survey, in Mentally Disordered Offenders: Perspectives From Law and Social Science. Edited by Monahan J, Stedman H. New York, Plenum, 1983, pp 247–295

Fitch WL: Competency to stand trial and criminal responsibility in the juvenile court, in Juvenile Homicide. Edited by Benedek EP, Cornell DG. Washington, DC, American Psychiatric Press, 1989, pp 145–162

Ford v Wainwright, 477 US 399 (1986)

Grisso T: Juvenile's competency to stand trial, in Forensic Evaluation of Juveniles. Sarasota, FL, Professional Resources Press, 1998a, pp 83–126

Grisso T: Juvenile's waiver of Miranda rights, in Forensic Evaluation of Juveniles. Sarasota, FL, Professional Resources Press, 1998b, pp 37–82

Grisso T: Preparing for evaluations in delinquency cases, in Forensic Evaluation of Juveniles. Sarasota, FL, Professional Resources Press, 1998c, pp 1–35

In re Gault, 387 US 1 (1967)

Kent v United States, 383 US 541 (1966)

M'Naughten's Rule, 8 Eng Rep 718, 8 Eng Rep 722 (1843)

Melton GB, Petrila J, Poythress NG, et al: Competency to stand trial, in Psychological Evaluations for the Courts, 2nd Edition. New York, Guilford, 1997, pp 119–155

Miller R: Criminal responsibility, in Principles and Practice of Forensic Psychiatry. Edited by Rosner R. New York, Chapman & Hall, 1994, p 199

Miranda v Arizona, 384 US 436 (1966)

People v Lara, 432 P2d 202 Cal (1967)

Puzzanchera CM: The youngest offenders, 1996 (fact sheet #87). Washington, DC, Office of Juvenile Justice and Delinquency Prevention, 1998

Schetky DH, Benedek EP: Clinical Handbook of Child Psychiatry and the Law. Philadelphia, PA, Lippincott Williams & Wilkins, 1991, pp 216–229

Shepherd RE: Rebirth of the Infancy Defense. Criminal Justice Magazine, Summer 1997 [http://www.abanet.org/crimjust/juvjus/12-2shep.html. Accessed March 8, 1999]

Stanford v Kentucky, 109 S Ct 2969 (1989)

Streib V: The juvenile death penalty today: death sentences and executions for juvenile crimes, January 1973–June 1999 [http://www.law.onu.edu/faculty/streib/juvdeath. htm. Accessed July 15, 1999]

Thompson v Oklahoma, 56 USLW 4892 (1988)

West v United States, 399 F2d 467 (1968)

PART VI

Legal Issues

Ms. Macbeth, an attorney, reviews important legal issues in the treatment of minors in Chapter 30—critical information for all clinicians. Awareness of these issues will help to keep clinicians out of court as defendants and provide knowledge on standard-of-care issues should they be asked to testify as experts in malpractice suits.

Drs. Brinich, Amaya, and Burlingame follow with Chapter 31 on the current state of psychiatric commitment of minors to inpatient and outpatient treatment, including recent court decisions. As noted by the authors, testifying in commitment hearings can improve or destroy rapport with a minor and his or her family. However, the skillful clinician may incorporate the commitment hearing into treatment planning and use it to confront the minor with reality.

In Chapter 32, the many special issues involved in dealing with mentally retarded people are discussed in depth by Dr. Harris. Mentally retarded persons deserve special consideration and forensic evaluations by experts knowledgeable about cognitive development and mental retardation. Problems with language, comprehension, abstract thinking, and eagerness to please affect the mentally retarded person's appreciation of the law and, in turn, issues of criminal responsibility. Dr. Harris discusses civil rights issues around educational mainstreaming, normalization, and entitlement to services. In addition, he covers issues of competency, management of sexuality, and legal issues related to medication.

Psychic trauma and civil litigation are covered by Drs. Schetky and Guyer, who discuss evolving case law, new areas of litigation, and the admissibility of expert testimony in Chapter 33. In terms of the forensic evaluation, they discuss important questions to ask, the differential diagnosis of posttraumatic stress disorder, and common errors made in doing these evaluations.

The text concludes with a look toward the future, with Dr. Merideth writing on the usefulness of telepsychiatry in Chapter 34. As the forensic clinician's practice is often characterized by too much to do in too little time, telepsychiatry may prove to be one additional tool in a therapeutic armamentarium by allowing the busy clinician to devote less time to travel and more to seeing patients. Even more importantly, it will encourage the use of consultation by forensic clinicians on difficult cases and in remote locales.

CHAPTER 30

Legal Issues in the Treatment of Minors

JoAnn Macbeth, J.D.

Psychiatrists who treat minors—children and adolescents—face the same legal issues and problems as psychiatrists who treat adults. However, the resolution of these problems may require a different approach and/or additional steps because of two factors that distinguish a treatment relationship and legal situation when the patient is a minor from that when the patient is an adult. These factors are 1) that the patient, a minor, has limited, if any, legal capacity and 2) that the mutual relationship between psychiatrist and patient must bend to accommodate a third party (or third and fourth parties)—the parent(s). This chapter reviews the legal issues and problems that derive from these differences, summarizes the situations in which they are most likely to be played out, and offers a framework for their resolution.[1]

Both the case and the statutory law in this area reflect a tension and a balance between 1) the presumptions that "natural bounds of affection" will lead parents to act in the best interests of their children[2] and that parents have the "maturity, experience, and capacity for judgment" that their child does not to make difficult decisions,[3] and 2) a recognition that children possess independent liberty interests and that experience suggests that parents do not always act in what would generally be understood to be the best interests of their children. In addition, an important overlay has developed to address the issues that arise because it is no longer uncommon for a minor to have parents who are separated or divorced and who may disagree about important decisions in the minor's life.

An introductory word of caution: this is an area of the law that has been changing relatively rapidly. Changes have tended to give minors—particularly adolescents—greater autonomy with regard to treatment and related decisions. Beyond this, generalizations about changes are not possible. It would be prudent for a practitioner to review periodically the basic statutes and regulations in this area. It may also prove useful to identify an attorney with expertise in these issues who could be consulted if a difficult case arises.

CONSENT TO TREATMENT: WHO MAKES MEDICAL DECISIONS FOR A MINOR?

As is the case with treatment provided to adults, a psychiatrist or other physician who provides treatment to a minor[4] without legally adequate consent risks suit and potential tort, or malpractice, liability. The physician will be responsible for any untoward consequences of, or damage caused by, such unauthorized treatment, even if the care was entirely appropriate and satisfied all applicable standards of care. As is also the case with adults, in order for the consent to treatment to be effective, it must be "informed." In other words, the consent must be given only after the decision maker has received a fair and reasonable explanation of the proposed treatment. The explanation must include an appropriate explanation of all the risks, as the decision maker cannot make a knowledgeable choice if he or she is not aware of all risks.

These basic principles apply whether the patient is a minor or an adult. However, in almost all circumstances involving adults, the person with the power to make decisions regarding treatment is the patient, that is, the person who can be expected to both enjoy the benefits of the treatment and suffer the side effects, risks, and other potential ill effects. The source of the challenges that this situation presents for the child psychiatrist is that in many situations, the individual with decision-making authority is not the patient—the individual who will be benefited or harmed by the treatment at issue.

General Principles

The law has traditionally considered minors to be incompetent for most purposes, for example, entering contracts, incurring of debts, and so forth. This has included the making of decisions about medical treatment. This reflects the judgment that, as a general matter, individuals younger than age 18 cannot fully appreciate the potential consequences of receiving or forgoing treatment. As such decisions must be made, the law has provided that those persons legally responsible for minors—in most cases, their parents—will make these decisions on their behalf.

Thus, as a traditional matter, for a physician to be protected against charges of battery or unauthorized treatment, a minor's parents (or legal guardian) have had to consent to the treatment in question. To the extent this general rule applies, it means both that the psychiatrist will be safe as a legal matter if he acts as directed by a minor's parents *and* that he will be at risk to the extent he follows the directions of the minor and they diverge from those of the minor's parents.[5]

Two caveats are in order. First, as discussed, there are many exceptions, both statutory and judicial, to this rule. These exceptions vary significantly from one jurisdiction to another, and it would be prudent for a psychiatrist to become familiar with the major relevant exceptions in her state or jurisdiction. However, although there are many potentially relevant exceptions, it would be inadvisable to assume in any given situation that it is safe to treat minors without obtaining parental consent. Particularly with young minors, unless the practitioner is aware of an exception, valid in the jurisdiction in which she has seen the patient, that is clearly applicable, she would be well advised to obtain the consent of the minor's parent. As is the case with adults, this is not merely general consent to treatment, but specific consent tailored to any particular intervention at issue, for example, medication, that provides sufficient information about potential risks, such as side effects, for the parent to make an informed decision.

Second, as stated, these principles reflect society as it used to be: most children lived with, and were cared for by, two parents. In these circumstances, the law was based on the presumption that parents were in accord as to decisions such as medical treatment or, at least, that there was agreement that one would make the decisions for both. As is discussed below, both society and the law have changed; a psychiatrist needs to stay alert to the possibility that he may be dealing with a *parent*, but that the parent may not have the legal right to make decisions regarding his or her child's treatment. This does not mean that the psychiatrist needs to investigate to make certain that he is dealing with an adult with decision-making authority. Although only a parent with legal custody has authority to consent to a child's treatment, without some information that calls into question the authority of the parent, there is no duty to affirmatively inquire about custody when a parent first brings a child for evaluation and/or treatment.

A psychiatrist's duties in this regard may well change if, during the course of treatment, she develops a reason to believe that the parent who brought the child for treatment does not have legal custody. This could result from statements made by the patient or the parent, from notification of changed living circumstances, from a subpoena attempting to secure the psychiatrist's testimony in connection with divorce or custody litigation, and so forth. Once the psychiatrist is put on notice that there may be some question as to the legal authority of the parent to consent to treatment on the child's behalf, she has the duty to clarify the situation. She will be required to take reasonable steps to determine which parent has legal custody and confirm the consent of this parent. If the psychiatrist receives conflicting information about this, she may even need to consider requiring some proof of custody, for example, a copy of the custody decree.

Treatment When Parents Are Divorced or Separated

As this suggests, a psychiatrist needs to be particularly careful about issues involving consent when a minor patient's parents are divorced or separated—or where there is reason to believe that they may be. In these circumstances, the psychiatrist should take reasonable steps to determine which parent has legal custody of the minor, and particularly whether the parent who consents to treatment has legal custody.

The situation may be even more difficult when a minor's parents have both been involved in the minor's treatment but separate or divorce during the course of treatment. It is probably safe for a psychiatrist to continue treatment when this occurs unless the psychiatrist is told by one of the parents to stop treatment. If this occurs, the psychiatrist should consult the parent continuing to request treatment and ask for some confirmation of authority to consent to treatment.

Treatment Without Parental Consent: Exceptions

Although it would be prudent for a psychiatrist to assume that he or she should obtain the consent of a custodial parent before undertaking treatment of a minor, there are a number of exceptions to this general rule. As the nature and availability of such exceptions vary significantly from one jurisdiction to another, it would be advisable for a psychiatrist who treats minors to become familiar with relevant exceptions in the jurisdiction(s) in which he or she practices. The following exceptions may be available.

Emergency Exception

In most jurisdictions, no consent is necessary if the situation is an emergency. The psychiatrist will not risk exposure if he proceeds to treat a child in such circumstances, regardless of who brought the child in for treatment. The exception reflects the assumption that if there were sufficient time to consult a parent, the parent would consent to the provision of emergency medical treatment.

Although this is a very common exception, the foundation of the exception as well as its contours vary. In a number of states, the rule that protects a physician who provides services to an adult in an emergency extends to minors as well. Courts have struggled to define what constitutes a sufficient emergency to proceed without consent, recognizing that an overly broad definition could subsume the informed consent doctrine, whereas one that was too narrow could leave physicians who respond to life-threatening situations at risk and, thus, potentially unwilling to provide such care. The resulting case law does not always seem consistent.[6]

The case law that specifically addresses the treatment of children in emergencies indicates that courts are especially willing to invoke this exception when obtaining or attempting to obtain consent would delay treatment and this delay would significantly increase the risk to the minor's life. In a number of jurisdictions, courts apply the exception more broadly, permitting treatment without parental consent when the delay would endanger the health of the minor.[7] There also seems to be a tendency to lower the gravity requirement and permit treatment in situations that are only semi-emergent when the minor is

older, is aware of the treatment, and cooperates with it.[8] As discussed below, this is particularly the case under some of the statutes that address emergency situations.

In addition to exceptions made by judges, many states have now enacted emergency statutes that are specifically applicable to minors. A few states will endorse proceeding without consent only in a "life-threatening situation."[9] Others permit emergency treatment without a parent's consent if the delay would endanger the health of the minor.[10]

Some states have also broadened the circumstances in which care can be provided without parental consent to situations that are not emergencies but in which the delay involved in securing parental consent would increase the risk of danger to the minor's health. For example, in the District of Columbia, there is a standard regulation authorizing the provision of emergency services to any person when the professional believes "that the giving of aid is the only alternative to probable death or serious physical or mental damage."[11] However, there is also a regulation that addresses only the provision of "health services" to minors of any age without parental consent. This requires only a judgment by the treating physician that the delay that would result from attempting to obtain consent would "substantially increase the risk to the minor's life, health, mental health, or welfare, or would unduly prolong suffering."[12]

Emancipated Minors

In most jurisdictions, parental consent is not necessary for the provision of treatment to an emancipated minor, that is, a minor who is no longer under the control of his or her parents. In deciding about emancipation—which may occur in the context of litigation contesting the physician's treatment—courts may base their decisions on an agreement between child and parent or on the conduct of child and parent.[13] Marriage, military service, and parenthood generally support a finding of emancipation. Financial independence is also an important factor. Emancipation will not necessarily be defeated by some financial assistance from parents if the minor is living on her own and managing her own financial affairs.[14]

Most states have also adopted legislation that identifies specific criteria that will be adequate to guarantee minors who satisfy them the right to make decisions about medical or mental health treatment.

Mature Minor Exception

An additional exception may be available to a minor who is "mature," even if he or she would not meet the test for being legally emancipated. The test is whether the minor is capable of appreciating (and does appreciate) the nature, extent, and consequences of the medical treatment to which the minor is giving consent. Again, there is significant variability in the circumstances in which this exception has been available to a minor. However, the case law that recognizes this exception frequently involves older minors, those whose parents were not available when the treatment decision was made, and/or treatments that were relatively low risk and clearly of benefit to the minor.

Cardwell v. Bechtol demonstrates the principle in operation. The case involved a 17-year-old girl who had gone to a family osteopath on her own. The treatment resulted in a herniated disc, bladder and bowel problems, and decreased sensation in her legs. Finding the girl able to give effective consent to treatment, the Tennessee Supreme Court explained that whether a minor is sufficiently mature "depends upon the age, ability, experience, education, training and degree of maturity or judgment obtained by a minor, as well as upon the conduct and demeanor of the minor at the time of the incident involved."[15]

Although relatively few states have adopted mature minor provisions, courts in recent years have seemed reluctant to hold a physician liable for treatment of an older minor who has consented to treatment. For a psychiatrist, the risks of providing treatment when only the minor patient consents are likely to be lower when only psychotherapy—as opposed to medication or electroconvulsive therapy—is involved. Even in jurisdictions that have explicitly recognized the exception, care should be taken in relying on it. The rule's subjective nature requires the psychiatrist to make judgments about the individual minor's capacity to comprehend the nature and purpose of the treatment in question. Psychiatrists who are considering proceeding in reliance on this exception should familiarize themselves with the contours of the rule in their state. Psychiatrists should also document in their records the basis of their conclusions that the minor satisfies the requirements.

Specific Consent Statutes

Increasingly, state legislatures are addressing the question of when minors should be able to consent to medical treatment by identifying specific kinds of treatment decisions that minors may make, rather than the characteristics of minors who may make the decisions (which is the case with emancipated or mature minor statutes). These frequently involve treatment that is necessary, in circumstances in which requiring parental consent would discourage the minor from receiving care. For example,

minors are likely not to tell their parents about drug problems or sexually transmitted diseases. If their parents must consent to treatment for such conditions—which inevitably requires that they know of the problem—the minors are much less likely to receive required treatment.

Who Pays?

As the above indicates, there are an increasing number of circumstances in which a minor can validly consent to the medical treatment that he or she wishes to receive. This ability protects the physician against charges of assault and battery, unpermitted touching, malpractice, and so forth. However, it may create situations in which the physician is unlikely to be paid for his or her services. If services are provided pursuant to the emergency exception, it is likely that a physician would, as a legal matter, be able to look to the parent or guardian for payment. In other circumstances, however, it is likely that the minor's ability to consent to treatment means that when he or she does so, it is to the minor that the psychiatrist must look for payment.

Some jurisdictions address this issue directly in their statutes or implementing regulations. For example, the District of Columbia regulations that authorize consent by minors in certain circumstances provide both that a minor who consents to the provision of health care services to himself or herself as permitted by the regulations will be liable for payment for the services and that the parents or legal guardian of a minor who consents to such services will *not* be liable for payment for those services unless they expressly agree to pay.[16]

Limits of Parental Authority: A Minor's Right to Refuse Treatment Arranged by or Consented to by Parents

The converse of the question of whether a minor may consent to treatment without parental consent or involvement is whether a minor may effectively refuse treatment requested or arranged by a parent with legal custody of the minor. Again, this is a question about which it is very difficult to generalize. Some states have addressed this question through legislation or regulations that relate to specific situations; others have decisional law that provides some guidance; and some have not yet addressed the issue.

Perhaps the only generalization that is possible is that states seem to be reluctant to permit a minor—even an older or "mature" minor—to refuse medical treatment requested by parent or legal guardian if that treatment is necessary to save the minor's life. The result is asymmetrical. In other words, while law may uphold or reflect the right of a minor to consent—without parental consent—to life-sustaining treatment, it is much less likely to permit the minor to refuse such treatment when the parent has requested it.

In re E.G.[17] involved a decision by a 17-year-old to refuse, on religious grounds, blood transfusions that were necessary to prevent her from dying of leukemia. Her mother acquiesced in this decision, also for religious reasons. When the case reached the Illinois Supreme Court, the court reached out to address an issue that was not before it: whether the minor's rejection of treatment would have been effective if the mother had wanted her to receive the treatment. In this situation, the court said, "If a parent or guardian opposes an unemancipated mature minor's refusal to consent to treatment for a life-threatening health problem, this opposition would weigh heavily against the minor's right to refuse."[18]

This asymmetry is reflected in statutory and regulatory provisions in a number of jurisdictions. For example, in Maryland, a minor has the same capacity as an adult to consent to a number of specific kinds of treatment, including treatment for drug abuse or alcoholism.[19] However, the Maryland Code specifically provides that the capacity of a minor to consent to this treatment "does not include the capacity to refuse treatment for drug abuse or alcoholism in an inpatient alcohol or drug abuse treatment program…for which a parent or guardian has given consent."[20]

CONFIDENTIALITY AND PRIVILEGE

Psychiatrists are both legally and ethically bound not to disclose information learned from a patient or information about a patient learned through, or in connection with, a treatment relationship. That duty is reflected in two overlapping, but distinct, areas of law that are frequently confused: privilege and confidentiality. Privilege rules are rules of evidence; they govern disclosure of information in judicial, quasi-judicial, or administrative proceedings. Information disclosed to a psychiatrist during treatment is "privileged," that is, absent some applicable exception, the patient may prevent the psychiatrist from disclosing it in such a proceeding. Confidentiality rules are much broader, barring disclosure of any information learned from the patient to any person not directly involved in the current patient's care. Privilege and confidentiality rules apply to the oral or written disclosure of information learned from patients as well as to the release of written notes, records, and so forth.

Confidentiality

Confidentiality is essential to the therapeutic relationship and effective treatment. Its importance is reflected in the double duty—ethical and legal—to maintain patient confidences. Unfortunately, the legal status of minors complicates the rather clear-cut rules that apply in the treatment of adults and results in countervailing duties running to different interested parties.[21] On one hand, it is clear both that a minor's parents generally are entitled to more information about the patient than family members of an adult patient would be and that they may make certain decisions about the release of information about the minor that would ordinarily only be made by the patient. On the other hand, it is also clear that minors possess certain independent, albeit relatively limited, rights of confidentiality, which must be considered and which will outweigh parental rights in certain situations. Thus, psychiatrists must proceed with care when parents seek information and minor patients resist disclosure.

Risks of Confidentiality Breach: General Principles

In most jurisdictions, what was solely an ethical obligation to keep patient information confidential is now also a legal duty. Suits for breach of confidentiality have been brought under various theories.[22] Patients have sued for invasion of privacy, tortuous breach of a duty of confidentiality, breach of an implied contract to maintain confidentiality, and breach of duties derived from state licensing statutes or testimonial privileges. Whereas not all such theories have been successful, the trend is very clearly in the direction of recognizing a legal duty and concomitant right of recovery, regardless of the legal theory on which this duty is based.[23] In addition, in recent years an increasing number of states have enacted statutes that provide for the confidentiality of information and records of mental health treatment and set out any exceptions to that rule.

It would be reasonable to assume that the rules governing who may authorize the release of confidential treatment information would derive from those governing who may authorize treatment and that when a parent controls consent to treatment, the parent also makes all decisions regarding waivers of confidentiality and the release of information. Although this is a good jumping-off place for analyzing confidentiality questions and this approach has been explicitly adopted in a number of situations (and seems to be implicitly followed in others), it will not always yield the right result. Assuming that it is universally followed could create exposure for the clinician. This is an area in which there may not be an easy legal answer; there may not always be a statute or regulation that sets out in what circumstances and at what age a minor enjoys independent confidentiality rights. Nevertheless, there are generally ways in which a clinician can control and minimize risk.

Release of Information to Custodial Parents

Generally. The issue of what information about the minor and his or her treatment may be released to the minor's parents is one of the questions that arises most frequently and is one of the more difficult confidentiality questions a psychiatrist faces. The closeness of the parent-child relationship, the anxiety a parent is likely to feel about a child in treatment, and the fact that the parent is likely to be paying for treatment lead many parents to ask for and expect complete information about a child in treatment.

As a strictly legal matter, unless there is a statute to the contrary—which is considerably more likely than it was 10 years ago—it is fair to assume that if a parent is legally entitled to authorize treatment for a minor child, that parent has a legal right to full information disclosed by the minor. This legal rule poses obvious clinical problems. Even when patients are young, many psychiatrists would feel uncomfortable if parents actually sought to exercise their right of full access to complete information about the treatment. The potential damage to the therapeutic relationship with the minor is the most obvious risk. In addition, certain disclosures may well exacerbate family problems.

To avoid such risks, when parents appear to have a legal right to full information—or to more information than the psychiatrist may feel it is appropriate to give them—it is advisable to lay out ground rules regarding confidentiality and disclosure at the outset of treatment. The psychiatrist should explain to the parents what he will tell them, what he will withhold, and his reasoning. Most parents will understand. If they elect to go forward with treatment, the psychiatrist may assume that they have agreed to those terms.[24]

The problem of disclosure to parents assumes even greater importance with adolescent patients. As discussed later, statutes frequently give adolescents greater authority regarding the release of information about them and their treatment. Even in the absence of such statutes, parents of adolescent children may well not be entitled to the same amount of information as are parents of very young minors. To begin with, as discussed earlier, in many circumstances and jurisdictions, it is likely that minors who are legally able to give effective consent to treatment will also be entitled to control the release of information about that treatment. The statutes of some states specifically link consent to treatment and disclosure authority. Even without such a statute, unless there is a statute or regulation specifically giving the parents control over disclosure, there is little risk in relying on an adolescent's consent to release confidential information when that adolescent was legally entitled to consent to the treatment in question.

When it is not clear that the adolescent controls consent to treatment, it is essential that the psychiatrist make disclosure rules clear to both the adolescent and his or her parents. The risks of not doing so are significant. If the matter is not discussed, the adolescent and parent each may well assume that he or she controls confidentiality. Both the adolescent and the parent should be informed at the outset of treatment to what extent the adolescent will control the disclosure of the information—including disclosure to the parents—and to what extent or in what situations information will be shared with the parents regardless of the adolescent's wishes.

The decision of where this line will be drawn should be informed by both ethical[25] and legal considerations. As a legal matter, a psychiatrist will be at risk if he or she withholds information that could enable parents to protect their adolescent from serious harm. When the interests involved are less vital, but the psychiatrist feels that certain information would benefit the family, he should attempt to arrange this disclosure without breaching confidentiality and, thus, endangering his relationship with the adolescent. First, the psychiatrist may be able to work with the adolescent, encouraging him to disclose the information to his parents himself. If the adolescent is unwilling to do this, he may be willing to permit the psychiatrist to do so. If the adolescent resists both options, the psychiatrist may be able to accomplish this purpose by discussing with the parents a general problem without disclosing anything the minor may have said about himself or any specific information about the minor.

State statutes and regulations. Much of the preceding discussion has been predicated on the assumption that there is no statute specifically addressing the confidentiality rights of minors, or at least no statute that speaks to the situation at issue. Increasingly, this is not the case. This has been an area of relative activity in state legislatures and regulatory bodies, and it may well be that a state that had not addressed the issue 5 years ago has done so now. It would be advisable for psychiatrists whose practices include minor patients to become familiar with any statutory or regulatory provisions relevant to these issues in the jurisdictions in which they practice.

Although there is still great variability in the legislative approaches of different jurisdictions, several approaches are common. As suggested earlier, a number of jurisdictions have adopted an approach under which, as a general matter, a minor's ability to control the release of information is coterminous with his or her ability to consent to treatment. For example, in Massachusetts, when a minor is able to consent to treatment, absent limited exceptions, all information is confidential between the minor and the psychiatrist.[26]

The District of Columbia's confidentiality rules reflect another common approach—one based on the age of the minor—and also have a consent to treatment overlay. The D.C. Mental Health Information Act provides that if a patient is between 14 and 18 years of age, both patient and parent must authorize, in writing, the disclosure of confidential information. Disclosures about a patient younger than age 14 may be authorized by a parent or legal guardian alone; however, if the parent has not consented to the minor's receipt of services, the minor alone may authorize the release of information.

In some jurisdictions, the parent or legal guardian is generally excepted from a requirement that the minor authorize the release of any mental health information. For example, New Mexico requires the minor to authorize the release of any information from which he or she could be identified and establishes clear rules as to who acts for the child if he or she is incapable of giving or withholding consent. (Parents may act for children younger than age 14; a treatment guardian must be appointed for older minors.) However, the statute provides that no authorization by the child is required if either 1) the disclosure is to the parent or legal guardian and is essential for the treatment of the child or 2) the disclosure is to the primary caregiver and is only of information necessary for the continuity of the child's treatment.

Even when minors appear to have a clear legal right to control the release of information, psychiatrists should be alert to exceptions that may either permit or require them to provide certain information to parents. For example, in Massachusetts, even if the minor in question is able to give consent and, thus, controls disclosure, a psychiatrist must notify parents of a medical condition so serious that "life or limb is endangered."[27] In Maryland, a minor has the same capacity as an adult to consent to treatment for a variety of conditions (including drug abuse, alcoholism, venereal disease, and pregnancy). Nevertheless, a physician, without the consent of the minor, or even over the express objection of the minor, may, but is not required to, give information to a parent or guardian about treatment needed by or provided to

the minor (other than abortion). In the District of Columbia, rather broad provisions permitting a physician to give information to parents are trumped by the D.C. Mental Health Information Act, discussed earlier. However, the District still requires providers to inform parents about treatment needed by a minor who is infected with a sexually transmitted disease and has refused treatment.[28]

Parental separation or divorce.   The divorce or separation of the parents of a minor patient further complicates the situation. Traditionally, the principles discussed above applied: the parent(s) with legal custody enjoyed whatever legal rights existed to obtain information about the minor's treatment, including information disclosed by the minor in the course of therapy. Increasingly, however, the law protects the interests of the noncustodial parent to such information. The provision of the Michigan Code is typical:

> Notwithstanding any other provision of law, a parent shall not be denied access to records or information concerning his or her child because the parent is not the custodial parent, unless the parent is prohibited from having access to the records or information by a protective order.[29]

Note that this does not give the noncustodial parent any greater right to information than he would otherwise have. That is, such a provision must be interpreted through the overlay of other provisions of state law that may limit even a custodial parent's right to information regarding a child.

Even in the absence of such a statute, a psychiatrist would be ill advised to treat the parent who does not have legal custody as an ordinary third party. Particularly if the parent has *actual* custody, arrangements should be made to provide the noncustodial parent with any information the psychiatrist believes essential, for example, information about medications, behavior that has signaled trouble in the past, and concerns about the minor's safety. If possible, consent should be obtained from the parent with legal custody. If the custodial parent is unwilling, the parent with the child can seek assistance from the court or guardian *ad litem*.

Release of Information to Third Parties

The rules that govern the release of information about minors to unrelated third parties—schools, researchers, insurers—are somewhat less clear. The principles discussed earlier would suggest that at least in the absence of specific statutory provisions addressing the situation, custodial parents may consent to such releases unless the minor controls the right to consent to the underlying treatment. However, both ethical and legal concerns suggest that this general rule needs to be tempered somewhat when the information is to be released to someone other than the minor's parents.

In addition, in this area in which statutory and regulatory provisions are proliferating, it is critical to determine whether there is a statutory provision on this point. Most of the statutes discussed earlier in the context of the release of information to a minor patient's parent have provisions that address the release of information to third parties. For example, as indicated, the New Mexico Code, which permits the disclosure of information to parents if it is essential to the minor's treatment or necessary for the continuity of treatment, provides that the minor controls the release of information in most other circumstances.

Even when the psychiatrist has authorization for the disclosure of information from the appropriate party, the psychiatrist has an ethical obligation to limit disclosures to those necessary in the particular situations.[30] Psychiatrists should be particularly sensitive to this obligation when the person authorizing the disclosure (the parent) is someone other than the person who may be harmed by the disclosures (the minor). Moreover, as the foregoing discussion indicates, increasingly, minors have some independent right of confidentiality. Although its contours are far from clear, courts may be less reluctant to protect this right when information is being withheld from third parties rather than from the minor's parents.

Particular caution should be exercised when the disclosures are to benefit someone other than the child. The psychiatrist who wants to write about the minor or use information about the patient in some other kind of research would be well advised to obtain the consent of both the parents and the minor.

Exceptions to Consent Requirement: Reporting Statutes and Other Public Safety Considerations

There are important exceptions to the requirement that confidential information be disclosed to third parties only with consent.

Reporting statutes.   *Child abuse reporting.*   Most psychiatrists, whether treating children or adults, are aware that they are obligated to report known or suspected abuse or neglect of children.[31] However, the exact circumstances in which this duty arises are often unclear, as is the approach to be taken in analyzing the situation.

Although child abuse statutes vary from one jurisdiction to another, there are some constants that underlie most: 1) a psychiatrists' duty to report child abuse gener-

ally derives from their licensure in a state, which makes their duties less clear if the abuse has occurred or the victim lives in a different state; 2) as statutes give little or no discretion regarding reporting, patients may need to be warned before they make disclosures; 3) reports must generally be made very quickly, that is, within 24 to 48 hours; and 4) because virtually all states also have statutes granting reporters immunity from civil liability for reports made in good faith, a psychiatrist who believes that abuse has occurred should not be dissuaded by the risk of a lawsuit by enraged parents or others reported. Beyond this, state legislative schemes vary, following one of several different approaches, and each psychiatrist should familiarize himself or herself with the basic elements of the scheme in the state(s) in which he or she practices.

Regardless of the approach, the determination of whether to report child abuse or neglect generally should be made through a two-step process:

1. First, the psychiatrist must determine whether the reported behavior constitutes abuse or neglect under the operative statute. Most statutes contain precise definitions of physical, emotional, and sexual abuse and of neglect. These should be reviewed in connection with any difficult questions, for example, whether corporal punishment would be considered abuse. Statutory definitions are also likely to control what "abuse" will have to be reported. In a number of states, for example, conduct that would otherwise qualify as abuse does not have to be reported as child abuse unless a parent, guardian, or caretaker inflicts the abuse or allows it to occur.[32]

2. If the psychiatrist determines that the alleged conduct would qualify as reportable child abuse, he or she must determine whether there is an actual duty to report. States take many different approaches to this issue. It is not unusual for a state to require reporting upon the receipt of any indication that there may have been abuse, even when the psychiatrist may have suspicions about the veracity of the reporter, for example, a young minor.[33] This approach appears to reflect the belief that children are optimally protected when a state investigative process, rather than the variable responses of individual professionals, is used to screen out unsubstantiated reports.

Many other states take a different approach, requiring reporting only when the reporter has "reason to believe" or "reasonable cause to suspect" that abuse has occurred. For example, in Washington State, a practitioner need report only when he or she "has reasonable cause to believe that a child...has suffered abuse or neglect."[34] This would appear to permit the exercise of some discretion, for example, when the practitioner believes that the report is false. Care should be taken in deciding not to report, however, and the reasoning for such a conclusion carefully documented.

Finally, although this may be less relevant for the psychiatrist who treats minors, some states make the decision to report contingent on whether the reporter has had professional contact with the alleged victim. In Wisconsin, for example, the duty to report arises only for "a physician…having reasonable cause to suspect that a child seen in the course of professional duties has been abused or neglected."[35]

Whether the decision is to report or not to report, once the question of possible child abuse has surfaced, the psychiatrist should carefully document the reasoning that led to his decision. State statutes can be very useful in this effort, offering a framework for analysis and the decisions that need to be made in order to make a decision about reporting.

Other reporting statutes. In some states, other statutes require the psychiatrist to report infectious diseases and other conditions that may affect children. The requirements vary significantly from state to state; psychiatrists should familiarize themselves with the law of the jurisdictions in which they practice. Statutes more recently adopted in a number of jurisdictions may have implications for psychiatrists who treat adolescents. These require a physician to report to state motor vehicle authorities the identity of patients suffering from certain disorders that might impair their driving. At their broadest, these statutes require the reporting of identified conditions if the condition is likely to impair the ability to control a vehicle and drive safely. The conditions are likely to include mental or emotional disorders and chronic abuse of substances that may impair motor skills.

Duties imposed by permissive reporting statutes. State confidentiality statutes sometimes authorize psychiatrists to breach confidentiality in order to warn of a danger posed by a patient. These statutes obviously apply to minors as well as to adults. Although these statutes are only permissive in nature, that is, they do not by their terms *require* reporting, psychiatrists should be extremely careful if they practice in a jurisdiction with such a statute. It is very likely that in the presence of such a statute, the common, or judge-made, law of such a jurisdiction would be interpreted as imposing a duty to warn.

Duties in the absence of specific reporting statutes. Even in the absence of statutes that impose, or are likely

to be interpreted as imposing, a duty to report, in most jurisdictions a psychiatrist will be at risk if she does not appropriately disclose information that suggests that another person is endangered by her patient, minor or adult. Most courts that have considered the issue have held not only that a physician *may* warn a third party of threatened harm but also that the physician can be held responsible for the consequences of not doing so. Similarly, as with adult patients, if a psychiatrist possesses information about a minor's suicidal intent, it must be disclosed as necessary and appropriate to prevent suicide. In both cases, the interests of the patient and the state in confidentiality are considered outweighed by the interest in preservation of life and safety.

Custody Disputes

The issues a clinician must consider when a minor's custody has been settled through a separation agreement or divorce decree have been addressed. When parents separate during the course of a minor's treatment, different problems may arise. It is not uncommon in such a situation for one, or even both, parents to seek the psychiatrist's assistance in the custody contest. As discussed below, the physician-patient privilege may permit one parent or the other to prevent this testimony. Even if it does not, and even if the psychiatrist has very clear opinions as to where the patient's custody interests lie, he should resist efforts to draw him into the case.

The risks are many. If the minor is aware of the psychiatrist's appearances in court, particularly if it is "in support of" one parent and "against" the other, it may seriously undermine the treatment relationship. Nor are the risks confined to the minor patient's reactions. One or both parents may resent the psychiatrist's expressed views and may refuse to continue to work with the psychiatrist or to pay for treatment. The psychiatrist should explain to the parent(s) seeking his help that the child is best served by the therapist remaining solely in a therapeutic role and that they can obtain an independent evaluation for purposes of the litigation. The following section on privilege will discuss how to proceed if the parent or his counsel persists and seeks to compel the psychiatrist's involvement.

Authorization to Release Information: Formalities of Consent

Regardless of who—minor, parent, both parents, other, or a combination—has the authority to consent to the release of confidential information, the psychiatrist should make certain that the consent on which he or she relies is legally valid. A psychiatrist should make certain that the authorization actually extends to the information in question and that it satisfies state confidentiality law requirements. A number of states now have mental health confidentiality statutes that specify the form and content of effective authorization.[36] Psychiatrists should familiarize themselves with the specifics, because there may be elements that they would not otherwise include, for example, a statement that the consenting party has the right to revoke consent at any time, a description of the use that may be made of the information released, and a statement that the consenting party has the right to examine any information disclosed.

As a general rule, these statutes require written authorization to release information. Even when there is no such statutory requirement, it is advisable to obtain written consent. The use of a consent form both encourages a patient to focus on the process and the rights being waived and serves as documentation of consent. This is particularly useful when children and adolescents are involved and consent may become a contentious issue between them and their parents.

Before releasing the information in question, a psychiatrist should satisfy herself that the patient's and/or parents' consent is informed.[37] Those authorizing disclosure should be aware of the nature of the information sought as well as what will be included in the information released. If release of the patient's medical record is at issue, the patient should be informed of the types and sources of information in the record. This is particularly important when the consent of a minor is involved, because the record is likely to include significant information from parents and other sources of which the patient is unaware.

Authorization for the release of information frequently comes indirectly from third parties—such as insurance carriers or schools—who have obtained written authorization from the patient or parent. If the psychiatrist believes that the patient or parent would not have consented if fully aware of the nature of the information involved or was not aware that the authorization would be used to obtain mental health information, the psychiatrist should contact the patient to discuss authorization and disclosure. The most effective consent is that made with knowledge of exactly what the psychiatrist will be disclosing. This would require the psychiatrist to make all disclosures in writing and to provide the patient a copy to review and approve prior to release.

Privilege

Privilege rules govern the disclosure of confidential information in judicial, quasi-judicial, or administrative pro-

ceedings. Privileges were created by statute in recognition that certain social values—the protection of certain kinds of relationships—were more important than the need for full disclosure. Privileges encourage full and frank communication in these relationships. The rationale for the physician-patient privilege is that without full communication between doctors and patients, effective treatment cannot take place.

Scope of the Privilege

The law of virtually every state includes a psychotherapist-patient or physician-patient privilege that applies to communications between psychiatrists and their patients, including minor patients. Whether or not particular information from or about the patient will be found privileged—and therefore, subject to exclusion by the patient (or the person legally authorized to exercise the privilege on the patient's behalf)—depends on a variety of factors that vary considerably from jurisdiction to jurisdiction. These state law rules will apply in proceedings in state courts or administrative bodies. Federal courts apply both state and federal laws, depending on the nature of the claim at issue. When entertaining a federal claim, federal courts will apply federal privilege law. Until recently, whether a patient enjoyed a privilege when federal law was applied depended on the jurisdiction. Whereas federal courts in some states recognized a federal psychotherapist-patient privilege, those in other states did not.[38]

This situation ended in 1996, with *Jaffe v. Redmond*, which recognized a federal psychotherapist-patient privilege. Reasoning that "[e]ffective psychotherapy...depends upon an atmosphere of confidence and trust in which the patient is willing to make a frank and complete disclosure of facts, emotions, memories, and fears," the U.S. Supreme Court held that "confidential communications between a licensed psychotherapist and her patients in the course of diagnosis or treatment are protected from compelled disclosure under [the federal rules of evidence]."[39]

Matters Protected by Privilege

In most jurisdictions, the privilege protects not only appropriate communications from the patient to the psychiatrist, but also any information learned in the course of examination and the psychiatrist's diagnosis and other conclusions about the patient and diagnosis.[40] The privilege is usually held to apply only to communications between the psychiatrist and patient that relate to the patient's treatment. This should cover virtually all information learned by a psychiatrist from a patient.[41]

An important issue in the treatment of children and adolescents is whether information disclosed in the presence of another person is privileged. The traditional rule was that such communications were not privileged—that there could be no expectation of privacy when a third person, including a parent, was present. However, this rule is under modification as courts examine and acknowledge the reality of child and adolescent therapy and other family treatment situations.

Another issue of importance in the treatment of children and adolescents is whether information received from a minor patient's parent, family members, and other third parties is protected by the privilege. Important interests are served by including this information within the privilege. Some of the most sensitive information about both the patient and the family—and the information most critical to successful treatment of the minor—may come from parents. If the confidentiality of such information is not assured, family members may not be willing to provide it to the psychiatrist. To date, although some courts have understood the importance of extending the privilege to such third-party communications, there is no uniformity on this point.[42]

Exceptions to the Privilege

Virtually every privilege statute contains significant exceptions—circumstances in which the privilege does not apply and the psychiatrist may have to testify regardless of the confidential treatment relationship. Courts have developed other "exceptions," reasoning that the patient has waived the privilege by various means. Commitment proceedings, will contests, and criminal matters are frequently excepted from the privilege. Particularly important to the psychiatrist who treats minors is the common abrogation of the privilege in proceedings relating to child abuse or neglect.[43] The scope of this exception varies from state to state, depending on the language of the state's statute and subsequent judicial interpretations. In some states, such as Alaska, the privilege is abrogated only in proceedings brought under the state's child abuse acts.[44] In other states, the exception is broader and courts have held that the privilege does not apply in civil proceedings unrelated to the state's child abuse act.

Some state statutes have created a possible exception in child custody cases. In these jurisdictions, a minor's treating psychiatrist can be compelled to provide testimony and disclose confidential information learned through treatment even over the objection of the minor patient and the minor's parents. However, some courts have recognized that there are countervailing interests and that the evidence can be obtained in other ways.

These courts have upheld the privilege, requiring an independent psychiatrist examination instead. In Massachusetts a psychiatrist's testimony will be permitted only if the judge determines after a hearing not only that the psychiatrist has significant evidence regarding the parent's ability to provide custody but also that the disclosure of the evidence is more important to the child's welfare than is the protection of the therapeutic relationship.[45]

Waiver

Explicit waiver. The physician-patient and the psychotherapist-patient privileges may be waived. If the patient or the person authorized to act on his behalf waives the privilege (does not choose to exercise it), the confidential information that would otherwise be privileged may be introduced into the judicial proceeding. Psychiatrists who treat children and adolescents face the uncertainty of whether a minor patient may decline to exercise (and therefore waive) the privilege. Although this depends on state statutes and case law, which differ from state to state, if the patient is a minor, the parent or legal guardian will ordinarily have the power to waive the privilege on behalf of the child.[46] If the parents are divorced or separated, the parent with legal custody traditionally has controlled the exercise of the privilege.

Although it is generally safe for a psychiatrist to rely on the waiver of one parent, he or she should be cautious if the minor's parents are separated or divorced or custody seems unclear. The most difficult questions arise in the context of custody disputes, in which the psychiatrist's testimony is likely to be central to the dispute and the parents frequently disagree abut whether the privilege should be exercised or waived. The law in this area varies dramatically from state to state. In *Nagle v. Hooks*,[47] Maryland's highest court held that when a child was too young to make decisions about the privilege himself, the decision in a custody dispute could not be made by either parent or even by both together. The court explained that a custodial parent has an inherent conflict of interest in acting on the child's behalf in asserting or waiving the privilege in the context of a continuing custody dispute. The court required that a neutral party be appointed to serve as guardian for the limited purpose of deciding whether or not to assert the privilege. The guardian was to be guided by what was in the child's best interests.

Implied waiver. Courts have also recognized implied waiver of the privilege in a variety of circumstances. These include cases in which the patient has testified about his treatment,[48] in which the patient has testified about his condition at the time of the communications in question or has called another physician to testify about his condition at that time, and in which there has been a waiver in another case or disclosure of the confidential information outside the courtroom.

The extent to which the privilege is held to be waived in these or other circumstances varies from one jurisdiction to another. Because the applicability of the privilege is often unclear, a psychiatrist should never disclose information in reliance on a litigant's or lawyer's representation that the patient has waived the privilege or waived confidentiality. Unless the psychiatrist is provided with a signed release from the patient (or person authorized to act on the patient's behalf), the psychiatrist should explain that he will not turn over any information without a subpoena and should follow the procedures outlined next for responding to a subpoena.

RESPONDING TO A SUBPOENA

Responding to a subpoena may be one of the most common legal problems or issues a psychiatrist faces. This is certainly the case with child psychiatrists, who have information that most divorce and custody lawyers are likely to believe is relevant, even critical, to their client's case. Although subpoenas frequently look quite formal and can be difficult to interpret, the rules for responding to them are straightforward. As a general matter, information sought by a subpoena can be provided if the patient—or the individual who controls the privilege on the patient's behalf—waives the physician-patient or psychotherapist-patient privilege, that is, consents to the information's release, or there has been a judicial determination that the privilege does not apply or has been waived by some conduct of the patient's.

As discussed earlier, privilege statutes and interpretive case law can be confusing, contradictory, and unclear. Nevertheless, a psychiatrist's obligation on receipt of a subpoena is simple: the psychiatrist should attempt to determine whether there has been a waiver by the patient and, unless it is completely clear that there has been such a waiver, should take necessary steps to protect the information within the context of responding to the subpoena and, as appropriate, securing judicial direction as to his or her obligations. These steps will depend to a certain extent on whether the subpoena is for trial or for deposition and/or document production.

Deposition and Document Subpoena

A subpoena for a deposition should first be reviewed to determine if written authorization or consent from the patient—or whoever controls the privilege—is included. Such authorization is not unusual. If the patient must waive the privilege in order to pursue the litigation, opposing counsel will generally have requested a release from the patient for this purpose. The subpoena should include the name, address, and telephone number of the attorney that has issued it. If an authorization is not included, a call or brief letter to the attorney may yield one. If not, the psychiatrist can contact the patient's attorney to determine if the patient consents to the deposition or document production.[49] If consent is not forthcoming from one source or another, the psychiatrist must contact the attorney who issued the subpoena to notify him or her that it will not be possible to provide any substantive information about the patient—including confirmation of treatment—without authorization by the patient or a court order. The attorney should then take steps to secure one or the other.

If the psychiatrist receives neither—or the issuing attorney makes it clear that she will not take steps to secure one or the other—the psychiatrist should make it clear that without a court order, he will appear as the subpoena requires, will provide information about himself and his practice, but will provide no information about the patient. In order to avoid a useless deposition session and the attendant waste of time and money, attorneys who are notified of this position are likely to take steps to secure consent or a court order before the deposition—or to cancel the deposition.

If the attorney insists on going forward with the deposition, the psychiatrist is obligated to appear unless she has taken steps to quash the subpoena herself.[50] At such a deposition, the psychiatrist should remember not to provide any information about a patient. If asked questions that seek such information, the psychiatrist should respond that the information is confidential and privileged. It is possible that another deposition will be scheduled after the issuing attorney has obtained a court order or consent.

Trial Subpoena

As with a subpoena for a deposition, when a psychiatrist receives a trial subpoena, the psychiatrist should attempt to determine whether the patient has authorized his or her testimony. Although subpoenas usually come from someone other than the patient, that is not always the case, particularly at trial.[51] If the subpoena has been issued by the attorney for the patient, a psychiatrist can assume that the patient has consented to the testimony sought. The situation when the patient is a minor is somewhat more complicated and is discussed later.

If the situation has not been resolved before the date on which the psychiatrist has been ordered to appear for trial, the psychiatrist should appear as directed. As at deposition, the psychiatrist can testify about matters that do not involve patient or confidential information, for example, his name and address, and credentials. When asked the first question that the answer to which would entail confidential information, the patient's attorney or opposing counsel may object on terms of the physician-patient or psychotherapist-patient privilege. If this occurs, the psychiatrist may follow the judge's subsequent decision and direction. To the extent a judge has considered a claim of privilege and ordered the testimony in question, the physician is protected. If there is no objection but the psychiatrist does not feel that there has been adequate consent or that the issue of privilege has been considered and resolved, the psychiatrist may raise the issue herself. It would be appropriate for the psychiatrist to state the concern (that it is her understanding that the information is privileged and confidential) and to ask whether she should testify.

Minor Patient

This discussion has focused on the issues all psychiatrists face when they receive a subpoena. As is the case with other issues discussed in this chapter, although the analytical framework remains the same, minor patients are likely to pose special challenges. The psychiatrist should not assume, as is the case with an adult patient, that the minor patient may authorize deposition and trial testimony. Instead, the rules discussed in the context of privilege will control. As there remains uncertainty in this area, the psychiatrist should be cautious about assuming that an authorization is valid.

As with other issues, the greatest uncertainty is in the custody area. To begin with, it is very common in a custody case for one parent to "consent" to disclosure and testimony and for the other parent to oppose it adamantly. As discussed previously, a psychiatrist is generally safe in relying on the consent of one parent, but it would be very risky to do so in the custody context unless the psychiatrist has confirmation that the consenting parent has sole legal custody of the minor patient. In any other case, if parental consent is to be the basis of the psychiatrist's disclosure, it must be the consent of both parents. The situation may be even more complicated when adolescents are involved. Because there is an increasing tendency to accord adolescents greater control over the release of information about themselves and their treatment, in contentious situations, the psychiatrist may need to consider proceeding as if there were no consent,

even when the parent with legal custody or both parents have authorized the psychiatrist's testimony.

For clinical reasons, even when there appears to be effective consent or waiver of the privilege, the psychiatrist should attempt to negotiate a solution that would allow him to restrict his role to treatment. The psychiatrist may be able to convince a minor's parents of the importance of protecting the treatment relationship with the child. Offering assistance in locating another psychiatrist or professional to evaluate the child may encourage them in this regard. It may also help to discuss these matters with the attorney(s) for the parent(s). To the extent the attorneys are looking for inexpensive expert testimony, they may be convinced to turn elsewhere for assistance if they understand that the psychiatrist will testify only to issues of fact, not opinion, and that any testimony will be given reluctantly. Most attorneys will not want to call experts who are reluctant to testify. If parents and their attorneys cannot be convinced, the psychiatrist may want to consider contacting the judge to urge the appointment of an independent psychiatrist to conduct an evaluation and testify in the custody proceedings.

NOTES

1. This chapter focuses on the legal issues facing psychiatrists who treat children and adolescents. However, central to the resolution of any such legal issues is the impact their resolution may have on the patient's treatment and status.

2. *Parham v. J.R.*, 442 US 584 (1979).

3. *Parham v. J.R.* at 602.

4. A psychiatrist should make certain as to the age of majority in the jurisdiction in which he or she practices. Although it is 18 in most states, it is higher (age 19 or 21) in a number of states.

5. The physician who provides services to a minor on the mistaken, though good-faith, belief that the minor is an adult is likely to be protected if that belief appears reasonable. A number of state statutes and regulations address this situation directly. For example, in the District of Columbia, "[i]f having acted in good faith, no physician…shall be held liable on the basis of a minor's representation" (Title 22 District of Columbia Municipal Regulations [DCMR] §602.3 [1995]).

6. For example, courts addressing the more limited question of when psychotropic medication can be provided under this exception have defined the emergency circumstances that justify the administration variously as 1) when it is "essential"…to prevent the death or serious consequences to a patient, *Rennie v. Klein*, 653 F2d 852 (1981); 2) when failure to medicate would "result in a substantial likelihood of physical harm to that patient, other patients or to staff," *Rogers v. Okin*, 478 F Supp 1342, 1365 (1979); and 3) when there is a "possibility of immediate, substantial, and irreversible deterioration of a serious

mental illness, [and] when even the smallest of avoidable delays would be intolerable," *In re Matter of Guardianship of Richard Roe III*, 421 NE2d 40, 55 (Mass 1981).

7. See, generally, annotation, *Medical Practitioner's Liability for Treatment Given Child Without Parent's Consent*, 67 American Law Reports (ALR) 4th 511 (1989) and Supp (1990).

8. See, for example, *Younts v. St. Francis Hosp. and School of Nursing*, 469 P2d 330 (Kan 1970).

9. See, for example, ND Cent Code §14-10-17.1 (1999).

10. For example, Fla Stat Ann §743.069 (1999) permits treatment when there is a medical emergency endangering the minor's health and it is not practical to contact the parents within the time available.

11. 22 DCMR §600.5 (1995).

12. 22 DCMR §600.4 (1995).

13. See, for example *Smith v. Selby*, 431 P2d 719 (Wash 1967), in which the court focused on the minor's conduct, including his completion of high school and his financial independence, in determining that he was emancipated and, thus, capable of consenting to a vasectomy without his parents' consent.

14. See, for example, *Carter v. Cangello*, 105 Cal App 3d 348 (Cal 1980).

15. *Cardwell v. Bechtol*, 724 SW2d 739 (Tenn 1987).

16. 22 DCMR §§600.1 and 601.2 (1995).

17. 549 NE2d 322 (Ill 1989).

18. Ibid.

19. Md Health Code Ann §20–102(c)(1) and (2).

20. Ibid.

21. See, for example, American Psychiatric Association (APA), *Principles of Medical Ethics With Annotations Especially Applicable to Psychiatry*, section 4, annotation 7 (Washington, DC, American Psychiatric Association, 2001).

22. See annotation, *Physicians' Tort Liability for Unauthorized Disclosure of Confidential Information About Patient*, 48 ALR 4th 668 (1986) and supp (1990).

23. In addition to potential civil liability, a breach of confidentiality may form the basis of a complaint to a psychiatrist's professional organization. The resulting investigation is likely to be time-consuming, expensive, and anxiety-provoking; negative findings may have to be reported to the National Practitioner Data Bank, licensing boards, insurance carriers, and so forth. Similarly, in states where breach of confidentiality is included within the definition of unprofessional conduct by the licensing authority, the psychiatrist is potentially subject to a licensure action.

24. Whereas obtaining written agreement to such conditions offers the greatest degree of protection, many psychiatrists are unwilling to go beyond an oral explanation to their patients' parents. An intermediate approach would be to develop a standard statement regarding confidentiality to go over with, and provide to, the parents.

25. The APA's *Principles of Medical Ethics With Annotations Especially Applicable to Psychiatry*, section 4, annotation 7 (see note 21 above), addresses the countervailing ethical interests as follows: "Careful judgment must be exercised by the psychiatrist in order to include, when appropriate, the parents or guardian in the treatment of a minor. At the same time, the psychiatrist must assure the minor proper confidentiality."

26. Massachusetts General Laws (MGL) chapter 112, §12F.

27. Ibid.

28. 22 DCMR §602.7 (1995).

29. Mich Stat Ann §25.312(10) (1999). In a state with such a provision, a psychiatrist would usually be safe in assuming that there is no protective order prohibiting disclosure to the noncustodial parent. As discussed above, however, if circumstances cause the psychiatrist to wonder whether there is such an order, the psychiatrist should undertake to clarify the situation and his or her responsibilities.

30. The APA's *Principles of Medical Ethics With Annotations Especially Applicable to Psychiatry*, section 4, annotation 5 (see note 21 above) provides: "Ethically, the psychiatrist may disclose only that information which is relevant to a given situation. He/she should avoid offering speculation as fact. Sensitive information such as an individual's sexual orientation or fantasy material is usually unnecessary."

31. Frequently, statutes that require the reporting of child abuse carry criminal penalties. Civil liability is less clear. At least one court has rejected an attempt to bring a civil action under such a penal statute. In *Fischer v. Metcalf* (543 So2d 785 [1989]), the court dismissed a suit brought on behalf of two children against the psychiatrist who had treated their father but had failed to report their abuse by the father to the state department of rehabilitation services. Nonetheless, there is authority to the contrary, even in Florida, and psychiatrists should realize that failure to report child abuse may subject them to civil liability there and in other jurisdictions.

32. See, for example, NY Fam Ct Act §1012 (1999).

33. Texas has relatively broad reporting requirements, extending the duty to cases when the reporter has concern about the child's future welfare. It requires reporting by "[a] person having cause to believe that a child's physical or mental health or welfare has been adversely affected by abuse or neglect…" (Tex Fam Code Ann §261.101 [1999]).

34. Wash Rev Code §26.44.030(l) (1999).

35. Wis Stat Ann §48.981(2) (1999).

36. See, for example, Ill Stat Ann chapter 91½, §805. These statutes should be consulted prior to the release of any patient information; they may preclude the release of certain information despite patient (or parent) consent.

37. This is advisable for ethical as well as for legal reasons. Section 4, annotation 2 of the APA's *Principles of Medical Ethics With Annotations Especially Applicable to Psychiatry* (see note 21) provides in part: "The continuing duty of the psychiatrist to protect the patient includes fully apprising him/her of the connotations of waiving the privilege of privacy."

38. See *Dickson v. City of Lawton, Oklahoma*, 898 F2d 1443, 1450 (10th Cir 1990).

39. 518 US 1 (1996).

40. This is the case even in most jurisdictions that refer only to patient communications. See, for example, *State v. District Court*, 218 NW2d 641 (Iowa 1974).

41. Communications made during the course of examinations undertaken for purposes other than treatment usually will not be protected. This exception would likely include examinations conducted pursuant to court order and evaluations required by a school.

42. See *Grosslight v. Superior Court*, 72 Cal App 3d 502, 140 Cal Rptr 278 (1977).

43. See generally, annotation, *Validity, Construction, and Application of Statute Limiting Physician-Patient Privilege to Judicial Proceedings Relating to Child Abuse or Neglect*, 11 ALR 4th 649 (1986) and supp (1990).

44. See *State ex rel D.M. v. Hoester*, 681 SW2d 449, 452 n 5 (Mo 1984) (en banc); Alaska Statute §47.17.060 (1990).

45. MGL Ann chapter 233, §20B(e).

46. See *Yancy v. Erman*, 99 NE2d 524, 532 (Ct Common Pleas, Cuyahoga Cty, 1951).

47. 295 Md 123, 460 A2d 49 (Md 1983).

48. See, for example, *Giamanco v. Giamanco*, 57 AD2d 564, 393 NYS 2d 453 (1977).

49. Although oral consent may be effective in some circumstances, it is preferable to obtain written consent. Unless there has been a judicial determination that the privilege has been waived or does not apply, written consent that conforms to statutory or regulatory specifications may be necessary in jurisdictions with such provisions.

50. Absent special circumstances, for example, an impending trial date or a deposition conducted by out-of-town counsel, deposition scheduling is generally flexible. Although the subpoena may specify a date and time, it is usually possible to negotiate a more convenient time. Opposing counsel may be helpful in this effort.

51. Trial counsel frequently issue subpoenas for witnesses they have worked with and who will be supporting their case. This permits the rescheduling of testimony should the witness not appear for some reason.

CHAPTER 31

Psychiatric Commitment of Children and Adolescents

Paul M. Brinich, Ph.D.

Marc Amaya, M.D.

W. V. Burlingame, Ph.D.

Case Example 1

Margie, a 14-year-old junior high school girl, was brought to the emergency room of a city hospital by emergency medical technicians who had been summoned to her junior high school by a guidance counselor. Margie's friends had told the counselor that she had ingested a large number of aspirin tablets after an over-the-counter pregnancy test had indicated that she was pregnant. The emergency room consulting psychiatrist concluded that Margie had impulsively attempted suicide because she feared her parents' reactions to the pregnancy. Now medically stable, Margie wanted to leave but refused to "contract" that she would not harm herself in the immediate future. Margie's parents were out of town, and she refused to tell anyone how they could be reached. Faced with a clinical impasse and the possibility that Margie might make another attempt on her life, the psychiatrist decided to petition for Margie's involuntary psychiatric hospitalization.

Case Example 2

Paul, a 15-year-old boy, came to his outpatient psychotherapy and family therapy appointments at a community mental health center only sporadically. His stepmother first brought him to the center due to a variety of conduct disturbances. These included running away, shoplifting, truancy, alcohol and marijuana use, defiance of parental rules and expectations, grade failure, and a pervasive oppositional stance toward adult authority. Prior to their divorce, Paul's biological parents had a highly conflicted marriage, and each also had significant difficulties with substance abuse.

When Paul refused to come to the mental health center, his father and stepmother met with Paul's therapist and reported that Paul recently had been involved in several quite serious delinquent acts. These included breaking and entering and joyriding in a stolen car. Paul's father and stepmother felt that he was beyond their control and said that Paul's mother and stepfather also felt powerless to help him.

Paul had been arrested for his recent delinquent acts. The juvenile authorities suggested to Paul's parents that prosecution might be avoided if Paul's parents would arrange for an inpatient evaluation and treatment. Faced with the possibility of detention in training school, Paul reluctantly had agreed to an inpatient psychiatric hospitalization. However, just as quickly, Paul had begun haggling with his parents over how long he might be hospitalized. Faced with willing parents but a highly resistant adolescent, Paul's therapist weighed the various options for inpatient hospitalization and/or residential treatment.

Case Example 3

Jenny, a 13-year-old girl, had struggled with significant separation difficulties since she began first grade. Her attendance record was very spotty throughout grammar school. After the Christmas holidays of her seventh-grade year, she absolutely refused to return to school. The remainder of the school year was taken up with outpatient psychotherapy, family therapy, medication, special class placement, behavioral regimens, and two brief psychiatric hospitalizations. All of these interventions appeared to have been fruitless, as Jenny began the following school year (her second attempt at seventh grade) by still refusing to go to school. Jenny's child psychiatrist, having struggled with this case for nearly a year, now suggested a long-term psychiatric hospitalization. He felt that the structure provided by an inpatient setting might help Jenny to contain her severe separation anxiety disorder.

HISTORICAL AND SOCIOPOLITICAL PERSPECTIVES

The Historical Context

Although the psychiatric hospitalization of children[1] is a comparatively recent phenomenon, the individual and social problems that lead to such out-of-home care have waxed and waned throughout recorded history and across the range of human cultures and societies.

Boswell (1988) has described how, in the Europe of Roman times, children whose parents were unwilling or unable to look after them were left to "the kindness of strangers." Such unwanted children were taken in by adults, who provided for their needs as best they could with interventions that tended to be individualized and personal. Most children who were abandoned or who were "donated" to religious organizations survived; some even prospered. Although some of these children must have suffered from disorders that today would be termed "psychiatric," such distinctions did not exist at the time.

The advent of the institutional care of children—the "foundling" homes of thirteenth-century Italy—meant that individualized care was replaced by group care, crowded living conditions, poor sanitation, and poor nutrition. Not surprisingly, up to 80% of the children placed in foundling homes died before they reached the age of 5 years. Adults who were "taken into care"—whether they were sent to the almshouses or to the "lunatik asylums" of the Middle Ages—fared little better.

Stavis (1995) points out that, throughout this period of history, "mental illness was not differentiated from other conditions such as idleness, drunkenness, homelessness, etc., which society condemned or sought to correct by the power of the state." During the sixteenth century both France and England passed laws which allowed the state to place its more unfortunate citizens in "houses of correction."

It was not until the nineteenth century that a distinction between mental illness and other types of social deviance began to be made. Although this distinction now is included in our legal system, the state's power to intervene in the lives of mentally ill people remains closely tied to the need to prevent social unrest and disruption (see "Legal Issues" later in this chapter). The state may restrict the freedom of mentally ill people when they appear to pose a danger to themselves or others.

Practically speaking, throughout much of the twentieth century the decision to commit a person to a psychiatric institution often was left to the vagaries of "expert" opinion. Physicians, psychiatrists, and psychologists were allowed to certify that a person required confinement due to mental illness.

The American civil rights movement of the 1960s and 1970s led to some important unintended consequences when it became clear that commitment laws often conflicted with individual constitutional rights. Many states opted to require judicial review of all psychiatric commitments, arguing that it was unconstitutional to deprive a person of his or her liberty without such due process. Although such arguments initially did not extend to minor children (cf. *Parham v. J.R.* 1979), the past two decades have seen a slow but steady evolution toward a perspective that grants at least some due process rights to minors.

Some might argue that efforts to protect citizens from the restrictions of liberty implied in involuntary commitment laws went too far. In 1975 the U.S. Supreme Court (*O'Connor v. Donaldson*) seemed to side with the argument that the state's power to restrict the freedom of its mentally ill citizens applied only to those people who posed a clear and present danger to themselves or others. Ironically, then, today's laws often require that a person be certified as "dangerous" in some increasingly vague sense of that word (Stavis 1995) before that person can be compelled to receive psychiatric treatment.

New Trends

Several additional competing and sometimes contradictory trends have played important parts in the evolution of social attitudes and legislation in the United States during the latter half of the twentieth century. These include at least the following:

- The growth of psychiatry and child psychiatry as medical subspecialties
- The optimistic attitude that social and/or medical intervention can prevent or cure many mental illnesses
- The willingness of a profit-driven health system to provide whatever services that health insurance plans

---

[1] "Children," as used in this chapter, includes all patients who have not reached the age of legal majority.

would reimburse (i.e., inpatient psychiatric treatment)

- The growing commitment to provide *all* children—regardless of their limitations—with a free public education in the least restrictive setting possible
- The continuing hope that psychopharmacology might provide medications able to effectively treat a wide range of mental illnesses
- The wish to minimize the intrusions of "big government" into the lives of individuals
- The wish to cut back on the public funding of a wide variety of social welfare programs (including those aimed at helping the mentally ill)

Emergence and Evolution of the "Youth-in-Trouble" Institutional System

Melton et al. (1998) open their chapter on residential treatment with a lengthy quote from an article titled "Trends and Issues in the Deinstitutionalization of Youths in Trouble," published in the journal *Crime and Delinquency* by Lerman (1980). Lerman described how, during the 1970s, "troublesome" adolescents were shifted from the juvenile justice system to the mental health system. Despite this shift, however, Lerman noted that

> …it would be misleading to conclude that deinstitutionalization has been achieved; for there have been offsetting changes in the use of private correctional facilities, residential treatment associated with child welfare, and psychiatric units of general and state hospitals. In effect, there has emerged in unplanned fashion a *new youth-in-trouble institutional system* that includes old and new institutions from all three fields: juvenile correction, child welfare, and mental health. (Lerman 1980, p. 282 [emphasis added])

The trend toward moving adolescents out of the juvenile justice system and into the child welfare and mental health systems persisted throughout much of the 1980s but was reversed during the 1990s. We now are seeing decreased lengths of stay for children and adolescents admitted to psychiatric facilities and increased numbers within our juvenile justice and correctional systems.

As we enter the new millennium, state and federal prisons are expanding at record rates while spending on child welfare and mental health remains stagnant. "Youths-in-trouble" bounce from one agency to another, each agency insisting that they belong to someone else. Which corner of the triangle—corrections, welfare, or mental health—a troubled (and troubling) child ends up in now depends as much on the youth's health insurance and family income as on the actual details of his or her disturbed (and disturbing) behavior.

As states have shifted the administration of their public health funds (e.g., Medicaid) toward managed care models, a new and often dominant factor has emerged: the case manager, armed with a "care map." Given the mandate to limit public spending on health services, case managers must refuse to authorize reimbursement of such services. Increasingly they rely on care maps to limit the kinds of care that may be provided to treat specific disorders. Children who in the past might have been well served by the mental health care system are denied such services and diverted into corrections or welfare services.

LEGAL ISSUES

Two Sources of the State's Power to Commit: Police Power and *Parens Patriae*

The state's right to commit an individual for confinement and/or treatment has generally been founded on one or both of two separate duties (Nurcombe and Partlett 1994; Stavis 1995). The first is the state's duty to *police* its citizens (i.e., to keep order and ensure their safety). The second is the state's duty to *protect and care for* those citizens who are unable to provide for themselves (i.e., to act as surrogate parents, following the legal principle of *parens patriae*).

While the psychiatric commitment of a child or adolescent might be based on either of these principles, commitments of children generally are founded more on *parens patriae* than on the police power of the state. Indeed, it is rare for a child to be committed to a psychiatric hospital unless the child has acted in a way that has left his or her caretakers feeling unable to care for the child. Under such circumstances the state may sanction the support and structure provided by an inpatient psychiatric setting as a way of providing needed resources to the child and his or her family.

In re Gault and *Parham v. J.R.*

Procedures governing the psychiatric commitment of children were, in the United States of the 1960s, ripe for reform. In its review *In re Gault* (1967), the U.S. Supreme Court overturned much of the procedural underpinnings of juvenile justice, holding that the doctrine of *parens patriae* had been unconstitutionally applied. The Court ordered broad procedural and due process protections for children whose liberty interests were at stake.

Over the ensuing decade, the Court's reasoning in *Gault* was applied to other instances of the psychiatric hospitalization of minors. Various suits alleged that children and adolescents confined in psychiatric institutions sometimes

- Had been admitted in error (with admitting officers tending to believe parents uncritically and to err on the side of caution)
- Failed to receive adequate and appropriate care
- Remained confined although treatment had been completed
- Were not considered for less restrictive placements
- Were unable to leave the institution due to the unavailability of less restrictive placements
- Suffered social stigmata and limitations as a consequence of institutionalization

All of these groups of youths were thought to have had their liberty interests compromised.

The trend begun by *Gault* ended in 1979 when the U.S. Supreme Court, in a controversial and much criticized decision (*Parham v. J.R.*), reversed its earlier course and left largely intact a Georgia statute that allowed parents and guardians to consent to the psychiatric commitment of their children (with, of course, the concurrence of hospital administrators and clinicians). In its attempt to balance the child's liberty interest, the parents' interests in having the child receive treatment, and the state's interest in the best utilization of its facilities, the Court did not mandate judicial or administrative review. However, the Court held that

> …the risk of error inherent in the parental decision to have a child institutionalized for mental health care is sufficiently great that some kind of inquiry should be made by a 'neutral factfinder' to determine whether the statutory requirements for admission are satisfied. (*Parham* 1979, p. 606)

This "neutral factfinder" could be the admissions officer who would conduct a careful inquiry, interview the child, and who had the authority to deny admission. The Court also required that

> …the child's continuing need for commitment [should] be reviewed periodically by a similarly independent procedure. (*Parham* 1979, p. 606)

This decision provided strong support for parental and professional authority regarding the psychiatric commitment of minors—this despite the fact that a number of states already had enacted or established much more stringent due process protections in response to earlier lower court decisions that ran counter to *Parham*.

Post-*Parham* Trends and the Subsequent Backlash

Growth of For-Profit Inpatient Psychiatric Facilities for Adolescents During the 1980s

In the first decade following *Parham*, the pace at which the states effected due process protections for minors in psychiatric hospitals slowed and admission rates—particularly to private adolescent psychiatric facilities—soared. Weithorn (1988) cited "skyrocketing" admission rates, primarily of "troublesome" youths who, she suggested, would have been referred as "delinquent" to the juvenile justice system a few years earlier. Weithorn noted that, while public facilities reduced their admission rates, private psychiatric hospitals increased their admission rates more than fourfold in the first 5 years following *Parham*.

Weithorn further contended that many of the adolescents admitted to private facilities during the 1980s were not those with severe and persistent mental illnesses, but those diagnosed as "conduct disorders," a term which she criticized as ambiguous and probably implying the same behaviors as those associated with "status offender" or "juvenile delinquent." The practice of admitting "conduct disordered" youths to psychiatric facilities thus facilitated the "transinstitutionalization" of youths from the juvenile justice system to the mental health system. Weithorn argued that these youths were only mildly disordered (if not simply struggling with some of the normal developmental processes of adolescence) and that community-based outpatient treatment would have been more effective were it available.

Containment of Health Care Costs by Denial of Services: Managed Care During the 1990s

Many of the concerns voiced by Weithorn in 1988 seemed remarkably irrelevant a decade later, as most of the for-profit psychiatric facilities whose practices she criticized have closed up shop, having been driven out of business by the refusal of insurance companies to reimburse them for their services. Managed care has been at the center of this change. As case managers have put increasing limitations on length of stay in psychiatric hospitals, the amount and kind of services provided have changed. Long-term inpatient treatment of DSM-IV-TR Axis II character problems (e.g., antisocial, borderline, or narcissistic personality disorders) is available only to those patients with very deep pockets. Long-term inpatient treatment of the various severe and persistent mental illnesses (e.g., schizophrenia and major mood disorders) is available only via the public mental health system (and a very few private institutions).

Managed care administrators have protected themselves against liability for the cost of care for serious and persistent mental illnesses by diverting such patients from the private sector to the public mental health system. State hospitals have become safety nets for private psychiatric hospitals—when a patient's insurance coverage is exhausted, the patient is transferred from the private to the state hospital. It then becomes the state hospital's responsibility to locate appropriate community-based aftercare resources. This is often one of the most labor-intensive, expensive, and frustrating aspects of the care of a seriously mentally ill patient. What's more, limitations in community-based services often mean that a hospitalized patient who is ready for discharge has no appropriate place to go for continued care. Gaps in the continuum of care end up lengthening the time that patients stay in restrictive facilities such as state psychiatric hospitals. This amounts to a kind of commitment by default—when both the private insurance sector and the community refuse to pay for needed posthospital services, the patient often remains confined in the hospital.

Statutory Criteria, Standards of Proof, "Medical Necessity," and Third-Party Criteria

State procedures for the voluntary admission of children and adolescents to psychiatric facilities have been summarized by Arambula and colleagues (1993), Burlingame and Amaya (1985), Knitzer (1982), Melton and colleagues (1998), Nurcombe and Partlett (1994), Weithorn (1988), and Wilson (1978). Because there is scarcely a constitutional "floor," state approaches to the issue tend to be diverse and constantly changing in the wake of local court decisions and legislative action.

As we have mentioned, *Parham* gave significant pause to jurisdictions that were contemplating due process protections; however, those that were already enacted have typically been left in place. Statutes vary widely: some empower the parent or guardian to admit a child without judicial or administrative review (Idaho), whereas others mandate a full-blown (and potentially adversarial) judicial proceeding for all admissions (North Carolina).

Statutes vary on a variety of other aspects as well. Some afford additional due process protections to youths in public facilities (California), whereas others require such protections in private and public facilities alike (North Carolina). Some offer additional protections to wards of the state (District of Columbia). Some require a preadmission hearing (Virginia); others defer the hearing for up to 10 days postadmission (North Carolina).

Some states initiate a hearing only on a child's refusal to consent to admission (several states) whereas others require a hearing in every case (North Carolina). Some states have experimented with an independent clinical/administrative review in lieu of an adversary court proceeding (Tennessee).

States differ in their approaches to the developmental abilities of children to participate in the legal processes of commitment. Some states allow youths of specified ages to seek due process protections (in Illinois, minors age 12 or older may request judicial review) or to participate in their admission (in New Mexico, juveniles as young as 12 years old may admit themselves; those younger than 12 must cosign the admissions document with their parent and may seek judicial review if they subsequently object to the hospitalization). Many states allow older adolescents to admit themselves, even over parental objection.

Statutory criteria for voluntary admission vary considerably. Some states provide ambiguous standards that can be attacked on the grounds of constitutional vagueness. For example, in Idaho, hospitalization by the parent or guardian must be "medically necessary," whereas in Arizona, a child must "benefit from care and treatment of a mental disorder" (Weithorn 1988). Given such statutory language, the courts often defer to professional expertise, particularly in contested cases in which the child and parent oppose one another.

When states have seen fit to embody criteria in statutes, they have tended to employ variations on the following three-pronged test:

1. The patient must suffer from a mental illness or mental disorder. (However, the definitions of these terms vary from the vague and circular to more rigorous itemizations of use of behavioral criteria.)
2. Treatment must be provided in the least restrictive or intensive setting. (However, this criterion is occasionally diluted by permitting continuing hospitalization if less restrictive appropriate settings are not available.)
3. The necessary treatment must be available in the hospital to which the patient is being committed. (This provides a measure of protection to patient and hospital alike in the case of overcrowded or otherwise compromised or limited facilities.)

At least one state (North Carolina) has additionally indicated in its voluntary admissions statute for minors that a finding of dangerousness is *not* necessary; this alerts judges and others that they need not employ the involuntary-commitment criterion of "dangerous to self or others" that they tend to be familiar with.

The standard of proof (i.e., the degree of certainty) that a judge must find in order to concur with either a parental request for admission or a finding of dangerousness (in an involuntary proceeding) also varies from state to state. Some states require the most rigorous standard (i.e., "beyond a reasonable doubt"). Others opt for the least stringent standard (i.e., "a preponderance of the evidence"). The U.S. Supreme Court has held that, when liberty is at stake, a more rigorous but intermediate standard is appropriate (i.e., "clear and convincing evidence").

Model Statutes, American Academy of Child and Adolescent Psychiatry Guidelines, and Care Maps

The major United States mental health professional associations provided amicus briefs to the U.S. Supreme Court in *Parham*. Although these briefs differed somewhat from one another, each recognized the need for checks on parental and professional authority; they also called attention to how adversarial proceedings could damage relationships between child and parent (as each recited his or her version of the events which led to admission) and/or between child and therapist (as the therapist presented his or her evidence for mental illness or disorder).

In the years following *Parham*, a number of model statutes have emerged (American Psychological Association 1984; Committee on the Civil Commitment of Minors 1998; Guidelines for the Psychiatric Hospitalization of Minors 1982; Wilson 1978). In common, these models call for an independent and neutral review process, typically carried out under court auspices and with legal representation for the child. This neutral review is intended to either ratify or overturn the decision to admit made by parents and professionals. Although the standards for commitment vary across the models, most tend to recognize the need for inpatient treatment for some conditions that do not necessarily meet a dangerousness standard.

Several professional associations and public interest groups also have approached the matter of the psychiatric hospitalization of children from the point of view of policy and professional ethics. One of the most comprehensive is the American Academy of Child and Adolescent Psychiatry's policy statement on "Inpatient Hospital Treatment of Children and Adolescents" (1989). The World Health Organization also has recently promulgated its own policy statement on "Mental Health Care Law" (Division of Mental Health and Prevention of Substance Abuse, World Health Organization 1996).

At present, however, it seems likely that the mental health care available to children in the United States will—for the next few years, at least—be influenced more by care maps than by laws and policy statements. Care maps—often developed by for-profit, proprietary organizations with a vested interest in minimizing health care expenditures—are built around treatments that have been empirically validated as the most effective interventions available for specific disorders. Whereas such epidemiological and statistically driven approaches make sense at the level of public policy, it still remains true that treatment is always provided to *individual patients* with their own variations. A child diagnosed with attention-deficit/hyperactivity disorder may be prescribed methylphenidate with little or no regard for the many other factors that may be playing a part in how his or her problems are expressed. A child admitted to a psychiatric facility after a suicide attempt may find that the care map used by his or her health insurance company allows for 5 days of "crisis stabilization" followed by outpatient follow-up—regardless of the environmental variables that may have played a crucial part in the emergence of the child's disturbance.

Special Cases: Minors Charged With Sexual and/or Violent Offenses

Over the past decade there has been growing public concern about youngsters who have been charged with sexual and/or violent offenses. These children illustrate in a particularly poignant way the blurring of boundaries between the correctional, child welfare, and mental health realms that led Lerman (1980) to coin the phrase, "youth-in-trouble institutional system."

When it comes time for out-of-home placement, children charged with sexual offenses are true "hot potatoes"; very few institutions feel competent to deal with their requirements for close supervision, their clinical needs for treatment (including family treatment), their frequent provocation and/or accusation of staff members, and the legal liabilities which follow in the wake of such children.

Likewise, children charged with extremely violent offenses (e.g., the murder of another child or of a parent) elicit strong reactions from many people and most institutions. It is common for people to take the attitude that a child "must be crazy" to have done such a harmful deed. Given the fact that such children often do well within the highly structured environment of an inpatient psychiatric facility, it is common for staff to find it hard to believe that the child would be capable of such a thing.

However, such children sometimes are neither crazy nor innocent.

What these children have in common is the fact that they often are unwanted in their home communities. They have been extruded into the "youth-in-trouble" system, and most members of their home communities prefer that they stay there. When such children end up in the mental health corner of the triangle they often remain there for a very long time, regardless of the terms of their commitment. This is especially true when, as is usually the case, the psychiatric hospital cannot force anyone in the community to take on responsibility for the care of the child.

CLINICAL ISSUES

Commitment

Admission Processes

Laws and procedures governing the psychiatric commitment of minors vary widely from state to state. Therefore, the remarks that follow will be general in character. We shall presume that most jurisdictions have defined a process for involuntary commitment, that the process utilized with minors may vary somewhat from that used with adults, and that judicial proceedings may uphold or deny a voluntary or involuntary psychiatric commitment.

Typically, these procedures require notarized or sworn written statements which attest to the circumstances, which a judge or magistrate must then evaluate to determine whether the relevant statutory criteria for commitment have been met. It therefore is critical that clinicians involved in these procedures be thoroughly familiar with the statutory criteria and that they personally verify the presence of behaviors and circumstances that meet the criteria. This requirement unfortunately but inevitably distorts clinical interviews and interventions, because the clinician must balance the need to provide psychological first aid and crisis intervention with the need to gather data in anticipation of administrative and/or legal reviews. Although hearsay rules often are applied less stringently in psychiatric commitments than in other legal proceedings, the clinician must be able to convince both himself or herself and the court that there is indeed sufficient reason for infringing on the liberty of the patient.

The evaluation of risk in a psychiatric patient is a demanding task under the best of circumstances. When faced with the possibility of commitment proceedings, the clinician must attend not only to the patient and his or her behavior, but also to reports by parents, guardians, law enforcement personnel, and others who may have been involved in bringing the patient to the clinical setting.

A careful clinician interviews not only the child and any family members who may be available but also talks with others who may possess relevant information or who witnessed the events leading to the referral for commitment. Needless to say, an authority-sensitive child already in conflict with important adults is hardly off to a good start in his hospitalization if he feels that he has been judged unfairly by a committing clinician.

Judicial Review

Judicial hearings and rehearings that follow admission present additional potential dilemmas. They may be the occasion for yet another clash between child and parents, or for a collision between a contesting child and the very clinician who is attempting to form an alliance with her. It often is best if a treating clinician is able to sidestep the testimony or court affidavits required by judicial review, leaving them to a colleague who is not thereby caught in a dual relationship that operates at the expense of the therapeutic alliance.

As in precommitment proceedings, the clinician must be careful to validate events; nothing plays into the defenses of a legalistic adolescent so much as inaccuracies that can then become the crux of his "case" and allow him to distract himself from the core issues.

In general, it is a good idea to prepare the child, his family, and any respective attorneys for both the court procedures and for the content of the anticipated testimony. The child should be told what will be said on the issue of mental illness or mental disorder; it often is helpful to discuss the possible disclosure of diagnoses beforehand, as this may prevent some potentially deleterious effects of these judicial proceedings. An aggressive public defender who is committed to defending his client's liberty interest may need to hear something from the clinician regarding "the best interests of the child." A little preparation of this sort may reduce the intensity of a contested hearing. A child who has been prepared for a commitment hearing by a clinician who reflects her own calmness, confidence, and integrity, despite the adversarial nature of the legal arena, is less apt to make the proceeding one more skirmish in his struggle with controlling adults.

There are many things to be said both for and against asking parents to testify in a commitment hearing. On the one hand, parents often are in the best position to document the child's behaviors and condition. On the other hand, such testimony may further stress an already damaged relationship and cause significant distress for one or more parties. Referring clinicians and prior caregivers often are in an excellent position to provide the court with information regarding their unsuccessful attempts to treat the child in less restrictive settings.

"Medical Necessity" and the Authorization of Reimbursement

Although it may seem odd to include a section titled "'Medical Necessity' and the Authorization of Reimbursement" in a chapter titled "Psychiatric Commitment of Children and Adolescents," it has been our experience that a patient's disturbed behavior sometimes clearly meets a state's legal criteria for commitment but still fails to meet the criteria used by an insurance reviewer who has been asked to authorize reimbursement for inpatient treatment. Over the past decade many managed care reviewers have required that a patient be in imminent danger of injuring himself or others (echoing *O'Connor v. Donaldson* 1975) before they will authorize inpatient treatment; lacking evidence of imminent danger, they claim that inpatient treatment is not "medically necessary."

This situation confronts clinicians, parents, and hospital administrators with some very difficult decisions. As soon as a seriously disturbed patient has been stabilized for a day or two, the case manager refuses to authorize any further reimbursement for inpatient care. The treating clinicians then are caught between a rock and a hard place. Although they may disagree with the case manager's judgment, and even though the case manager's decision to deny reimbursement in no way abrogates their continuing clinical and ethical duties toward the patient, the clinicians usually have no legal standing in this conflict between the patient and his insurance carrier. Although clinicians certainly have an ethical responsibility to assist parents in appealing a decision to deny reimbursement, generally speaking only parents (or other legal guardians) may initiate such appeals.

Parents also feel torn; whereas they may wish to take their child home, they may feel unable to care for her safely. Parents may want and need the help available from the clinicians and the hospital; but they also may be frightened by the possibility of huge bills that they fear will not be covered by their health insurance.

Hospital administrators may be concerned about a patient's welfare and about the fact that the hospital might be found to have some legal liability should the patient harm himself or others following discharge; on

the other hand, the hospital may be unable to provide services to a patient who cannot pay for them.

It turns out, then, that sometimes a commitment is *not* a commitment. That is, when a case manager refuses to authorize the reimbursement of inpatient treatment, a patient who meets a state's legal commitment criteria may leave the hospital nonetheless. Ironically, in most cases the case manager who decides that there is no medical necessity for such treatment has no medical training, has never seen the patient, and is immune from any liability associated with the patient's nonadmission or discharge from the hospital.

Clinical Phenomena Associated With Conflicts Regarding Commitment

Burlingame and Amaya have written at some length regarding some of the clinical phenomena associated with judicial review of voluntary admissions (Amaya and Burlingame 1981; Burlingame and Amaya 1985). Their list of danger points is a lengthy one (Amaya and Burlingame 1981, p. 766):

- the stress of a hearing may overtax the child or adolescent's resources, precipitating a psychotic episode, regression, withdrawal, or aggressive acting out;
- severe declines in self-esteem may occur in response to testimony regarding diagnosis, personality structure, or dynamics;
- substantial anxiety and the utilization of excessive ego defense may occur in response to the premature revelation of personality dynamics, unconscious content, or family secrets;
- the already tenuous or damaged relationship between youth and parents may be further eroded in response to the open collision and conflict in court;
- the fragile relationship between youth and therapist may be ruptured by the court encounter in which the therapist opposes release and marshals suitable but threatening evidence;
- considerable amounts of treatment time may be lost as the child or adolescent prepares his defense, putting emotional energies into securing release rather than addressing pathology;
- the authority and stature of treatment personnel and parents may be undermined, particularly for smaller children, by a confusing process in which important adults conflict with one another;
- treatment personnel may be intimidated, blackmailed, or compromised by the threats of youth, such that limits may not be set, rules may not be enforced in the milieu and living areas, and the patient's [feelings of] omnipotence may not be addressed;
- younger children, youth with defective reality testing, and those with primitive conscience formation may perceive themselves as on trial for all varieties of actual transgressions or other fantasized sins or misdeeds;

- the adolescent with a delinquent orientation and pathological [feelings of] omnipotence, who also denies personal responsibility and attributes causation for his dilemma to others, may be able to continue to attempt to manipulate others and avoid a necessary day of reckoning;
- the respective attorneys may debate procedural details and technicalities, which obscures the relevant behavioral and personality issues or provides the very unfortunate message that such issues do not matter;
- and, perhaps of greatest concern, there is considerable possibility that a seriously troubled youth may be unexpectedly and abruptly released without a plan or placement, through accident, judicial ignorance, or whimsy, a technicality, or the inexperience or lack of preparedness on the part of treatment personnel.

This list does not include the delay of treatment that occurs when a hearing is continued (perhaps because some necessary witness was not available); a continuance provides no closure, anxiety continues unabated, and the patient has good reason to continue using his defenses to ward off any engagement in treatment. Such events demonstrate how poorly legal time frames fit with treatment needs.

We have also seen instances in which an attorney affiliates emotionally with a contesting child and lends his own affective fuel to the process. Such an alliance provides unexcelled opportunities for "splitting" on the part of patients with such propensities (i.e., patients pit their allies—those who argue against commitment—against their enemies—those who argue in favor of commitment). Some inpatient facilities avoid such difficulties by simply refusing to admit or retain contesting youth; unfortunately, such policies reduce the treatment opportunities available to some of the most severely troubled patients.

Having detailed many of the things that can go wrong in such hearings, we should add that many hearings are relatively uneventful and some are actually useful from a therapeutic standpoint. It can be helpful, for example, when an irritated judge responds decisively to the narcissism, omnipotent feelings, or denial of an acting-out adolescent. The judge's actions may breach the adolescent's defenses in a way that allows treatment to begin. At other times, a judge's positive statements regarding his experience with the treatment unit and its professionals may help the child and family to engage in treatment. Although the negative outcomes are always more memorable than the positive, in those states (like North Carolina) in which hearings are routine, most children do not choose to contest their hospitalization and most hearings are fairly benign.

ASPECTS OF THE COMMITMENT PROCESS REQUIRING SPECIAL ATTENTION

Documentation and Supporting Testimony

The failure to verify incidents that demonstrate dangerousness or the presence of a mental disorder requiring treatment represents a major error on the part of the clinician. Commitment documentation should include clear descriptions of specific behaviors that illustrate why it is important for the state to intervene by temporarily limiting the liberty of the patient. Any use of hyperbole or exaggeration in the documentation serves only to undermine the credibility of the clinician—both in the eyes of the court and in the eyes of the child patient. Citing behavior that violates parental or community standards but which does not relate to issues of dangerousness or psychopathology (e.g., sexual promiscuity or addiction to cult music) will not strengthen the argument in favor of commitment. Likewise, using technical terminology or jargon is not usually useful in that the court often ends up rendering a "man on the street" judgment as to the need for hospitalization.

The failure to review, verify, and document behavioral data and events probably contributes more than any other substantive item to the release of patients by courts. It is especially helpful when people who have witnessed the events that precipitated the referral for commitment are available to give their testimony. In addition to describing these events, they also can describe general patterns of behavior that may illustrate the child's psychopathology and make clear why alternatives to commitment are not realistic.

When a child has stabilized in the treatment setting and no longer meets commitment criteria tied to dangerousness, the clinician must be careful to demonstrate if and how the treatment and the structure of the treatment program remain crucial to maintaining therapeutic gains.

Technical Errors

A variety of technical errors in the commitment process sometimes leads to the release of youths who actually meet commitment criteria. Some of these errors may be as blatant as the child or adolescent having been brought for admission by a person not holding legal custody (e.g., a grandparent). Other errors occur if adequate notice of the commitment hearing is not given, if a signature is misplaced on the commitment form, or if a form is signed by someone who does not hold an appropriate license or qualification. Such errors would seem to be avoidable, but they often are a product of the turmoil surrounding a commitment. However they occur, if they constitute an abridgement of due process, they may establish a basis for denying or dissolving a commitment and releasing the child.

Clinical Issues and Liabilities

Some of the clinical issues associated with commitment have been described previously in "Clinical Phenomena Associated With Conflicts Regarding Commitment." The child and family who have been well prepared for the commitment hearing, who know who will say what during the testimony, who are prepared for a redisclosure of traumatic incidents, and who are prepared for testimony regarding diagnosis and the presence of mental illness, will generally tolerate the proceeding with no serious disruption in clinical treatment. The adolescent whose clinician deals with him openly and without defensiveness or anger is less likely to experience the commitment process as one more circumstance in which he has been victimized by a powerful adult. A clinician who includes in his testimony some of the positive things about the child and his treatment gains may thereby neutralize some of the harshness of the testimony that argues in favor of commitment.

Clinicians rarely are sued because of their involvement in commitment proceedings. In most jurisdictions they are protected by "good faith" presumptions, which hold that, when acting in good faith (rather than acting vindictively or capriciously) in the discharge of their official duties, clinicians are immune from suit, even if error is found.

The most common form of error or malfeasance occurs when a beleaguered clinician, faced with overwhelmed parents and a child who has no other place of safety to go, bends statutory criteria to make a case for commitment on the basis of dangerousness. Other parties to the commitment process, particularly those with no responsibility for the child, often recognize such distortions. When such distortions become obvious, the court may be forced to deny or dissolve a commitment; the child then must be returned to the custody of his already overwhelmed family (i.e., to the very people who requested the child's commitment). Although such distortions of the commitment process may not lead to suit, they create distrust and resentment within the continuum of care and may become the basis for irritated clinicians bringing ethics complaints against their colleagues.

Clinical Sequelae of the Commitment Process

We have described some of the most common disturbances in treatment resulting from untoward commitment hearings (see "Clinical Phenomena Associated With Conflicts Regarding Commitment"). The following clinical vignette provides a particularly helpful illustration of some of the issues and problems that can emerge from the commitment process. Most of these difficulties have to do with the fact that commitment hearings have the potential to force a clinician into multiple and contradictory roles vis-à-vis his or her patient.

> An adolescent patient who was treated by a trainee under my supervision decided to contest his admission and commitment in court. I represented the hospital at the hearing and the judge ruled in favor of the boy's continued treatment. The whole event was quite distressing to the patient and he attempted to run away when he reentered the court's waiting room. He then threw an ashtray and had a physical altercation with the technicians who tried to subdue him.
>
> Two months later I became this boy's therapist when the trainee's placement ended. We spent several sessions dealing with his still intense feelings regarding the court hearing. He remained angry that I had written negative things about his behavior and testified that he was mentally ill. He also was embarrassed that I had witnessed his outbursts following the hearing. It was remarkable to me that, two months later, his memories of the hearing remained so vivid and continued to constitute a significant barrier to the development of a therapeutic relationship.
>
> We eventually were able to work through the situation; however, given the short-term nature of our treatment, it was unfortunate that we were forced to give so much time to dealing with his reaction to the court hearing. It was clear that the events surrounding the hearing constituted one more assault on his damaged self-esteem. In fairness, many patients proceed through the court process with few complications. However, there also have been occasions when I have had to "mop up the mess" therapeutically with patients who experienced the court process as a loss of control, a public humiliation, or an adversarial interaction—not just with the judicial system, but with their therapists and other treatment team members as well. In particular, it is extremely difficult to write a court document that will be specific and decisive enough to ensure a favorable ruling from the judge, yet still be benign enough to be heard by the patient without negative reactions. (A. Margolis, personal communication, June 1990)

CASE EXAMPLE EPILOGUES

Case Example 1

Margie's impulsive suicide attempt seemed intended to provide an escape from the wrath she anticipated from her parents regarding her pregnancy. By refusing to identify her parents and by continuing to hint that she intended to harm herself, she created a situation in which the consulting psychiatrist felt compelled to petition for involuntary commitment in view of Margie's "imminent danger to self." A magistrate and a second physician concurred and (in Margie's home state) this allowed her to be placed in the hospital's locked psychiatric unit for up to 10 days. At that point a court hearing would be held to determine whether the commitment should be extended or not. Thus Margie was detained and provided with short-term treatment despite the fact that she did not agree to such treatment and her parents were initially unavailable to provide their consent. This procedure is typically referred to as an "involuntary commitment" or "involuntary hospitalization." It is common throughout the United States and is used with children, adolescents, and adults alike, given a finding of "imminent danger to self or others." In Margie's case, the hospitalization gave clinicians time to locate and contact her parents, to engage Margie and her parents in family treatment, and to make some inroads on the estrangement between Margie and her parents.

Margie's dysthymia remitted quickly, and outpatient resources were located which could provide continuing treatment to Margie and her parents. Once it appeared that it was safe for Margie to return home, she was discharged in the custody of her parents. Because the discharge occurred less than 10 days after her initial commitment, there was no need for a second commitment hearing.

Case Example 2

In the case of Paul, the 15-year-old boy with conduct disorder who was willing to consider inpatient evaluation and treatment only because he wanted to avoid his other option, prosecution within the juvenile justice system, the clinician arranged for his admission for an extended evaluation on an inpatient psychiatric unit specializing in the treatment of adolescent conduct disorders.

Paul's parents agreed to and supported this plan. However, in North Carolina such a voluntary admission (voluntary not in Paul's eyes, but in those of his parents) still requires ratification by the court. The judge agreed with the clinicians and granted a 30-day commitment, at the end of which time the court would review Paul's situation and either continue or terminate his commitment.

In some other jurisdictions a parent or guardian may consent to the inpatient treatment of a minor *without* such judicial review, even when the child objects and even when there is no "imminent danger to self or others."

In still other jurisdictions an older child (age 12, 14, or 16 years) may herself consent to hospitalization, either alone or in concert with a guardian.

Each of these admissions would be considered voluntary, although this term is obviously a misnomer when the child objects or when the guardian has not been involved in the decision.

Case Example 3

For Jenny, the 13-year-old with a disabling separation anxiety disorder, the treating child psychiatrist recommended long-term inpatient treatment. In her home state, however, Jenny's parents' decision to request inpatient treatment was not enough. Even though her psychiatrist and hospital staff supported the parents' decision, her admission still required judicial review. Several professionals who had worked with Jenny (both in her school and in outpatient treatment) testified regarding the details of her severe and disabling separation anxieties, their unsuccessful attempts to help Jenny with these anxieties, and their conviction that Jenny's problems required this level of restrictive treatment. Although Jenny and her attorney argued against this position, claiming that she had overcome her difficulties and deserved another chance to prove herself, the court agreed that the preponderance of the evidence lay on the side of those requesting her commitment.

Jenny's lengthy treatment (9 months) was punctuated by several more such hearings, and the court could have chosen to order her discharge at any point along the way. However, since Jenny's clinicians were able to demonstrate both the severity of her disturbance and the progress that she was making as a result of her confinement in the inpatient treatment setting, the court chose to continue Jenny's commitment. Interestingly, these repeated hearings were not all that disruptive to Jenny's treatment. Although she certainly continued to protest against her confinement, the fact that the court took her arguments seriously and required the clinicians treating her to demonstrate why the commitment should continue seemed to reassure Jenny. Her right to liberty—a precious right to anyone, but especially an adolescent—was being protected by due process.

ACTION GUIDELINES

General Principles

A. Clinicians involved in the psychiatric commitment of minor patients should be thoroughly familiar with both the *procedures* and the *criteria* mandated by statutes governing voluntary and involuntary commitments in their jurisdiction.
B. Clinicians should be prepared to articulate for the court the additional clinical principles on which they base their decision of whether or not to support the commitment of a child. Two common principles are "the best interests of the child" and "the least restrictive appropriate placement."

Unfortunately, Voltaire's observation that "the best is the enemy of the good" often holds true in the area of child placement. Solnit and colleagues (1992) have argued that attempts to find the best placement for a child often founder because of limited resources. They propose the "least detrimental" placement as a more realistic alternative.

Similarly, the least restrictive placement is not necessarily an appropriate placement. For some children the only *appropriate* placement is one that is *highly restrictive*—an inpatient psychiatric hospital.

Principles Relevant to the Commitment Hearings

Document Completely

Traditional clinical documentation often does not suffice. The clinician also must gather data specifically relevant to the statutory criteria for commitment of a minor. Incidents that the clinician intends to use in court documents and testimony should be verified. It is especially helpful to include corroborative reports from schools, departments of social service, and juvenile justice authorities. It also is important to document prior attempts to treat the child in less restrictive settings and how these attempts failed.

Document Clearly

Avoid the use of technical terms or jargon. When they are necessary, be prepared to translate them into lay terms. Tie all diagnostic conclusions to examples from the child's behavior and make clear how inpatient treatment may be helpful to the specific problems that led to the referral for commitment.

Avoid Value Judgments

If the court concludes that the commitment statutes are being used to try to control behavior that some consider immoral or illegal, it is likely that commitment will be denied. The clinician must make clear the links between the child's troublesome behavior and the underlying psychopathology that might be expected to respond to inpatient treatment.

Protect the Therapeutic Alliance

When possible, it is best that direct testimony regarding a child's need for inpatient commitment be provided not by the child's therapist but by another clinician or administrator. This testimony should include mention of the child's assets and strengths as well as his or her problems and weaknesses. It is especially helpful to include any indications of progress during treatment (when the child has been committed for some time already).

Minimize Adversarial Aspects

It is important to prepare the child for court. This preparation should include an explanation of the procedures as well as a brief review of anticipated testimony and recommendations. When parents are involved, they also should be prepared for what is to occur and what is to be said. If they intend to testify, it is helpful to go over with them what they intend to say.

Clinicians who plan to testify in favor of a child's commitment should consult with the attorney who will represent the hospital prior to the hearing. It also is sometimes possible to meet with the attorney who will represent the child. Opportunities to educate the child's attorney regarding the child's need for treatment should be welcomed.

Follow Up After the Hearing

It is wise to provide for catharsis, ventilation, and debriefing following court proceedings. Ward staff should be alerted when the child has been upset by the outcome of the hearing. Clinicians should assure the child that they will advocate for the child's release as soon as the goals of hospitalization have been achieved and transition to a less restrictive setting is appropriate.

Miscellaneous

It is crucial that clinicians who are involved in the psychiatric commitment of minor patients take an active role in matters of public policy regarding this special application of the power of the state. By doing so they will demonstrate to their patients, to the courts, and to the public that they are using the powers granted to them in ways that are sensitive to *both* the psychological welfare and the individual liberties of their patients.

Examples include the following:

1. Advocate for responsible advertising on the part of hospitals offering inpatient treatment for children and adolescents.
2. Educate judges, attorneys, and legislators regarding current gaps in the continuum of mental health care for children and problems in current commitment procedures.
3. Acknowledge the conflicts of interest that can occur in the use of commitment, and seek periodic formal independent review of the individuals and institutions involved in such proceedings.

4. Alert members of the public, employers, and legislators to the fact that managed care case managers frequently interfere with commitment proceedings by refusing to authorize reimbursement for inpatient care that has been judged necessary by both clinicians and courts.

REFERENCES

Amaya M, Burlingame WV: Judicial review of psychiatric admissions. J Am Acad Child Adolesc Psychiatry 20:761–776, 1981

American Academy of Child and Adolescent Psychiatry: Inpatient hospital treatment of children and adolescents. Washington, DC, American Academy of Child and Adolescent Psychiatry, 1989 [http://www.aacap.org/publications/policy/ps16.htm]

American Psychological Association: A Model Act for the Mental Health Treatment of Minors. Washington, DC, American Psychological Association, 1984

Arambula D, DeKraai M, Sales B: Law, children, and therapists, in Handbook of Psychotherapy With Children and Adolescents. Edited by Kratochwill T, Morris RJ. Boston, MA, Allyn & Bacon, 1993, pp 583–619

Boswell J: The Kindness of Strangers: The Abandonment of Children in Western Europe From Late Antiquity to the Renaissance. New York, Pantheon, 1988

Burlingame WV, Amaya M: Psychiatric commitment of children and adolescents, in Emerging Issues in Child Psychiatry and the Law. Edited by Schetky D, Benedek E. New York, Brunner/Mazel, 1985, pp 229–249

Committee on the Civil Commitment of Minors, Division of Child, Youth, and Family Services of the American Psychological Association: A model act for the mental health treatment of minors, in No Place to Go: The Civil Commitment of Minors. Edited by Melton GB, Lyons PM, Spaulding WJ. Lincoln, NE, University of Nebraska Press, 1998, pp 163–180

Division of Mental Health and Prevention of Substance Abuse, World Health Organization: Mental health care law: ten basic principles (with annotations suggesting selected actions to promote their implementation). Geneva, Switzerland, World Health Organization, 1996 [http://www.who.int/msa/mnh/mnd/legal.htm]

Guidelines for the psychiatric hospitalization of minors. Am J Psychiatry 139:971–974, 1982

In re Gault, 387 US 1 (1967)

Knitzer J: Unclaimed Children. Washington, DC, Children's Defense Fund, 1982

Lerman P: Trends and issues in the deinstitutionalization of youths in trouble. Crime and Delinquency 26(3):281–298, 1980

Melton GB, Lyons PM, Spaulding WJ: No Place to Go: The Civil Commitment of Minors. Lincoln, NE, University of Nebraska Press, 1998

Nurcombe B, Partlett DF: Child Mental Health and the Law. New York, Free Press, 1994

O'Connor v Donaldson, 422 US 563 (1975)

Parham v J.R., 442 US 584 (1979)

Solnit AJ, Nordhaus BF, Lord R: When Home Is No Haven: Child Placement Issues. New Haven, CT, Yale University Press, 1992

Stavis PF: Civil commitment: past, present, and future. Unpublished paper presented to the national conference of the National Alliance for the Mentally Ill, Washington, DC, July 1995 [http://www.cqc.state.ny.us/cc64.htm]

Weithorn L: Mental hospitalization of troublesome youth. Stanford Law Review 40:773–838, 1988

Wilson JP: The Rights of Adolescents in the Mental Health System. Lexington, MA, Lexington Books, 1978

SUGGESTED RESOURCES

American Academy of Child and Adolescent Psychiatry
http://www.aacap.org
American Psychiatric Association
http://www.psych.org
American Psychological Association
http://www.apa.org
National Alliance for the Mentally Ill
http://www.nami.org
National Association of Social Workers
http://www.socialworkers.org
National Guideline Clearinghouse
http://www.guideline.gov/index.asp
National Institute of Mental Health
http://www.nimh.nih.gov

CHAPTER 32

Legal Aspects of Mental Retardation

James C. Harris, M.D.

Case Example 1

William, a 19-year-old mildly mentally retarded male who lives at home with his parents, has been referred for evaluation after being convicted of fire setting. His attorney is concerned about his enthusiasm in confessing not only to these fires but also to a series of other fires that took place in areas where he is not known to have access. Furthermore, although he was seen in the area where the first fires occurred (those he was convicted of setting), there were no witnesses to the fire setting. He has a history of aggressive behavior with his father and of two brief hospitalizations that took place following outbursts of temper and aggressive behavior. When interviewed, he talks rapidly in the initial part of the examination about how the family television set caught on fire many years ago. When he thinks about the television set burning, he gets excited and feels the need to exercise to settle himself down.

Case Example 2

Raymond, a 19-year-old profoundly mentally retarded male with cri du chat syndrome, is referred for evaluation of self-injury (hand biting), sleep disturbance, and genital self-stimulation. He is a short, dysmorphic, nonverbal adolescent male who shows aggressive behavior toward both parents. When not attended to, he falls to the floor and attempts to masturbate through his clothing. His mother is embarrassed by his behavior and also expresses concern that he may harm himself. She reports that he roams the house at night keeping the family awake.

He is admitted to the hospital for treatment of his symptoms but fails to respond to behavioral treatment; he continues to be constantly preoccupied with finding objects to use for masturbation. A trial of an antilibidinal agent, Provera, is recommended, but staff members raise questions about his legal rights regarding informed consent for the use of this medication.

Case Example 3

David, a 24-year-old male who is mildly to moderately mentally retarded and has brain damage (mental age 9–10 years), is seen for evaluation after killing the owner of a convenience store where David had worked part-time. After stealing merchandise from the store, he got in an argument with the owner over the theft. He then went to his family home and returned to the store with a gun, killing the owner after a second argument ensued. Is he competent to stand trial and participate in his own defense? The death penalty is a particular concern for his family, and they ask if the death penalty can be applied to a mentally retarded person.

MENTAL RETARDATION

Definition of Mental Retardation

Mental retardation refers to significantly subaverage intellectual function along with concurrent deficits or impairments in present adaptive functioning (i.e., the person's effectiveness in meeting the standards expected for his or her age by his or her cultural group, in at least two of the following skill areas: communication, self-care, home living, social/interpersonal skills, use of community resources, self-direction, functional academic skills, work, leisure, health, and safety). The onset is before age 18 (American Association on Mental Retardation [AAMR] 1992; American Psychiatric Association 2000). The DSM-IV-TR (American Psychiatric Association 2000) and AAMR classifications should be consulted for further details regarding definition. This chapter uses the term *mental retardation* because it is the current usage in the AAMR and DSM-IV-TR classification systems. However, the terms *intellectual disability* and *developmental cognitive disability* are increasingly used, and one of these terms may become the preferred usage.

Significantly subaverage general intellectual functioning refers to the ability to learn and is measured by the intelligence quotient. Subaverage intellectual functioning is defined as an IQ of below 70 with a variation in measurement error of approximately 5 IQ points. However, the intelligence test alone is not an adequate assessment, because an individual may come from deprived circumstances and the test itself could be culturally biased. More specifically, IQ tests do not accurately measure how an individual may function in society, although they may predict educational progress. The deficits in adaptive behavior are included to indicate that IQ tests alone are not an accurate measure of a mentally retarded person's functioning. Adaptive behavior has been defined as "insignificant limitations in an individual's effectiveness or the degree with which the individual meets the standards of maturation, learning, personal independence and/or social responsibility expected of his age and cultural group" (Grossman 1983, p. 11). This includes the areas of social skills and responsibility as listed.

Mental retardation is not a disease or illness in itself. In those individuals classified as mentally retarded, thinking is not characteristically disordered and perception is not distorted unless there is a concurrent mental disorder. Mental retardation is made up of a heterogeneous group of conditions that range from genetic and metabolic disorders to functional changes that follow trauma to the nervous system at birth or later in the developmental period. Because of this heterogeneity, each case must be considered independently according to whether or not there is an associated syndrome (e.g., Down syndrome) or an associated etiology (e.g., head trauma).

Although the mentally retarded person may also have a diagnosis of a major psychiatric condition, his or her day-to-day problems ordinarily relate to difficulties in developmental functioning. Depending on the degree of cognitive ability, there may be deficits in abstract thinking, in social judgment, and in his or her fund of general information. Difficulties in these areas, if appropriate to the person's cognitive level, are not evidence of a mental disorder. (At the time of examination, it should be ascertained whether the individual was previously functioning at a higher level and has lost skills and regressed.) The mentally retarded person will develop over time and pass through the same developmental stages as a non–mentally retarded person but will not reach the higher levels of cognitive functioning. Abilities are reduced in all areas of functioning, including language, language communication, memory, attention, self-concept, suggestibility, knowledge base, control of impulsivity, moral development, and overall motivation. From a legal perspective, difficulty in logical thinking, planning strategies for action, and foresight are among the most important deficits. Furthermore, there is an intellectual rigidity associated with mental retardation, which may be seen as an impaired ability to learn from mistakes and difficulty in mentally generating a range of options to choose from in a new situation, particularly when stressed. A mentally retarded adult with a mental age of 6 years may show less flexibility in thinking than a non–mentally retarded 6-year-old. However, the mentally retarded adult will have more life experience on which to base his or her options than a child of equivalent mental age.

Levels of Severity of Mental Retardation

Mental retardation is divided into four degrees of severity reflecting the amount of intellectual impairment: mild, moderate, severe, and profound. Although an intelligence test is not the sole basis for determining if someone is mentally retarded, these tests are the accepted standard to measure the degree of severity of mental retardation. Profound mental retardation is an IQ of less than 20 (adult mental age less than 3 years), severe is an IQ of 20 to 34 (adult mental age 3 to less than 6 years), moderate is an IQ of 35 to 49 (adult mental age 6 to 8 years), and mild is an IQ of 50 to 69 (adult mental age 8 to 11 years) (World Health Organization 1992). Intelligence scores are based on the assessment of a variety of relatively specific skills. Although these skills generally develop together, there may be wide discrepancies between subtest scores (Jones et al. 1988) (e.g., language functioning may be low and performance on tests of visuospatial skills much higher). Because of this scattering of skills, the test profile must be considered with regard to adaptive functioning. Moreover, if there are large discrepancies between verbal and performance scores, the full-scale IQ may not adequately reflect true ability level. In these cases neuropsychological testing may be needed to clarify cognitive functions. Tests of adaptive behavior that are used in conjunction with intelligence tests include the AAMR Adaptive Behavior Scale and the Vineland Adaptive Behavior Scales. The overall occurrence of mental retardation (Bregman and Harris 1995) is estimated to be approximately 3% of the school-age population. In the adult population, the occurrence of mental retardation is about 1%, because many mildly mentally retarded persons may adapt in society following an appropriate education and the more severely mentally retarded persons who have medical complications may not survive into adulthood. Of the mentally retarded population, 85% fall into the mildly mentally retarded range, and the remaining 15% are moderately, severely, or profoundly mentally retarded. Those persons who function in the mildly mentally retarded range are the ones most likely to be involved in criminal proceedings and may be found to be legally competent.

Multiaxial Classification

DSM-IV-TR includes mental retardation on Axis II, the designated developmental axis. Mental disorders occurring in mentally retarded persons are coded on Axis I, and multiple psychiatric diagnoses may be listed. Medical conditions that relate to mental retardation are classified on Axis III. Psychosocial complications that commonly occur in the lives of mentally retarded persons are coded on Axis IV, and global adaptive functioning is coded on Axis V. This multiaxial approach allows for the diagnosis of mental retardation, mental disorders that may be associated with mental retardation, and physical conditions that may be etiologically important regarding mental retardation. In program planning, the multiaxial classification is of particular importance, as it designates each of the areas that are important in treatment planning and highlights those areas that are of most importance in evaluating the overall function of the mentally retarded person. The AAMR (1992) uses a multidimensional approach with four dimensions: 1) intellectual functioning and adaptive skills, 2) psychological/emotional considerations, 3) physical/health/etiology considerations, and 4) environmental considerations.

Normalization—The Developmental Model

Mental retardation is a permanent condition and is not curable, although the degree of habilitation that can be accomplished for the mentally retarded person can be substantial. Deficits in current adaptive functioning are major targets for intervention. During the past 20 years, a focus on a developmental model that acknowledges the capability for growth, of developing independence in social skills, and of new learning has been emphasized. The developmental model specifically addresses the fact that the mentally retarded person's level of functioning is not static and that an individual's adaptive behavior may be improved through habilitation. Because a mentally retarded person is capable of learning and adapting, legal approaches need to take into account that the mentally retarded person, although he or she may require additional education and instructional effort, can learn new information.

The focus on normalization (Wofenberger 1972) for mentally retarded persons has emphasized as important that mentally retarded persons are entitled to services that are as culturally normative as possible in order to help them establish and maintain more appropriate personal behavior. Normalization emphasizes that mentally retarded persons should live in the community, go to regular schools, seek competitive employment, and behave as closely as possible to the standards of non–mentally retarded persons at a comparable developmental age. They should be responsible for their own behavior, and others should not assume that because they are mentally retarded, they lack that capability. Their differences and their need for individual assessment must be recognized to guarantee that services are provided (Simpson 1998). For normalization it is proposed that not only must social competence be a critical focus in treatment programs but that an ethical approach that recognizes interests, desires, and preferences of the individual is also needed (Simpson 1998). One risk is excessive programming for an individual, with a lack of allowance for personal choices.

Sexuality in Mental Retardation

Mentally retarded persons may be stereotyped regarding the expression of sexuality (Abram et al. 1988; Bregman and Harris 1995; Harris 1998). On one hand, they may be thought of as sexually uninhibited; on the other hand, they may be considered eternal children or asexual and not having sexual interests and needs. Because of the former assumption, as well as concerns about heritability, sterilization of mentally retarded persons was practiced in the past, and some states still have such legislation. Although this has not been the case, it was feared that mentally retarded individuals would procreate indiscriminately, leading to an increase in the incidence of mental retardation. Consequently, involuntary sterilizations (Appelbaum 1982; Denekens et al. 1999) have been performed and marriages between mentally retarded persons were often prohibited. In some circumstances, a mentally retarded person was denied the opportunity to socialize and develop an intimate relationship with someone of the opposite sex.

It is ordinarily after puberty that sexual interest becomes apparent; however, puberty may be delayed in some mentally retarded persons secondary to the disorder that underlies the retardation. Regardless of the age at pubertal onset, profoundly and severely mentally retarded individuals may show little interest in sexual behavior toward others. However, mildly mentally retarded individuals and many moderately mentally retarded persons may have normal pubertal development, demonstrate appropriate sexual interests, and establish sexual identities.

When their expressions of sexual interest are denied, sexual activity may be a response used to demonstrate a sense of self-importance and be aimed at gaining acceptance from others. Sexual status may be important for their peer group, just as it is for those who are not mentally retarded. The encouragement of a relationship with another person and the learning of social skills are essential and must precede specific instructions about sexual activity.

Mentally retarded persons, particularly women, may be exploited sexually. Their knowledge of sexuality is often not fully developed because the usual sources of information may not available to them. Peer relationships, printed reading material, and sex education in school are often limited or unavailable for mentally retarded persons. Furthermore, family members may be reluctant to review sexual matters with them. Mildly and moderately mentally retarded adolescents frequently lack basic information on sexual anatomy, contraceptive issues, and venereal disease. Their knowledge of sexuality often is related more to life experience and opportunity than to intelligence level.

LEGAL ISSUES

Scope of Psychiatric Involvement

The forensic examiner may be called on to evaluate mentally retarded persons in a variety of situations that have legal implications. To properly conduct these assessments, background information is needed regarding the nature and etiology of mental retardation, an understanding of the legal rights of mentally retarded persons, recognition that mental retardation is a vulnerability factor in mental illness, and awareness of developmental issues that relate to mental retardation (e.g., attachment, sexuality, aggression, moral development, attention processes, and memory formation). The issue of brain damage in mental retardation and its relationship to aggression and social disinhibition, the use of psychotropic drugs and their complications (Reiss and Aman 1998), and the recognition of the heterogeneity of mental retardation syndromes (e.g., Down syndrome, fragile X syndrome, XYY syndrome, and so on) must be considered.

Psychiatrists may evaluate mentally retarded persons in a variety of settings: emergency rooms, where aggression toward self or others may present or where abuse of the mentally retarded person is questioned; forensic evaluations, in which there may be questions of competency to stand trial, to act as a witness, or to serve on juries; the clinic, in circumstances when an assessment of parenting skills or a diagnostic evaluation may be requested; and the school, where questions are raised about the least restrictive environment for education. Questions of legal rights are common (e.g., access to education, participation in decisions about medical treatment, access to medical records by mentally retarded adults, and the utilization of a guardian to guarantee the rights of an incompetent mentally retarded person). To adequately conduct these evaluations, the psychiatrist needs to be aware of the legal rights legislation that relates to mentally retarded individuals as well as the more traditional forensic concerns that relate to competence.

The forensic examiner must consider the special case that arises when a person who has been in an institution for much of his or her lifetime is deinstitutionalized and commits a criminal act without knowing that it is against the law. The person has not learned the law during his or her institutional stay (Bregman and Harris 1995). Furthermore, during the institutional stay, there may have been no opportunity to be involved in an illegal action.

The Insanity Defense and Culpability

Formulations of the insanity defense traditionally base the defense on "mental disease or defect," the latter referring to mental retardation, which can be used as a basis for the insanity defense (Menninger 1986). Ordinarily, the culpability of persons with mental retardation can be considered as reduced, so mental retardation can be considered to be a mitigating circumstance. Mental disorder and mental retardation both must be considered in decisions regarding the insanity defense. The distinction between them is clearly made in international classifications of disorders and diseases. However, this distinction is sometimes blurred in the courts. This blurring may occur because cases brought for criminal action may involve both mental retardation and a mental disorder, which both must then be taken into account in the assessment process.

In cases involving mentally retarded individuals, the insanity defense is most frequently considered in murder cases in which the question of the culpability of a mentally retarded person is raised. Culpability refers to the capacity of the accused to distinguish right from wrong. As noted in Chapter 29, "State-of-Mind Assessments: Competency and Criminal Responsibility," the M'Naughten Rule (1843) has been replaced in federal courts and many jurisdictions by the American Law Institute standard, which states: "A person is not responsible for criminal conduct if at the time of such conduct as a result of mental disease or defect, he lacks substantial capacity either to *appreciate* the criminality (wrongfulness) of his conduct or to conform his conduct to the requirements of the law [emphasis added]." The difference in wording focuses on substituting the word appreciate, which suggests both emotional and cognitive awareness, for the word know. Knowing that an act is wrong may indicate only surface knowledge of its wrongfulness without a full appreciation of why it is wrong (Menninger 1986). Furthermore, even if they know an act is wrong, because of excessive impulsiveness, enhanced suggestibility, or acquiescence to authority, mentally retarded persons may have difficulty in conforming their conduct to the law (Luckasson 1988).

Competency

In addition to competency to stand trial, which is covered in Chapter 29, "State-of-Mind Assessments: Competency and Criminal Responsibility," forensic assessments may be requested regarding competency to be a witness or juror, to manage one's own affairs, to care for oneself, and to parent. Basic elements of competency include 1) the ability to understand information presented regarding the consequences of the decision that is made, 2) the ability to consider alternatives before making a decision, 3) the manner in which the decision is made (weighing the alternatives and expressing a preference), and 4) the nature of and degree of commitment to the final decision (Kaplan et al. 1988). A competent decision requires comprehension of the issues, autonomy in decision making, a rational, reasoned process, an awareness of the future consequences of the decision, and the judgment to make choices despite uncertainty of the outcome. An accused person should not be allowed to waive a competency examination, and all parties involved in the process have a duty to raise the issue of competency if there is any doubt (*Pate v. Robinson* 1966).

Competency to Stand Trial

Persons accused of a crime cannot be tried for that crime unless they understand both the charge that is made against them and the consequences if they are convicted (Buescher and Dinerstein 1999; Curran 1972; *Dusky v. United States* 1960; Golding et al. 1984; Heller et al. 1981; see also Chapter 29 of this text). Furthermore, the individual must be able to aid his lawyer in his defense. A mentally retarded person may have difficulties in each of these situations because of limited ability to understand the charges or their consequences due to reduced intelligence, lack of life experience, inadequate educa-

tion, a tendency to be overly concerned with pleasing others, or a fear of the authorities.

In most states a defendant in a criminal trial who is thought to be incompetent is committed to a mental hospital for further assessment. If he is found to be incompetent, he will stay in the hospital for assessment, after which he may be released or committed on civil grounds. There is the expectation that the individual may become competent at a later date when the illness is resolved. For mentally ill persons who are not mentally retarded, this may be the case; however, the acquisition of later competence is more complicated in the case of mental retardation. Consequently, mentally retarded persons have been committed to institutions for life after being accused of offenses that are minor. Had they been tried for them and convicted, they may not have been incarcerated at all. The U.S. Supreme Court considered that situation in *Jackson v. Indiana* (1972), a case that involved a deafmute mentally retarded man who was charged with stealing a coat. The determination was that Jackson's lengthy hospitalization was not justified on the grounds of restoring the mentally retarded person to competency. The court noted that due process requires that the nature and duration of commitment bear a relationship to the purpose for the commitment. It ruled that if an individual is committed because of his incapacity to proceed to trial, he cannot be held more than a reasonable time in order to determine if there is a substantial probability that he will obtain that capacity in the foreseeable future. If he cannot achieve competency, the state must institute customary civil commitment proceedings, as would be the case for other citizens, or release the defendant. If it is thought that the individual will be able to stand trial, continued commitment must be justified by evidence that progress is being made toward accomplishment of that goal.

Competency to Testify

In certain circumstances, a mentally retarded person may be asked to testify for the prosecution in a criminal case. The defense may argue that she is not competent to be a witness and raise questions about her reliability. A witness is not specifically disqualified by law simply because she is mentally retarded, but an individual assessment of her competency to testify may be required. To do so, the prospective witness must understand that she may be punished for not telling the truth. She must be able to demonstrate the ability to recall and to report past events accurately. In this instance, the assessment of the mentally retarded person to testify will require an evaluation of her language and memory capabilities, her personal understanding of the meaning of the alleged crime, the pressures exerted by others on her, and her capacity to differentiate reality from fantasy. The final determination of credibility of the mentally retarded witness will be up to the court and jury. The evaluation of a mentally retarded potential witness should include whether or not there is a past history of compulsive reporting of fantasy stories regarding the issue in question. The impact on her of testifying on the witness stand should also be considered, particularly if testimony is directed toward a family member or guardian who has a supervisory role for the mentally retarded person (Bregman and Harris 1995).

Confessions

Mentally retarded persons are at risk of giving a nonvoluntary confession (Praiss 1989). In confessions it is important to measure understanding and suggestibility in defendants (Everington and Fulero 1999). A criminal confession in response to questioning while in custody cannot be used in evidence unless the defendant voluntarily, knowingly, and intelligently waived Miranda rights. These rights ensure that when a person is taken into custody he is informed of his Fifth Amendment right to remain silent and to have counsel retained or appointed before an admissible confession can be obtained. A mentally retarded person requires a thorough explanation of these rights. Because of adaptive problems and intellectual limitations, care is needed in determining whether the waiver of rights is valid. Because of a mentally retarded person's special needs, counsel should be sought as early as the precustodial stage. A mentally retarded person's waiver is best protected, and more likely to be voluntary, with early access to an attorney and a familiar person.

Partial Competency and Guardianship

Mentally retarded persons may be competent to carry out some but not all of their affairs. A person who is mentally retarded and who has difficulty in managing financial affairs (Kapp 1981; Mesibov et al. 1980) but can handle other activities may have a guardian appointed to decide only financial matters. The view is that the mentally retarded person is partially competent in handling his affairs. The assignment of a guardian may be determined by the degree of mental retardation (O'Sullivan 1999). Mildly and moderately mentally retarded individuals need to be judged on the basis of their adaptive functioning and not their IQ scores alone. However, severely and profoundly mentally retarded individuals will usually need to have a guardian assigned to them when they reach maturity.

Parental Competency

The ability to care for a child on a day-to-day basis, to make future plans for his or her child, and to consistently set limits on behavior must be evaluated in the mentally retarded parent (Feldman 1986; Keltner 1999). Mentally retarded adults may be overrepresented among neglectful parents but not necessarily among abusive parents (Schilling et al. 1982; Seagull and Scheurer 1986; Tymchuk et al. 1999). Mental retardation, per se, is not automatically considered evidence for lack of competency in child care, although it is increasingly evident that successful parenting by a mentally retarded person is fraught with difficulty, particularly in the care of children beyond infancy (Whitman and Accardo 1990). Children of mentally retarded parents are at risk for mental retardation, but a substantial number—60% to 70%—studied by Accardo and Whitman (1990; Whitman and Accardo 1989) were not mentally retarded. Factual evidence of competence is necessary for mildly and moderately mentally retarded parents; however, if the parent is severely or profoundly mentally retarded, then the child will ordinarily require placement. Considerable efforts may be needed to teach parenting skills to mentally retarded adults. This may be attempted either through group or individual instruction with the additional provision of ongoing home support services. In some settings, both the parent and the child may be placed in a foster home. Here the foster parents can assume overall responsibility for the child's care, and the natural parent can assist them as he or she learns new skills. Issues of parenting by a mentally retarded person are of particular importance when there are multiple children in the home and when the mentally retarded person has a child of normal intelligence. The adolescent who is not mentally retarded may have particular difficulties in relating to a mentally retarded parent.

Rights of Incompetent Persons

Some mentally retarded individuals will be mentally incompetent from birth, and the protection of their constitutional rights is an ongoing consideration throughout their lifetime. The issues that come up most often relate to procreation, sterilization (Appelbaum 1982; Denekens et al. 1999), rights regarding involuntary institutionalization, giving consent to sexual activity (Stavis and Walker-Hirsch 1999), and the right of others to initiate medical intervention (Brakman and Amari-Vaught 1999; Sundram 1988; Wong et al. 1999) or to terminate life-sustaining treatment. A mentally incompetent, developmentally disabled individual is generally unable to exercise these rights. The procedural safeguards necessary to guarantee his rights even though he is incompetent are important to consider. How best to preserve the mentally retarded person's autonomy despite his incompetence has been considered in several ways. Legislation focusing on the best interests test is one recent standard. This standard is contrasted with the substituted judgment test.

An incompetent mentally retarded person cannot function normally in society or voluntarily give consent regarding decisions about his well-being; others must make decisions for him. These include the choice to undergo or terminate life-sustaining treatment; the right to reproduce; and the right to remain in the community and not be institutionalized. These rights have been considered constitutionally protected (Roesch and Golding 1979). However, the right of self-determination is exercised not by the mentally retarded person but by another person—a parent or guardian appointed by the state through the courts.

The approach to the right of self-determination for incompetent individuals includes the best interests test and the substituted judgment test. In the best interests test, the focus is primarily on the needs of an incompetent person. His expressed desires or intentions are considered but may be disregarded depending on the circumstances. In the substituted judgment test, the court renders the decision for the developmentally disabled person that it believes the person would render for himself if he were competent. The substituted judgment test has been questioned, as it may lead to excessive involvement of the courts in matters that can be handled more personally and expeditiously by a guardian or family member. The best interests procedure may lead to better accountability and avoids the abstractions inherent in the court's assumption of how a person who has never been competent would make a decision.

Procedural safeguards that are available to protect the rights of the incompetent individual include the appointment of a guardian *ad litem*, an adversarial hearing, and limits on the control by the court. A mandatory due process hearing may be required for specific issues regarding the mentally retarded person (e.g., sterilization). In the due process hearing several issues must be addressed, including the opportunity to be heard and to question and cross-examine witnesses and the right to offer evidence. Such hearings may be necessary when there is a question as to whether a family is acting in the best interests of their mentally retarded member and whether that mentally retarded person's constitutional rights are being protected.

Regarding the role of the court, the judge must weigh the overall circumstances with regard to determining both the rights of an incompetent litigant and those of family members. Family stability must be considered in reviewing the constitutional rights of the mentally retarded person. For example, a family might not be able to control a very aggressive child or may not be able to provide for the person's basic physical needs, such as dressing, toileting, and transporting the mentally retarded juvenile or adolescent family member. The court would need to balance the constitutional interests of the child and the reasonable interests of the family who cannot properly care for the child at home.

Sterilization and Antilibidinal Agents

Legal issues regarding the use of antilibidinal agents (Clarke 1989) may come to the attention of the court in relation to legal rights and in cases in which sexual deviancy is at issue. The sterilization of mentally retarded persons has also been an area of continuing concern (Webster 1985). The Mental Health Law Project has recommended standards (Rousso 1984). These standards require representation by a disinterested guardian *ad litem*, independent evaluation of the individual, and the finding that the individual is not capable of and not able to develop the capacity to make an informed judgment. The individual also must be physically capable of procreation, likely to engage in sexual activity, and permanently incapable of taking care of a child. Furthermore, there must be no alternatives to sterilization. The major concerns are to protect the individual's rights and to follow due process.

Responsibility in Capital Crimes—Murder

The U.S. Supreme Court has indicated that mental retardation must be considered as a mitigating circumstance in capital crimes. However, the Court has not ruled out the possibility that a mentally retarded person could be given the death penalty. The issue is most likely to arise with a mildly mentally retarded person. Deliberations in *Penry v. Lynaugh* (1989) (Keyes and Edwards 1997; Keyes et al. 1998) suggest that the death penalty most likely would not be applied to severely or profoundly mentally retarded persons. The *Penry* case was reconsidered by the U.S. Superior Court in 2001 after Penry was found guilty of murder a second time (*Penry v. Johnson*) following the initial U.S. Supreme Court decision. The Supreme Court vacated the second trial because of inadequate jury instruction, stating that a sentence must be allowed to give *full* consideration and *full* effect to mitigating circumstances. The jury must be given "a vehicle for expressing its reasoned moral response to the evidence in rendering its sentencing decision so that we can be sure that the jury has treated the defendant as a uniquely individual human being and has made a reliable determination that death is the appropriate sentence" (*Penry v. Johnson* 2001). Moreover, the sentence imposed must "reflect a reasoned moral response to the defendant's background, character, and crime."

Because mental retardation is a mitigating circumstance, efforts may be made by an attorney to demonstrate that a person whose IQ is in the borderline range functions adaptively in the mentally retarded range. Finally, evaluation of the specific profile on psychological tests and formal assessment of adaptive functioning may be critical in the assessment because test scatter makes it difficult to assess IQ accurately.

The AAMR's position is that no mentally retarded person should be sentenced to death or executed. They suggest that such executions serve no purpose penologically, are disproportionate to the mentally retarded person's culpability, do not consider degree of moral blameworthiness in mentally retarded persons, and are a cruel and unusual punishment for someone who is developmentally disabled.

Since 1976, when the U.S. Supreme Court reinstated the death penalty, 33 men with mental retardation have been executed in the United States. Currently, 13 state laws and a federal law prohibit the execution of people with mental retardation (Keyes et al. 1998), and such legislation is pending in several other states. Keyes and colleagues (1998) found that defense lawyers did not raise the issue of the defendant's mental retardation as a mitigating factor in almost one-third of capital cases in which that evidence was pertinent to the case.

CLINICAL ISSUES

Forensic Assessment

It is a basic right of a mentally retarded person to be responsible for himself and to be held accountable for his own behavior (Bregman and Harris 1995). Suggesting incompetence based on intelligence alone, without considering adaptive ability, diminishes the mentally retarded person as an individual. In criminal cases, the opportunity to stand trial offers the chance for probation, whereas being found incompetent may lead to an indeterminate sentence. When brought in for a forensic assessment, a mentally retarded person may be overwhelmed, particularly if there are legal proceedings that he does not understand. Time and patience by the clinician will be needed to establish a sense of trust and rap-

port and to gain the developmentally disabled person's assent to continue with the assessment. A mentally retarded person may not understand the officer's recitation when his rights are read to him, may not understand the nature of the offense that he is accused of, may not appreciate the consequences of the accusation, and may not know how to defend himself. A more gradual and considered approach that acknowledges his disability may render the individual competent. If one makes the necessary initial efforts at gaining the mentally retarded person's confidence, the assessment can be direct and detailed. The focus is on his self-care skills, his comprehension of the meaning of others' social behavior, and his facility in interpersonal communication. The comprehensive psychiatric examination deals with all these issues, co-occurring psychiatric diagnosis, and the specific legal questions of competency to stand trial as well as those regarding the kind of service programs needed by the individual. This added detailed information about therapeutic programming can then be used by the court in making the final disposition.

Mentally retarded persons, rather than being self-referred, are ordinarily referred for psychiatric assessment by their caretakers. Because they often have difficulty in verbal expression, may have problems in memory, and are generally dependent on the caretaker, the history the caretaker provides is of paramount importance. A variety of special approaches may be needed in interviewing the mentally retarded person; they include devices to augment communication (e.g., communication boards, computers, signing) and interviewing methods used for establishing therapeutic contact with younger children of normal intelligence (e.g., drawings, stories, structured settings). In assessing the mentally retarded person, one must consider, for example, her capacity to understand basic explanations for medical procedures, her degree of credibility and her ability to exercise independent decision making, the ability to advocate for her own rights, her ability to postpone immediate gratification for subsequent benefits, and her knowledge of managing her financial affairs. A past history of ability to carry out these activities is central and should be confirmed in the examination.

It is necessary to use several sources for the history in addition to the family and mentally retarded person herself (e.g., schools, community programs, sheltered workshop staff, job coaches). When eliciting historical information, one must consider not only the specific behaviors of concern but also the circumstances under which the behavior is said to have taken place and how others responded to it. The caretaker's relationship with the mentally retarded person must also be taken into account. The extent of parental recognition of the disability and its meaning to them must be considered in the assessment. Their ability to see the referred person's strengths as well as her weaknesses should be investigated.

Parental Competence

Assessment for parental competency requires a careful review of the individual's personal history and an evaluation of their child or children (Whitman and Accardo 1989). If homemakers have been in the home, information needs to be gathered from the social agency regarding how the homemaker was received. It is important to verify whether or not a homemaker who was placed to help with the children and the mentally retarded adult is aware of the issues of mental retardation and to verify the degree of sensitivity shown toward the parents' ability and efforts. The parents may be familiar with how to provide physical care; however, they may have difficulty with judgment when there are unexpected illnesses or when other new situations arise. The mentally retarded parents' ability to appreciate the unique needs of a child and understand that the child's misbehavior may be a developmental issue en route to greater independence rather than a challenge to their authority will need to be considered. Some mentally retarded parents will be able to provide adequate physical care and nurturance for an infant but may have more difficulty with an older child, particularly an adolescent. The family system evaluation needs to consider what alternatives there are within the family for other family members to assist. This assessment must evaluate whether or not it is in the child's best interests to be placed outside the home at an early age or at a later age, when the parents' caregiving abilities are more strained.

Criminal Liability

The majority of individuals with mental retardation are not prone to criminal or violent behavior. Those that are frequently have multiple risk factors, as pointed out by Lewis et al. (1988). Statistics show that mentally retarded persons may have a higher likelihood of being arrested for criminal behavior, especially for minor delinquent behavior (President's Committee on Mental Retardation 1991). Crimes involving impulsive acts may be disproportionately more common among mentally retarded individuals. One study found no increase in fantasy aggression among mentally retarded offenders but suggested possible difficulties in inhibiting impulses (Silber and Courtless 1968), a finding that bears replication.

Fire setting has also been associated with mental retardation (Foust 1979; Kearns and O'Connor 1988; Yesavage et al. 1983). Rather than a specific cause of criminal behavior, mental retardation and its associated features are risk factors for legal difficulty. It is not mental retardation, per se, but the higher rate of associated behavioral and emotional problems in the mentally retarded population that is of particular concern (Feinstein and Reiss 1996). The likelihood of emotional and behavioral problems is enhanced by frequent psychosocial adversity and central nervous system dysfunction. This increased prevalence of mental disorder further increases mentally retarded persons' vulnerability to acting antisocially. The issue of stigma must also be considered, because "being different" and "being mentally retarded" are factors that influence attitudes in the community. Often, mentally retarded persons are the first ones suspected of delinquency in their neighborhoods because of these attitudes in the community. Yet, in criminal proceedings, mental retardation may be a mitigating circumstance that may lead to a reduction of the offender's personal culpability and moral blameworthiness for the act committed.

Confessions

Clinically, the mentally retarded person may be considered to be a normalized individual with limited learning capacity and problems in adaptation. Characteristics of mental retardation may impede voluntary and intelligent constitutional waiver of rights by a mentally retarded person. Competency must also be considered regarding the reliability of a confession to a crime made by a mentally retarded person (Praiss 1989). A mentally retarded defendant who has pleaded guilty may be referred to a psychiatrist to determine whether he was competent to do so. In some instances, mentally retarded persons have insisted that they were guilty and should be in prison. In these cases, the individual may be responding to the attention accorded them at the time of the examination with the hope that this recognition might elevate their standing in the community; they may feel their self-esteem as individuals is enhanced by the proceedings. Thus it is important to carefully assess the degree of understanding and extent of suggestibility found in mentally retarded persons (Everington and Fulero 1999).

A mentally retarded person may be compliant, seek approval, have a desire to be accepted, and demonstrate easy suggestibility. In this way, a compliant mentally retarded person is not a major problem for the police, but the police, in the process of interrogation, may be a major problem because the mentally retarded person may not understand police proceedings. Although there is no specific correlation between mental retardation and criminal behavior, a large number of mentally retarded persons have been incarcerated. Despite the 2% to 3% of the general population who are mentally retarded, up to 10% to 25% of the prison population has tested in the mentally retarded range. In some instances, mentally retarded people may be easily apprehended but may be less often paroled. When they are apprehended, they may assume blame to please their accuser. Mentally retarded persons may also be implicated and used by others who have encouraged them.

Mental retardation does not necessarily preclude the ability to understand the constitutional rights to remain silent and to obtain legal counsel (Buescher and Dinerstein 1999). To reach the appropriate level of comprehension, rights must be slowly and carefully explained in terms that could be understood at the appropriate developmental level. Moreover, adaptive impairments can cause mentally retarded persons to become confused and more dependent in stressful circumstances. This may further inhibit their ability to understand new concepts and make independent decisions. Consequently, a police officer's recitation of the standard Miranda warning may not be understood and the mentally retarded person may not appreciate or have a requisite understanding of his rights and the consequences of waiving them; nor will the person necessarily be able to make a voluntary decision to waive those rights. A further complication is that even if police officers are trained to identify mentally retarded persons and provide an appropriate setting and explanation of their constitutional rights and the consequences of abandoning them, the creation of a favorable environment of warmth and friendliness may, in itself, result in the mentally retarded suspect making a voluntary confession or being induced to make an nonvoluntary confession after waiving his rights. Consideration must also be given to the family and their perspective regarding confession (Cockram et al. 1998).

Psychiatric Diagnosis in Mental Retardation

Vulnerability to Mental Disorder

A mentally retarded and mentally ill defendant raises concerns regarding the relationship between the legal and mental health systems (Williams and Spruill 1987). The prevalence of psychiatric disorders in the mentally retarded population is three to five times that found in the general population (Bregman and Harris 1995). The more severely mentally retarded the child, the greater the likelihood of disturbed behavior and interpersonal relationships (Szymanski and Tanguay 1980). The term *dual diagnosis* has been used in describing psychiatric

disorders in mentally retarded individuals. The mildly mentally retarded individual is prone to the same range of psychiatric disorders as seen in the general population, but their vulnerability is increased as a result of cognitive deficits and their difficulty in social adaptation. Severely and profoundly mentally retarded children are more likely to be vulnerable due to brain disorders that are often associated with genetic syndromes and metabolic diseases. Seizure disorders are the most common neurological problem seen in the mentally retarded population. However, birth trauma is also of considerable importance. Brain dysfunction is a vulnerability factor that increases the likelihood of behavioral and interpersonal difficulties, but not all behavior problems can be ascribed to brain dysfunction.

Mentally retarded persons are just as likely as others in the population to be diagnosed with major mental illnesses, such as depression and schizophrenia (Feinstein and Reiss 1996). Pervasive developmental disorders, which include autism and other forms of pervasive developmental disturbances in language and social behavior, are particularly important to recognize. Services for those with these disorders must include intensive training in social skills because this is the major deficit. The American Academy of Child and Adolescent Psychiatry has published practice parameters for the treatment of mental illness in mentally retarded persons (Szymanski and King 1999) as a guide to more effective practice. Dykens and Hodapp (2001) provide a recent review of psychopathology and pertinent family issues.

THE PROBLEM OF PSYCHOSIS

Of major concern is the diagnosis of psychosis in mentally retarded persons. The application of the diagnosis of psychosis disorder for any disorganized behavior whose etiology may be unclear to the evaluator creates particular concerns. For example, talking to oneself, self-injury, self-stimulation, and unexplained aggression have been attributed to psychosis. Furthermore, the stereotypies and behavior mannerisms that are commonly seen in mental retardation syndromes, particularly in the autistic disorder group, have been misinterpreted as symptoms of psychosis in the past. Historically, a special term, *propfschizophrenie*, was introduced to describe these manifestations. More recent investigations have demonstrated that standard diagnostic criteria can be used in the differential diagnosis of psychosis in mentally retarded persons. Although it may be difficult to differentiate particular subtypes of psychotic presentations, such as schizophrenia in the nonverbal mentally retarded, moderately and mildly mentally retarded persons who are verbal can describe symptoms such as delusions and hallucinations. For the nonverbal group, disorganized behavior and substantial difficulties in interpersonal relations may require the use of atypical or not otherwise specified diagnostic categories. The prevalence of psychotic conditions in mentally retarded persons requires further research.

One must consider the diagnoses of brief psychotic episodes and schizophreniform disorder in mentally retarded persons. Individuals with brain dysfunction are more likely, under severe stress, to show these forms of psychotic manifestation, conditions that might resolve with appropriate supportive interventions. Stress leading to acute panic may result in substantial disorganization, which may result in the misdiagnosis of schizophrenia. These potentially transient psychotic episodes and the manifestations of posttraumatic stress in mentally retarded persons need to be appreciated to avoid unnecessary labeling with a major mental disorder when in fact the episode is an acute reactive one. Mentally retarded persons may not necessarily require any more time to recover from an acute psychotic episode than a non–mentally retarded person.

The diagnosis of schizophrenia may lead to referral to a mental hospital when in fact the individual may actually have one of the other diagnoses mentioned. This may lead to longer periods of incarceration. When mentally retarded defendants are identified, they have the same right to treatment for a diagnosed psychosis as do others who are not mentally retarded. To be found legally competent, treatment for the mental illness is necessary as well as training in the legal system routines and basic courtroom procedures. With treatment for the mental illness and with preparation for testimony, the mentally retarded person may be found to be competent. However, the training period should not begin until the acute psychotic symptoms are resolved. Therefore, mentally retarded, mentally ill defendants may require longer periods of time than non–mentally retarded persons to be found competent or incompetent to stand trial. The condition of mental retardation may require additional due process considerations in the courtroom, but it should not be automatically assumed that a mentally retarded person will remain incompetent to stand trial indefinitely. The majority of mentally retarded defendants, most of whom are mildly mentally retarded, can achieve a basic understanding of courtroom procedures such that they can present themselves favorably and assist their counsel.

MOOD DISORDERS

Mood disorders, particularly depressive disorders, are often not recognized in mentally retarded persons. In the past, it has sometimes been assumed that mentally retarded persons do not become depressed because they lack the cognitive capacity to show self-blame. Furthermore, it was assumed that mentally retarded individuals did not develop low self-esteem because they were unaware of environmental expectations. In fact, mildly and moderately mentally retarded persons often have low self-esteem. Major affective disorders can be diagnosed using modifications of the standard diagnostic criteria for depressive disorder or bipolar disorder. Modifications in the assessment procedures must be made because difficulties in expressive language and difficulty in finding words to describe feelings may be associated with mental retardation. Diagnostic criteria may be difficult to apply, because some require verbal reflection and others assume normal functioning prior to the suspected depression. However, mood disorders may be demonstrated by sad expression, loss of interest in usual activities, and the characteristic changes in appetite and sleep. Unfortunately, individuals who are mentally retarded and depressed may go undiagnosed if their behavior is not disruptive in the home or school setting. Individuals with Down syndrome may be more likely to develop depressive disorders (Harris 1988).

The recognition of low self-esteem in higher functioning mentally retarded persons and the degree of demoralization that these individuals experience is one consideration. Besides the recognition of mood disorders, it is particularly important to identify antisocial behavior associated with mood changes. Irritability and agitation are early signs of a mood disorder that may go unrecognized or be mislabeled as bad behavior. The vulnerability to mood disorders and the fact of low self-esteem in many mentally retarded individuals may be factors in their confessing to crimes that they did not commit. If they are stressed when incarcerated, subsequent stress in prison may provoke a mentally retarded person to act in a self-destructive manner. Suicide is the most important complication of depression in mentally retarded persons.

Manic episodes may also occur in mentally retarded individuals and be associated with antisocial behavior and sometimes with sexual dysfunction. Although the classic manic symptoms (e.g., flight of ideas, grandiosity, spending sprees, and delusions) may not be demonstrated because of a lack of verbal skills, behavioral symptoms such as agitation, hyperactivity, self-injury, aggression, weight loss, sleep disturbance, and mood lability may be recognized.

ATTENTION-DEFICIT/ HYPERACTIVITY DISORDER

Attention-deficit/hyperactivity disorder is another condition that occurs in the mentally retarded population and may go unrecognized if it is assumed that mentally retarded people are necessarily impulsive and hyperactive. Symptoms of impulsivity, distractibility, and hyperactivity need to be assessed in view of the person's developmental level. The extent and intensity of impulsivity and distractibility noted is a diagnostic consideration of importance, because an impulsive act may be an antisocial one. Attention-deficit/hyperactivity disorder—or the diagnosis that is more commonly used in mentally retarded persons, undifferentiated attention-deficit disorder—is an additional vulnerability factor. It may interact with adverse psychosocial situations to contribute to aggressive and antisocial behavior.

PERVASIVE DEVELOPMENTAL DISORDER

Pervasive developmental disorder represents a range of clinical conditions characterized by developmental disturbances, with particular deficits in language and social communication. Both autistic disorder and a general category of pervasive developmental disorder not otherwise specified are listed in the DSM-IV-TR classification. The majority of individuals with the diagnosis of an autistic disorder, 75% to 80%, fall within the mentally retarded range on cognitive testing. It is particularly important to recognize an autistic disorder or autistic features in the mildly mentally retarded person because the deficits in language communication, and particularly in social interaction, may contribute to legal difficulties.

DELIRIUM, DEMENTIA, AND OTHER COGNITIVE DISORDERS

The diagnosis of dementia requires that memory impairment and other cognitive deficits are linked to a specific decline from a documented previous higher level of func-

tioning. For young children the diagnosis of dementia may not be indicated until the child is 4 to 6 years of age (American Psychiatric Association 2000). For those younger than age 18, a diagnosis of dementia is made only if the presentation is not fully characterized by a diagnosis of mental retardation. Delirium may occur in mentally retarded persons from causes such as metabolic insults, and following head trauma.

SEXUALITY IN MENTAL RETARDATION

A minority of mentally retarded individuals may show socially unacceptable sexual behavior that brings them into conflict with the legal system. Early studies of criminology reported an increase in sexual offenses by mentally retarded persons. These studies, however, are questionable on methodological grounds. From a legal point of view, important issues that have to do with the rights of the individual include sterilization (*In re Grady* 1979) and the use of antilibidinal drugs (Clarke 1989). Pharmacological agents, particularly Provera, have been used to reduce libido in mentally retarded individuals (e.g., when excessive masturbation has prevented participation in programming and in cases of sexually deviant behavior). Authors working in this area have suggested that a small reduction in sexual drive may be sufficient to enable a patient to avoid acting on an impulse that would lead to unacceptable behavior. Treatment with antilibidinal drugs in addition to psychotherapy is more effective than treatment with antilibidinal agents alone. The drug treatment will reduce the intensity of the drive but will not alter the direction of the drive.

RIGHTS OF MENTALLY RETARDED PERSONS

Legislation providing for the right of mentally retarded persons to self-determination has increased substantially in the past 20 years. The Education for All Handicapped Act (also called Individuals With Disabilities Education Act, or IDEA), the Americans With Disabilities Act, reimbursement provisions under Title XIX, and amendments to the Vocational Rehabilitation Act have addressed restrictive treatment plans and focused on elimination of discrimination and provision of protections similar to those for other citizens. Guidelines for assessing decision-making capacities for research have been proposed by the American Psychiatric Association (1998).

PITFALLS

Inadequate Assessment of Mental Age

The determination of the features of mental retardation requires individual testing and interpretation of results on tests, such as the WISC III. Assessment of adaptive functioning may not be routinely carried out. Pitfalls include reliance on the group administration of tests rather than one-to-one testing and general descriptions of adaptive functioning when more formal measures, such as the AAMR Adaptive Behavior Scales (Lambert et al. 1993) or the Vineland Adaptive Behavior Scales (Sparrow et al. 1984), are indicated.

Failure to Understand the Law and Failure to Provide Counsel at an Early Stage

The Mentally Retarded Person

Understanding of the law by the mentally retarded person is a major issue. It is of particular importance that the developmentally disabled person understands the Miranda warnings at the time of arrest. One way to avoid this pitfall is to provide for the presence of a familiar person, and legal counsel should be available at an early stage to ensure that the mentally retarded person is provided a requisite understanding of his constitutional rights to remain silent and to retain counsel before these rights can be waived. There is a need for effective safeguards for these constitutional rights so that a mentally retarded citizen will not be vulnerable to misunderstandings about the justice system.

The Professional

Failure by the professional (e.g., attorneys, police, physicians, social workers) to understand the nature of mental retardation or to understand issues related to competency and to legal rights legislation takes on special importance regarding the presentation of Miranda warnings and confessions.

Attitudes Toward Mental Retardation

Mentally retarded persons may be stigmatized because of their appearance, social habits, and history of behavior with others in the community. Efforts are continually needed to educate professionals and the public that, with normalization, behavioral difficulty can be reduced.

CASE EXAMPLE EPILOGUES

Case Example 1

William's assessment demonstrates that when he agreed to charges of fire setting, he did not understand the implications of his confession. In order to please the authorities, he had confessed as an attention-seeking maneuver and told them what he thought they wished to hear. Although he admitted to becoming excited by fires when he saw them, there was no evidence that he set them. As he had already been found guilty, the charges could not be reversed. However, a community program was developed with the eventual goal of a supervised placement. In addition, a behavioral treatment program was implemented to help him deal with his anxiety about fires and to address issues of fire safety.

Case Example 2

A meeting was held with Raymond's parents, his treating staff, and the unit social worker. The psychiatrist explained the rationale for antilibidinal treatment and reviewed the medical literature regarding its effects on sexual arousal and its potential side effects. The parents, who were his legal guardians, and every member of the treatment team signed a statement that outlined the risks, the benefits, and the risk-benefit ratio in choosing to use this medication. Antilibidinal treatment with Provera was then initiated prior to hospital discharge and after obtaining informed consent from both parents; they were deemed to be acting in his best interests because his masturbation prevented him from participation in a habilitation program. The parents and the patient's siblings were trained in behavioral overcorrection procedures, which were to be used when he became aggressive at home. A bedtime behavioral program was instituted along with the periodic utilization of sleep medication. The use of Provera was associated with a reduction in sexual drive and elimination of his attempts to fall to the floor to masturbate during the day. The new program was successfully instituted at his school as well.

Case Example 3

David, whose mental retardation is related to brain damage at birth and who currently has an IQ of 60 (mental age 9–10 years) on standard testing, was found competent to stand trial and his confession was considered to be voluntary. On the Vineland Social Maturity Scale and the AAMR Adaptive Behavior Scale, he was found to be adapting in the same mental age range as his IQ. The psychiatrist testified that David was able to appreciate the wrongfulness of his behavior and able to distinguish right from wrong. No specific mental illness was diagnosed, and he was considered to be sane at the time of the crime. He was found guilty of murder, but because of the mitigating circumstance of his mental retardation, the death penalty was not considered and he was given a life sentence with the possibility of parole.

ACTION GUIDELINES

A. Mental retardation—essentials

1. Be familiar with the definitions of mental retardation.
2. Remember that assessment of adaptive function is a crucial aspect for evaluation.
3. Consider variability in cognitive profile on IQ tests, language functioning, and the presence of neurological conditions.
4. Keep in mind that mental retardation includes a heterogeneous group of individuals who range from mildly to profoundly mentally retarded and includes specific syndromes as well as retardation secondary to traumatic head injury occurring during the developmental period.
5. Be cognizant of developmental level as well as IQ test data
6. Record data using a multiaxial classification.

B. Competency in relation to the mentally retarded population

1. Consider the level of mental retardation in competency assessment.
2. Be aware of the definitions of competency and culpability as they relate to criminal responsibility.
3. Consider the stresses that may be involved when a mentally retarded person is asked to testify.
4. Carefully consider the circumstances in the elicitation of confessions.
5. Utilize all means to facilitate communication (e.g., communication boards, speech synthesizers, drawings) at the appropriate mental age level.
6. Be aware of the legal rights of incompetent mentally retarded persons.
7. Consider the following regarding competency: lack of life experience, inadequate education, problems with over- or undercompliance, fear of authority, and associated defects.

C. Mentally ill/mentally retarded persons

1. Consider all DSM-IV-TR diagnoses that may be pertinent on Axis I.
2. Appreciate how diagnostic criteria may require modification for the mentally retarded person.
3. Utilize all five DSM-IV-TR axes.

4. Remember to consider features of mental retardation when evaluating for suspected psychosis. Exercise caution in the diagnosis of schizophrenia.

D. Forensic assessment

1. Find and make careful use of multiple informants for data collection.
2. Be aware of issues of stigma in mental retardation.
3. Consider cognitive and adaptive limitations of mentally retarded persons.
4. Remember that there may be considerable variability in profile.
5. Use specific measures of adaptive functioning.

REFERENCES BY TOPIC AREA

General

Bregman J, Harris J: Mental retardation, in Comprehensive Textbook of Psychiatry, 6th Edition. Edited by Kaplan HI, Sadock BJ. Baltimore, MD, Williams & Wilkins, 1995, pp 2207–2241

Harris JC: Mental retardation, in Developmental Neuropsychiatry, Vol 2: Assessment, Diagnosis, and Treatment of Developmental Disorders. New York, Oxford University Press, 1998, pp 91–126

President's Committee on Mental Retardation: Citizens With Mental Retardation and the Criminal Justice System. Washington DC, U.S. Department of Health and Human Services, 1991

Reiss S, Aman MG (eds): The International Consensus Handbook: Psychotropic Medications and Developmental Disabilities. Columbus, OH, Ohio State University, Nisonger Center for Mental Retardation and Developmental Disabilities, 1998

Simpson MK: The roots of normalization: a reappraisal. J Intellect Disabil Res 42:1–7, 1998

Wofenberger W: The Principle of Normalization in Human Service. Toronto, ON, National Institute on Mental Retardation, 1972

Definition and Classification of Mental Retardation

American Association on Mental Retardation: Mental Retardation: Definition, Classification, and Systems of Support, Special 9th Edition. Washington, DC, American Association on Mental Retardation, 1992

American Psychiatric Association: Diagnostic and Statistical Manual of Mental Disorders, 4th Edition, Text Revision. Washington, DC, American Psychiatric Association, 2000

Feinstein C, Reiss AL: Psychiatric disorder in mentally retarded children and adolescents: the challenges of meaningful diagnosis. Child Adolesc Psychiatr Clin North Am 5:827–852, 1996

Grossman HK: Manual on Terminology and Classification in Mental Retardation, Revised Edition. Washington, DC, American Association on Mental Deficiency, 1983

Jones JM, Barnet RW, McCormack KJ: Verbal/Performance splits in inmates assessed with multidimensional aptitude battery. J Clin Psychol 44:995–1000, 1988

Lambert N, Nihira K, Leland H: AAMR Adaptive Behavior Scales. Austin, TX, Pro-Ed, 1993

Sparrow SS, Balla DA, Cicchetti DV: Vineland Adaptive Behavior Scales, Interview Edition. Circle Pines, MN, American Guidance Service, 1984

World Health Organization: International Classification of Diseases, 10th Revision. Geneva, Switzerland, World Health Organization, 1992

Considerations in Forensic Assessment

M'Naughten Case, 8 Eng Rep 718, 8 Eng Rep 722 (1843)

Menninger K: Mental retardation and criminal responsibility: some thoughts on the idiocy defense. Int J Law Psychiatry 8:343–357, 1986

Yesavage JA, Benezech M, Ceccaldi P, et al: Arson in mentally ill and criminal populations. J Clin Psychiatry 44:128–130, 1983

Competency

Buescher M, Dinerstein RD: Capacity and the courts, in A Guide to Consent. Edited by Dinerstein RD, Herr SS, O'Sullivan JL. Washington, DC, American Association on Mental Retardation, 1999, pp 95–107

Curran WJ: Competency of the mentally retarded to stand trial: new rules from the Supreme Court. N Engl J Med 287:1184–1185, 1972

Dusky v United States, 362 US 401 (1960)

Golding SL, Roesch R, Schreiber J: Assessment and conceptualization of competence to stand trial: preliminary data on the interdisciplinary fitness interview. Law Hum Behav 8:321–334, 1984

Heller MS, Traylor WH, Ehrlich SM, et al: Intelligence, psychosis, and competency to stand trial. Bulletin of the American Academy of Psychiatry and the Law 9:267–274, 1981

Jackson v Indiana, 406 US 715 (1971)

Kaplan KH, Strang JP, Ahmed I: Dementia, mental retardation, and competency to make decisions. Gen Hosp Psychiatry 10:385–388, 1988

Pate v Robinson, 383 US 375 (1966)

Wong JG, Clare ICH, Gunn MJ, et al: Capacity to make health care decisions: its importance in clinical practice. Psychol Med 29:437–446, 1999

Parenting

Accardo PJ, Whitman BY: Children of mentally retarded parents. Am J Dis Child 144:69–70, 1990

Feldman MA: Research on parenting by mentally retarded persons. Psychiatr Clin North Am 9:777–796, 1986

Keltner BR, Wise LA, Taylor G: Mothers with intellectual limitations and their 2-year-old children's developmental outcomes. Journal of Intellectual and Developmental Disability 24:45–57, 1999

Schilling RF, Schinke SP, Blythe BJ: Child maltreatment and mentally retarded parents: is there a relationship? Ment Retard 20:201–209, 1982

Seagull EAW, Scheurer SL: Neglected and abused children of mentally retarded parents. Child Abuse Negl 10:493–500, 1986

Tymchuk AJ, Llewellyn G, Feldman M: Parenting by persons with intellectual disabilities: a timely international perspective. Journal of Intellectual and Developmental Disability 24:3–6, 1999

Whitman BY, Accardo PJ: When a Parent Is Mentally Retarded. Baltimore, MD, Brookes Publishing, 1989

Criminal Liability/Death Penalty

Cockram J, Jackson R, Underwood R: People with an intellectual disability and the criminal justice system: the family perspective. Journal of Intellectual and Developmental Disability 23:41–56, 1998

Foust LL: The legal significance of clinical formulations of fire-setting behavior. Int J Law Psychiatry 2(3):371–387, 1979

Keyes DW, Edwards WJ: Mental retardation and the death penalty: current status of exemption legislation. Ment Phys Disabil Law Rep 21:687–696, 1997

Keyes DW, Edwards WJ, Derning TJ: Mitigating mental retardation in capital cases: finding the "invisible" defendant. Ment Phys Disabil Law Rep 22:529–539, 1998

Lewis DO, Pincus JH, Bard B, et al: Neuropsychiatric, psychoeducational, and family characteristics of 14 juveniles condemned to death in the United States. Am J Psychiatry 145:584–589, 1988

Penry v Lynaugh, 109 S Ct 2934 (1989)

Penry v Johnson (No 00-6677) (2001), US Lexus 4309, 69 USLW 4402

Silber DE, Courtless TF: Measures of fantasy aggression among mentally retarded offenders. American Journal of Mental Deficiency 72(6):918–923, 1968

Confessions

Everington C, Fulero SM: Competence to confess: measuring understanding and suggestibility of defendants with mental retardation. Ment Retard 37:212–220, 1999

Praiss DM: Constitutional protection of confessions made by mentally retarded defendants. Am J Law Med 14:431–465, 1989

The Incompetent Cognitively Disabled Person

Brakman SV, Amari-Vaught E: Resistance and refusal: a case study. Hastings Cent Rep 29(1):22–23, 1999

O'Sullivan JL: Adult guardianships and alternatives, in A Guide to Consent. Edited by Dinerstein RD, Herr SS, O'Sullivan JL. Washington, DC, American Association on Mental Retardation, 1999, pp 7–35

Sundram CJ: Informed consent for major medical treatment of mentally disabled people: a new approach. N Engl J Med 318:1368–1373, 1988

Psychiatric Diagnosis

American Psychiatric Association: Guidelines for assessing the decision-making capacities of potential research subjects with cognitive impairment. Am J Psychiatry 155:1649–1650, 1998

Dykens EM, Hodapp RM: Research in mental retardation: toward an etiologic approach. J Child Psychol Psychiatry 42:49–71, 2001

Harris JC: Psychological adaptation and psychiatric disorders in adolescents and young adults with Down syndrome, in The Young Person With Down Syndrome: Transition From Adolescence to Adulthood. Edited by Pueschel SM. Baltimore, MD, Brookes Publishing, 1988, pp 35–51

Kearns A, O'Connor A: The mentally handicapped criminal offender: a 10-year study of two hospitals. Br J Psychiatry 152:848–851, 1988

Luckasson R: The dually diagnosed in criminal justice, in Mental Retardation and Mental Health: Classification, Diagnosis, Treatment, Services. Edited by Stark JA, Menolascino FJ, Albarelli MH, et al. New York, Springer-Verlag, 1988, pp 354–361

Szymanski LS, King BH: Practice parameters for the assessment and treatment of children, adolescents, and adults with mental retardation and comorbid mental disorders. American Academy of Child and Adolescent Psychiatry Working Group on Quality Issues. J Am Acad Child Adolesc Psychiatry 38 (12 suppl):5S–31S, 1999

Szymanski LS, Tanguay P: Emotional Disorders of Mentally Retarded Persons. Baltimore, MD, University Park Press, 1980

Williams W, Spruill J: The criminal justice/mental health system and the mentally retarded, mentally ill defendant. Soc Sci Med 25:1027–1032, 1987

Rights of the Mentally Retarded

Kapp MB: Protecting the personal funds of the mentally retarded: new federal regulations. Hospital and Community Psychiatry 32:567–571, 1981

Mesibov GB, Conover BS, Saur WG: Limited guardianship laws and developmentally disabled adults: needs and obstacles. Ment Retard 18:221–226, 1980

Roesch R, Golding SL: The treatment and disposition of defendants found incompetent to stand trial: a review and a proposal. International Journal of Law and Psychiatry 2:349–370, 1979

Sexuality

Abram PR, Parker T, Weisberg SR: Sexual expression of mentally retarded people: educational and legal implications. Am J Ment Retard 93:328–334, 1988

Appelbaum PS: The issue of sterilization and the mentally retarded. Hospital and Community Psychiatry 33:523–524, 1982

Clarke DJ: Antilibidinal drugs and mental retardation: a review. Med Sci Law 29:136–146, 1989

Denekens JPM, Nys H, Stuer H: Sterilization of incompetent mentally handicapped persons: a model for decision making. J Med Ethics 25:237–241, 1999

In re Grady, 170 NJ Super 98 405 A2d 851 (1979)

Rousso A: Sterilization of the mentally retarded. Med Law 3:353–362, 1984

Stavis PF, Walker-Hirsch LW: Consent to sexual activity, in A Guide to Consent. Edited by Dinerstein RD, Herr SS, O'Sullivan JL. Washington, DC, American Association on Mental Retardation, 1999, pp 57–65

Vick L, Webster F: A report on voluntary sterilization with special reference to minors and women who are intellectually disabled. Clinical Reproduction and Fertility 3:99–106, 1985

SUGGESTED READINGS

Kebbell MR, Hatton C: People with mental retardation as witnesses in court: a review. Ment Retard 37:179–187, 1999

McAfee JK, Gural M: Individuals with mental retardation and the criminal justice system: the view from states' attorneys general. Ment Retard 26:5–12, 1988

McCreary BD, Thompson J: Psychiatric aspects of sexual abuse involving persons with developmental disabilities. Can J Psychiatry 44:350–355, 1999

U.S. Supreme Court remands execution of man with mental retardation. Ment Phys Disabil Law Rep 13:334–338, 1989

CHAPTER 33

Psychic Trauma and Civil Litigation

Diane H. Schetky, M.D.

Melvin J. Guyer, J.D., Ph.D.

Case Example 1

LaTanya, a shy, overweight 14-year-old African American, was a passenger in a motorboat that collided with another boat. She was thrown overboard, became entangled in the propeller, and lost consciousness. She suffered extensive facial lacerations and nerve damage to her right arm and spent 2 weeks in the hospital. Her attorney, who is filing suit for physical damages, wonders if she might also have a case for psychic trauma and seeks psychiatric consultation.

Case Example 2

Jesse was 10 when he was repeatedly fondled by a male teacher at school. Psychiatric consultation is sought 5 years later during pending litigation against the school. Questions have to do with causality, effects of the abuse, and treatment needs. Jesse gives a very convincing and detailed account of the abuse. His subsequent course has been stormy, with academic failure, substance abuse, self-abuse, and conflicts around his sexual identity. His mother, who is single, portrays him as a model child prior to the abuse and minimizes the role of family or preexisting problems in Jesse's current psychopathology.

Case Example 3

Ahmed, age 5, was attacked by his neighbor's pit bull and required plastic surgery for his face. On return home from the hospital, he developed nightmares, was afraid to play alone outdoors, and became fearful whenever he saw a dog. His parents, Mr. and Mrs. Hussain, promptly took him to a child psychologist, who initiated play and behavioral therapy. The Hussains state they have no intention of suing but want their neighbor to pay for Ahmed's treatment. The referring attorney requests recommendations regarding Ahmed's treatment needs.

LEGAL ISSUES

Tort Law

Definition

A *tort* is a claim of wrong done to another person that has a remedy in law, typically a monetary award to the injured party. The term derives from the Latin word *tortus*, which means twisted, and the French *torquere*, which means to torture. For an act to be a tort it must be demonstrated that there has been a breach of a duty owed by the defendant to the plaintiff, the injured party. Further, it must be established that the plaintiff suffered compensable damage and that the damage resulted from breach of the duty. In many instances, the plaintiff may be required to show that the harm suffered was a *foreseeable* consequence of the breach of the duty of care (negligence) owed to the plaintiff.

Intentional Torts

An intentional tort occurs when an individual deliberately sets out to harm another through acts of omission or commission. Examples might be intentional infliction of emotional distress, slander, and in some cases, "undue familiarity" suits. In these cases, the plaintiff has the burden of demonstrating the intent or state of mind of the defendant. Other intentional torts may include the taking of someone's goods or property, such as when an employee or business partner wrongly takes money from the till.

Unintentional Torts

This category includes acts that are negligent but not willful, such as medical malpractice and personal injury cases. Negligence is defined as "conduct which falls below the standard of care established by law for the protection of others against unreasonable harm" (Keeton 1989). The standard of care is held to be that which would be expected from a reasonably careful and prudent person under the circumstances. In medical malpractice cases the standard refers to the standard of practice within that community, although increasingly courts are moving toward accepting a national standard of practice for medical professionals.

Purpose

Generally, the sole remedy provided by a tort claim is a monetary award to the plaintiff, which is intended to compensate the victim for injuries suffered or to help restore the victim to his or her prior level of functioning. Damages may be broken down into 1) compensatory damages for pain and suffering; 2) special damages for medical and psychiatric care, property damage, and loss of income; and 3) punitive damages, which may be awarded in an intentional tort (e.g., against manufacturers of a defective product that caused harm). Compensatory damages are the most difficult to determine; how does one put a price tag on the grief and loss sustained by a child in a suit that claims wrongful death of her parents? Lost wages, loss of consortium damages, and exemplary damages may also be awarded when circumstances require.

Contributory and Comparative Negligence

Awards may be limited if the plaintiff is found to be partially at fault, that is, has assumed unreasonable risk, contributed to his or her own injury or the negligence, or failed to mitigate his or her own damages.

Preexisting Conditions

The concept of the "eggshell plaintiff" deals with predisposing conditions that might render a plaintiff more vulnerable than the average person to certain stresses. Literally, it refers to a case such as the child with osteogenesis imperfecta (so-called brittle-bone disease) who suffers a skull fracture when another child at school throws a basketball at his head. Under law, the defendant is held liable for the disproportionate harm that the eggshell plaintiff suffers. In other words, the defendant must take the plaintiff as he finds him. If a plaintiff has a psychological vulnerability, he or she may be entitled to recover for damages related to trauma that should not affect an ordinary person.

Evolution of Case Law

It is only recently that courts have allowed recovery for damages that are purely psychic in nature. In the past, it was feared that recovery for psychological suffering would open the floodgates to fraudulent claims. In the early twentieth century, recovery for psychic trauma was permitted for the first time—but only if there were concomitant physical losses. This then gave way to the "zone of danger" principle, which permitted recovery by plaintiffs who were at risk for physical injury owing to their proximity to a dangerous circumstance yet only suffered psychic trauma. The next extension of this was to allow recovery by a person who had a special relationship to the injured or killed party if they witnessed the trauma but were not in the zone of danger. Thus, in *Dillon v. Legg* (1968), a mother and daughter who witnessed the negligent death of another daughter, even though they were not in danger, were allowed to recover for psychic injuries even though they suffered no physical injuries.

New Areas of Litigation

Suits Brought About by Third Parties Against Therapists

One of the first suits brought by a third party against a physician occurred in 1974 in the case of *Molien v. Kaiser Foundation Hospitals*. The issue involved Mr. Molien's suing a physician and hospital that wrongly diagnosed his wife as having syphilis. As a result of this misdiagnosis and the suspicions it engendered, the couple divorced. The claim alleged negligent infliction of emotional distress as a result of the erroneous diagnosis. The court held that the effect of the negligent diagnosis was foreseeable and that the physician had a duty to the husband.

The well-known case of *Ramona v. Isabella* (1994), also in California, brought the issue to bear on psychotherapists. Ramona sued his daughter Holly's therapist, alleging negligent and intentional infliction of emotional distress. He alleged that the therapist had suggested memories of sexual abuse to Holly through the use of amobarbital sodium interviews and by inferring that her bulimia was caused by sexual abuse and, hence, was proof of sexual abuse. Ramona further alleged that the therapist encouraged Holly to confront him and that the therapist participated in this confrontation. The jury found in his favor and awarded him $500,000. Another troubling case, *Althaus v. Cohen* (1998) in Pennsylvania, raised the issue of whether a treating psychiatrist has a duty to the parents of her adolescent patient. The court held that the defendant, Dr. Cohen, had a duty of care not only to Nicole Althaus, whom she was treating for alleged sexual abuse by her father, but also to Nicole's parents, who were directly affected by Dr. Cohen's alleged failure to properly diagnose and treat Nicole. Further, it held that by virtue of Dr. Cohen's involvement in related court proceedings, it was reasonably foreseeable that the Althauses would be harmed by Dr. Cohen's negligent diagnosis. Ironically, Nicole was not in her parents' custody at the time Dr. Cohen was treating her, and the parents had declined to meet with Dr. Cohen. Dr. Cohen, who had based her assessment on a prior forensic evaluation done elsewhere, did not view her role as that of an investigator or forensic psychiatrist. Nonetheless, the court faulted her for not pursuing a more vigorous investigation and for not being more skeptical of her patient's allegations. Dr. Cohen appealed the verdict but lost, and the case was then heard by the Pennsylvania Supreme Court in 1999. The supreme court reversed the appellate court decision and opined that a duty of care to the parents would create a conflict of interests and destroy the doctor-patient relationship (*Althaus ex rel Althaus v. Cohen* 2000; Weiss 2001).

Appelbaum and Zoltek-Jick (1996) argue that these decisions that expect therapists to be detectives have a chilling effect on psychotherapy and may affect the willingness of therapists to treat alleged victims of childhood sexual abuse. They ask, "How can therapy continue when the therapist is, in effect, competing with a person outside of therapy for the allegiance of the patient?" For instance, if a therapist urges an adolescent to leave an abusive home or reports suspected abuse, will the therapist be sued for alienating the patient from his or her family? However, in most instances, mandatory reporting acts provide immunity to the reporter. Issues of confidentiality of medical records arise if a third party brings suit and demands them as part of discovery. Note Appelbaum and Zoltek-Jick (1996); the mere threat of suit could effectively bring therapy to a halt.

False and Repressed Memory Suits Against Therapists

The *Ramona* case has fueled subsequent claims against therapists for implanting false memories of abuse, and further momentum for these suits has come from The False Memory Syndrome Foundation. The American Bar Association estimates that there are about 800 to 1,000 pending suits against therapists relating to this issue. In contrast to *Ramona*, many of these suits have been brought by former patients who now side with their parents in saying the abuse never happened. Expert witnesses may be brought into these cases to review the standard of care as well as to educate jurors on the claimed phenomenon of repression. In many instances,

these cases have involved questionable therapeutic techniques under the guise of "memory work," including guided imagery, age regression, hypnotherapy, dream work, and exposure to allegations of other "survivors" in group therapies prior to determining if indeed the patient had been sexually abused. Some therapists have erroneously attributed the absence of early childhood memory to repression of a traumatic event or attempted to attribute a host of maladies from eating disorders to trouble with interpersonal relationships to childhood sexual abuse. On the other hand, Brown (1998) asserts that many recanters of memories of sexual abuse have been influenced by posttherapy suggestions, such as those made by the media and false memory syndrome advocates, and that recanters are likely to be highly suggestible. The clinical field has become very polarized regarding the existence of repressed memories. The clinician needs to strive to keep an open mind regarding this issue, which has not been scientifically resolved.

Suggestibility of Child Witnesses

The 1980s saw a spate of cases alleging sexual abuse of children in day care settings. Much hysteria erupted over these cases; subsequently, there has been much criticism over how investigations were conducted and the techniques used to interview the children involved. Subsequent sophisticated psychological research has addressed the issue of the suggestibility of children, and these studies have been used in often successful attempts to overthrow those early trial decisions. Some appellate court appeals of trial court convictions, such as *New Jersey v. Michaels* (1994), have been successful, whereas a few others, such as *Massachusetts v. Amirault LeFave* (1998), have not. Trial Judge Borenstein, who reviewed Amirault LeFave's appeal for a new trial, which was based on tainted evidence and new research findings that would show the unreliability of the children's earlier testimonies, ruled that the complainant children had been hopelessly tainted by the early investigative interviews and could not be witnesses in any future trial.

Judge Borenstein further opined that the newly discovered evidence entitled the defendant to a new trial. Amirault LeFave, who had already served 8 years, remained free until the appellate court ruled that the issue of suggestibility had been adequately addressed in the initial trial in the 1980s and ordered her back to prison. In this case, Dr. Maggie Bruck testified about new research on the suggestibility of child witnesses and critiqued the evaluations that had been done on the young children. Dr. Diane Schetky, a coauthor of this chapter, testified as to the acceptability of the new research within the professional community. The case finally achieved some closure in 1999, when the prosecutor and defense reached an agreement that precluded further prison time in exchange for Amirault LeFave's agreement to not pursue any future claims and to avoid television interviews.

Negligent Evaluation or Treatment of Children

Both criminal and civil lawsuits have been brought against child and adolescent therapists for failing to diagnose or erroneously diagnosing sexual abuse, for using unconventional therapy techniques, and for the misuse of psychiatric hospitalization. Negligent evaluation charges frequently arise in child custody and sexual abuse evaluations in which bias of the investigator is often an issue. Experts may be retained to critique these evaluations and comment on the standard of care.

Nonsexual Boundary Violations

Complaints about these types of boundary issues are increasing, whereas complaints about sexual boundary issues are declining. Nonsexual boundary issues may involve business deals with patients, pursuing social relationships with patients, or in one case, a psychiatrist who adopted his adolescent patient. Although, thus far, most of these complaints tend to involve adult patients, there is no reason not to encounter them with child and adolescent patients whose parents may bring complaints on their behalf.

New Developments Regarding Admissibility of Expert Testimony

The admissibility of expert testimony under *Frye* and *Daubert* is covered in Chapter 5, "Testifying: The Expert Witness in Court." As noted there, under the 1993 *Daubert* decision, the court gave guidelines to trial judges that were to assist them in their new roles as gatekeepers over scientific opinion testimony. These included whether the opinions were derived from the use of an empirically tested methodology, known error rates, and/or other indications of the validity and reliability of the methods employed. Left unclear was the issue of how the court should handle nonscientific expert testimony that might involve specialized knowledge. However, this question was decided in the 1999 U.S. Supreme Court decision in *Kumho Tire Co., Ltd. v. Carmichael*. This case, which involved a civil action against a tire manufacturer, alleged that a defective tire design had caused a fatal automobile accident. The question arose as to whether the nonscientific testimony of an expert on tire

failure would survive a *Daubert* challenge of admissibility. The court ruled that the various reliability factors set out in *Daubert* could be employed by the trial judge regarding the admissibility of expert testimony.

It remains to be seen what effect this decision will have on the admissibility of mental health or psychiatric testimony. What is clear is that there will be new and more stringent challenges to the admissibility of clinical expertise, especially when it is founded on mere claims of special knowledge and experience. Opponents of such testimony will seek *Daubert* hearings, which place a burden on clinical experts to demonstrate the reliability of their methodologies and the known error rates of their predictions. Questions are likely to arise about the reliability of clinical diagnoses based on the DSM-IV-TR (American Psychiatric Association 2000) taxonomy, the efficacy of treatment interventions, and the reliability of predictions of dangerousness. The *Kumho* decision is likely to challenge the foundation of clinical judgments and, hopefully, may serve to improve the methodologies and empirical bases from which forensic opinions are derived.

Issues for the Plaintiff

Statute of Limitations

The statute of limitations refers to the time period in which an action must be brought in order to avoid being dismissed for staleness. By limiting the time period to file a complaint, the defendant is in a better position to defend himself or herself, and presumably evidence and the memories of witnesses have not yet faded. The statutory limit usually begins at the time the injury is discovered and runs until the period of limitations, which varies from state to state and with type of action, has expired. The statute is tolled for minors and does not begin to run until they reach the age of majority ("tolling" means to stop the clock on the time allowed to file a suit). Some states have now extended the statute of limitations for cases involving alleged sexual abuse. Other conditions that may extend or toll the statute include insanity, imprisonment, and incompetence, including being comatose.

Costs

The plaintiff who brings suit is liable for the cost of the suit, in contrast to criminal proceedings in which the state is the moving party. In many cases, plaintiff attorneys will accept a case on a contingency fee if there appears to be a good chance of recovery.

Standard of Evidence

As is discussed in Chapter 2 ("Introduction to the Legal System"), in civil litigation a lower standard of proof—preponderance of evidence—is used than in criminal proceedings. The burden of proof lies with the plaintiff, who is obligated to prove the case he or she has brought.

Tendering Records

If a plaintiff introduces his or her mental or physical health as an issue, the plaintiff waives claims of confidentiality regarding his or her medical records. The plaintiff's relevant medical records will be made available to the defendant's attorney in order to assist in the defense of the case.

CLINICAL ISSUES

This section will focus on issues unique to civil litigation. For information on the forensic evaluation in general and the written report, the reader is referred to Chapter 4 ("Introduction to Forensic Evaluations").

Questions to Be Asked

Degree of Impairment

The forensic examiner needs to determine whether the plaintiff is suffering from a mental disorder or impairment. Sometimes the effects of abuse may be subtle, such as inability to trust or feeling damaged or conflicted about sexuality. These effects taken alone do not constitute a mental disorder but may be grounds for seeking compensation. In contrast, some plaintiffs may demonstrate full-blown symptoms of posttraumatic stress disorder (PTSD), which are easily recognized, following a trauma. The clinician should be mindful that many abused persons report few if any lasting negative consequences. Lawsuits tend to lead to exaggerated symptom reports. However, the defendant's attorney may argue that these symptoms are purely subjective and imply that they could be malingered or, alternatively, that they are attributable to a trauma unrelated to the case being litigated.

Causality

If impairment is established, the next step is to determine whether there is a proximate relationship between the trauma being litigated and the symptoms reported or observed. It is useful to ask: "But for this trauma, would the patient have developed these symptoms?" Hoffman

and Spiegel (1989) caution that the relationship between severity of trauma and ensuing harm is not necessarily linear. A severe reaction to a minimal trauma may occur if the injury is sudden and unexpected, defensive action is blocked, and the injury occurs in a safe, familiar environment. Symptoms may also be modified by constitutional factors, prior experience, the family and community's responses, and the plaintiff's need to be looked after.

Credibility

Credibility may be affected by the plaintiff's conscious or unconscious wish for secondary gain. Symptoms may be exaggerated or held onto because they engender attention or because of the hope of financial gain. The latter is unusual for children, but they may be influenced by parental attitudes. Plaintiffs or parents may give a skewed history, minimizing the impact of other traumas or emotional problems in their life and exaggerating current claims. Hoffman and Spiegel (1989) point out that it is not the history of prior conditions that prejudice the plaintiff's claim so much as it is the attempt to conceal them. Credibility is enhanced by consistency in the telling of the history over time, corroboration of findings, symptoms that seem understandable in the context of the trauma, and generally, the ability to give details. Exceptions to the latter include children who undergo multiple investigatory interviews and may begin to embellish their stories or confabulate. Clinicians should recognize that "credible" does not mean "true."

Posttraumatic Stress Disorder in Children

The diagnosis of PTSD is one of the few DSM-IV-TR psychiatric diagnoses that require exposure to a known etiologic event. Specifically, the threshold necessary to qualify for this diagnosis requires that 1) "the person experienced, witnessed, or was confronted with an event or events that involved actual or threatened death or serious injury, or a threat to the physical integrity of self or others," *and* 2) "the person's response involved intense fear, helplessness or horror" (American Psychiatric Association 2000, p. 467). DSM-IV-TR does not recognize a separate category of PTSD for children, yet it notes that children with this disorder may present differently from adults. To meet the criteria for the diagnosis of PTSD, the individual must have symptoms in each of three categories: 1) reexperiencing, 2) avoidance or numbing, and 3) increased arousal. Children must have at least one reexperiencing symptom, three avoidance or numbing symptoms, and two symptoms of increased arousal (American Academy of Child and Adolescent Psychiatry 1998).

Children with PTSD are more likely than adults with PTSD to have sleep disturbances and are quite susceptible to the responses of adults around them. Somatic complaints, reluctance to go to school, and regression to younger behaviors are common following trauma. As noted by Quinn (1995), children may have more difficulty than adults in verbalizing the numbing symptoms of this disorder. Very young children may be unable to articulate any symptoms, many of which require verbal descriptions of internal states. However, children often manifest their distress in play, during which they may exhibit repetitive and monotonous acting out of the trauma to which they are not able to find resolution. Symptoms of heightened arousal, disorganization, and aggression in these children may be mistaken for attention-deficit/hyperactivity disorder or be confused with conduct disorders. Terr (1983, 1991) has described cognitive and memory changes that may be associated with trauma in children, including time shortening, experiencing omens, misidentifying the perpetrator, minimizing or omitting the threat to life, and belief in a foreshortened future.

It is known that rates of PTSD are higher following traumatic acts caused by others as opposed to natural disasters (Green 1995). Separation from parents, as occurs in a kidnapping or due to physical trauma necessitating hospitalization, will heighten the child's stress and sense of helplessness. Cultural factors may also affect how PTSD is manifested (McGruder-Johnson et al. 2000; DiNicola 1996; Jenkins and Bell 1994). Debate exists as to whether children are more or less susceptible to the effects of trauma than adults. Factors that have been found to consistently mediate the development of PTSD in children include temporal proximity to the trauma and parental trauma–related distress (Foy et al. 1996). Data on severity of exposure to the trauma as a mediator of symptom formation are conflicted. Symptoms of PTSD may spontaneously remit, but for many the course may be chronic (American Academy of Child and Adolescent Psychiatry 1998).

Differential Diagnoses

In considering the source of a plaintiff's complaints, it is useful to consider other possible disorders, including the following:

Conversion disorder. The forensic examiner needs to ask whether or not the child's presentation is consistent with a recognized medical or psychiatric disorder. Persons with conversion disorders are usually compliant, dependent, cooperative with evaluators, and highly suggestible.

Symptoms in conversion disorders are symbolic, triggered by an unconscious psychological conflict, are not under voluntary control, and become a source of secondary gain. The picture may be complicated if the psychic trauma being litigated has triggered the conversion disorder. For instance, hysterical seizures may occur as a sequela to childhood sexual abuse. The important distinction to make in such a case is that the child's distress is real but is psychic not physical in origin.

Malingering. The malingerer consciously feigns illness, often resists examination, may exaggerate symptoms or call attention to them, and is consciously using symptoms for secondary gain. Like the symptoms of persons with conversion disorders, their symptoms often do not fit any known diagnostic entity. However, in contrast, there is no alteration in physical functioning. Typically there will be a discrepancy between alleged complaints of functional impairment and what the plaintiff is actually able to do. Observations made by others, including detectives, may be useful in this regard.

Factitious disorder. The patient with a factitious disorder has a need to be in the sick role and will intentionally feign symptoms or induce physical findings. In contrast to malingering, economic gain is not an issue. In Munchausen syndrome by proxy (also known as factitious disorder by proxy), a parent will induce symptoms in a child for his or her own gratification. Because these parents have a lot invested in having a sick child, they are unlikely to litigate. The forensic clinician is more likely to encounter these cases in the context of murder trials, dependency and neglect hearings, or terminations of parental rights. Children who are victims of Munchausen syndrome by proxy may go on to develop factitious disorders.

Somatoform pain disorders. In these disorders, complaints of pain may have an important psychological basis with or without an underlying physical disorder. However, the pain is real and not feigned. For further discussion of this and factitious disorder, the reader is referred to Feldman and Eisendrath (1996).

Implications of Injury on Ensuing Development

Traumas need to be understood in the context of the child plaintiff's development. For instance, a 4-year-old boy who witnesses his mother being raped is likely to confuse violence with sexuality, feel guilty about not protecting her, and perhaps develop problems separating from her because in his fantasies he imagines repeated assault. Without help, these issues may interfere with his entering into latency, his ability to focus in school, and his development of a healthy male identity. Children who are sexually assaulted may experience reactivation of the trauma on reaching puberty when they have to deal with their own sexuality and sexual identity. Thus, some children may require therapy not only at the time of the trauma but also at subsequent critical points in their lives. There is no empirical research that informs us about reactivation effects; rather, knowledge is based on clinical impressions and individual case studies.

Treatment Needs, Prognosis, and Cost

Assessing the need for treatment involves taking into consideration prior functioning; predisposing, contributing, and perpetuating conditions; the child's level of development and current functioning; the nature of the traumas; and the response from the child's environment. As noted by Quinn (1995), traumas that are severe in intensity, duration, suddenness, and personal impact are likely to have a more prolonged course. Chronic courses are often associated with multiple traumas and numerous losses of life. How supportive the child's environment is will also affect outcome. For instance, children whose mothers believe their allegations of abuse fare better than those whose mothers do not (Everson et al. 1991; Gomes-Schwartz et al. 1990). The plaintiff's strengths as well as weaknesses, diagnosis, availability of treatment, and likelihood of utilization all must be taken into consideration. Familiarity with long-term studies on the outcome of PTSD is also helpful (see Green 1995). The cost of future therapy can be estimated based on prevailing rates in the area where the plaintiff resides, taking inflation into consideration. However, the variability among persons is so great that these estimates are necessarily speculative.

Effects of Litigation on Therapy

It is commonly believed that patients in litigation would hold onto their symptoms in order to gain compensation for them, although this notion has been challenged (Mendelson 1985). There is little evidence bearing on this issue in the child and adolescent psychiatry literature. A second concern has been that therapy might improve the plaintiff's symptoms and diminish his or her chances for recovery in court. Unfortunately, many attorneys continue to defer getting treatment for their clients until the case has been tried or settled. This does a great disservice to children and their families, many of whom cannot afford psychiatric help. Typically, years may pass before these cases settle, and untreated symptoms may interfere with the child's ensuing development. A second reason for seeking therapy early on is to provide the child with support to help him or her deal with the litigation and the disruptive effect it has on the child's life. For instance, a study by Runyon et al. (1988) on sexually abused children concluded that testifying in juvenile court might be beneficial to the child, whereas testifying in protracted criminal proceedings may have an adverse effect on the child. Debate continues among professionals as to whether testifying is harmful or beneficial to children and more data are needed.

The downside to treating a patient under the shadow of litigation is that it may sidetrack therapy and prevent the child from dealing with other issues. However, the issues related to a forthcoming trial may also serve as a catalyst, because the child once again must deal with issues of trust, guilt, and lack of control over his or her life. Having to confront the alleged offender in court may exacerbate symptoms of PTSD but may also help the child begin to combat his or her fears. (This, of course, presumes that the alleged offender is actually the offender. Innocent people are sometimes tried for crimes they did not commit.) Litigation may enable the child to direct anger to where it belongs and to have his or her feelings validated. However, there is also risk that if the child's side does not prevail, the child may feel that he or she is not believed. A further risk is that the therapist may be subpoenaed to testify as to damages, thereby threatening confidentiality and trust, which are the cornerstones of psychotherapy. The child who claims damages in civil action will be subject to an independent medical exam arranged by opposing counsel.

Testifying Against Other Clinicians

Being an expert witness in a malpractice case and having to testify regarding the professional conduct of another clinician is not a comfortable position to be in, and one may even face the scorn of colleagues for doing so. However, if we fail to advocate for patients who have been mistreated by clinicians, then who will uphold the standards of practice? The expert should avoid testifying either for or against clinicians with whom he or she has any sort of professional or social relationship or with whom he or she may be in economic competition. Potential problems might arise in testifying about boundary violations of someone from a different discipline unless the expert familiarizes himself or herself with that discipline's code of ethical behavior.

PITFALLS

Failure to Consider Other Stressors

A common mistake in taking a history is to attribute all of a child's symptoms to the trauma in question without taking a thorough past history, which could unveil other sources of trauma and stress. The defense attorney will have left no stone unturned in this regard and may confront the plaintiff's expert in court with potentially embarrassing material that the expert has failed to consider. The net effect is to undermine the expert's credibility and the thoroughness of the evaluation. If confronted with new, *significant* information in court, the expert may need to be prepared to alter his or her opinion.

Misuse of Psychiatric Diagnoses

Inexperienced clinicians and some experts may hear a trauma history and automatically assume the patient/plaintiff has PTSD. They may also err in discounting the threshold of trauma necessary to meet the diagnosis of PTSD in DSM-IV-TR. Thus, for example, sexual harassment in school, although distressing, might not qualify as a severe enough trauma to cause PTSD. Another pitfall is when clinicians invoke syndrome testimony such as "the sexually abused child syndrome" to prove that the child was abused. Their logic tends to run along the lines that "she looks like a sexually abused child, therefore, she must be one." Such overly simplistic thinking ignores the fact that the so-called syndrome includes many nonspecific symptoms and that it is not officially recognized as a diagnosis because it lacks scientific foundation.

Failure to Consider Other Diagnoses

A forensic examiner may fail to diagnose PTSD if he or she underestimates the plaintiff's pathology or assumes it is a normal reaction to the event in question. Inadequate time spent with the plaintiff may also result in missing the diagnosis. Another source of error is confusing preexisting psychopathology with recent-onset PTSD. As noted, heightened arousal may also be seen in children with attention-deficit/hyperactivity disorder and in children who have been exposed to domestic violence or other traumas in their lives.

Credibility

The forensic examiner needs to consider other possible explanations for a child's behavior or symptoms and to explore any contradictions in the history or the child's statements. Having done so will fortify the examiner's convictions about his or her ultimate opinion and will prepare the examiner to answer questions in court about whether he or she has considered malingering. Corroborating discovery material is important along with psychological test results to support one's findings. The forensic examiner should be proactive in seeking records and documents that will test or corroborate the plaintiff's presented history.

The Subjective Nature of Posttraumatic Stress Disorder

Defense attorneys may be quick to point out the subjective nature of PTSD and suggest that it is easy to malinger this condition. This is less likely in cases involving children, as it would be difficult for them to malinger the behavioral manifestations of PTSD. Nonetheless, psychological testing may go a long way toward fortifying a diagnosis and may be perceived by juries as more objective than the psychiatrist's findings. Because PTSD is, to a large extent, diagnosed by child or parental reports, independent corroboration of symptom severity and onset is even more important. Memory of symptoms readily repositions itself when litigation is pending. It is not unusual for individuals who are claiming psychic injuries to present with distorted autobiographical recollections of when their symptoms began. Thus, symptoms of long duration and problems that predated the alleged traumatic event are inaccurately recalled as having had their onset only after the event and so, in reconstructed memory, are wrongly ascribed as flowing from the event that is the basis of the lawsuit. Persons may report that they had no school or medical or emotional or employment problems until the traumatic event occurred. A check of independent records may show that all of the supposedly trauma-caused problems predated the alleged trauma.

Issues for the Treating Therapist

Therapists of plaintiffs may be subpoenaed into court to testify concerning damages and treatment needs. How to deal with this situation is discussed in Chapter 3 ("Forensic Ethics") and Chapter 4 ("Introduction to Forensic Evaluations"). Another peril is that in some cases of PTSD, defense attorneys have tried to attribute the plaintiff's symptoms to therapy or imply they have been induced or suggested by the treating therapist rather than to the trauma per se.

CASE EXAMPLE EPILOGUES

Case Example 1

LaTanya remained unconscious in the hospital for several days and on awakening had no recollection of the accident. Her friends and family rallied around her, and her parents noted that she seemed to be more outgoing than before her accident. In spite of her nerve injury, she returned to play basketball, counter to predictions. She has been dealing well with her facial disfigurement and has decided to postpone plastic surgery. The forensic examiner found no evidence for PTSD or other symptoms of emotional distress related to the accident. She told the attorney that in the absence of memory, there is no basis for the development of PTSD symptoms and in her opinion there is no basis for a claim for psychic trauma. The attorney agreed and did not pursue the claim for psychic trauma.

Case Example 2

It was not until his deposition that the forensic examiner learned from the defense attorney that Jesse had been treated for enuresis prior to the sexual abuse and had also been diagnosed with a conduct disorder. Two siblings have substance abuse problems, an area about which the expert neglected to inquire. Although these facts did not alter his opinion about Jesse's credibility, they did put more weight on a contributory role of ongoing family problems and a conduct disorder in Jesse's behavioral problems.

Case Example 3

Ahmed entered therapy; within 6 months his symptoms remitted, and he acquired a puppy. He continued to do well until he entered first grade, where he had difficulty keeping up. Psychological testing documented a learning disorder that seemed unrelated to the dog bite. Your report reflected that Ahmed developed acute PTSD after a dog bite, that he responded well to therapy, and that he has a good prognosis. The case settled out of court, and the owner of the pit bull agreed to pay for the cost of Ahmed's related medical and psychiatric care.

ACTION GUIDELINES

A. *Be thorough.* Shortcuts and premature conclusions can only lead to embarrassment down the line.
B. *Maintain objectivity.* Keep an open mind, be receptive to new information, and strive for an objective stance that weighs all possibilities. Test your hypotheses throughout your work.
C. *Don't get too invested in the outcome.* This is easier said than done when one has invested hours in a case. The risks of overinvolvement are that of losing objectivity and appearing as too much of an advocate on the witness stand.
D. *Consider the value of psychological testing to help with diagnosis and fortify your opinions.*
E. *Keep current with the literature.* There is a burgeoning literature on PTSD, including information on neurophysiological factors that may account for the chronic and episodic nature of symptoms as well as long-term studies. These data are relevant to diagnosis, prognosis, and treatment recommendations.

REFERENCES

Althaus v Cohen, 710 A2d 1147 (Pa Sup Ct 1998)

Althaus ex rel Althaus v Cohen, 756 A2d 1166 (Pa 2000)

American Academy of Child and Adolescent Psychiatry: Practice Parameters for the Assessment and Treatment of Children and Adolescents With Posttraumatic Stress Disorder. Washington, DC, American Academy of Child and Adolescent Psychiatry, 1998

American Psychiatric Association: Diagnostic and Statistical Manual of Mental Disorders, 4th Edition, Text Revision. Washington, DC, American Psychiatric Association, 2000

Appelbaum P, Zoltek-Jick R: Psychotherapists' duties to third parties: Ramona and beyond. Am J Psychiatry 153:457–465, 1996

Brown D: False memory lawsuits: the weight of the scientific and legal evidence. Guttmacher Award lecture presented at the annual meeting of the American Psychiatric Association, Toronto, ON, Canada May/June 1998

Massachusetts v Amirault LeFave, 424 Mass 618 (1998)

Dillon v Legg, 68 Cal2d 728 (1968)

DiNicola V: Ethnocentric aspects of posttraumatic stress disorder and related disorders among children and adolescents, in Ethnocultural Aspects of Posttraumatic Stress Disorder: Issues, Research and Clinical Application. Edited by Marsella A, Friedman M, Gerrity E, et al. Washington, DC, American Psychological Association, 1996, pp 389–414

Everson M, Hunter W, Runyan D, et al: Maternal support following disclosure of incest. Am J Orthopsychiatry 59:197–227, 1991

Feldman M, Eisendrath A: The Spectrum of Factitious Disorders. Washington, DC, American Psychiatric Press, 1996

Foy D, Madvig B, Pynoos T, et al: Etiologic factors in the development of posttraumatic stress disorder in children and adolescents. Journal of School Psychology 34:133–145, 1996

Gomes-Schwartz B, Horowitz JM, Cardarelli AP: Child Sexual Abuse: The Initial Effects. Newbury Park, CA, Sage, 1990

Green B: Recent research findings on the diagnosis of posttraumatic stress disorder: prevalence, course, comorbidity and risk, in Posttraumatic Stress Disorder in Litigation: Guidelines for Forensic Assessment. Edited by Simon R. Washington, DC, American Psychiatric Press, 1995, pp 13–30

Hoffman B, Spiegel H: Legal principles in the psychiatric assessment of the personal injury litigant. Am J Psychiatry 146:304–310, 1989

Jenkins E, Bell C: Violence among inner city high school students and posttraumatic stress disorder, in Anxiety Disorders in African Americans. Edited by Friedman S. New York, Springer, 1994

Keeton WP (ed): Prosser and Keeton on the Law of Torts, 5th Edition. St Paul, MN, West Publishing, 1984, pp 772–773

Kumho Tire Co, Ltd v Carmichael, 119 S Ct 1167 (1999)

McGruder-Johnson AK, Davidson ES, Gleaves DH, et al: Interpersonal violence and posttraumatic symptomatology: the effects of ethnicity, gender, and exposure to violent events. Journal of Interpersonal Violence 15:205–221, 2000

Mendelson G: Compensation neurosis. Med J Aust 142:561–564, 1985

Molien v Kaiser Foundation Hospitals, 27 Cal3d, 616 P2d 813 (Cal 1974)

New Jersey v Michaels, 625 A2d 579, 642 A2d 1372 (1994)

Quinn K: Guidelines for the psychiatric examination of posttraumatic stress disorder in children and adolescents, in Posttraumatic Stress Disorder in Litigation. Edited by Simon R. Washington, DC, American Psychiatric Press, 1995, pp 85–98

Ramona v Isabella, 61898 Napa Cty (Cal Sup Ct 1994)

Runyon E, Emerson M, Edelsohn G, et al: Impact of legal intervention on sexually abused children. J Pediatr 113:647–653, 1988

Terr L: Chowchilla revisited: the effects of psychic trauma four years after a school bus kidnapping. Am J Psychiatry 140:1542–1550, 1983

Terr L: Childhood traumas: an outline and overview. Am J Psychiatry 148:10–20, 1991

Weiss K: A duty to the parents of an allegedly abused child? *Althaus v. Cohen.* J Am Acad Psychiatry Law 29:238–240, 2001

SUGGESTED READINGS

American Academy of Child and Adolescent Psychiatry: Practice parameters for the forensic evaluation of children and adolescents who may have been physically or sexually abused (AACAP Official Action). J Am Acad Child Adolesc Psychiatry 36:423–442, 1997

Cohen J, Mannarino A: Factors that mediate treatment outcome in sexually abused preschoolers. J Am Acad Child Adolesc Psychiatry 35:1402–1410, 1996

Daubert v Merrill Dow Pharmaceuticals, Inc, 113 S Ct 2786 (1993)

Eth R: Developmental perspectives on psychic trauma in childhood, in Trauma and Its Wake. Edited by Figley C. New York, Brunner/Mazel, 1985, pp 36–52

Frye v United States, 293F 1013, 34 ALR 145 (DC Cir 1923)

Grudzinskas A: Kumho Tire Co, Ltd v Carmichael. J Am Acad Psychiatry Law 27:482–488, 1999

Hoffman B: How to write a psychiatric report for litigation following a personal injury. Am J Psychiatry 143:164–169, 1986

McLeer S, Deblinger E, Henry D, et al: Sexually abused children at high risk for posttraumatic stress disorder. J Am Acad Child Adolesc Psychiatry 31:875–879, 1992

Schetky D: Child victims in the legal system, in Trauma and Memory: Clinical and Legal Controversies. Edited by Appelbaum P, Uyehara L, Elin M. New York, Oxford, 1997, pp 496–510

CHAPTER 34

Forensic Telepsychiatry

Philip Merideth, M.D., J.D.

Telemedicine has changed the delivery of health care services in psychiatry and other medical specialties. The technology that makes telemedicine possible has existed for decades, but it was not until about 1990 that health care providers and organizations began efforts to use the technology on a large scale. The Institute of Medicine has defined telemedicine as "the use of electronic information and communication technologies to provide and support health care when distance separates the participants" (Field 1996). Although telemedicine encompasses many forms of electronic communication, the technology discussed in this chapter is limited to live, two-way interactive video, also known as videoconferencing. Psychiatric interviews conducted by videoconferencing appear to be generally reliable (Frueh et al. 2000).

DEFINITION OF FORENSIC TELEPSYCHIATRY

As a subcomponent of telemedicine, forensic telepsychiatry has been defined as "the use of telecommunications technology to provide mental health services in a medicolegal context" (Merideth 1999). Like other forms of telemedicine, forensic telepsychiatry currently is underused. However, forensic psychiatrists and the legal system should be aware that forensic mental evaluations of adults and children, and court testimony, may be performed efficiently and reliably by telepsychiatry.

APPLICATIONS OF FORENSIC TELEPSYCHIATRY

The American Psychiatric Association's (APA's) resource document on telepsychiatry recognizes that telepsychiatry is appropriate in courts, prisons, and other forensic settings such as civil commitment proceedings (American Psychiatric Association Committee on Telemedical Services 1998). However, the APA's recognition of appropriate applications for forensic telepsychiatry does not define the limits of the technology's use. With correct application of the technology, telepsychiatry's use in forensic settings should be limited only by its acceptance by the legal system. As the technology improves and as forensic psychiatrists' experience with telepsychiatry increases, the legal system's acceptance of forensic telepsychiatry surely will follow.

Civil Commitment

The greatest potential use of forensic telepsychiatry is in civil commitment proceedings. In that setting, it is possible for a psychiatrist to evaluate a child or an adult and testify about the need for civil commitment without leaving the office. Conducting civil commitment hearings by telepsychiatry also offers the advantage of having family members present to testify and to give emotional support when they might otherwise be unable to attend (Zarate et al. 1997).

This chapter contains material adapted from Merideth P: "Forensic Applications of Telepsychiatry." *Psychiatric Annals* 29:429–431, 1999. Used with permission.

Prior to the court hearing, the psychiatrist should ensure that the state's laws permit civil commitment evaluation by telepsychiatry. Unless explicitly forbidden by a court decision or a statute, an examination for civil commitment done by telepsychiatry should be as valid as a face-to-face examination. In support of this position, proponents have shown that simultaneous face-to-face and telepsychiatric evaluation of the need for civil commitment has resulted in perfect agreement between raters (Bear et al. 1997).

Competence and Sanity Evaluation

Competence to stand trial and the insanity defense are mental health issues encountered frequently in the criminal courts. Evaluation of these issues makes necessary an in-depth examination of the defendant's mental state at the time of the evaluation and at the time of the alleged offense, which may be done by using telepsychiatry. However, examiners should be aware that laws on competence and sanity are jurisdiction-specific and may vary significantly among federal and state courts. Therefore, one must be familiar with the legal definitions of competence and sanity in the jurisdiction where the accused person faces criminal proceedings.

The telepsychiatric interview process for conducting forensic mental evaluations for the criminal courts is essentially the same as a face-to-face evaluation. The defendant must be notified of the limits of confidentiality of the evaluation. The examiner also should ensure that the defendant has received adequate notice of the evaluation and should explain the defendant's constitutional right not to make incriminating statements.

Published studies about forensic telepsychiatry are rare. One study found comparable reliability with the use of a structured instrument (the MacArthur Competence Assessment Tool) in a simultaneous face-to-face and interactive video evaluation of competence to stand trial (Lexcen et al. 1998).

Civil Litigation

Forensic telepsychiatry is also useful in civil litigation involving children and adults. Mental health issues that frequently arise in civil litigation and that are amenable to telepsychiatric evaluation include posttraumatic stress disorder, infliction of emotional distress, psychiatric disability, and medication complications such as tardive dyskinesia. Consultation with psychiatrists who have expertise in such areas may be facilitated by the use of telepsychiatry. When evaluating movement disorders, psychiatrists may prefer to use telepsychiatry systems with bandwidths of 384 kilobytes per second (kbps) or

greater, as higher bandwidths provide better picture resolution, which makes possible a more reliable assessment (Zarate et al. 1997). However, a system that provides a bandwidth of 128–256 kbps is adequate for most forensic psychiatric evaluations. Telepsychiatry certainly has a role to play in the forensic evaluation of a wide variety of mental health issues in civil litigation, in which the legal protections afforded to defendants in the criminal courts (e.g., the right to remain silent) are not a factor.

Pretrial Conference and Court Testimony

After the completion of a forensic mental evaluation, the attorney who requested the evaluation may wish to have a pretrial conference with the psychiatrist. Telepsychiatry offers the attorney and the psychiatrist the opportunity to interact in a time-efficient manner. Likewise, pretrial depositions may be taken by using telepsychiatry.

For the psychiatrist, court testimony is one of the most time-consuming aspects of a forensic mental evaluation. At times, irreconcilable conflicts occur between court dates and the psychiatrist's schedule. Such conflicts can be resolved by the use of teletestimony. Teletestimony is an area of litigation support that uses satellite or other interactive video technology to bring live testimony into the courtroom. Satellite teletestimony involves the use of a satellite hookup that allows trial participants to see, hear, and interact with a witness located at a remote site. Attorneys and litigation support specialists agree that teletestimony offers an efficient solution to the problem of scheduling trial appearances for busy professionals.

Use of satellite technology for teletestimony has been preferred because of its television-like picture quality. However, the expense and effort required to employ satellite technology are limitations on its use in teletestimony. Advances in the technology of video telephones and desktop computer videoconferencing have made teletestimony a readily available, affordable option.

This author conducted jury research on the effectiveness of satellite teletestimony following its use in a tort suit in 1996. At the time of the trial, the defendant's psychiatric expert was scheduled to make a presentation at a national meeting in Puerto Rico. To resolve this scheduling conflict, the defense attorney arranged for the psychiatrist's live testimony to be transmitted via satellite from a Puerto Rican television station to a Mississippi courtroom. Seven of the 14 jurors and alternate jurors responded to a posttrial questionnaire. Six of the 7 jurors who responded were of the opinion that the use of teletestimony did not make that witness seem more important or more credible than the other witnesses.

Regarding the use of video equipment in the courtroom, all 7 jurors agreed that the teletestimony was presented in a professional manner. None of the 7 jurors indicated that the use of teletestimony affected their decision in the case (P. Merideth, unpublished data, 1997).

Consultation and Education

The workforce in forensic psychiatry is relatively small, as there were only 1,384 board-certified forensic psychiatrists in the United States in 2001. However, many forensic psychiatric evaluations are performed by general psychiatrists with no formal forensic training. Telepsychiatry provides an opportunity for general psychiatrists to employ expert consultation on difficult forensic cases.

Telepsychiatry also has an important role in teaching forensic psychiatry to adult psychiatry residents, child and forensic psychiatry fellows, and other mental health professionals. For example, forensic psychiatric educators may use telepsychiatry to conduct teaching conferences or to supervise forensic evaluations done by trainees at distant sites. As its educational uses increase, telepsychiatry has great potential to alleviate the workforce shortage in forensic psychiatry and to improve the quality of forensic psychiatric evaluations.

Correctional Psychiatry

The most frequent use of forensic telepsychiatry is in providing mental health services to correctional institutions. Thirty percent of all telemedicine consults in 1998 occurred in correctional settings (Chin 2000). Telepsychiatry offers the opportunity for mental health services, which often are concentrated at large urban medical centers and teaching hospitals, to be provided to distant prisons and jails where mental health resources are often scarce. Providing mental health services by telepsychiatry decreases the costs and security risks associated with the transport of detainees. Telepsychiatry also has been employed to provide consultation to juvenile justice programs (Ermer 1999).

Forensic psychiatric patients at the King County Correctional Facility in Seattle reported no significant difference in the level of satisfaction with an evaluation done by interactive televideo versus a face-to-face evaluation (Brodey et al. 2000).

The Federal Bureau of Prisons also has found high inmate and clinician satisfaction with telepsychiatry (Magaletta et al. 2000).

Child and Adolescent Forensic Psychiatry

Most forensic mental health issues regarding children and adolescents are amenable to evaluation and consultation by telepsychiatry in a manner similar to that for adults. For example, parental competence evaluations, assessment of juveniles for waiver to adult court, and school violence risk assessments all may be accomplished by telepsychiatry.

However, telepsychiatry in its current form is not well suited to the performance of child custody evaluations regarding young children. Young children, especially hyperactive ones, are frequently too mobile to allow the camera to capture the subtleties of their parental attachments. The degree of interpersonal interaction required between the evaluator, parent, and child also precludes the use of telepsychiatry in custody evaluations of young children except in extraordinary circumstances, such as geographic barriers that cannot reasonably be overcome.

In spite of this current limitation, telepsychiatry is useful and appropriate for providing mental health services to children and adolescents for nonforensic purposes (Ermer 1999). The use of telepsychiatry to evaluate and treat minors for forensic and nonforensic purposes can be expected to increase with further advances in technology and with increasing awareness of telepsychiatry's efficiency.

LEGAL AND PRACTICAL ISSUES

More than in any other area of psychiatry, forensic telepsychiatry requires a clear delineation of roles and responsibilities among persons who use the technology. The evaluator's role as a forensic evaluator and not a therapist should be explained clearly to the evaluee (American Psychiatric Association Committee on Telemedical Services 1998). The forensic evaluator also should ensure that the technology employed is sufficient to achieve the purpose of the evaluation. In order to withstand a challenge to the introduction of a telepsychiatric evaluation in a legal proceeding, the quality of the evaluation should not be compromised by the use of telepsychiatry.

Because the use of telepsychiatry for forensic purposes may be a new concept for some courts, the attorney who plans to introduce the results of an evaluation conducted by telepsychiatry would be well advised to seek the agreement of the judge and opposing attorney in advance. Thus far, the federal judiciary has taken the lead in bringing videoconferencing into the courts, because its use is permitted by the federal procedural rules. The use of videoconferencing in the courtroom has withstood constitutional challenges in the federal courts (*United States v. Baker* 1995; *Edwards v. Logan* 1999).

Informed consent should be obtained from the evaluee prior to performing a forensic evaluation by telepsychiatry. Prior to the telepsychiatric evaluation of a minor, consent should be obtained from a parent or other legally authorized decision maker. Children and adolescents should be given a developmentally appropriate explanation of the nature and purpose of the evaluation and the use of the technology. Some evaluees, especially children, may need reassurance that the evaluation is not being broadcast on television. The evaluee should be informed of the limits of confidentiality involved in a forensic evaluation done by telepsychiatry. The evaluee also may be given the option of not participating in a telepsychiatric evaluation.

In the case of court-ordered evaluations, such as civil commitment, competence to stand trial, and the insanity defense, the evaluee may be required to participate in an interview done by telepsychiatry. However, forensic telepsychiatrists have an ethical obligation to consider the interests of the evaluee (American Psychiatric Association Committee on Telemedical Services 1995). Respect for the evaluee's wishes should be given consideration, especially if the use of telepsychiatry may negatively affect the evaluee or compromise the quality of the examination. In such cases, the advantages of conducting a forensic evaluation by telepsychiatry may have to give way to the concern for maintaining rapport with the evaluee.

Forensic psychiatry evaluations often require review of medical records and other documents. A second camera, for the video transmission of documents, is helpful. Otherwise, documents may be sent by fax, mail, or overnight courier.

Telepsychiatry makes it possible to conduct forensic psychiatric evaluations across state lines and internationally. This offers the advantage of decreasing travel time, but it also raises other issues. Since 1994, at least 26 states have enacted laws or regulations affecting the practice of telemedicine (see Table 34–1). Most of the states that have addressed the issue of interstate telemedicine require out-of-state physicians to obtain a full and unrestricted medical license before practicing telemedicine in the state of the evaluee (Hinton 1998). Therefore, psychiatrists who plan to practice telepsychiatry across state or national borders may consider checking with the medical licensing agency of the state or nation in which they propose to practice (American Psychiatric Association Committee on Telemedical Services 1998). Telepsychiatrists may also need to be credentialed at the distant facility if they provide treatment there.

Liability issues are also of concern in the practice of forensic telepsychiatry. It is widely accepted that the person proposing to use telepsychiatry as an evaluation tool bears the risk of a transmission failure (American Psychi-

TABLE 34–1. States that regulate telemedicine

Alabama	Indiana	Oklahoma
Arkansas	Kansas	Oregon
California	Mississippi	South Dakota
Colorado	Montana	Tennessee
Connecticut	Nebraska	Texas
Florida	Nevada	Utah
Georgia	New Hampshire	West Virginia
Hawaii	North Carolina	Wyoming
Illinois	North Dakota	

Source. Center for Telemedicine Law: "Telemedicine-Related State Licensure Laws." *Quarterly Telemedicine Licensure Update* 2(2):15–18, 2000. Used with permission.

atric Association Committee on Telemedical Services 1998). Courts have not yet considered standards of care for this relatively new technology, so the scope of liability for professional negligence in telepsychiatric encounters has not been determined.

Psychiatrists who practice telepsychiatry across state lines may seek to limit their obligation to respond to a lawsuit in a distant state by having a contractual agreement with the person who retained their services, stating that the psychiatrist may be sued only in the psychiatrist's state of residence. However, some states may find such agreements unenforceable. Practitioners of telepsychiatry also may consider notifying their malpractice insurance provider regarding the use of telepsychiatry, as a malpractice insurance policy may be interpreted not to include coverage for telepsychiatry unless it is stated explicitly in the policy that it does (Hinton 1998).

SUMMARY

Telepsychiatry is useful and appropriate for the forensic evaluation of minors and adults in a wide variety of mental health issues in civil and criminal law. Research studies and case reports have shown favorable results in the use of telepsychiatry for forensic purposes. By using telepsychiatry, the legal system may gain access to the expertise of forensic psychiatrists located in distant states or nations. Telepsychiatry is also a valuable tool in forensic psychiatry education.

Forensic telepsychiatry has a promising future. Further advances in forensic telepsychiatry will depend on improvements in technology, an increasing awareness of its advantages, and its increasing acceptance by the legal system.

There is a need for further study of forensic telepsychiatry to verify the initial findings regarding its efficiency and reliability. There is also a need for a leader in the field to promote the development of telepsychiatry as a practice modality in forensic settings and to develop guidelines for the practice of forensic telepsychiatry (Grinfeld 1998; Merideth 1998; Rothchild and Zaylor 1999).

REFERENCES

American Psychiatric Association Committee on Telemedical Services: Position statement on the ethical use of telemedicine, December 1995 [http://www.psych.org/pract_of_psych/tp_position.cfm]

American Psychiatric Association Committee on Telemedical Services: APA resource document on telepsychiatry via videoconferencing, July 1998 [http://www.psych.org/pract_of_psych/tp_paper.cfm]

Bear D, Jacobson G, Aaronson S, et al: Telemedicine in psychiatry: making the dream reality (letter). Am J Psychiatry 154:885, 1997

Brodey BB, Claypoole KH, Motto J, et al: Satisfaction of forensic psychiatric patients with remote telepsychiatric evaluation. Psychiatr Serv 51:1305–1307, 2000

Center for Telemedicine Law: Telemedicine-related state licensure laws. Quarterly Telemedicine Licensure Update 2(2):15–18, 2000

Chin T: Telemedicine use growing, but slowly. American Medical News, July 31, 2000, p 31

Edwards v Logan, 38 F Supp 2d 463 (WD Va 1999)

Ermer DJ: Experience with a rural telepsychiatry clinic for children and adolescents. Psychiatr Serv 50:260–261, 1999

Field MJ (ed): Telemedicine: A Guide to Assessing Telecommunications in Health Care. Washington, DC, National Academy Press, 1996

Frueh BC, Deitsch SE, Santos AB, et al: Procedural and methodological issues in telepsychiatry research and program development. Psychiatr Serv 51:1522–1527, 2000

Grinfeld MJ: Telepsychiatry: the vision emerges. Psychiatric Times 15(4):45–46, 1998

Hinton M: Telemedicine: the next generation of care? Rx for Risk 6(2):6–10, 1998

Lexcen F, Hawk G, Blank M, et al: Televideo-assisted evaluation of trial competence. Paper presented at the annual meeting of the American Psychological Association, San Francisco, CA, August 1998

Magaletta PR, Fagan TJ, Peyrot MF: Telehealth in the Federal Bureau of Prisons: inmates' perceptions. Professional Psychology: Research and Practice 31:497–502, 2000

Merideth P: Telemedicine committee proposed (letter). American Academy of Psychiatry and the Law Newsletter 23(2):25, 1998

Merideth P: Forensic applications of telepsychiatry. Psychiatric Annals 29(7):429–431, 1999

Rothchild E, Zaylor C (eds): Telepsychiatry (special issue). Psychiatric Annals 29(7), 1999

United States v Baker, 45 F3d 837 (4th Cir 1995)

Zarate CA Jr, Weinstock L, Cukor P, et al: Applicability of telemedicine for assessing patients with schizophrenia: acceptance and reliability. J Clin Psychiatry 58:22–25, 1997

Index

Page numbers in **boldface** type refer to figures or tables.